introductory pediatric nursing

j. b. lippincott company

philadelphia

with the consultation of
joan c. jordan, r.n., b.s.n.
instructor in practical nursing, st. louis board of education, st. louis, missouri

introductory pediatric nursing

third edition

violet broadribb, r.n., m.s.

formerly assistant professor of pediatric nursing, university of oregon school of nursing, portland, oregon

Sponsoring Editor: Paul R. Hill
Manuscript Editor: Helen Ewan
Indexer: Ruth Elwell
Art Director: Tracy Baldwin

Designer: Arlene Putterman
Production Assistant: Barney Fernandes
Compositor: Bi-Comp, Incorporated
Printer/Binder: The Murray Printing Company

Third Edition

6 5 4 3 2

Library of Congress Cataloging in Publication Data

Broadribb, Violet.
    Introductory pediatric nursing.

    Rev. ed. of: Foundations of pediatric nursing.
2nd ed. [1973]
    Includes index.
    1. Pediatric nursing.   I. Jordan, Joan C.
II. Title.   [DNLM: 1. Pediatric nursing.   WY 159
B863i]
RJ245.B764   610.73′62   81-23611
ISBN 0-397-54330-1   AACR2

The author and publisher have exerted every effort to ensure that drug selection and dosage set forth in this text are in accord with current recommendations and practice at the time of publication. However, in view of ongoing research, changes in government regulations, and the constant flow of information relating to drug therapy and drug reactions, the reader is urged to check the package insert for each drug for any change in indications and dosage and for added warnings and precautions. This is particularly important when the recommended agent is a new or infrequently employed drug.

preface

Caring for children and their families demands a wide range of skills and knowledge from today's nurse. Emphasis has shifted from acute care of the hospitalized child to care of the child at home and ongoing maintenance of health. To be effective, nursing care must consider the total needs of the child—physical, emotional, mental, and spiritual—at each stage of growth and development within the family and community environment. More than therapeutic and comfort measures, nursing care means teaching parents and children how to meet their own health needs.

When acute illness or accident requires hospitalization of the child, the goal of care is to restore the child to maximum health and function as quickly as possible with minimum interruption in normal development. Although the physiologic effect of illness may be brief, separation, strangeness, loneliness, and discomfort may cause severe and lasting consequences in the life of a child. Nursing care that recognizes the potential impact of illness can help avoid problems and contribute to the growth of the child and the strengthening of the family unit.

In light of the new challenges and responsibilities that confront today's pediatric nurse, this text has undergone extensive revision. As the new title implies, its major function is to provide an *introduction* to pediatric nursing, the basic principles of growth and development and the prevention and treatment of common childhood health problems. The text has been thoroughly updated and reorganized in four units: "A Child Is Born," "A Child Grows," "A Child Enters the Hospital," and "A Child Faces Chronic or Terminal Illness."

The first unit discusses life before birth, the normal newborn, the high-risk newborn, and the newborn with special needs. New material includes preparation for childbirth and parenthood, parent–infant attachment, and grief that accompanies fetal or neonatal death or birth of a child with a defect.

The second unit opens with a chapter on the child and the family, followed by chapters on the infant, toddler, preschooler, school-age child, and adolescent. Two chapters are devoted to each age group; the first discusses normal growth and development, and the second, health problems common to that age group. This unit includes new material on autism, learning disorders, child abuse, diabetes mellitus, asthma and allergies, alcohol and other drug abuse, anorexia nervosa, obesity, and Crohn's disease.

The third unit describes current concepts and procedures for care of hospitalized children and their families. New discussions include preoperative teaching, laboratory tests, and care of the patient with spinal cord injuries and other mobility problems.

The fourth unit comprises two totally new chapters on the child with a chronic health problem and the dying child.

Chapters open with a list of key vocabulary terms, and conclude with up-to-date references and bibliography and new study questions. The vocabulary terms are defined in the new glossary. New tables, photographs, and drawings have been added throughout to clarify and reinforce information.

Despite extensive revisions, the book's primary objective remains unchanged: to provide the student nurse with the essential knowledge and skills to offer competent, compassionate care for children and their families. Instructors and students who use this text can help assure its usefulness in future editions by sharing their comments and suggestions.

Many persons have assisted in making this new edition

possible. Special thanks are due R. R. Wieczorek and J. N. Natapoff for permission to use many illustrations and tables from their text. Sincere appreciation is given to Marian Langer, R.N., M.S., whose thorough review of the material on diabetes mellitus, asthma, and allergy helped make those vital discussions more complete and up-to-date than ever before. To all other individuals and organizations whose support and encouragement were part of the total effort, deep gratitude is expressed. Foremost among these are David Miller and Paul R. Hill of the J. B. Lippincott Company. To Maggi Speer, whose diligence and dedication transformed the roughest of drafts into the most polished of manuscripts, are offered enduring appreciation and affection.

Violet Broadribb, R.N., M.S.

introduction
care of children and families:
changes, challenges, controversies

Nurses preparing to care for today's and tomorrow's children and families face vastly different responsibilities and challenges than did the pediatric nurse of two or three decades ago. Nurses and other health professionals are becoming increasingly concerned with much more than the care of sick children. Health teaching, prevention of illness, and promotion of optimal (most desirable or satisfactory) physical, developmental, and emotional health are all part of modern nursing (Table I–1).

Scientific and technologic advances have reduced the incidence of communicable disease and helped to control metabolic disorders such as diabetes. Much of health care takes place outside the hospital, either at home or in clinics or doctors' offices. Prenatal diagnosis of birth defects, transfusions, and other treatments for the unborn fetus as well as improved life-support systems for premature infants are but a few examples of the remarkable progress in child care.

In 1978 the world's first "test-tube" baby was born, the result of *in vitro fertilization*, a process developed to permit infertile couples to have children. In this process, ova are removed from the mother-to-be, fertilized by the father's sperm in a laboratory dish, and then reimplanted into the mother's uterus.

Such advances have given medical scientists and health-care consumers greater control over when children are born and how they are cared for. Some individuals and organizations regard these advances as potentially dangerous and unethical; others consider them landmarks in the progress toward better health.

Controversy continues about choices in family planning. In January, 1973, a Supreme Court decision declared abortion legal anywhere in the United States. In 1981, efforts were made to convince Congress that legislation should be passed to make all abortions illegal on the alleged grounds that the fetus is a person and therefore has the right to life. Bitter debate between pro-life and pro-choice groups seems likely to continue, at least until this legislation is passed or defeated.

Tremendous sociologic changes have affected attitudes toward, and concepts in, child health. American society is largely urban, with a population of highly mobile individuals and families. The women's movement has focused new attention on the needs of families in which the mother works outside the home. Escalating divorce rates and changing attitudes toward sexual roles have increased the number of single-parent families. Many people have come to regard health care as a right, not a privilege, and expect fair value received for their investment.

The reduction in communicable and infectious diseases has made it possible to devote more attention to such critical problems as child abuse, learning and behavior disorders, developmental disabilities, and chronic illness. Research in these areas continues, and as these findings become available, nurses will be among the practitioners who will help translate this research into improved health care for children and families.

Despite remarkable advances in many areas of maternal and child health, the maternal and infant mortality statistics are still grim. Infant mortality has declined steadily since 1960, even though the birthrate is beginning to climb after a leveling off period during the early 1970s (Fig. I–1).

Both infant and maternal mortality rates are much higher among nonwhite populations, a fact that studies repeatedly attribute to lack of adequate prenatal care and an increased birthrate among women 15 to 19 years of age, a high-risk group.

TABLE I–1. PREVENTIVE HEALTH SERVICES NECESSARY FOR WOMEN AND CHILDREN

Services for Infants, Children, and Youth	Services for Girls and Women of Childbearing Age
Health appraisal	Preconceptional care
History	Nutrition education and service
Screening	Family planning
Health examination	Prenatal care
Nutrition education and service	Health appraisal
Immunizations	Counseling
Safety and accident prevention	Early identification of health problems
Dental examination	Dental health
Early identification of health problems	Special care of high-risk women
Counseling and health education	Intrapartum care
	Postpartum care
	Interconceptional care
	Genetic diagnostic studies and counseling
	Abortion
	Sterilization
	Care of infertility
	Counseling and health education, including family life education and sex education; and prenatal counseling

(After Wallace H, Miller CA: A national health program for infants, children and youth. Health Care Management Review, 3, No. 4: 14, 1978)

development of child health care

Pediatrics is a comparatively young medical specialty, developing only in the mid-1800s. The first children's hospital opened in Philadelphia in 1855. Until that point in Western civilization's development, children were not considered important except as contributors to family income, and in hospitals had been cared for as adults were, often in the same bed.

Concern over hordes of homeless children brought about the formation of the Children's Aid Society in New York City in 1853. In 1876, the Society for the Prevention of Cruelty to Children (SPCC) was organized, years after the Society for Prevention of Cruelty to Animals had been formed.

Enforceable laws regulating child labor came very late in the United States. Not until 1938 did the Fair Labor Standards become federal law, finally providing for the enforcement of laws to abolish child labor for many, but not for all, children.

CHILDREN'S BUREAU

Little had been done to lower the death rate of infants and young children. Although no accurate statistics were kept, a study made as late as 1913 estimated that of 2,500,000 babies born each year in the United States, 300,000 died before their first birthday: a ratio of approximately 124 deaths per 1,000 live births (more than 10 times as many as in 1979).

Mothers had only the most elementary knowledge about infant care, and small children in orphanages or in-

fant homes received little care or attention. Public dismay mounted and indignation grew, and in 1903, Miss Lillian Wald, founder of the Henry Street Settlement, began working toward national action on the problem. Eventually she was able to interest President Theodore Roosevelt in the problem of infant mortality, and together they worked to mobilize public opinion.

In 1909, President Roosevelt called a conference to consider how the nation could best serve its children. The major recommendation from this first White House Conference was for the formation of a Children's Bureau.

In 1912, the Children's Bureau finally came into being. Its first task was a nationwide study of the high infant-mortality problem. After the fact-finding came wide dissemination of expert advice on child care, advice that was desperately needed. The Bureau eventually became the chief agency for dispensing financial and technical aid for the betterment of child welfare.

WHITE HOUSE CONFERENCES

Since 1909, White House Conferences have been called every 10 years by the President of the United States. These conferences have provided useful opportunities for discussing child-related problems on a nationwide scale. Recommendations for action are carried back to individual states by their representatives. Some of the conferences have been especially noteworthy. For instance, the 1950 White House Conference focused on the emotional development of the child, and at this conference the Pledge to Children was written (see boxed material).

The Golden Anniversary Conference on Children and

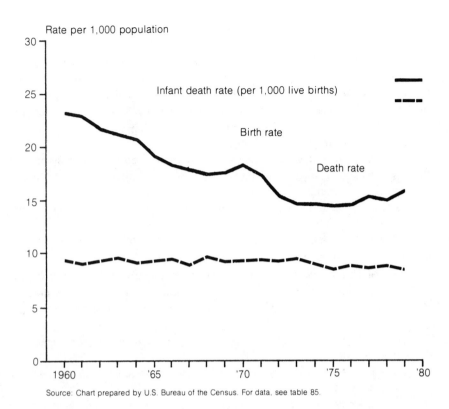

Rate per 1,000 population

Infant death rate (per 1,000 live births)

Birth rate

Death rate

FIG. I–1. Birth and death rates—1960 to 1979. (Redrawn from U.S. Bureau of the Census, Statistical Abstracts of 1980, Washington DC, 1980)

Source: Chart prepared by U.S. Bureau of the Census. For data, see table 85.

Youth in 1960 was attended by more than 14,000 persons, among whom were 1400 college- and high-school-age youths. Its theme was to promote opportunities for children and youth so that they could realize their full potential for a creative life in freedom and dignity.

The 1970 to 1971 White House Conference (perhaps the last national one) comprised two series of meetings—the Children's Conference (dealing with children ages 0–13) and the Youth Conference (dealing with issues relevant to adolescents and young adults). Specific recommendations emerged from both conferences and were submitted to the President. Delegates to the Youth Conference included many young persons between the ages of 14 and 24, whose concerns included drugs, environmental issues, military service, poverty, minorities, values, and ethics.

The 1980 to 1981 White House Conference was postponed because of the controversial values and issues surrounding family structure. Wieczorek and Natapoff indicated, "To have a single female head of household leading the conference was politically unacceptable."[1] Following the postponement, Secretary of Health and Human Services Richard Schweiker suggested that conferences held at the state level might be more productive and responsive to the specific needs of consumers.

President Jimmy Carter called a 1980 White House Conference on Families to "examine the strengths of American families, the difficulties they face and the ways in which family life is affected by public policies." Characterized by controversy throughout, this conference was not even able to agree upon a definition of what precisely constitutes a family. Pro-life factions argued that only persons related by blood, marriage, or adoption constitute a family; other more liberal groups suggested that homosexual couples or people living together out of wedlock also constitute a family. This sharp controversy typifies the emotional climate surrounding the dramatic changes occurring in American family lifestyles during the past two decades.

ADMINISTRATION FOR CHILDREN, YOUTH AND FAMILIES

In 1978, the Office of Child Development was replaced by a new agency, Administration for Children, Youth and Families (ACYF). It has three principal divisions: the Children's Bureau, the Head Start Program, and the Youth Development Program, and coordinates all children's programs within the federal government.

SELECT PANEL FOR THE PROMOTION OF CHILD HEALTH

Beginning in 1979, a Select Panel for the Promotion of Child Health conducted an 18-month study mandated by congressional action. Their findings were submitted to Congress and the Secretary of Health and Human Services in December, 1980, in a four-volume report, Better Health for Our Children: A National Strategy. The report announced that the government must assure universal access to three kinds of services: prenatal and maternity care, comprehensive care for children from birth through age five, and family-planning services. It called for creation of two new federal agencies: a new Maternal and Child Health Administration within the Public Health Service

PLEDGE TO CHILDREN

To you, our children, who hold within you our most cherished hopes, we, the members of the Midcentury White House Conference on Children and Youth, relying on your full response, make this pledge:

From your earliest infancy we give you our love, so that you may grow with trust in yourself and in others.

We will recognize your worth as a person and we will help you to strengthen your sense of belonging.

We will respect your right to be yourself and at the same time help you to understand the rights of others, so that you may experience cooperative living.

We will help you develop initiative and imagination, so that you may have the opportunity freely to create.

We will encourage your curiosity and your pride in workmanship, so that you may have the satisfaction that comes from achievement.

We will provide the conditions for wholesome play that will add to your learning, to your social experience, and to your happiness.

We will illustrate by precept and example the value of integrity and the importance of moral courage.

We will encourage you always to seek the truth.

We will provide you with all opportunities possible to develop your own faith in God.

We will open the way for you to enjoy the arts and to use them for deepening your understanding of life.

We will work to rid ourselves of prejudice and discrimination, so that together we may achieve a truly democratic society.

We will work to lift the standard of living and to improve our economic practices, so that you may have the material basis for a full life.

We will provide you with rewarding educational opportunities, so that you may develop your talents and contribute to a better world.

We will protect you against exploitation and undue hazards and help you grow in health and strength.

We will work to conserve and improve family life and, as needed, to provide foster care according to your inherent rights.

We will intensify our search for new knowledge in order to guide you more effectively as you develop your potentialities.

As you grow from child to youth to adult, establishing a family life of your own and accepting larger social responsibilities, we will work with you to improve conditions for all children and youth.

Aware that these promises to you cannot be fully met in a world at war, we ask you to join us in a firm dedication to the building of a world society based on freedom, justice, and mutual respect.

So may you grow in joy, in faith in God and in man, and in those qualities of vision and of the spirit that will sustain us all and give us new hope for the future.

---

and a National Commission on Maternal and Child Health. Primary emphasis is on reorganization of health services to stress prevention and primary care. It is likely that the recommendations of the Select Panel may not meet with the favor of the budget-slashing Congress and the Reagan administration, even though the recommendations may be sound and the services sorely needed.

INTERNATIONAL CHILD HEALTH

Although, overall, the United States has excellent pediatric medical care, there are gaps in its service to many of its people. Sweden has one half the infant mortality rate of the United States, whereas many Latin American countries have infant mortality rates 2.5 times that of the United States. The infant mortality rates are a good index of any country's health and should be studied carefully because they are a total figure of general health. They would not, for example, show a tribal difference in Uganda, a racial difference in Great Britain, or a sex differ-

ence in a primitive culture. It is necessary to study the statistics carefully to follow the differences in mortality rates and the access to health care among groups in any country.

The World Health Organization (WHO), the primary health agency of the United Nations, was established in 1948. Its primary objective is to help all peoples attain the highest possible level of health. WHO is an authority on international health care, and its many functions for health include the promotion of maternal–child health and welfare. It has done great work in decreasing the incidence of infectious diseases, a great killer of infants and children, and is a very important source for hygiene, health, and preventive education throughout the world.

As the 20th century world becomes increasingly industrialized, there is more access to health care for children even in the developing nations. Progress in development and availability of a service, however, does not always mean better health care. The high mortality rate of infants in the Third-World countries even with the modern invention of prepared milk formulas is an example of the large gap between progress and availability. In places where infants had been breastfed for long periods, modern, sanitized prepared formulas were introduced, but they were diluted with unsterile water (causing serious gastrointestinal infections) to further extend the supply (diminishing the nutrients), and kept in unhygienic conditions (not refrigerated when opened). For obvious reasons infant-mortality rates increased.

In May, 1981, WHO voted to support a voluntary commercial code to ban advertising and restrict marketing of commercial baby-formulas in Third-World countries. Those supporting this code said that it might save as many as 1 million infants who die each year from diseases related to poor feeding practices. This step was taken to encourage breastfeeding among Third-World mothers, because breast milk contains important antibodies that help protect infants against infection, and breastfeeding strengthens the psychological bond between mother and child. Nursing also acts as a functional contraceptive by delaying the return of the menstrual cycle after pregnancy. Ironically, the United States was the only member nation opposing this code, because, according to some sources, baby-formula is big business—$2 billion annually.

The United Nations International Children's Emergency Fund (UNICEF) was created in 1946 to serve a worldwide need for emergency aid in crises such as earthquakes, floods, and other disasters.

Canada and the United States have made an outreach to the rest of the world with the Canadian University Students Overseas (CUSO) and the United States's Peace Corps. Both organizations send skilled people, chiefly to developing countries, to teach, to nurse, to demonstrate, and to provide counsel and care for countries that request their services. Both organizations are also responsive to teaching about health and to meeting the health needs of children. The American Peace Corps is now under the organizational umbrella of ACTION.

Project Hope is another example of American outreach to the needy of the world. For many years it operated as a ship called *Hope,* which based itself in a needy, developing area, provided health care and treatment in that area, and taught citizens of developing countries how to improve their own health care. The ship no longer sails for this purpose but the project is actively functional, still with the dual service of medical care and teaching. In 1981, International Nursing Interchange was established at the Project Hope Health Sciences Education Center in Millwood, Virginia, to enhance nursing's contribution to improving world health, and thereby advance nursing practice, education, and research worldwide.[2]

changing concepts in child health care

INSTITUTIONAL CARE

Unfortunately, early institutions for children were notorious for their unsanitary conditions, neglect, and lack of proper infant nutrition. Well into the 19th century, mortality rates were commonly 50% to 100% among institutionalized children, whether in asylums or hospitals.

During the early 1900s a primary cause of death in children's institutions was the intractable diarrhea the majority of these children developed. Initiation of the simple practice of boiling milk and isolating children with septic conditions lowered the incidence of diarrhea.

Following World War I, a period of strict asepsis began. Babies were placed in individual cubicles, and the nurses were strictly forbidden to pick up the children except when absolutely necessary. Crib sides were draped with clean sheets, leaving infants with nothing to do but stare at the ceiling. The importance of toys in a child's environment appears not to have been recognized; besides, it was thought that such objects could transmit infection. Only parents were allowed to visit for half an hour or perhaps an hour each week. They were forbidden to pick up their children under penalty of having visiting privileges taken away entirely.

Despite these precautions, the high infant mortality continued. One of the first to suspect the cause was Joseph Brennaman, a physician of Children's Memorial Hospital, Chicago. Writing in 1932, he suggested that the infants suffered from a lack of stimulation; other concerned child specialists became interested. In the 1940s, Rene Spitz published the results of studies that supported his contention that deprivation of maternal care caused a state of dazed stupor in an infant. He believed this condition could become irreversible if the child were not returned to his mother promptly. He termed this state *anaclitic depression.* He also coined the term *hospitalism,* which he defined as "a *vitiated* condition of the body due to long confinement in the hospital [vitiated—feeble or weak]." Later it came to be used almost entirely to denote the harmful effects of institutional care on infants. Another physician, Bakwin, found that infants hospitalized for a long period of time actually developed physical symptoms, which he attributed to a lack of emotional stimulation and a lack of feeding satisfaction.

John Bowlby of London explored the subject of maternal deprivation thoroughly, working under the auspices of WHO. His report in 1951 received worldwide attention. His study revealed the negative results of the separation of a child from his mother because of hospitalization. His work, together with that of John Robertson, an associate, led to a reevaluation and liberalization of hospital-visiting policies for children.

Marshall Klaus and John Kennell, physicians at Rainbow Babies and Childrens Hospital, Cleveland, did important studies in the 1970s and 1980s on the effect of separation of newborns and parents. They established that this early separation can have long-term effects on family relationships, and that offering the new family an opportunity to be together at birth, and for a significant period after birth, can provide benefits that last well into early childhood (Fig. I-2). These findings have also helped to modify hospital policies.

Hospital regulations have changed slowly, but gradually have begun to reflect the human needs of patients and

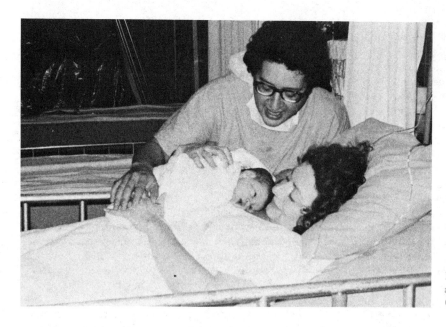

FIG. I–2. A new family together immediately after birth. (Courtesy of Nancy and Richard Guiterrez)

parents. Isolation practices have been relaxed for children who do not have infectious diseases; children are encouraged to ambulate as early as possible and to visit the playroom where they can be with other children. Nurses at all levels who work with children are prepared to understand, value, and use play as a therapeutic tool in the daily care of children.

Visiting hours are flexible for parents. Many parents are encouraged to stay with their child and participate in his care; some hospitals allow and even encourage siblings to visit. No longer is the parent "the visitor," but a family member and a partner in care.

The strange austerity of the hospital, with all its frightening apparatus, was made more threatening by the nurse's presence in a stark white uniform and cap. To many children, white represents doctors, needles, and things that are painful. To help overcome this fear, many pediatric nurses now wear colored uniforms, or even street clothes, and have omitted the cap.

FAMILY-CENTERED CARE

Family-centered nursing is a new and broadened concept in the health-care institutions of the United States. No longer are child-patients treated as clinical cases with attention given exclusively to their medical problems. Instead, caregivers recognize that children have at least one parent, belong to a family, a community, and a particular way of life or culture, and their health is influenced by these and other factors (Fig. I–3). Separating children from their background means that their needs are met only in a superficial manner, if at all. Even if nursing takes place entirely inside hospital walls, family-centered care pays attention to every child's emotional, developmental, social, and scholastic needs as well as his physical ones.

REGIONALIZED CARE

During the past three decades there has been a definite trend toward centralization and regionalization of pediat-

ric services. To provide high quality medical care in pediatrics necessitated moving the child-patient to medical teaching centers with the best resources for diagnosis and treatment.

To avoid duplication of services and equipment, the most intricate and expensive services and the most highly specialized personnel were made available in the centralized location: pediatric neurologists, adolescent allergy specialists, pediatric oncologists, nurse play therapists, child psychiatrists, pediatric nurse practitioners, and clinical nurse specialists. Here are found geneticists, neonatal intensive-care units, computerized tomography (CT) scanners, and burn-care units.

Regionalized care often takes the child-patient far from home. It is a longer distance for his parents and family to travel in order to visit than it would be for them to travel to the local suburban hospital. Family-centered care becomes even more important under these circumstances. Measures are always taken to keep the child's hospitalization as brief as possible, keep him as ambulatory as possible, and keep his family as close to him as possible. For the child to be separated from his family is traumatic and may actually retard recovery.

OTHER INNOVATIVE CHILD HEALTH-CARE PROGRAMS

Many pediatric hospitals have home-care programs for children with chronic illness such as leukemia, hemophilia, and cystic fibrosis. Between hospitalizations, the child's condition is monitored at home by the hospital's nurses, offering continuity of care.

Some pediatric hospitals have *primary nursing,* a system whereby one nurse plans the total care for a child and directs the efforts of nurses on the other two shifts. The primary nurse is responsible for his care at all times and will often make home visits to the child after discharge and before readmission.

Many children are now being cared for in Health

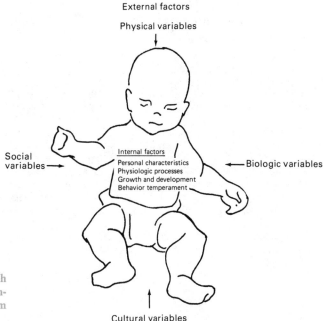

FIG. I–3. Internal and external factors that influence the health and illness pattern of the child. (Wieczarek RR, Natapoff JN: A Conceptual Approach to the Nursing of Children: Health Care From Birth to Adolescence. Philadelphia, JB Lippincott, 1981)

Maintenance Organizations (HMOs). These are professional groups of physicians, laboratory service people, nurse practitioners, nurses, and consultants who care for the health of a family on a continuing basis and are geared to health care and disease prevention. The family pays a set fee for total care; any necessary hospitalization is covered by that fee. Emphasis is on health and prevention, rather than on the acute-care, cure-oriented pediatric medical center (Fig. I–4).

In some private practices and in many clinic settings, the child is cared for by a pediatric nurse practitioner (PNP), a professional nurse, prepared at the postbaccalaureate level, to give primary health care to children and families. PNPs use pediatricians or family physicians as consultants but offer day-to-day assessment and care.

Nurses at all levels are legally accountable for their actions. As they increase their education, nurses can assume new responsibilities and accountability. Nurses at all levels and in all functions must keep their education current and maintain an up-to-date awareness of how to help their young patients and where to direct families for help, when other resources are needed (Table I–2).

THE NURSE'S CHANGING ROLE

In addition to helping children achieve optimal health, the nurse is also a teacher, advisor, and resource person who must know where and how to turn for assistance in various problems. It is important that information and advice be correct, pertinent, and useful to the person in need.

For example, Mrs. J asks advice concerning her retarded child. "He cannot learn; he is under foot all day long, getting into every form of mischief known. The neighbors are complaining, but what can I do? I don't want to put him in an institution," she says.

The nurse must be informed enough to tell her about public school classes for retarded children, and the re-

markable adjustments her child can make with the help of these classes. She should know whether transportation is provided for the children to and from school.

The nurse may also hear, "I am so completely exhausted with the new baby and the other small children. I know I am not giving the care they need, but if I could only have a little time to rest away from it all. . . ."

Anemia	3,000,000	
Mental retardation	2,800,000	
Speech impairment	2,200,000	
Crippling impairments (cardiovascular, cerebral palsy, epilepsy, diabetes, asthma)	1,700,000	
Emotional disturbances	1,500,000	
Learning disabilities	750,000	
Deafness	500,000	
Blindness	200,000	

FIG. I–4. Health problems that preventive services may curtail. (Data from Report of the Harvard Child Health Project Task Force. Toward a primary medical care system responsive to children's needs. Cambridge, Ballinger, 1977)

TABLE I–2.   TYPES OF HEALTH-CARE PROVIDERS AND THEIR MAJOR ROLES IN THE HEALTH-CARE SYSTEM

Health-care Providers	Major Roles
Nurses	Supervise health programs, teach children's health care, provide health-care treatments and procedures, assess health, offer nursing diagnosis, assist in health planning, and refer health problems to multidisciplinary teams
Pediatricians	Diagnose, treat problems, write prescriptions, supervise children's medical progress, make referrals to other specialists
Social workers	Provide guidance and referrals in familial, social, political, and economic health-care areas
Psychiatrists, psychologists, and mental health consultants	Treat emotional problems of children and families through appropriate therapy plan based on individual needs and diagnoses
Medical specialists (e.g., pediatric cardiologists, allergists, surgeons, and neurologists)	Provide consultation (medical or surgical) and therapy for specialized illnesses or deviations from normal
Clinical nurse-specialists, pediatric nurse-practitioners, and community health nurses	Specialize in specific health needs of children, offer health care involving nursing supervision in institutions, homes, and communities
Play therapists and recreation therapists	Develop the special needs of sick children through therapeutic use of the play process, help children express their feelings, attitudes, and beliefs about their health and treatment regimens
Laboratory technicians (e.g., hematologists, x-ray, EEG, and ECG technicians)	Administer prescribed tests or procedures to children as an aid in making diagnoses or in evaluating treatment plans
Speech and hearing therapists	Evaluate speech and hearing problems in children, aid in diagnosing these problems, establish and implement individualized treatment plans
Rehabilitation therapists	Assist handicapped children to reach their maximum level of performance based on their particular disability, help children with temporary loss of function to regain abilities based on their expected level of performance and past achievements
Hospital teachers	Work in hospitals to assist children with their academic needs during their separation from community schools
Nutritionists	Plan children's nutritional therapy based on their diagnoses, age, cultural and religious backgrounds, and state of health
Dentists	Care for the teeth and gums of children by preventing decay and malocclusion, fill and clean teeth, and make referrals for malocclusions
Optometrists	Examine children's visual acuity, measure vision errors, and prescribe glasses to correct visual defects

(Wieczorek RR, Natapoff JN: A Conceptual Approach to the Nursing of Children: Health Care From Birth Through Adolescence. Philadelphia, JB Lippincott, 1981)

The nurse who knows about Homemaker Service and other available resources may be of genuine assistance.

Nursing's image has changed and the horizons and responsibilities have broadened tremendously. Child care now involves surveillance of growth and development, anticipatory guidance about maturational and common health problems, teaching and follow-up about immunization and health teaching as well as treatment of disease and physical problems.

COMMUNITY RESOURCES

Too often the distraught parent does not know where to turn to find help, or perhaps does not even know that help is available. The well-informed nurse can be the guide to better health and living. Today, there are multiple sources of help for families in need of guidance or physical care. Government-sponsored resources are now available in every state, in both city and rural areas. Specialized cen-

ters and clinics, usually functioning through government grants and private contributions, are able to give free or inexpensive help. In addition, private organizations interested in child health and welfare usually are easily available in most areas. City or state funds and private donations help keep these agencies solvent.

The United States Department of Health and Human Services has provided grants to large numbers of community-health projects in the cities and rural areas of all states. Among these are children and youth projects, neighborhood health centers, maternal and infant care, mental retardation projects, crippled children projects, and migrant health projects.

Nearly all of the projects help with transportation by providing carfare or reimbursing the cost of private means, or by picking up the children at their homes or schools. A few projects provide babysitting services for the mother while she takes some of her children for health care.

HOMEMAKER SERVICE

Any family may be caught by circumstances that make it temporarily impossible for a parent to care for the children. A mother may be ill and require hospitalization; she may have an ill or disturbed child who requires so much attention that she has little time or strength to care for the rest of the family. Or, she may need help and guidance in meeting the family's many needs.

Homemaker service offers help in these and other crises. Homemaker workers receive training in such subjects as health practices, behavior problems, and housekeeping. This preliminary training is given by public health nurses, social workers, nutritionists, and when on an assignment the worker frequently meets with a member of the agency staff.

The professional homemaker may come into a home for a few hours to relieve the parent and allow her to get much needed rest, or to help her meet other problems. Some agencies are able to provide 24-hour service. Charges for services are on a sliding scale, according to the ability of the client to pay.

One example serves to illustrate this needed service: Mrs. S was a blind mother of a young baby; there was no father in the home. She lived in an upper flat with an outside stairway, in a poor area of the city. A professional homemaker came daily to teach her how to care for the child; Mrs. S was a proud woman who learned quickly.

When a visiting nurse came into the home she found an 18-month-old baby, spotlessly clean, well-nourished and cared for. The flat was neatly kept. Mrs. S had progressed to the point that the homemaker needed only to visit the home once a week to see if all was going well.

FOSTER GRANDPARENT PROGRAM

In 1971, a federal agency called ACTION was established for the purpose of providing opportunities for all Americans to serve their communities through volunteer work. ACTION operates in all of the states; one of its successful programs is the Foster Grandparent Program.[3]

The Foster Grandparent Program provides part-time volunteer opportunities for older persons to render supportive person-to-person services to children with special needs in health, education, and related areas. The program focuses primarily on a continuing relationship between an older person and a child with special needs. Thus, it is a mutually beneficial relationship for both child and adult that can serve in many settings: hospital pediatric departments; institutions or schools for physically, emotionally, or mentally handicapped children; correctional facilities; daycare settings; and, if circumstances warrant it, private homes. This service is available to children through age seventeen.

The volunteer foster grandparent must be sixty years or over. Generally the grandparent has a low income, but must be physically and mentally able, be understanding of a child's needs, and have a desire to help children. After a 40-hour period of special training, they work 4 hours daily, 5 days a week. Each volunteer usually serves two children each day; activities may include personal care for a child, such as bathing, dressing, feeding, or just holding the child. Volunteers may assist a child in learning or in therapy sessions; they may read to him, talk, or just listen.

Individual supervision, additional continuing instruction for 4 hours a week, and support and counseling are given to the volunteers when requested or needed. All foster grandparents receive a stipend, which supplements their low income.

Although not available in every community, the service has been both successful and rewarding to the children and to the volunteer grandparents. There are many children the nurse will discover in practice who could use this valuable service.

HEAD START PROGRAM

The Head Start program is based on the premise that all children share certain needs, and that children of low-income families, in particular, can benefit from a comprehensive developmental program to meet these needs. It is aimed particularly at stimulation of the preschool child so that he has a healthy start at the beginning of the school years. The primary goal for the Head Start program is to bring about a greater degree of competence in the child's everyday effectiveness in dealing with responsibilities in school and in life. This includes the following:

- Improvement of the child's health and physical abilities
- Correction of any physical and mental problems
- Working toward the goal of an adequate diet for the child
- Offering help to the child's family toward improvement of future health care and physical abilities of the child

Head Start seeks to involve the entire family of a child, as well as the community. Parents are assisted in providing developmental experiences in their homes, and some programs are entirely home-based if this is indicated.

Head Start operates as a preschool project, but some programs have been continued into kindergarten and first grade, for the purpose of enabling these children to experience continuity of development as they transfer from Head Start into school programs.

All Head Start programs encourage and provide opportunities for the use of volunteers, in addition to the regular staff.

One facet of the Head Start program is the Head Start Services to Handicapped Children. It is mandated to serve children with a broad range of handicaps such as mental retardation, deafness, speech or visual impairment, emotional disturbances, crippling conditions, and other health impairments.

The majority of Head Start programs enroll handicapped children in full-year programs. Most of these provide special equipment or materials for these children. Staff members serving handicapped children have additional preparation for working with the handicapped.[4]

WELL CHILD CLINICS

Well child clinics are sometimes called Child Health Conferences, and they are designed to maintain the health of the child, give guidance, and help with problems of development. They offer a ready resource for information and counseling for parents. Supervised playrooms are available in many clinics. Most projects accept children from birth to 18 years of age. Activities include screening for vision and hearing problems, dental care, as well as teaching dental hygiene, nutrition, and social services, and many more.

summary

Nursing care of infants and children has made tremendous strides during the last half of the twentieth century. New knowledge, techniques, and technology are available to improve health care for all children. Staying in step with changing practice and procedures, keeping current with the nursing literature, and remembering always to consider the total needs of the child and the family present a continuing challenge. Meeting that challenge offers tremendous personal and professional satisfaction.

references

1. Child health panel releases report; sees larger RN role. Am J Nurs 81:275–276, 1981
2. International Nursing Interchange established by Project HOPE. Image 13, No. 2:43, 1981
3. Foster grandparent program: operations handbook for sponsors. U.S. Department of Health, Education, and Welfare, 1974
4. Head Start program. Performance standards. Head Start policy manual. U.S. Department of Health, Education, and Welfare, 1975

bibliography

Barnes FEF: Ambulatory Maternal Health Care and Family Planning Services. Washington, DC, American Public Health Association, 1978

Healthy People: The Surgeon General's Report on Health Promotion and Disease Prevention, 1979. Department of Health, Education, and Welfare (PHS) Pub. II-79-55071. Washington, DC, U.S. Government Printing Office, 1979

Jensen MD, Benson R, Bobak IM: Maternity Care: The Nurse and the Family, 2nd ed. St Louis, CV Mosby, 1981

Kalisch BJ: From medical care helper to health care provider: Perspectives on the development of maternal child nursing. Am J Mat Child Nurs 5:377–382, 1980

March of Dimes Birth Defects Foundation. Toward Improving the Outcome of Pregnancy: Recommendations for the Regional Development of Maternal and Perinatal Health Services. White Plains, The Foundation, 1977

Phillips CR: Family-centered Maternity Newborn Care. St Louis, CV Mosby, 1980

Shearer MH: The effects of regionalization of perinatal care on hospital services for normal childbirth. Birth and the Family Journal 4:4, winter 1977

Sprague HA, Taylor JR: The Health Impact of Maternity and Infant Care Programs. Report of Michigan Public Health Services, 1979.

Whaley L, Wong D: Nursing Care of Infants and Children. St. Louis, CV Mosby, 1979

Wieczorek RR, Natapoff JN: A Conceptual Approach to the Nursing of Children: Health Care From Birth to Adolescence. Philadelphia, JB Lippincott, 1981

contents

unit two: a child grows

unit three: a child enters the hospital

unit four: a child faces chronic or terminal illness

introductory pediatric nursing

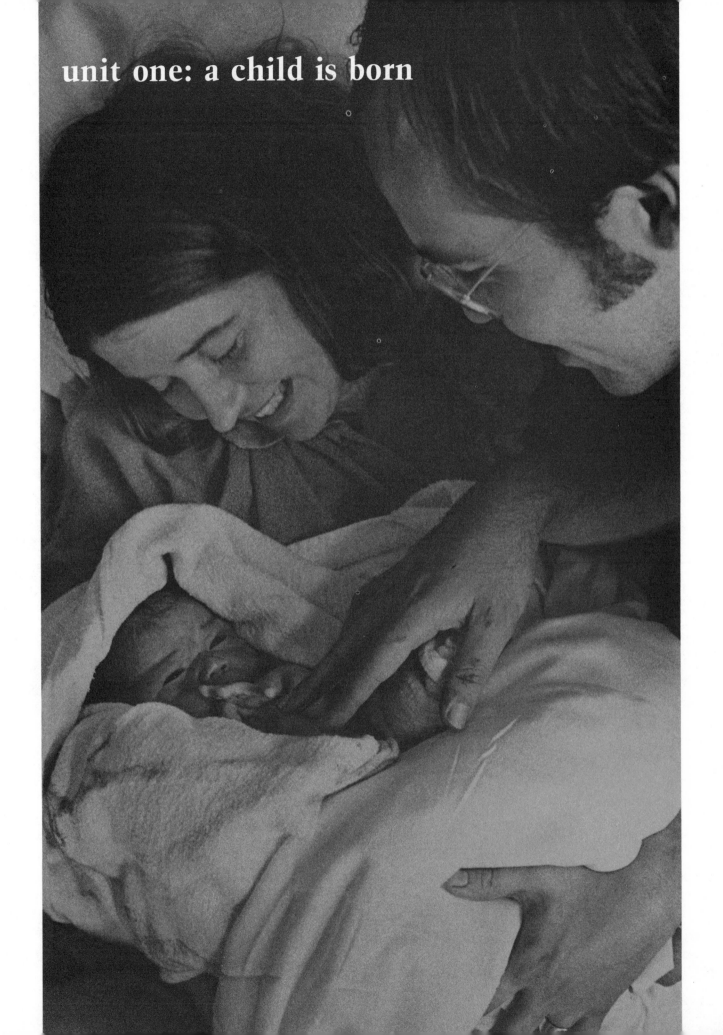

unit one: a child is born

life before birth

prenatal growth and development
gestation
genetic influences
karyotypes
determination of sex
determination of inherited traits
genetic counseling
environmental influences
maternal age
maternal nutrition
maternal infections
chemicals
radiation
mechanical factors
education for parenthood
prenatal care
prepared childbirth
summary
review questions
references
bibliography

student objectives

The student successfully attaining the goals of this chapter will be able to

1 Define the following vocabulary terms:

amniocentesis   birthing room   chromosome   embryo   fetus   genotype
karyotype   mutation   teratogenesis   zygote

2 Identify the three stages of prenatal development that occur during the first eight weeks following conception.

3 Describe a karyotype and explain two ways in which it can be used.

4 List three maternal habits that may be harmful to the fetus.

5 Discuss the effects of maternal age on the potential outcome of a woman's pregnancy.

6 List three primary goals of genetic counseling.

From the moment of conception until full maturity, human life proceeds in an orderly pattern of growth and development. This pattern and the individual that results are shaped by various factors that precede and follow conception. Genetic influences help determine a child's physical and intellectual characteristics, as do environmental influences. Once conception has occurred, a child's genetic heritage cannot be changed. The environment can be altered, however, with either positive or negative effects on the child and the family. Fortunately a great deal of knowledge is now available to prospective parents to help them to provide a favorable environment in which their child can grow and develop.

prenatal growth and development

Conception occurs when a sperm cell reaches and penetrates an ovum. This process is also called fertilization, and it produces a fertilized ovum, or *zygote*. During the first 10 days to 2 weeks of life, the zygote becomes implanted in the lining of the uterus. Once implanted, the growing organism is referred to as an *embryo*. After it acquires a human likeness, usually about the eighth week of life, it is termed a *fetus*.

At no other time in a person's life is growth more rapid than during the intrauterine period. The microscopic zygote increases in size more than 200-billion times during the 9 months before birth. Two distinct but related processes take place during the transformation of zygote to infant: growth and differentiation. *Growth* is the result of cell division and is marked by an increase in size and weight. *Differentiation* changes the dividing cells, creating specialized tissues necessary to form an organized, coordinated individual.

GESTATION

The normal time required for a child to grow from a single cell to a newborn infant is 9 calendar months or 10 lunar months (Fig. 1–1). A baby that is born before the sixth month is considered at risk and may not survive, even with the special life-support systems available in modern intensive care nurseries. The earliest gestational age at which a fetus can survive outside the uterine environment is called *viability*. Deviation in the gestational age of new-

born babies is normal, but the closer the infant comes to the full 9 months gestation, the greater the chances are for a healthy neonatal period.

TRIMESTERS

Gestation is divided into trimesters. *Organogenesis*, the process by which cells differentiate into major organ systems, commences shortly after conception and is almost completed by the end of the eighth week. Even the 4-week-old embryo (Fig. 1–2) shows evidence of beginning organs and organ systems. After the eighth week of life, the major changes are the growth and development of organs and organ systems. The first trimester is the time when the fetus is most vulnerable to any hazard in the intrauterine environment.

The second trimester is a period of continuing growth and development. All reflexes are present by the end of the fourth month, except for functional respiration and vocal response. All nerve cells are present by the fifth month, although not functionally mature.

If circumstances cause premature birth during the third trimester, the child has developed sufficiently to survive, provided he receives constant, expert care. During this last trimester, the fetus stores iron for postnatal use, and develops subcutaneous fat, which will enable it to begin independent life. Figure 1–3 summarizes the month-by-month growth and development of the fetus.

INTRAUTERINE ENVIRONMENT

The child develops within the protection of a fluid environment surrounded by the *amniotic sac*. This strong, translucent membrane is large and elastic enough to permit the fetus to move about and turn at will during most of its intrauterine life. The amniotic sac usually contains about 1000 ml of amniotic fluid, which is a clear, neutral to slightly alkaline (*p*H 7.0 to 7.25) liquid. This fluid protects the fetus from direct impact upon the mother's abdomen, separates the fetus from the membranes, aids symmetric growth and development, helps to maintain a constant body temperature by preventing heat loss, provides oral fluid for the fetus, and acts as an excretion collection system.

Studies of amniotic fluid have provided a wealth of knowledge such as fetal sex, state of fetal health, and fetal

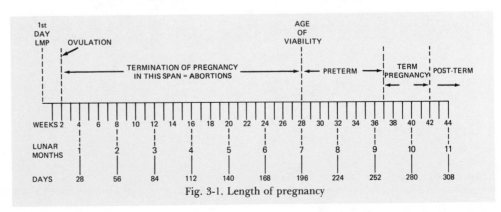

FIG. 1–1. Length of pregnancy. (Bethea DC: Introductory Maternity Nursing, 3rd ed. Philadelphia, JB Lippincott, 1979)

Fig. 3-1. Length of pregnancy

maturity. *Amniocentesis* is a recently developed procedure in which a sample of amniotic fluid is withdrawn for early diagnosis of possible abnormalities such as mental retardation, blood disorders, or respiratory problems. Performed under local anesthesia, the procedure is done by inserting a needle through the abdominal and uterine walls into the amniotic sac. A small amount of fluid is removed (about 20 ml) and placed in a special medium where it is allowed to grow for 3 to 4 weeks. At the end of this time the fluid is analyzed, and any abnormalities are reported to the prospective parents. Because this procedure holds some risk to mother and fetus, it is not performed unless the physician believes a problem exists. Later in pregnancy, this test may also be used to determine fetal lung and kidney maturity prior to early cesarean delivery or induction of labor.

During intrauterine development, the *placenta*, or what will be the afterbirth, links the fetus to the mother. This marvelous organ performs four functions for the developing fetus: respiration, nutrition, excretion, and protection. The placenta is a reddish, disc-shaped organ, connected to the fetus by the *umbilical cord* (Fig. 1–4). The cord is relatively stiff owing to the pulsating blood carried in its two arteries and one vein, it is long enough to allow the fetus to move freely. Blood from the placenta brings food, oxygen, hormones, and protective antibodies to the fetus by way of the umbilical vein. The umbilical arteries carry deoxygenated fetal blood and waste products back to the placenta. Only at birth when the umbilical blood flow diminishes and stops is the cord flexible enough to be hazardous to the infant, and at that time there is usually someone present to assist the delivery. The placenta normally emerges soon after delivery of the baby, hence the term *afterbirth*.

Many drugs, viruses, and infections cross the placental barrier from mother to fetus. These hazards to the developing fetus are discussed under "Environmental Influences."

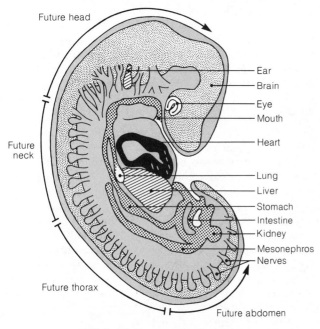

FIG. 1–2. Four-week-old embryo.

1st Lunar Month
1. *Length* 0.75–1 cm. (0.3–0.4 inch)
2. Trophoblasts imbed in decidua.
3. Chorionic villi form.
4. Foundations formed for nervous system, genitourinary system, skin, bones, and lungs.
5. Buds of arms and legs begin to form.
6. Rudiments of eyes, ears, and nose appear.

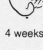

4 weeks

2nd Lunar Month
1. *Length* 2.5 cm. (1 inch)
   Weight 4 gm.
2. Fetus is markedly bent.
3. Head is disproportionately large, owing to brain development.
4. Sex differentiation begins.
5. Centers of bone begin to ossify.

8 weeks

3rd Lunar Month
1. *Length* 7–9 cm. (2.8–3.6 inches)
   Weight 5.20 gm.
2. Fingers and toes are distinct.
3. Placenta is complete.
4. Fetal circulation is complete.

3 months

FIG. 1–3. Fetal growth by month. (Reeder SJ, Mastroianni Jr L, Martin L: Maternity Nursing, 14th ed. Philadelphia, JB Lippincott, 1980)

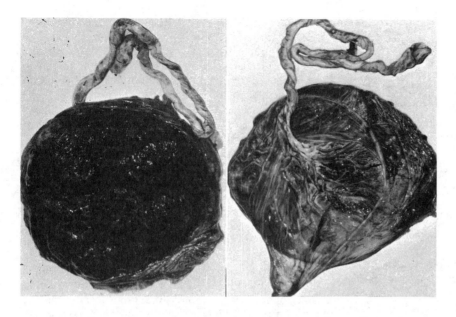

FIG. 1–4. (*Left*) The maternal surface of the placenta is rough and irregular. (*Right*) The fetal surface is smooth and shiny. (Bethea DC: Introductory Maternity Nursing, 3rd ed. Philadelphia, JB Lippincott, 1979)

4th Lunar Month
1. *Length* 10–17 cm. (4–6.7 inches)
   Weight 55–120 gm. (1.9–4.2 oz.)
2. Sex is differentiated.
3. Rudimentary kidneys secrete urine.
4. Heart beat is present.
5. Nasal septum and palate close.

4th month

5th Lunar Month
1. *Length* 30 cm. (12 inches)
   Weight 280–300 gm. (9.9–10.6 oz.)
2. Lanugo covers entire body.
3. Fetal movements are felt by mother.
4. Heart sounds are perceptible with fetoscope.

5th month

6th Lunar Month
1. *Length* 28–34 cm. (11.2–13.4 inches)
   Weight 650 gm. (1.4 lb.)
2. Skin appears wrinkled.
3. Vernix caseosa appears.
4. Eyebrows and fingernails develop.

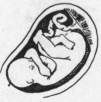

6th month

7th Lunar Month
1. *Length* 35–38 cm. (13.8–15 inches)
   Weight 1200 gm. (2.6 lb.)
2. Skin is red.
3. Pupillary membrane disappears from eyes.
4. If born, infant cries, breathes, but usually expires.

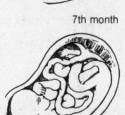

7th month

8th Lunar Month
1. *Length* 38–43 cm. (15–17 inches)
   Weight 2000 gm. (3.5–4.2 lb.)
2. Fetus is viable.
3. Eyelids open.
4. Fingerprints are set.
5. Vigorous fetal movement occurs.

8th month

9th Lunar Month
1. *Length* 42–49 cm. (16.5–19.3 inches)
   Weight 1700–2600 gm. (3.7–5.7 lb.)
2. Face and body have loose wrinkled appearance due to subcutaneous fat deposit.
3. Lanugo disappears.
4. Amniotic fluid decreases somewhat.

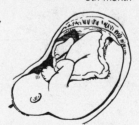

9th month

10th Lunar Month
1. *Length* 48–52 cm. (18.9–20.5 inches)
   Weight 3000–3600 gm. (6.6–7.9 lb.)
2. Skin is smooth.
3. Eyes are uniformly slate-colored.
4. Bones of skull are ossified and nearly together at sutures.

genetic influences

The science of genetics studies the ways in which normal and abnormal traits are transmitted from one generation to the next. The basic principles of genetics were discovered in 1865 by an Austrian monk named Gregor Mendel, through experimentation with common garden peas. Only within the 20th century have Mendel's principles been rediscovered and employed in science and medicine.

Before Mendel's time it was believed that the characteristics of parents were blended in their children. Mendel's experiments proved that this blending does not occur, but rather that the parent's individual characteristics could reappear unchanged in later generations.

All living organisms are composed of living cells that contain all the material necessary for the maintenance and propagation of the particular species. Each cell contains a number of small bodies called *chromosomes*. Chromosomes are threadlike structures, occurring in pairs; each pair is attached at the center by a *centromere*. Threaded along these chromosomes are *genes*, the units that carry genetic instructions from one generation to another. Like chromosomes, genes also occur in pairs. The instructions they carry are called the *genetic code*, the blueprint for the development of the individual organism. Each person's individual set of genes is called his *genotype*.

Each human cell contains 46 chromosomes, consisting of 23 essentially identical or homologous pairs. One member of each pair will be contributed by the father, and one by the mother, to the single cell formed by the union of sperm at conception, which determines the sex and inherited traits of the new organism.

Twenty-two of these pairs are alike in both the male and the female, and are called *autosomes*. The remaining pair is a pair of *sex chromosomes*, which differ in the male and the female. When the form or number of autosomes are altered, birth defects or abnormalities result.

KARYOTYPES

Modern technology has made it possible to photograph the nuclei of human cells and enlarge them to show the chromosomes. The chromosomes are cut from the photographs, matched in pairs, and grouped. The resulting picture is a *karyotype*, and is used to locate chromosomal malformations and translocations (the change in position of a segment of chromosome to another location on the chromosome or to another chromosome). Karyotypes of normal chromosomes are properly paired (Fig. 1–5). In some abnormal conditions, translocations occur. In others, such as in trisomy 21 (Down's syndrome, or mongolism), three chromosomes occur in the 21 or 22 position (Fig. 1–6), producing a total of 47 chromosomes instead of the normal 46.

DETERMINATION OF SEX

All egg cells from the female carry a pair of female chromosomes called the *X chromosomes*. Sperm cells, however, carry one X(female) and one Y(male) chromosome. It appears to be a matter of chance whether or not the egg, which always has an X chromosome, will be fertilized by a sperm carrying an X chromosome or by one carrying a Y. In the former case, the offspring is a girl (Figs. 1–7; 1–8). The Y chromosome is dominant over the X, so that if the Y enters into the union, the result is always a male child (Figs. 1–7; 1–9). In any event, it is the father's sex cell that determines the child's sex.

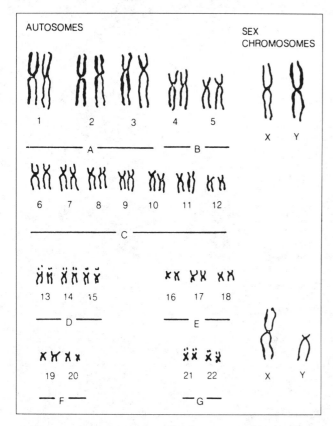

FIG. 1–5. Arrangement of normal chromosomes into a standard karyotype.

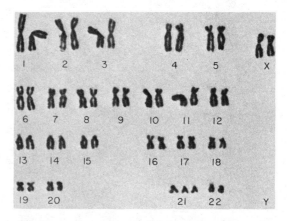

FIG. 1–6. Karyotype showing Trisomy 21. Note 3 chromosomes in 21 position. (Courtesy of Dr. Kurt Hirschhorn)

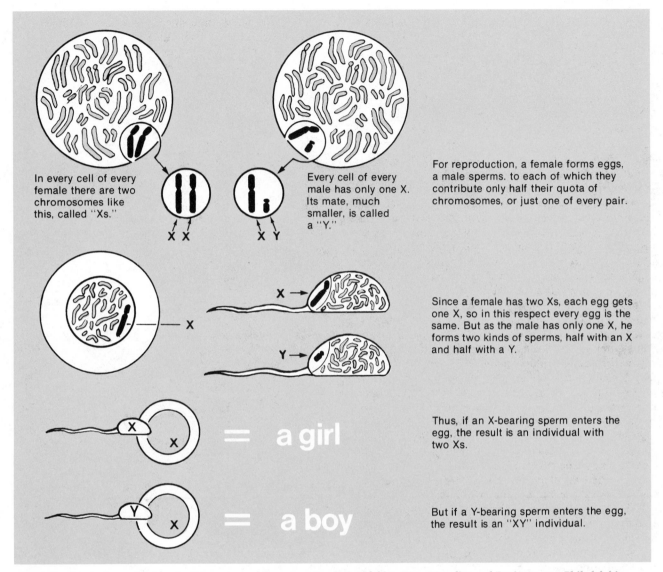

In every cell of every female there are two chromosomes like this, called "Xs."

Every cell of every male has only one X. Its mate, much smaller, is called a "Y."

For reproduction, a female forms eggs, a male sperms. to each of which they contribute only half their quota of chromosomes, or just one of every pair.

X X

X Y

Since a female has two Xs, each egg gets one X, so in this respect every egg is the same. But as the male has only one X, he forms two kinds of sperms, half with an X and half with a Y.

X

X

Y

= a girl

Thus, if an X-bearing sperm enters the egg, the result is an individual with two Xs.

X   X

= a boy

But if a Y-bearing sperm enters the egg, the result is an "XY" individual.

Y   X

FIG. 1-7.   Sex is determined at the time sperm and ovum unite. (Scheinfeld A: Your Heredity and Environment. Philadelphia, JB Lippincott, 1965)

FIG. 1-8.   Normal female karyotype. (Courtesy of Dr. Kurt Hirschhorn)

FIG. 1-9.   Normal male karyotype. Compare sex chromosomes (*right*) with those of female in Fig. 1-8. (Courtesy of Dr. Kurt Hirschhorn)

Cells reproduce by division; each parent cell produces two daughter cells, each of which in turn produces two new cells. In this manner the single cell produced by the union of sperm and ovum eventually multiplies to produce a human infant.

DETERMINATION OF INHERITED TRAITS

The ultramicroscopic bodies called genes carry genetic instruction from one generation to another with mathematic regularity. Any gene can be altered, however, by mutation or chromosomal rearrangement. *Mutation* in a gene means that a fundamental change has taken place in its structure, resulting in the transmission of a trait different from that normally carried by the particular gene. Much remains to be learned about the causes of mutations, most of which result in undesirable traits.

When any two members of a pair of genes carry the same genetic instructions, the person carrying these genes is said to be *homozygous* for that particular trait. When each member of a pair of genes carries different instructions, the person is *heterozygous* for the trait. One member of a heterozygous pair of genes will be the dominant gene. Thus a trait or condition appearing in a heterozygous person will be called an *autosomal dominant trait.* A gene carrying different information for the same trait that is not expressed (*e.g.*, blue eyes vs brown eyes) is called a *recessive* gene. Inheritance patterns for autosomal recessive traits are shown in Figure 1–10. However, if both parents express the recessive trait, all their children will have the same trait or condition, because each parent must have two genes for the trait and the children cannot possibly escape inheriting two also. Some examples of recessive diseases are thalassemia and cystic fibrosis.

A dominant gene may be defined as one that is expressed in only one of a chromosome pair. A recessive gene is only detectable when present on both chromosomes. One example of a dominant inheritance is the condition of osteogenesis imperfecta.

In autosomal dominant inheritance, the affected parent will usually trasmit the dominant allele* to half his children, who will be affected. This, however, may not *always* be the ratio of 1:1.

GENETIC COUNSELING

Knowledge about genetics and the causes of specific birth defects continues to increase rapidly. One of the benefits of this increased knowledge is *genetic counseling.* In many parts of the U.S., particularly in large cities, couples can consult a genetic counselor before deciding to have children. The counselor, a geneticist, studies the family history of both partners and may perform tissue analysis to determine chromosome patterns. This is particularly important to persons who may think they are carriers of such heritable disorders as Tay-Sachs disease or sickle cell

---

* Allele—forms of a gene found at the same locus on homologous chromosomes.

---

anemia. It is also helpful to persons whose family history includes one or more mentally retarded individuals.

Genetic counseling has three primary goals: the first is to identify malformations and diseases that can be trans-

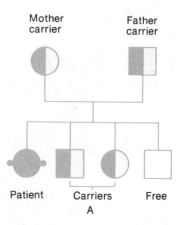

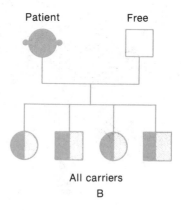

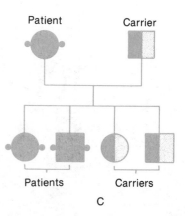

FIG. 1–10. Autosomal recessive pattern inheritance. (*A*) Both parents carriers—ratio of one patient, two carriers, one free from disease. (*B*) One patient—one parent free from disease, all children carriers—no clinical disease. (*C*) One parent carrier, one parent has disease—ratio of two children with disease, two carriers.

mitted genetically, and determine the probability of their recurrence; the second goal is to identify potential problems for the fetus or neonate and to assure early diagnosis and management; and, the third goal is to ultimately reduce the number of children born with heritable disorders. Health professionals can only provide information and support; the final decision concerning whether or not to have a child remains with one or both members of the couple.

environmental influences

Although it is recognized that the genetic material furnishes the building blocks for a new person, the old controversy concerning the importance of heredity versus environment (nature vs. nurture) has lost its significance, at least in relation to intrauterine life. Current knowledge indicates that heredity and environment influence and modify each other.

Because the mother's body is the environment for the developing fetus, nothing is more important to the successful outcome of a pregnancy than the mother's health, both physical and emotional. Though we no longer believe that a mother who attends concerts and art exhibitions will have a child who appreciates music and art, we do know that some of her reactions can influence the child. Emotions such as fear or anxiety cause adrenalin to be released into the bloodstream, which passes through the placenta to the fetus, triggering a physical reaction similar to the mother's. Extreme, prolonged stress in the mother may cause an autonomic imbalance in the unborn child, which will be reflected as irritability and emotional insecurity after birth.

MATERNAL AGE

Statistics indicate that the most favorable time for a woman to bear children is between the ages of 20 and 34. Mothers younger than age 20 experience such difficulties as excessive weight gain, toxemia, and prolonged labor more often than do older mothers. Teenage pregnancies produce infants of low birth weight, increasing the risk of neonatal morbidity and mortality. In addition to the physical problems encountered by teenage mothers, emotional and often financial complications occur. A young adolescent still has growing and maturing of her own to do, and may very much resent the pregnancy. This resentment may be reflected in neglect of her own health and, later, in neglect or in abuse of the infant. Very young couples are often limited in their earning capacity and the additional expense of a baby may be actually unwelcome.

The unmarried teenage mother presents very special problems. Frequently she has no one to support her emotionally or financially, nor anyone with whom to share the wondrous changes that are happening within her body. She may fail to obtain the prenatal care and advice necessary for a normal birth and healthy development of the infant. Should she decide to give her baby up for adoption, she may not have the counseling and guidance she needs to rebuild her changed life. It is important that nurses who care for these young women do so in a nonjudgmental manner so as not to contribute to their guilt and emotional insecurity.

Women who become mothers after age 35 are also subject to possible complications during pregnancy. This age group shows a higher incidence of hypertension, toxemia, uterine inertia, malposition of the fetus, and pelvic disproportion. Spontaneous abortion occurs more frequently in this age group as does the birth of children with Down's syndrome and other congenital anomalies. For example, the incidence of Down's syndrome is four times as great for mothers over age 35 as for those aged 20 to 29. The reasons for these problems are not completely understood. This is an important area of research, however, because motherhood is becoming increasingly common after age 35 as women choose to work longer before beginning their families.

MATERNAL NUTRITION

The unborn child has a comfortable nutritional arrangement with his mother. Generally speaking, a prospective mother who follows a sensible diet, and augments it correctly to fit the needs of the child, provides adequately for both herself and her child.

During the first part of pregnancy the average woman requires about 2000 to 2100 calories per day, which should be increased by 300 calories during the latter part of pregnancy, and by 500 calories during lactation. Women who are very active or nutritionally deficient might need as much as 3000 calories to fulfill energy and nutrient demands. The pregnant woman's calorie intake should comprise nutritious foods, selected from the basic-four food groups, and ample liquids, including 6 to 8 glasses of water each day.

Maternal dietary allowances of protein, iron, vitamins A, B, C, and D, and calcium need to be increased during pregnancy. The infant needs to receive sufficient iron to build up his iron store for the first few months after birth. All of the nutritional needs of the fetus will be met, as much as possible, to the detriment of the mother's health if her own nutrition is inadequate.

MATERNAL INFECTIONS

A mother's infections represent distinct hazards for the unborn child. The outstanding example is that of maternal rubella (German measles). Although a mild disease in adults, it produces a high percentage of congenital malformations in the fetus when the mother is infected during the first trimester. Congenital cataracts, deafness, mental retardation, and congenital heart disease are abnormalities resulting most often from this virus.

A live-virus rubella vaccine is now used to vaccinate young children, and should result in a marked decline of this disease in future generations. This vaccine is not given to girls or women of childbearing age because its possible effect on a developing fetus is not yet known.

Another virus encountered with increasing frequency is herpes simplex virus, hominus type II. A venereal disease that is almost impossible to cure, herpes type II causes painful lesions on the mother's vulva and vagina, and requires cesarean delivery of the infant for its survival.

CHEMICALS

As mentioned earlier, the placenta makes possible the transfer of food and oxygen from mother to developing child. But the placenta is not selective in the materials transferred. Therefore, many of the drugs—either prescribed or purchased over the counter—taken by the mother also reach the fetus, and can produce birth defects. Alcohol and nicotine are commonly used chemicals in today's society. Research indicates that their use by pregnant women can cause serious damage to the fetus.

When the prenatal growth processes are disrupted, resulting in a physical defect in the child, this is referred to as *teratogenesis* (from the Latin *terato*, monster, and *genesis*, meaning, birth). Any substance that can produce such a defect is called a *teratogen*. The effect of a teratogen depends on when it enters the fetal system and in what stages of differentiation the various organs and organ systems are at that time. Generally the fetus is most vulnerable to teratogens during the first trimester.

PRESCRIPTION AND OVER-THE-COUNTER MEDICATIONS

Studies have shown that certain medications taken by the mother during the first 12 weeks of pregnancy can produce structural changes in the embryo. The thalidomide tragedy of the 1960s focused international attention on this problem. This drug had been used widely in Germany and other parts of Europe for only a few years when its teratogenic effects became tragically apparent. In Germany alone, more than 4000 children were born with severe malformations of the extremities (phocomelia or amelia), as well as abnormalities of the face, heart, and viscera.

During 1980, controversy surfaced in the news media concerning the possible teratogenic effects of Bendectin, a drug commonly prescribed for pregnant women who experience "morning sickness." This controversy has not been resolved, but has prompted further investigations of Bendectin.

Hormones have also been suspected of causing fetal abnormalities. Since they are often administered as drugs, in addition to being present in both mother and fetus, the increased supply may cause a harmful imbalance or interaction with other drugs. The best advice for any pregnant woman is to ask her physician's advice before taking *any* medication, even those she has been accustomed to taking, including aspirin.

ALCOHOL AND OTHER MOOD-ALTERING DRUGS

During recent years, alcohol consumption has increased among the U.S. population, and particularly among those under age 25. Studies suggest that heavy consumption of alcohol during pregnancy can retard fetal growth and produce fetal alcohol syndrome. This syndrome is characterized by a flat facial profile, short eye slits, a smaller brain, and is sometimes associated with limb and cardiovascular defects.

Infants born to mothers who are addicted to heroin or morphine have been shown to be generally impaired, suffering withdrawal symptoms, convulsions, and even death. Early studies of the effects of lysergic acid diethylamide (LSD) were inconclusive but there was evidence of convulsions, stunted growth, skeletal defects, and chromosomal damage as possible effects.

Every woman of childbearing age needs to understand the potential damage that her use of alcohol and other drugs can inflict on her unborn child, because often the most serious damage can occur during the first 4 weeks of life before pregnancy is suspected.

SMOKING

Most women are aware that cigarette smoking is hazardous to their health but not all of them know that smoking may be even more hazardous to the fetus. Research evidence continues to build concerning the harmful effects of smoking during pregnancy. These hazards include increased risk for spontaneous abortion, perinatal death, abruptio placentae, placenta previa, bleeding during pregnancy, and prolonged and premature rupture of the membranes.[1]

Cigarette smoke contains more than 1000 drugs, including nicotine.[2] Nicotine has been shown to contribute to prematurity and low birth weight, and to have a depressant effect on the fetal heart rate and blood pressure, reducing the availability of oxygen. Evidence has been found of impaired physical and intellectual development in the offspring of women who smoke. The damage to the fetus seems to be dose-related, so that even if the mother does not stop smoking entirely, it is helpful to reduce the number of cigarettes she smokes.[3]

Many organizations provide educational materials that point out the hazards of smoking during pregnancy. Among these are the National Foundation of the March of Dimes and The American Lung Association.

RADIATION

Since the atomic bombs fell on Hiroshima and Nagasaki, evidence has clearly shown that radiation can cause genetic mutation and birth defects. Irradiation of the abdomen of a pregnant woman may arrest embryonic development and cause malformations. Because the most sensitive period of organogenesis begins within a week or two after conception, radiographic examination of the abdomen of any woman of childbearing age should be done only during the first two weeks after a regular menstrual period.

MECHANICAL FACTORS

Moving freely within the fluid of the amniotic sac, the fetus is protected from physical trauma. During the latter part of pregnancy, however, the fetus may be large enough to crowd the uterine cavity, which can result in certain positional abnormalities such as metatarsus varus (clubfoot), torticollis, and dislocation of the hip.

Occasionally bands of amniotic tissue can constrict fetal limbs and inhibit growth. If the production of amniotic fluid decreases as intrauterine space becomes more limited, malformations of the jaw, asymmetry of the head, and compression marks on the body can result.

Though the fetus is safeguarded within the uterus, its protection is not perfect. If the mother suffers severe abdominal trauma, it can cause spontaneous abortion, premature delivery, or a handicapping injury to the child.

education for parenthood

Parenthood is probably one of the most difficult tasks anyone can assume. Today its difficulties are more complex than ever. Despite our "affluent" society, the U.S. still has a high infant mortality rate, a large number of mentally retarded infants and children, a continuing breakdown in family structure, many culturally deprived families, increasing neglect or abuse of children, and a rising number of illegitimate pregnancies. Education for parenthood thus becomes a prime need.

Much of the education for parenthood focuses on prenatal care of the mother and on the mechanics of the birth process. These are and should be paramount concerns because they are the foundation from which the child grows. Complete education for parenthood must be an ongoing venture, helping parents cope with children at all stages of development. Nurses are providing more and more of that education as they assume an increasingly important role in the care of children and families.

PRENATAL CARE

As stated earlier, proper prenatal care is the best method to protect the health of the mother and her infant. Ideally prenatal visits to her physician or clinic should begin soon after the last menstrual period. These visits should be monthly until the 32nd week, every 2 weeks until the 36th week, and weekly thereafter until delivery.

The health care provider in prenatal care has the following goals: to assure that the pregnancy is proceeding normally, to answer questions and concerns of patient and family, and to teach parenting skills. Continuing care permits diagnosis of any maternal-health problems that existed before the pregnancy or that develop during gestation, and to monitor the growth and health of the fetus.

PRENATAL CLINICS

Too often, those in greatest need of prenatal care and other preparation for parenthood have the least awareness about the need for or the availability of such services. National attention has been directed toward the importance of locating and assisting women in the "high-risk" pregnancy group. These are women in particular need of prenatal care because of socioeconomic factors, poor health, history of previous difficulties in childbirth, lack of knowledge of prenatal hygiene, just to mention a few reasons.

Particular attention has been focused on providing adequate prenatal clinics. A prenatal clinic is inadequate if it cannot serve the population for which it is intended.

An adequate prenatal clinic should be located in the area where it is needed. The amount of money and time involved in reaching a clinic some distance away discourages early and regular attendance.

A clinic is inadequate if it is too small or deficient in personnel. Women are not encouraged to attend if they need to wait hours for attention, an attention too often routine, impersonal and inadequate.

Successful clinics need adequately trained personnel representing the various disciplines involved in healthy childbearing. One expects to find competent obstetricians and registered nurses. Are there nutritionists, social workers, family counselors as well? Is there a human, personal atmosphere, a genuine interest in people?

PREPARED CHILDBIRTH

Pregnancy affects more than the prospective mother; it touches the lives of the father-to-be, other children in the family, grandparents, and other relatives. Although it is often a time of joyous anticipation, it holds potential problems for everyone involved. "Pregnancy is more than simply a biologic event; it is a time of crisis for those involved, a time when identities are changing and new roles are being explored."[4] Each person reacts in a unique way, based on individual needs and interpretations of the event.

Preparation for childbirth includes consideration of total family involvement, particularly the "pregnant" father. He should be included in as much of the prenatal activity as possible, especially classes concerning prenatal care and hygiene, fetal development, and the mechanics of birth. These classes are offered under varying sponsorships in many communities.

NATURAL CHILDBIRTH

Never has more knowledge about pregnancy, labor, and birth been available to prospective parents. Many couples have taken advantage of this information, and have come to regard pregnancy and birth as natural, rather than pathologic processes. These couples often choose "natural" childbirth, that is, birth unassisted by maternal anesthesia, because they are aware that no drug can be considered completely safe for the unborn baby. They attend classes that emphasize the Lamaze or other prepared childbirth methods, including pain control through proper breathing (Fig. 1–11). Fathers learn how to coach the mothers during labor, and how to more effectively support the emotional and physical needs of their mate throughout the pregnancy. These classes offer couples the opportunity to share experiences, feelings, and concerns with each other as well as with the instructor. Two of the principal organizations fostering these kinds of prenatal education programs are, ICEA (International Childbirth Education Association) and ASPO (American Society for Psychoprophylaxis in Obstetrics).

CESAREAN BIRTH

Not all women have the option of natural childbirth or even a vaginal delivery in the traditional delivery room. Certain maternal problems such as a contracted pelvis, a weak or defective uterine scar, pre-eclampsia, eclampsia, placental disorders, difficult labor, pelvic tumors, gonorrhea, or herpes type II infections necessitate cesarean delivery (delivery of the infant through a uterine incision). Some of these problems may be apparent early in the pregnancy and the couple is therefore aware that cesarean delivery is a certainty. This couple has as great a need for

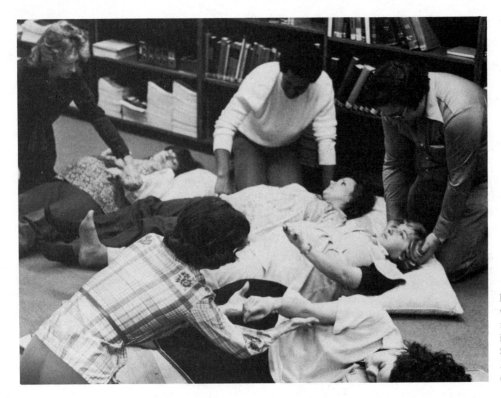

FIG. 1–11. Couples practicing various methods of pushing, muscle relaxation, and breathing in preparation for labor. (Reeder SJ, Mastroianni Jr L, Martin L: Maternity Nursing, 14th ed. Philadelphia, JB Lippincott, 1979)

educational preparation for their particular birth experience as does the couple planning natural childbirth. Classes for these parents have been slower developing, but they are being offered in greater numbers, and often are taught by women who have experienced cesarean delivery.

When cesarean delivery is performed as an emergency procedure owing to fetal or maternal distress, there is no time to psychologically prepare the couple. In many hospitals, the father will not be permitted in the operating room to witness the birth. This can lead to feelings of inadequacy and disappointment for the mother and feelings of exclusion for the father. This couple needs post-delivery counseling and reassurance to be sure that they understand the reason for the cesarean delivery.

ALTERNATIVE SETTINGS FOR BIRTH

Many couples are choosing to gain more control over the circumstances surrounding the birth of their children. Many fathers want to be present throughout labor and birth; and, in some hospitals, this is not permitted. These factors have led to a dramatic increase in the number of births at home during the last 10 years and to the development of homelike birth centers ("birthing rooms") within and outside of hospitals. Birthing rooms offer a setting conducive to genuine family-centered maternity care, such as colorful drapes and wallpaper, plants, pictures on the wall, and sometimes, the music of the parents' choice. Following birth, the family remains in the birthing room for a time of togetherness, sometimes as long as 24 hours (Fig. 1–12).

Birth at home or in a birth center is not without risk, even though 85% to 90% of pregnant women deliver without complications. Women who choose these non-traditional settings for birth should be low-risk, having had a healthy, normal pregnancy and thorough educational preparation for what to expect and what to do during labor and birth.

The following patients are *not* suitable for delivery at home:

1. High-risk patients (fetal or maternal jeopardy)
2. Women with a history of premature or postdate delivery in their previous pregnancy
3. Women with serious medical or surgical complications in this or prior pregnancies
4. Women who cannot be transferred easily to a hospital should the need arise
5. Women opposed to home delivery
6. Women with inadequate home facilities[5]

One of nursing's important roles is to help provide prospective parents with adequate, up-to-date information to use when making informed choices about where and how to give birth.

BREASTFEEDING

Closely associated with the return to natural childbirth and home birth is an increase in the number of women who choose to breastfeed their infants. Although breastfeeding is natural infant nutrition, it can present problems for the mother if her initial efforts are unsuccessful or if her choice is not supported by her partner. Again, it is important that the mother's choice be an informed choice. She needs to know the advantages and disadvan-

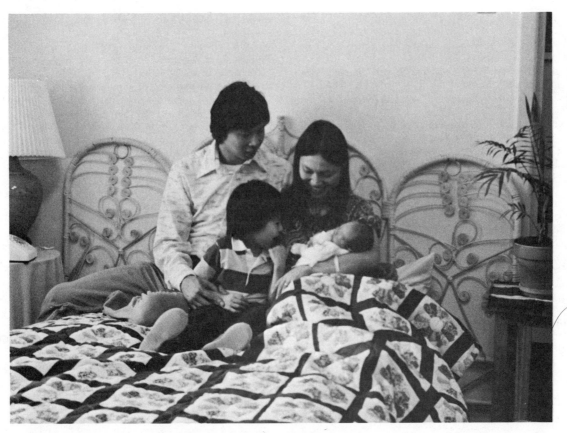

FIG. 1–12. An increasing number of hospitals offer homelike birthing rooms, or birth centers, so the new family can be together during and after birth. (Photo by Elaine Levy. Mt Zion Hospital and Medical Center. San Francisco, CA)

tages and she should be supported in whatever method she chooses without being made to feel guilty or inadequate if, for instance, she elects not to breastfeed.

The organization most instrumental in encouraging breastfeeding is La Leche League, International. Chapters are located in most larger communities offering direct support and counseling to new mothers. Breastfeeding is discussed more fully in Chapter 2.

summary

Life before birth is a time of remarkably rapid growth and differentiation. From zygote to embryo to fetus to infant, the child is shaped by the interaction of genetic and environmental influences. A healthy infant begins with healthy parents who understand the changes occurring in that new life and in their own lives. Nurses who care for and about children and families can help to build that understanding through sharing their knowledge.

review questions

1. Explain differentiation.
2. What is meant by the term viability?
3. What is organogenesis?
4. What are the six functions of amniotic fluid?
5. How many arteries are in the umbilical cord? How many veins?
6. Differentiate between the terms homozygous and heterozygous.
7. List the goals of genetic counseling.
8. Discuss why teenage pregnancies are considered "high risk."
9. Discuss the effects of smoking, chemicals, radiation, alcohol, and mood-altering drugs on the embryo.
10. Why is education for parenthood a fundamental need?

references

1. Meyer MB, Tonascia JA: Maternal smoking, pregnancy complications and perinatal mortality. Am J Obstet Gynecol 128:494–502, 1977
2. Kline, J, et al: Smoking: A risk factor for spontaneous abortion. New Engl J Med, 297:793–795, 1977
3. U.S. Office on Smoking and Health: The Health Consequences of Smoking, 1977–1978. Washington, DC, 1978
4. Colman AD, Colman LL: Pregnancy: The Psychological Experience. New York, Herder and Herder, 1971
5. Jensen MJ, Benson R, Bobak IM: Maternity Care: The Nurse and the Family, 2nd ed. St Louis, CV Mosby, 1981

bibliography

Apgar V, Beck J: Is My Baby All Right? New York, Simon and Schuster (Pocket Books), 1974

Boyd ST, Mahon P: The family-centered cesarean delivery. Am J Mat Child Nurs 5:176–180, 1980

Carlson B, Sumner PE: Hospital "at home" delivery: A celebration. JOGN 5:21–22, 1976

Cirz D: Nurses and the future in childbirth, JOGN 7:25–26, 1978

Devitt N: The transition from home to hospital birth in the U.S., 1930–1960. Birth and the Family Journal 4:47–58, 1977

Dick-Read G: Childbirth Without Fear: The Principles and Practice of Natural Childbirth, 4th ed. New York, Harper and Row, 1978

Donovan B: The Cesarean Birth Experience: A Practical, Comprehensive and Reassuring Guide for Parents and Professionals. Boston, Beacon Press, 1977

Ingalls J, Salerno C: Maternal and Child Health Nursing, 4th ed. St Louis, CV Mosby, 1979

Jensen MD, Benson R, Bobak IM: Maternity Care: The Nurse and the Family, 2nd ed. St. Louis, CV Mosby, 1981

Kramer R: Giving Birth: Childbearing in America Today. New York, Contemporary Books, 1978

Maloni JA: The birthing room: Some insights into parents' experiences. Am J Mat Child Nurs 5:5, 314–319, 1980

Moore, KL: Before We Are Born, rev reprint. Philadelphia, WB Saunders, 1977

Nilsson L: Behold Man. Boston, Little Brown, 1973

Phillips C, Anzalone J: Fathering: Participation in Labor and Birth. St Louis, CV Mosby, 1978

Ritchie CA, Swanson LA: Childbirth outside the hospital—The resurgence of home and clinic deliveries. Am J Mat Child Nurs 1:372–377, 1976

Stewart D, Stewart L: Safe alternatives in childbirth. Chapel Hill, National Association of Parents and Professionals for Safe Alternatives in Childbirth, 1976

Sumner P, Phillips C: Birthing Rooms: Concept and Reality. St. Louis, CV Mosby, 1981

Waechter EH, Blake FG: Nursing Care of Children, 9th ed. Philadelphia, JB Lippincott, 1976

Whaley L, Wong D: Nursing Care of Infants and Children. St Louis, CV Mosby, 1979

Wieczorek RR, Natapoff JN: A Conceptual Approach To the Nursing of Children. Philadelphia, JB Lippincott, 1981

Wiggins JD: Childbearing: Physiology, Experiences, Needs. St Louis, CV Mosby, 1979

Worthington-Roberts BS, Vermeersch J, Williams SR: Nutrition in Pregnancy and Lactation, 2nd ed. St Louis, CV Mosby, 1981

the normal newborn

student objectives

The student successfully attaining the goals of this chapter will be able to

1 Define the following vocabulary terms:

   Apgar score   attachment   cephalhematoma   engrossment   fontanel   lanugo
   meconium   milia   phenylketonuria   phimosis   vernix caseosa

2 Describe at least four reflexes of the normal newborn.

3 Explain the Apgar scoring system.

4 List four processes by which the newborn may lose body heat and explain the importance of
   the prevention of heat loss in the newborn.

5 Describe the attachment process and explain its importance to the family.

6 Describe the patient teaching the nurse should provide for the mother who plans to
   breastfeed her newborn.

Birth is hard work for mother and baby; therefore, calling it *labor* is very accurate. As the uterus prepares for birth, the infant's movements become restricted, and he is slowly squeezed against the bony areas of the mother's pelvis. Uterine contractions propel the infant down, into, and around through the birth canal with the head serving as a dilator. The head pushes repeatedly against the mother's perineum before finally emerging.

After 9 months in the warm, dark security of the uterus, the newborn suddenly enters a strange, bright, cold world. Is it any wonder that he cries? The cry fulfills a biological need: by drawing air into the lungs with the first breath, the breathing process is initiated, which is one big step for the infant toward maintaining life.

Though totally helpless in comparison to other baby mammals, the human infant is physically equipped to survive outside the uterus—to regulate temperature, to eat, sleep, and respond to certain stimuli—provided someone else is ready to meet all his needs.

The newborn is also ready to develop social relationships, usually with his parents first. Research has shown that the first hour after birth is critically important to future family relationships. Many health professionals have responded to this new knowledge by making it possible for the father to be with the mother and baby during delivery and for at least a 1-hour recovery period.

transition period

The transition period from intrauterine life to extrauterine existence is a period of instability. During the first 24 hours of life, the infant is highly vulnerable, and needs intensive observation, because this is the time when many of the physiologic adjustments required for extrauterine life are completed (Table 2–1).

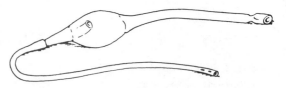

FIG. 2–2. DeLee mucus trap.

RESPIRATION BEGINS

Secretions of mucus and amniotic fluid fill the nose and mouth of the newborn. As soon as the head is delivered, the secretions should be gently suctioned with a bulb syringe, first from the mouth, and then from the nose (Fig. 2–1). After delivery is completed, the neonate should be held for a few seconds with his head lower than his body to facilitate drainage.

Failure to breathe within 1 minute after birth is an indication that some method of resuscitation is needed. The most frequent respiratory problems encountered in the delivery room are those of airway obstruction and central-nervous-system depression. Signs of respiratory distress include delayed respiration or irregular, gasping breath, sternal retractions, and cyanosis. Central-nervous-system narcosis produces anoxia and a slow, irregular, gasping breath. Narcosis is a state of stupor or insensibility, usually induced by the administration of anesthetics or other drugs to the mother during labor. This practice persists despite the many expert opinions that excessive drug in-

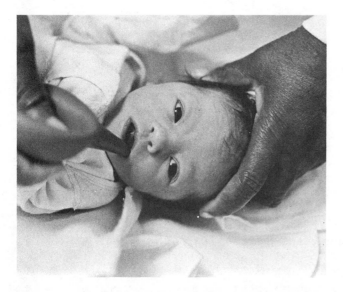

FIG. 2–1. A bulb syringe is used to gently clear secretions from the infant's mouth and nose. (Photo by Marcia Lieberman; Waechter EH, Blake FG: Nursing Care of Children, 9th ed. Philadelphia, JB Lippincott, 1976)

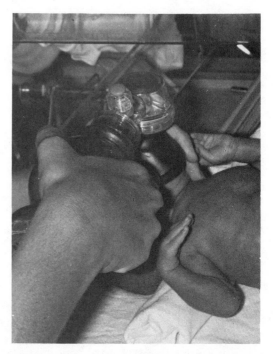

FIG. 2–3. Use of Ambu-bag portable resuscitator may be necessary when respirations are delayed or depressed. (Oehler JM: Family-Centered Neonatal Nursing Care. Philadelphia, JB Lippincott, 1981)

TABLE 2–1. CHANGES OCCURRING IN FETAL METABOLISM AFTER BIRTH

Fetal Period	Neonatal Period
Environmental	
Warm, stable, watery, fluid absorber of shock.	Bright, noisy, dry atmosphere.
Stable temperature, twilight lighting.	Temperature changes, much sensory
Minimal sensory stimulation.	stimulation.
Circulatory	
Ductus venosus—arterialized blood from umbilical vein goes to inferior vena cava.	Ductus venosus becomes occluded and is known as the ligamentum venosum. Anatomic closure completed at end of 2 months.
Ductus arteriosus—blood from right ventricle by-passes lung into descending aorta.	Ductus arteriosus becomes occluded, is known as ligamentum arteriosum. Functional closure within 3–4 days; anatomic closure completed by 3 weeks.
Foramen ovale—permits major portion of oxygenated blood entering the heart to go directly from the right atrium to the left atrium, left ventricle, and out the ascending aorta.	Foramen ovale closes, but closure is reversible for several days. Pulmonary circulation increases and more blood is returned from the lung to the left atrium.
Umbilical blood supply	
Oxygenated blood travels to fetus by way of the umbilical vein—returns to placenta via the umbilical arteries.	Placental circulation ceases when cord is tied. Umbilical vein becomes obliterated.
Blood composition	
High numbers of red cells and high hemoglobin level necessary to provide adequate oxygenation in utero.	Fall in red cells and hemoglobin during first days of life.
Respiratory	
Respiratory movements begin during 4th month of fetal life. Amniotic fluid moves in and out of lungs as result of these movements. Lungs are collapsed, oxygenation via placental circulation.	Lungs start to expand at first breath, full expansion takes several days. Placental oxygenation ceases with severance of umbilical cord.
Neurologic	
Fetus responds to stimulation as a whole. Neurologic activity seen at about 8 weeks gestation; isolated muscular reactions seen in response to stimulation. By 9 weeks, swimming motions and some spontaneous movements are present. By 13–14 weeks, movement may be perceptible to mother.	Infant responds to stimulation by certain discrete reflexes, such as rooting, plantar, moro reflexes.

tervention contributes to the disturbingly high infant-mortality rate in the U.S.—thirteenth among developing nations.

In the case of airway obstruction, after secretions are cleared from the nose and mouth, gentle stimulation, such as rubbing the infant's back or flicking the soles of his feet, may be helpful. If further measures are required, suctioning, possibly with a DeLee mucus trap, may be instituted (Fig. 2–2).

When respirations are delayed or depressed, the use of an Ambu bag may be helpful (Fig. 2–3). Measures used for the relief of serious respiratory problems are intubation, oxygen, and mouth-to-mouth resuscitation. These measures require the serious attention of the physician, anesthesiologist, and obstetric team. Infants manifesting severe distress are transferred to the newborn intensive-care unit (ICU).

CIRCULATION CHANGES

During fetal life, the lungs are inactive, requiring only a small amount of blood to nourish their tissues. Blood is circulated through the umbilical arteries to the placenta where waste products and carbon dioxide are exchanged for nutrients. The blood is then returned to the fetus through the umbilical vein.

At birth, the umbilical cord is cut, and the infant establishes his own independent system. *Certain fetal circulatory bypasses, such as the ductus arteriosus, the foramen ovale, and the ductus venosus* are no longer necessary after birth. They close and atrophy, although probably more gradually than had formerly been supposed (Fig. 2–4).

The foramen ovale closes with the first breath but the closure is reversible for the first few days of life. The ductus arteriosus closes within 3 to 4 days, but the ductus venosus does not achieve complete closure until about the end of the second month of life.

In the nursery the cord stump is examined to determine the presence of one vein and two arteries. If only one artery is present, this indicates that the newborn should be further examined for congenital defects of the internal organs.

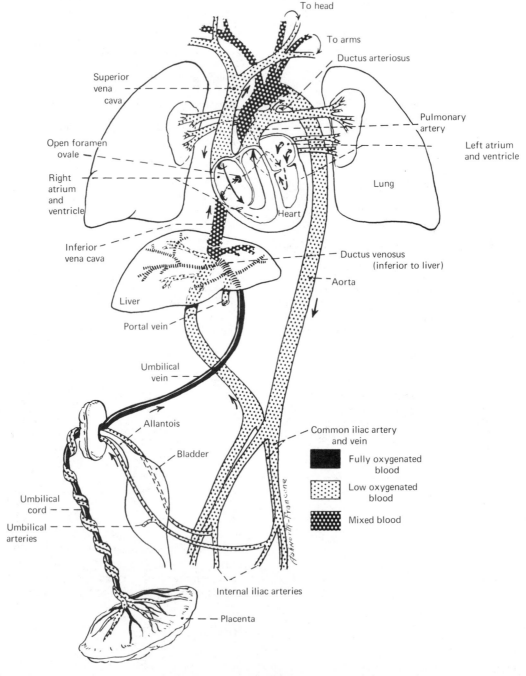

FIG. 2–4. Diagram of fetal circulation.

care in the delivery room

IMMEDIATE CARE

APGAR SCORE

Within 60 seconds after birth, and again 5 minutes later, the general condition of all infants should be assessed according to the Apgar score, an evaluation developed by the late Virginia Apgar, a physician (Table 2–2). The infant is given a score of 0, 1, or 2 for each of the five specific signs: heart rate, respiratory rate, muscle tone, reflex irritability, and color. A score of 10 indicates that the infant is in the best possible condition. With a score of 5 to 10, he usually requires no special treatment. A score below 5 calls for immediate attention and treatment, as well as careful and continuous observation in the intensive-care nursery.

This score is attached to the infant's chart for immediate availability as a reliable index of the condition at birth and as an important guide for subsequent care.

CORD CARE

The umbilical cord is clamped shortly after birth. Some physicians prefer to wait a few minutes until blood ceases to flow through the cord, providing the infant with additional iron-rich blood from the placenta. The cord is clamped with two clamps, then it is cut between the two clamps. The end attached to the infant is clamped with a cord clamp, or tied; the maternal clamp is then released. The cord appears to contain no nerve endings, as neither mother nor infant show any discomfort when it is cut. The stump is left without a dressing, and should be inspected daily until it falls off.

EYE CARE

Prophylactic eye treatment against gonococcal ophthalmia neonatorum is mandatory throughout the U.S. Because gonorrhea in a woman may be asymptomatic, this disease was formerly a frequent cause of neonatal blindness, infecting the infant during passage through the birth canal of the infected mother.

The drug of choice that is instilled into the eyes of the neonate is 1% silver-nitrate solution. Penicillin or antibiotic ophthalmic ointment is used in some hospitals when permitted by state law.

Because of the sensitive parent–infant attachment (bonding) period during the early hours after birth, some authorities recommend waiting 1 hour before instilling silver nitrate. Some state health codes, however, direct that instillation take place "immediately" after birth. Additional studies need to be done to provide more conclusive evidence.

Before the eyedrops are instilled, the infant's eyelids should be cleansed with sterile cotton moistened in sterile water. A separate pledget should be used for each eye, sponging from the nose outward until all blood or mucus is removed.

Next, the infant's eyes should be opened, one at a time, using gentle pressure on the upper and lower lids. One or two drops of solution should be dropped into each eye onto the conjunctival sac, never onto the cornea. The eyelids are held open for 30 to 60 seconds to allow the solution to flow from the inner to the outer aspect of the eye. A mild conjunctivitis can follow the use of silver nitrate, but clears up quickly without treatment.

At one time, the practice was to flush the eyes with sterile water or sterile saline solution following the instillation of silver nitrate. This practice has been discontinued in many hospitals because studies showed that the rinse did not reduce conjunctival irritation, and may have diluted the effectiveness of the prophylactic drops. The Committee on Ophthalmia Neonatorum of the National Society for the Prevention of Blindness issued a statement that it does not recommend irrigation of the eyes following instillation of silver nitrate. This statement was endorsed by the American Academy of Pediatrics.

IDENTIFICATION

Before the infant is transferred from the delivery room or birthing room, an identification bracelet identical to the one on the mother's wrist is placed on the baby's wrist. In some hospitals, handprints and footprints are also taken and become part of the infant's chart, sometimes with the addition of the mother's right index fingerprint.

If the father has not been permitted in the delivery

TABLE 2–2. APGAR SCORING CHART

Sign	0	1	2
Heart rate	absent	below 100	above 100
Respiratory rate	absent	slow, irregular	good, crying
Muscle tone	limp	some flexion of extremities	active motion
Reflex irritability	no response	grimace	cough or sneeze
Color	blue, pale	body pink, extremities blue	completely pink

(Developed by Dr. Virginia Apgar)

room, it is important that he have the opportunity to see and touch his infant before transfer to the nursery, if possible.

At birth, the infant is subject to severe heat loss through four processes: evaporation, radiation, conduction, and convection. From a stable intrauterine temperature of 98.6° F, the neonate emerges, wet and shivering, into a world nearly 30 degrees cooler. *Evaporation* of the amniotic fluid that covers the infant causes heat loss, so it is imperative that the infant be dried rapidly and gently with a warm towel and placed into a warm environment. In settings where skin-to-skin contact between infant and mother is encouraged, an overhead radiant warmer may be used to reduce heat loss. Some hospitals and birthing rooms use stockinette caps on neonates because much heat is lost through the top of the head. If the infant is not placed skin-to-skin with his mother, he should be wrapped in a soft, warm blanket and either given to his mother to hold or placed in a warm crib or infant warmer. When the Leboyer method (immersion of the newborn into a basin of warm water immediately after delivery to minimize the abruptness of the changes in environment) is used, the infant is dried with a warm towel after the bath and placed on the mother's abdomen.

Heat loss through *radiation* means that heat is lost to cooler solid objects that are not in direct contact with the infant. The temperature of the surrounding air has no effect on heat loss through radiation; therefore, the infant should not be examined until he is moved as far as possible from the walls of the delivery room.

Conduction heat loss occurs when the skin is in direct contact with a cooler solid object. To avoid this, the infant should be placed on a padded surface, and should be insulated with clothes and blankets.

Convection heat loss is similar to conduction but is increased by moving air currents. Transporting the infant in a crib with solid sides will reduce convection heat loss.

OBSERVATION AND DOCUMENTATION

During this critical transitional period, close observation of the infant is essential. In addition to the Apgar score,

the nurse records the exact time of birth, the skin condition, the quality of the infant's cry, the presence of any congenital anomalies or evidence of birth injuries, and the type of forceps used to extract the infant. Weight and length of the infant are noted before transfer from the delivery room, or immediately upon admission to the nursery. The first urination and defecation must be noted and recorded; usually this happens after transfer to the nursery or the mother's room. Failure to urinate during the first 24 hours or to defecate during the first 36 hours can indicate a serious problem.

physiologic characteristics of the newborn

Approximately 95% of newborn infants born at term weigh between 2.5 kg to 4.6 kg (5½ to 10 lb), and measure 45 to 55 cm (18 to 23 inches) in length. Normal head circumference measures about 33 cm to 35 cm (12 to 14 inches). Crown-to-rump measurements average 31 cm to 35 cm and are about equal to the head circumference.

HEAD AND SKULL

The six bones of the newborn skull are not united but can mold and overlap, to permit the large head to pass through the birth canal. These bones are divided by narrow bands of connective tissue called *sutures*. At the juncture of these bones are triangular spaces called *fontanels*. At birth the two palpable fontanels, or soft spots, are the *anterior fontanel* at the juncture of the frontal and parietal bones, and the *posterior fontanel* at the juncture of the parietal and occipital bones (Fig. 2–5).

During delivery, the head has molded along the suture lines, and may appear to be asymmetrical or elongated (Fig. 2–6). Usually normal shape is assumed after a few days. The sections of the bony skull calcify and join during the first months of life. The posterior (triangle-shaped) fontanel closes in about 1½ to 3 months of life; the anterior fontanel (diamond-shaped) closes between 12 and 18 months.

The brain is covered with a tough membrane, making it difficult to injure the child's head through the fontanels by

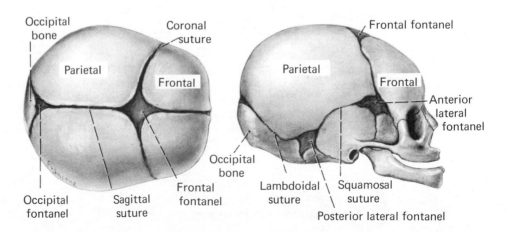

FIG. 2–5. Infant skull showing fontanels and cranial sutures.

ordinary handling. Mothers need to be reassured that the baby's scalp can be washed with soap and water (*not* baby oil) over these areas without harm, and ordinary cleansing can be helpful to prevent *cradle cap* (seborrheic dermatitis). Cradle cap is an accumulation of oil, serum, and dirt, which frequently forms on an infant's scalp.

CHEST

The chest of the newborn has a smaller circumference than the head. The breasts of both male and female may be engorged as a result of maternal estrogens in the bloodstream, and a pale, milky fluid called *witches' milk* may be secreted. This condition disappears within 4 to 6 weeks. In the meantime, the breasts should be handled gently and not manipulated in any way.

BONY STRUCTURE

The arms and legs of the newborn are short in comparison to the trunk. Prenatal development proceeds in a cephalocaudal (head to toe) progression and in a proximal to distal sequence (Fig. 2–7). This means that the head and trunk are well-developed, but the distal areas develop later. Development always proceeds from the general to the specific, the gross muscles coming under the control of the finer muscles.

BODY TEMPERATURE

At delivery, the infant's body temperature is generally the same as the mother's but drops rapidly after entering the cooler environment. As mentioned earlier, a warm, stable environment is necessary until the neonate has adjusted to independent living. In the delivery room, the infant is usually wrapped in a warm blanket, or placed in a heated crib. Body temperature varies after birth according to the environment, with a range of 36.4° C to 37° C (97.5° F to 98.6° F), owing to the immature nervous sytem. It usually stabilizes in a few days. Normal newborn axillary temperature, after stabilization, varies between 36° C and 37.2° C (96.8° F to 99° F).

   The newborn's temperature may be taken by rectum or axilla. In many newborn nurseries, the first temperature is taken rectally to determine the patency of the anal opening. There may be a shallow opening in the anus, however, with the rectum ending in a blind pouch. In this case, ability to insert a thermometer into the rectum does not signify a patent rectum. If a temperature is measured rectally, care must be taken to insert the thermometer only just beyond the bulb of the thermometer (see Fig. 2–18).

RESPIRATORY SYSTEM

The first and most important task of the neonate is to oxygenate his own red-blood cells, which he does with his first cry. Although respiratory movements appear in fetal life, there is no *functional* respiration before birth. Breathing in the healthy newborn is quiet and shallow, but variations in rate and rhythm are normal. In normal infants, the rate may vary from 20 to 100 per minute, according to whether the infant is sleeping or awake, crying, lying passively, or vigorously moving arms and legs. As the rate fluctuates rapidly, the respirations should be

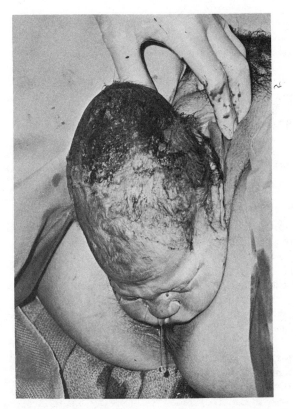

FIG. 2–6. The head of this newborn is elongated owing to the pressure applied by forceps.

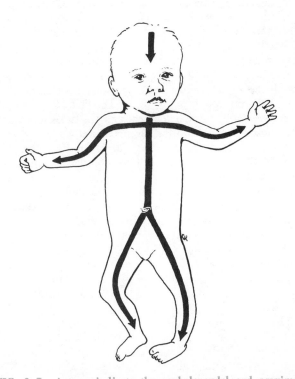

FIG. 2–7. Arrows indicate the cephalocaudal and proximal-distal progress of infant development.

counted for 1 full minute. The overall rate for the period of 1 minute is usually 30 to 50 breaths per minute. Persistent rates over 60 per minute or under 30 per minute should be called to the physician's attention as it may indicate cardiac or pulmonary difficulty. Sternal retractions are considered abnormal and should also be reported.

The newborn infant's breathing is diaphragmatic–abdominal, so respirations can be counted most easily by watching the rise and fall of the abdomen, rather than the chest. Mothers should be informed of this to prevent any alarm over what may seem to them to be abnormal breathing.

CIRCULATORY SYSTEM

The changes that occur in the circulatory system at birth are primarily due to the oxygenation of blood through the pulmonary system, and to discarding the placenta, umbilical vein, and arteries. Shortly after birth, the blood flows through the infant's circulatory system in the same manner as that of an adult. It is normal for the hands and feet to be slightly cyanotic, or blue. Whenever the infant cries, however, his color becomes rosy red.

At birth, the infant's heart rate may reach 180 per minutes, then fall to 100 to 120 per minute. Usually by the second day of life, the pulse varies between 90 and 160 per minute, depending on whether the infant is asleep or awake and active. Blood pressure is difficult to measure in the newborn and is not generally taken unless specifically ordered. When ordered, it can be measured with the Doppler blood pressure device.

GASTROINTESTINAL TRACT

The gastrointestinal tract is functional at birth and meconium is usually passed within 8 to 24 hours. *Meconium* is a sticky, greenish-black substance composed of bile, mucus, cellular waste, intestinal secretions, fat, hair, and other materials swallowed during fetal life, together with amniotic fluid. The time of the first stool should be noted and recorded in order to confirm anal patency. If no stool is passed during the first 24 hours after birth, some obstruction may exist in the intestinal tract, and should be called to the physician's attention.

The neonate is able to digest the fat, protein, and carbohydrates in breast milk, or in a modified formula. *Regurgitation,* spitting up of small quantities of milk, occurs rather easily in the young infant and is different from vomiting. It may be caused by an air bubble in the infant's stomach, too rapid nursing, or overfeeding.

Vomiting is differentiated from regurgitation in that there is an expulsion of an appreciable amount of fluid. Although this also may result from rapid feeding or inadequate bubbling, frequent or persistent vomiting may signal an abnormal condition and should be reported to the physician.

The neonate hiccoughs easily; this is most likely caused by too rapid feeding. However, he has been known to hiccough before birth. Bubbling the infant to bring up swallowed air or letting him nurse for another minute will usually control the hiccoughs. In any case, they will eventually stop without treatment.

GENITOURINARY TRACT

The kidneys secrete urine before birth and some urine collects in the bladder after birth. A record of the first urination is important to confirm adequate kidney function and the absence of severe constrictions somewhere in the urinary system.

The male testes are usually descended into the scrotum at birth, but occasionally one or both are in the process of descending, or remain in the abdomen. These testes usually descend spontaneously during the first year of life.

The prepuce of the penis in the male newborn child is normally tight. *Phimosis,* or adherence of the foreskin to the glans penis, is normal in early infancy. Forceful retraction should not be attempted. If minor irritations develop, soap and water cleansing is all that is necessary. One danger of forceful retraction of the foreskin during early infancy is that the elastic fibers at the tip of the foreskin may tear and bleed. The result will be that the foreskin heals by scarring, perhaps making circumcision necessary later.

Circumcision of the newborn male is performed frequently for religious reasons, and there is some controversy concerning the medical reason for this surgery. Circumcision does prevent the accumulation of the secretions collectively called *smegma,* and some authorities believe that this smegma may contain a virus that can cause cancer of the cervix in the sexual partner of an uncircumcised male. If the foreskin of the newborn male is so tight that it obstructs the urinary system, circumcision is performed at once. Normally the foreskin is retractable by age three; if not, circumcision may be considered, but is rarely needed for this reason.

In the female neonate, the labia are prominent owing to the effect of the mother's estrogens during intrauterine life. The infant may have a slight red-tinged vaginal discharge called *pseudomenses,* which results from a drop in the hormonal level compared to the higher concentration in the maternal hormone environment. Unless the mother understands why this happens, she can naturally become very alarmed. She should be told that although it does not appear in all newborn female infants, it is a natural manifestation resulting from hormonal transfer, and it will disappear in a few days. It should be particularly emphasized that this is not due to any trauma or infection.

NERVOUS SYSTEM

The neonate exhibits a number of reflexes triggered by his immature nervous system. Research evidence indicates that infants follow their reflexes for the first 3 months of life. For example, all newborns smile, even if they are blind, and all infants tightly grasp objects placed in their palms. Most of the reflexes disappear during the first year of life, but are normal for the neonate. Infants should be tested for the most common ones, as their absence may indicate a disturbance in the nervous system.

ROOTING REFLEX

This reflex is present at birth. The infant turns his head toward any warm object that touches his cheek, and actively seeks the nipple. Thus, when the mother or the nurse places a hand on his cheek to turn his head toward the breast, he turns instead towards the person's hand.

SUCKING REFLEX

This is so well developed at birth that personnel in the delivery room are often startled by the loud sucking noises coming from the newborn's crib.

GAG REFLEX

Present at birth, this reflex continues throughout life. Any stimulation of the posterior pharynx by food, suction, or passage of a tube will cause gagging.

GRASP REFLEX

Pressure on the palms of the hands or soles of the feet near the base of the digits causes flexion of hands and toes. The palmar grasp is so strong in a healthy infant that the infant can be lifted off the examining table (Fig. 2–8). The palmar grasp diminishes after 3 months; the plantar grasp persists until 9 to 12 months of age.

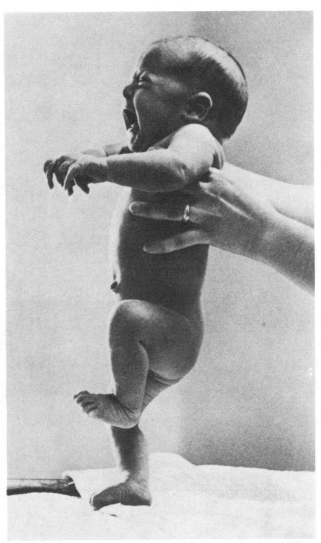

FIG. 2–9. Step, or dance, reflex simulates walking when infant is held so that the sole of the foot touches examining table. (Courtesy Mead Johnson Laboratories, Evansville, Ind.)

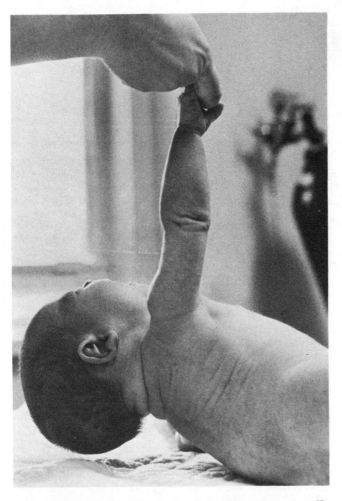

FIG. 2–8. Grasp reflex present in all normal newborns is sufficiently strong to lift them from the examining table. (Courtesy Mead Johnson Laboratories, Evansville, Ind.)

BABINSKI (PLANTAR) REFLEX

When the lateral plantar surface is stroked, the toes flare open. This usually disappears by the end of the first year.

STEP, OR DANCE, REFLEX

Until 6 weeks of age, most normal infants when held in an upright position will make stepping movements (Fig. 2–9).

MORO REFLEX

Any sudden jarring or abrupt change in equilibrium elicits this reflex in the normal newborn. It consists primarily of abduction and extension of arms. All digits extend except finger and thumb, which are flexed to form a C-shape (Fig. 2–10). If the response is not immediate, bilateral, and symmetric, possible injury to the brachial plexus, the humerus, or the clavicle may be present. If this reflex

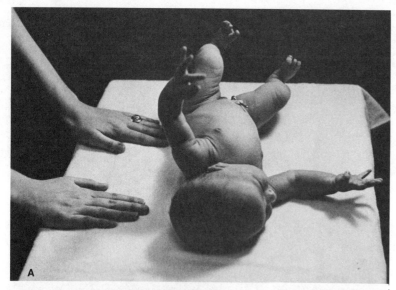

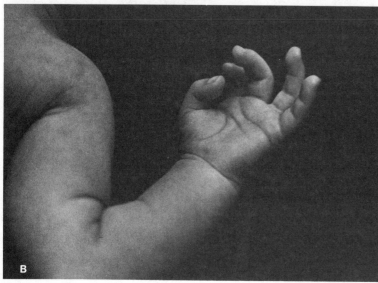

FIG. 2–10.   Moro reflex is elicited by sudden jarring or change in equilibrium. (*A*) Arms abduct at the shoulder and extend at the elbow. (*B*) All digits extend except finger and thumb, which curve into a C-shape. (Courtesy Mead Johnson Laboratories, Evansville, Ind.)

persists beyond 6 months of age, it may indicate brain damage.

STARTLE REFLEX

Similar to the Moro reflex, the startle reflex follows any loud noise and consists of abduction of the arms and flexion of the elbows. Unlike in the Moro reflex, hands remain clenched. Absence of this reflex may indicate hearing impairment.

TONIC NECK REFLEX

Not always apparent during the first weeks of life, this reflex can be observed when the infant lies on his back. He turns his head to one side, extends the arm on that side and flexes the opposite arm in a fencing position (Fig. 2–11). Normally this reflex disappears between 6 and 8 months of age.

SPECIAL SENSES

SIGHT

Research has shown that the unborn baby is able to distinguish light from dark, and that he can see at birth. The rod cells in the retina of the eyes, which are responsible for light perception, are functional at birth; but the retina, the newborn's special organ of visual perception, is not fully developed until about 16 weeks of age. The neonate will turn his head toward a light, and will blink and close his eyes at a bright light. He will follow a bright moving object momentarily, but coordination fixation comes much later. The nerves and muscles that control focusing and coordination are not completely developed until the 6th month, accounting for the crosseyed look that babies sporadically show. The mother does not have cause for alarm if the infant's eyes are not coordinated occasionally in their movements, but if lack of focusing remains at 4 months, she should alert her pediatrician.

Tears are produced constantly at birth, but are completely disposed of through the nasolacrimal duct, until around 2 or 3 months of age, when tear production increases.

Newborns have approximately 20/500 vision, as compared with a normal-seeing adult's vision of 20/20. This means that most distant objects appear very fuzzy. Close vision is much better, and the infant can see most of the features of a human face clearly at a distance of 7 to 15 inches (17.78–38.10 cm). This is one reason why the *en face* position that permits caregiver–infant eye contact in the same vertical plane is so important to parent–infant attachment during the period immediately after birth.

HEARING

A newborn will stop crying momentarily at the sound of a soothing voice; and as mentioned earlier, will startle and cry at a loud noise. Immediately after birth, the infant can distinguish the mother's voice from that of a male physician. The sense of hearing certainly contributes to the infant's emotional reactions to fear and to comforting. It is not known exactly how early the infant hears soft voices and other faint sounds, but infants 2 or 3 days old will stop crying momentarily when talked to soothingly.

SMELL

The sense of smell is poorly developed at birth, but the newborn infant does turn toward his mother's breast, seemingly because of the smell of breast milk.

TASTE

Because much of taste depends on the sense of smell, it is likely that the infant's sense of taste is also poorly developed at birth. Some studies have shown, however, that breathing, sucking, and swallowing patterns are different when infants are fed formula, than when they are fed breast milk.

TOUCH

Sensitivity to touch is present from birth, particularly in the lips and tongue. The sense of pain is also present at birth; but, like adults, infants vary in their sensitivity to pain. Newborns react to painful pinpricks. Sensitivity appears to increase during the first few days of life as part of individual development. The infant will cry lustily when suffering gastrointestinal discomfort.

SKIN
NORMAL APPEARANCE

Sluggish peripheral circulation and vasomotor instability are manifested in the deep red color the infant acquires when he cries, as well as in the pale hands and feet of many newborns. The skin is usually red and should feel elastic when picked up between the examiner's fingers.

Fine, downy hair, called *lanugo* covers the skin of the fetus. It is usually not present in a full-term infant, but may be seen on an infant born prematurely.

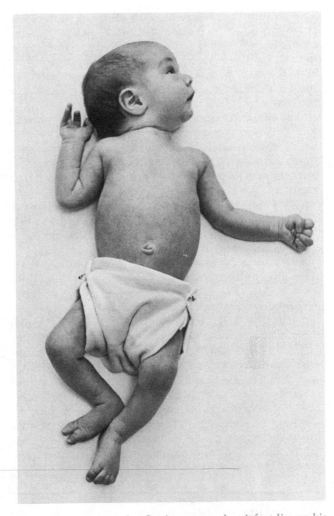

FIG. 2–11. Tonic neck reflex is present when infant lies on his back with his head turned to one side, with arm and leg on the same side extended, and arm on the opposite side flexed. (Courtesy Mead Johnson Laboratories, Evansville, Ind.)

A greasy, cheeselike substance called *vernix caseosa* protects the skin during fetal life. Vernix caseosa is an oil and water mixture containing cells flaked from the skin, and fatty substances secreted by the sebaceous glands. At birth, vernix may cover the skin or remain only in the folds of the skin. In most hospitals, not all of the vernix is removed with the first bath, but it is left on as a protective agent. It eventually is absorbed or rubs off.

SKIN BLEMISHES

Many temporary skin blemishes are not uncommon. One of the most common ones is a *vascular nevus*, known as a "strawberry mark." A *nevus* is defined as a circumscribed new growth of the skin of congenital origin; it may be either vascular or nonvascular. The strawberry mark is a slightly raised, bright-red collection of blood vessels that does not blanch completely on pressure. It may be present at birth, or may appear during the first 6 months of life.

This blemish may enlarge during the first 6 months of life, but eventually when it ceases to grow, fibrosis replaces the capillaries and the lesion shrinks. Treatment is not usually indicated as most of these regress and disappear by 10 years of age. If the lesion is so large as to cause emotional trauma in the child, the physician may suggest removal of the blemish.

Vascular nevi are sometimes present in *cavernous hemangiomas*, subcutaneous collections of blood vessels with bluish, overlying skin. Although these are benign tumors, they may become so large and extensive as to interfere with the functions of the body part on which they appear.

Milia are pearly white cysts appearing on the faces of about 40% of newborn infants. They are usually retention cysts of sebaceous glands or hair follicles, and disappear in a few weeks without treatment.

Forcep marks may be noticeable on the infant's face if the delivery was assisted with use of forceps. These ordinarily disappear in a day or two. After a difficult delivery, bruises and edema may be present on the head or scalp, or, if a breech delivery, on buttocks and genitalia. Though these gradually clear up without treatment, such bruises can be very distressing to the parents, who may not understand the relative insignificance of these marks. The nurse can carefully and simply explain that they are minor bruises and will fade quickly. Occasionally the infant's head is misshapen by its passage through the birth canal. The mother is naturally distressed and needs to know that this is temporary, owing to the ability of the head to accommodate to the narrow passage. It will acquire a normal rounded shape in a few days.

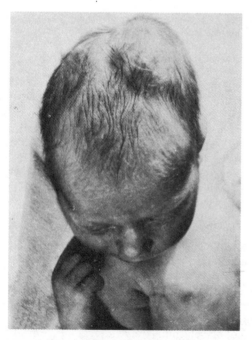

FIG. 2–12. Cephalhematoma of left parietal bone.

Caput succedaneum is an edematous swelling of the soft tissues of the scalp caused by prolonged pressure of the occiput against the cervix during labor and delivery. The edema disappears in a few days.

Cephalhematoma is a collection of blood between the periosteum and the skull (Fig. 2–12). The swelling of the overlying scalp is usually not visible until several hours after birth. This too may frighten the mother who may think some injury has occurred. Most cephalhematomas are reabsorbed within 2 weeks to 3 months, depending on their size. As the only serious complication can be the introduction of infection, then aspiration, incision, or any other treatment is contraindicated.

Physiologic jaundice (*icterus neonatorum*) occurs in a large number of newborn infants, has no medical significance, and is believed to be the result of the breakdown of fetal red cells. It must, however, be carefully observed and reported, in an effort to distinguish it from a serious jaundice condition. Physiologic jaundice, with yellowing of the skin, does not show until after the second day of life. *Any jaundice appearing during the first 3 days should be promptly called to the physician's attention.*

newborn–parental behavior

NEWBORN ACTIVITY

The healthy newborn, if placed face down, will lift or turn his head to one side to clear the airway. He exercises in uncoordinated, random movements, involving the entire body in the activity. The muscles are taut and it is difficult to manually extend the extremities. The infant will momentarily cease activity at the sound of a nearby voice.

The newborn can sneeze to clear his nasal passages; yawn, hiccup, stretch, blink, and cough. He learned to suck and swallow before he was born.

The infant's only way of expressing his tension from hunger, cold, pain or other discomfort is by crying. Prompt comforting and attention to his needs will usually restore his composure and alleviate the discomfort.

MOTHER–INFANT INTERACTION

Even though infant and mother have been physically inseparable for 9 months, their emotional togetherness and the beginning of mutual love and attachment start after delivery, ideally in the first few hours. Many babies are very alert for a short time after delivery, offering a good opportunity for sensory contact with the mother.

Pioneering research by Drs. Klaus and Kennell indicates that early attachment activities (originally called *bonding*) have a significant effect on the long-term parent–child relationship.[1] This does not mean that early attachment guarantees a satisfactory lifetime relationship, or that lack of opportunity for early attachment threatens seriously the family's chances for a strong relationship. It simply indicates that the family relationship is given the best possible start if mother, father, and infant can be together during this early sensitive period in their new life as a family.

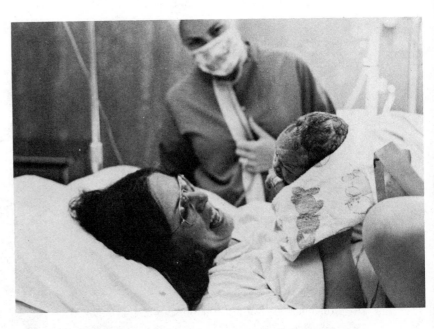

FIG. 2–13. Attachment. Touch is important in the attachment process. (Hawkins JW, Higgins LP: Maternity and Gynecological Nursing. Philadelphia, JB Lippincott, 1981)

Touch is a highly significant part of the attachment process. Many hospitals and birthing rooms offer the opportunity for skin-to-skin contact between mother and infant (and sometimes father and infant). Shortly after delivery, the nude infant is placed on the mother's abdomen and chest, and in some instances, is held to the mother's breast (Fig. 2–13). Touching provides warmth, comfort, and a sense of security—all very real needs of the vulnerable newborn.

Studies have shown that the mother is likely to follow a predictable pattern of touching her new baby, first using only the finger tips to touch the extremities, then gradually moving her fingers over the infant's entire body, and finally using her entire hand to massage the trunk of the body. Next, she will try to reposition herself and the baby in the *en face* position (mother and infant establish eye contact in the same vertical plane). It is also referred to as *mutual gazing.*

The attachment process is affected by many factors, among them the mother's physical and emotional condition after labor, the infant's condition and behavior, the comparison of the real infant with the "fantasy" infant that the mother has imagined since she became aware of her pregnancy. If the mother has had a difficult labor or heavy sedation, she may not be alert enough to participate effectively. If the infant has a problem that requires immediate transfer to the neonatal ICU, there will be no time for early attachment.

Every pregnant woman imagines what her baby will look like, how he or she will act, what the child will eventually accomplish, and how she and others in the family will be affected by this new person. This imaginary baby is likely quite different from the real infant she meets soon after delivery.

At first sight, the infant seldom presents the chubby, well-formed baby pictured by the world in general. The head is large in proportion to the body, and may be mis-

shapen by the process of being born. Blood and vernix still cling to his body, and he probably is crying. Is this the baby she has dreamed about and planned for? He appears so completely self-centered, so displeased over his introduction to the world. Such a first impression can summon feelings of guilt that she does not feel the expected gush of love and tenderness. If the baby is quiet and passive and she had imagined an awake, alert, active child, she may be somewhat disappointed, giving less attention and stimulation than she would to an infant who more closely resembles the imagined child. It is important that both parents understand that each infant is unique, with individual characteristics and developmental potential. Studies have shown that pointing out to parents their child's unique characteristics can help develop a more positive attitude, reduce feeding and sleeping problems, and bring about greater activity and alertness in the infant. One widely used guide for assessing neonatal activity is the Brazelton Neonatal Behavioral Assessment Scale (Fig. 2–14).

FATHER–INFANT INTERACTION

Only recently have the relationships of fathers and their infants been studied. In reporting a significant study of new fathers and their reaction to seeing their infants immediately after birth, Greenberg refers to this involvement as *engrossment.*[2] The dictionary defines *engross* as, "to occupy wholly, as the mind or attention." In this instance, engrossment refers to a sense of absorption and interest in the infant.

The father's attachment behavior is similar to that of the mother: touching; holding the infant in the *en face* position; observing the beauty of the child, particularly any features that resemble the father; and feelings of elation and satisfaction (Fig. 2–15). In Greenberg's study, most of the fathers indicated that they wanted to share with their wives the responsibility of raising the baby.

Some cultures dictate that men not show emotion; thus,

BRAZELTON SCALE CRITERIA

1. Response decrement to light
2. Response decrement to rattle
3. Response decrement to bell
4. Response decrement to pinprick
5. Orientation response—inanimate visual
6. Orientation response—inanimate auditory
7. Orientation—animate visual
8. Orientation—animate auditory
9. Orientation—animate-visual and auditory
10. Alertness
11. General tonus
12. Motor maturity
13. Pull-to-sit
14. Cuddliness
15. Defensive movements
16. Consolability with intervention
17. Peak of excitement
18. Rapidity of buildup
19. Irritability (to aversive stimuli: uncover, undress, pull-to-sit, prone, pinprick, TNR, Moro, defensive reaction)
20. Activity
21. Tremulousness
22. Amount of startle during exam
23. Lability of skin color
24. Lability of states
25. Self-quieting activity
26. Hand to mouth facility
27. Smiles

FIG. 2–14. Brazelton Neonatal Behavioral Assessment Scale. (Clinics in Developmental Medicine 50, England, Spastics International Publications, 1974)

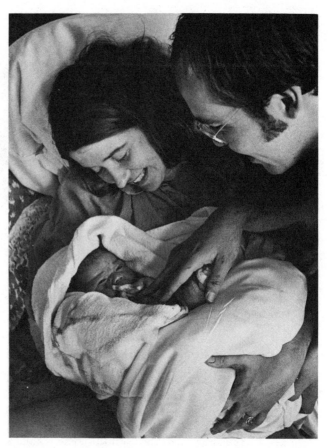

FIG. 2–15. Where rooming-in facilities are available, parents and infant can become acquainted before the baby is taken home.

some fathers may need encouragement to express their feelings about their infant. Nurses should reinforce any positive attachment behavior displayed by either parent, and should show, whenever necessary, the soothing effect of cuddling, stroking, and rocking the baby.

care in the hospital nursery or the mother's room

After a careful assessment of the newborn has been made and the family has had time together, the infant is transferred either to the newborn nursery or to the mother's room. Many maternity units now have a receiving or recovery nursery in which the infant is cared for and carefully watched for the first hours of life. Other units may set aside a portion of the general newborn nursery as a receiving area.

Prematurely born infants are transferred to a premature or intensive care unit. Here infants with serious congenital anomalies or birth defects also receive special care. Infants of diabetic mothers may be placed in the ICU,

because they need to be carefully observed, even though they are generally large for gestational age.

Every maternity unit must have an isolation unit available for infants who have been exposed to any sort of infection before, during, or after birth. Infants born on the way to the hospital are usually kept in this isolation unit.

ROOMING-IN

A growing number of mothers are choosing to keep their babies with them in the hospital, referred to as *rooming-in*. After the infant's condition has stabilized, he stays in a bassinet beside his mother who actively participates in his care.

Rooming-in has the following advantages:

1. It provides maximum opportunity for maternal–infant interaction while still in the care of maternity personnel.
2. It fosters infant feeding on a permissive (demand) schedule.
3. It offers a fine opportunity to teach mother and father about infant care and gives supervised experience in caring for their infant.
4. It reduces the incidence of cross-infection.

ADMISSION TO THE NURSERY

Upon admission, the infant's identification is verified, his Apgar score reported, cord stump inspected, and delivery room record reviewed. The infant is placed on his side in a bassinet or isolette to facilitate mucus drainage from nose and mouth. Some physicians have the foot of the bassinet elevated at a 15° to 20° angle to permit additional drainage. Others omit this procedure unless strictly necessary because of possible increased intracranial pressure.

The infant's temperature is taken, vital signs assessed, and he is allowed to rest. Bathing, weighing, and dressing may be postponed until his condition and temperature are stabilized. However, he is watched closely, and vital signs are assessed at 15 to 30 minute intervals (Fig. 2–16). The nursery temperature should be approximately 75° F, the humidity below 50%. When stable, the infant can be weighed, sponge bathed, and dressed.

DAILY NURSING CARE

Newborns are highly susceptible to infection. Removed from the protection of the uterus, they have not developed any defenses against disease; therefore, particular care should be used when handling the infant. All care except weighing is given inside the bassinet—bathing, examinations, taking temperatures. The nursery scale should be covered with a disposable liner that is discarded after one infant is weighed. The scale is sprayed with a germicidal, fungicidal spray, and covered with a fresh liner before the next infant is put on the scale.

HANDWASHING

Undoubtedly, the most important of all precautions is that of handwashing before handling any infant. This applies to all nurses, physicians, laboratory personnel, parents, or anyone handling a newborn child.

Before entering the nursery, remove any wristwatches, rings, and bracelets. After entering the handwashing area, clean under the fingernails with an orangewood stick. Wash hands under running water, using an antiseptic detergent. Wash between fingers, the palms and backs of hands, the wrists and arms up to the elbows for 2 minutes. Rinse and dry with paper towel. Between handling babies, wash thoroughly for 30 seconds. In most nurseries, attendants must wear scrub gowns.

Anyone suffering from any respiratory condition, intestinal upset, skin rash or cuts, elevated temperature, or any sign of illness should not enter the nursery or participate in care of the infants.

When the infant is rooming-in, parents also should use a thorough handwashing technique. Fathers or visitors should don long-sleeved gowns over their clothing. Wash basins, soap, clean towels, or paper towels should be available in the room as well as clean gowns. Directions for handwashing and donning gowns should be displayed prominently over the washbasin.

BATHING

Daily sponge baths are given using warm water, and, if needed, a bland soap. As with all infants, cleansing pro-

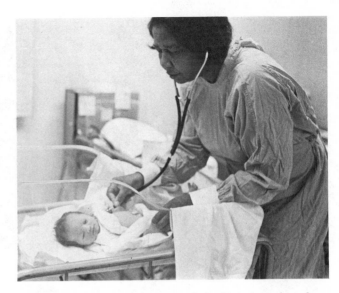

FIG. 2–16. Heart sounds, rate and rhythm are evaluated periodically after admission to the nursery. (Photo by Marcia Lieberman; Waechter EH, Blake FG: Nursing Care of Children, 9th ed. Philadelphia, JB Lippincott, 1976)

ceeds from the head downward. If the scalp needs cleansing it should be washed with water and soap, then rinsed with the washcloth, taking care not to get water in the infant's eyes.

Hexachlorophene is no longer used routinely for sponging newborn babies as it may be neurotoxic. The diaper area is cleansed after each bowel movement. In some nurseries complete sponge baths are given every other day instead of daily.

The umbilical stump is inspected daily for infection while the infant is undressed. It may be painted daily with an antiseptic to prevent infection, or may be cleansed daily with 70% alcohol, which also promotes antisepsis and has a drying effect. The stump is exposed to the air to allow it to dry.

If the infant has been circumcised, the area should be checked for bleeding. Sterile gauze with sterile petroleum-jelly may be applied to the area. Retraction of the foreskin should not be attempted as phimosis is normal in the newborn.

TEMPERATURE

The infant is weighed once daily in most nurseries, although some physicians prefer that it be done every other day. At this time the infant's temperature is taken, preferably by axilla, as harm to the rectal mucosa can occur if the thermometer is inserted too far (Fig. 2–17). If the temperature is to be taken rectally, lubricate the bulb end of the rectal thermometer. Place the infant flat on his back, and, grasping the ankles in one hand, raise the legs toward the head with knees bent outward. This will expose the rectum so that the end of the thermometer can slip in easily. The thermometer should not be inserted more than 2 cm (0.8 in). Continue to hold the infant's legs and the

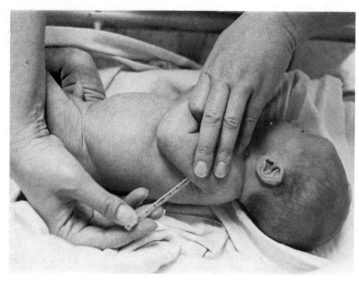

FIG. 2–17. Taking axillary temperature in the newborn. (Photo by Marcia Lieberman; Waechter EH, Blake FG: Nursing Care of Children, 9th ed. Philadelphia, JB Lippincott, 1976)

thermometer for about 1 minute (Fig. 2–18). Normal rectal temperature for a neonate is 37.0° C to 37.8° C (98.6° F to 100° F).

PKU TESTING

Laboratory screening for phenylketonuria (PKU) is mandatory in most states for all newborn infants. A simple procedure is used where the heel is pricked and three drops of blood are placed on filter paper, which is all that is necessary. However, the test is not valid until the infant has had an adequate intake of milk for a full 4 days. Testing too early, vomiting, or delayed feeding can cause false–negative results.

PKU testing is essential to prevent the mental retardation that can occur owing to a congenital lack of an enzyme necessary for the metabolism of phenylalanine, an essential amino acid. Once detected, this disorder can be completely corrected by dietary regulation.

feeding the newborn

Feeding time is an occasion providing stimulation and confidence. The infant makes eye-to-eye contact with his mother, touches her, while the mother looks, touches, explores, and talks to him. The infant learns to trust through repeated touch, fondling, and warm physical comfort. The infant's response to her comforting care gives the mother a sense of satisfaction and confidence. Eventually, when the infant learns that his signals of need are answered promptly, he is able to wait after his cry for the response. He should not be made to wait long; his newly developed sense of trust is fragile if it is not reinforced soon.

At one time, mothers were told, "Put the baby on a feeding schedule and never deviate from it. When he cries, check to see if there is anything disturbing him; then put him down and let him cry." Unfortunately, the infant did

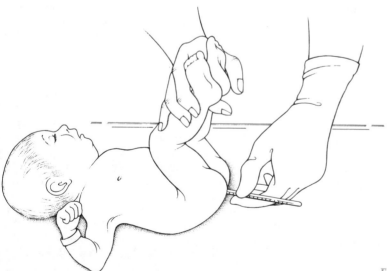

FIG. 2–18. Taking a newborn's temperature rectally.

TABLE 2–3. ADVANTAGES AND DISADVANTAGES OF BREASTFEEDING

Advantages	Disadvantages
Mother's milk is ideal food for human infants—proper proportion of nutrients	Mother must be available on a regular basis, although supplemental bottles can be used
Milk is pure, clean, and free of contaminating bacteria	Diet must contain adequate fluids, nutrients and calories
Milk is easily digested, fewer disturbances (i.e., colic, diarrhea, constipation)	Mother must learn methods of increasing and monitoring supply, since mental strain of mother affects milk supply
Provides better resistance to infection	Must have physician, family, or friends as support system to encourage mother to breast-feed
Child less likely to develop allergies	Must purchase vitamin and mineral supplements as recommended by physician or health center
Simple and convenient: correct temperature, immediately available	
Assists mother in resting and saving time, since there is no formula to measure, mix, or heat	
Emotionally satisfying experience for both mother and child	

(Courtesy Endres JB, Rockwell RE: Food, Nutrition and the Young Child. St Louis, CV Mosby, 1980)

not know he was being trained to conform to a schedule. He only knew that his hunger demanded satisfaction. His discomfort and sense of aloneness needed comfort and reassurance. Routine did nothing to satisfy his needs, but it did potentially shake his trust and belief that the world was a safe and caring place.

BREASTFEEDING

Breastfeeding is the ideal form of infant nutrition. Whether to breastfeed or formula feed, however, is the decision of the mother or the couple, unless there is a valid reason against either method. Many mothers will have already decided during pregnancy, but if there is any question or uncertainty, the nurse can cite the advantages and possible disadvantages of breastfeeding (Table 2–3).

If breastfeeding is chosen, the infant may be put to breast shortly after birth in the delivery room, so long as the mother is not under heavy sedation or deep anesthesia. The infant's suckling promotes early secretion of milk, is a source of security and comfort to the infant, a satisfaction to the mother, and a stimulant of uterine contractions.

After a period of rest for both mother and child, the infant may be permitted to nurse whenever he indicates his need. Although some physicians may still desire a certain period of time to elapse before the infant is put to breast, the trend is toward allowing the child to nurse when his body demands to be fed. This is easier to accomplish during rooming-in than in the traditional hospital nursery.

If this is the mother's first child, she will probably need help and support when she first attempts to nurse her infant. At first it is usually easier for the mother to nurse while lying flat with a pillow under her head and cradling the infant's head. The nurse can instruct the mother to turn to one side, place her nipple between her index and third finger, and bring it toward the infant's mouth. The nurse should caution the mother not to try to turn the infant's face toward her breast as the rooting reflex will cause him to turn toward her hand. As she brushes her nipple near his lips, he will actively seek it (Fig. 2–19).

A considerable portion of the areola should be drawn into the infant's mouth as he suckles because this stimulates the mammary glands and helps prevent sore nipples. If her breasts are large and soft, the infant's nose may be obstructed by pressing against the breast as he tries to nurse. The mother can be shown how to press her breast away from his nose with her finger so that he can breathe comfortably (Fig. 2–20). Later, when she regains some of her strength, she may find it more comfortable to nurse the infant while sitting upright in bed or in a chair.

Nearly all mothers experience some discomfort when the child is first put to breast. The nurse can reassure the mother that this discomfort is normal and will not last.

For the first 2 or 3 days the mother's breasts secrete *colostrum*, a yellowish, watery fluid, which has a higher protein, vitamin A, and mineral content, and a lower fat and carbohydrate content than breast milk. It also contains antibodies that may play a part in the immune mechanism of the newborn child. Its laxative effect helps promote evacuation of meconium from the infant's bowel.

Until lactation begins, both breasts should be used at each feeding, to stimulate secretion of milk. Later, when the breasts are full, one breast is generally sufficient at a feeding. A reminder of which breast to use each time may be needed, such as a safety pin on the brassiere strap of the side to be used next. It is important that a breast be emptied at one feeding to stimulate refilling.

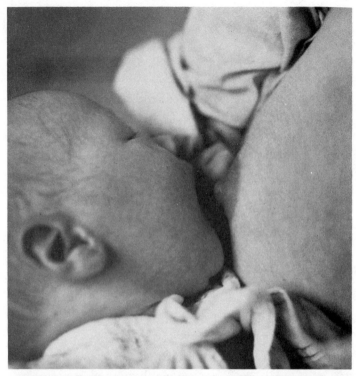

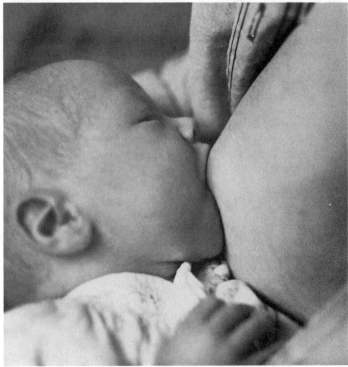

FIG. 2–19. When offered a nipple, the newborn responds immediately and vigorously owing to the rooting and sucking reflexes. (Photo by Imaginique Productions; Waechter EH, Blake FG: Nursing Care of Children, 9th ed. Philadelphia, JB Lippincott, 1976)

The nurse should inform the mother that a weight loss of 5% to 10% in the infant normally occurs during the first few days of life. That is to be expected, and should be regained within about 2 weeks (Table 2–4).

Whether the infant is breast or formula fed, he will swallow some air while nursing, and will need "burping" or "bubbling" to help him eructate (belch) the swallowed air. After feeding, he may be held up on his mother's shoulder and his back gently rubbed, or he may be sat upright on her lap with his head supported, while she rubs his back gently (Fig. 2–21). Some infants who nurse eagerly may need more than one bubbling during a feeding.

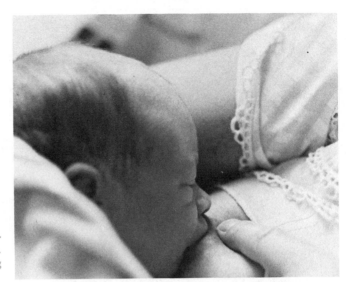

FIG. 2–20.   The mother presses her breast away from the infant's nose so he can breathe more comfortably while feeding. (Photo by Marcia Lieberman; Waechter EH, Blake FG: Nursing Care of Children, 9th ed. Philadelphia, JB Lippincott, 1976)

FORMULA FEEDING

If the mother does not breastfeed her infant, for whatever reason, she can still provide all the necessary nutrients through a formula (Table 2–5). She can also furnish the same comfort and security as she holds the infant (Fig. 2–22). The mother should be discouraged from "propping" the bottle. This practice deprives the infant of the comfort and security of being held, and can cause aspiration if the infant is left unattended. Infants who nurse from propped bottles become more prone to develop middle ear infections.

nurse's responsibility for patient teaching

It is an accepted fact that nurses have a responsibility for patient teaching, so it is of the utmost importance that they are well-informed. Usually new mothers are very eager to learn all they can about their responsibility. Many realize suddenly that they have taken on a tremendous task, that of raising a healthy, well-adjusted child. Although many will have attended prenatal classes, the situation has changed from a theoretical study to serious business.

Some of the mothers who have older children may have valuable contributions to make to a nurse's knowledge. Others may want to review and update on infant care. Many mothers have definite ideas about how they want to care for their infants, so nurses should be objective in the way they present information to the mothers.

The most effective teaching frequently occurs on a one-to-one basis when the nurse and the mother are together with the infant. In addition to determining how much the mother already knows, the nurse needs to know what anxieties the mother has, and perhaps any misunderstandings and misinformation that need to be corrected. The rooming-in situation is ideal for this, offering both parents a chance to care for their child under the guidance of the nurse.

In hospitals where maternity patients are taught as a group, ample time should be allowed for questions and

TABLE 2–4.   GROWTH DURING THE FIRST WEEK OF LIFE

Weight	Height
birth weight: 7½ lb average range: 5½ lb to 10 lb physiologic weight loss during first week of life: due to loss of body fluid and inadequate intake—up to 10% (normal loss)	birth height: 20 in average range: 18 in to 22 in grows approximately 6 in to 7 in

(See table on Normal Growth and Development in chapter on Infant Growth and Development)

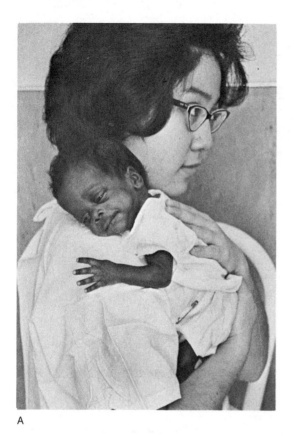

A

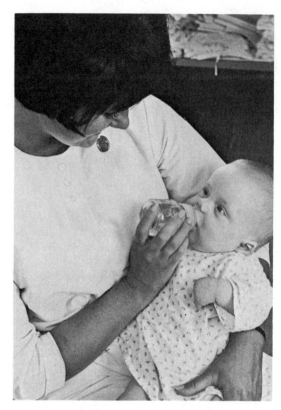

FIG. 2–22. Formula-fed babies need the warmth and closeness of the mother or other caregiver.

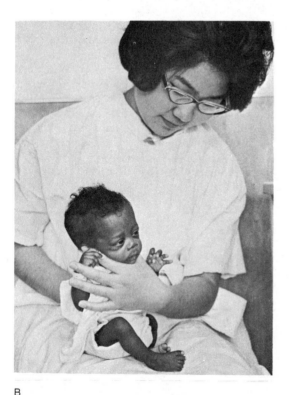

B

FIG. 2–21. (*A*) Bubbling a baby against the shoulder. (*B*) Bubbling a baby sitting upright.

discussion, as well as demonstration and teaching. The discussion will be even more valuable if it can be held at a time when fathers can be present as follows:

DISCUSSION

Leader: I am Miss D, a nurse in the newborn nursery. It will help us get acquainted if you each will tell

1. Your name.
2. Whether your baby is a boy or a girl and the name (if given).
3. Whether you have other children and, if so, their ages.
4. What special arrangements you've made for care of the new baby—diaper service, furniture, etc.
5. What is most important to you for discussion or demonstration here today.

It will be helpful to put these suggestions for discussion on a blackboard. Also assure members of the group that they may ask questions and offer suggestions of things they have found helpful.

Have all equipment that will be needed for home use readily available. It will probably be better to use an infant-size doll rather than a live baby for demonstration to a group, so that any member who desires may practice any of the procedures shown.

TABLE 2–5. APPROXIMATE COMPOSITION PER LITER OF BREAST MILK, COW'S MILK, AND SELECTED PROPRIETARY FORMULAS

Examples of Products	Human Breast Milk*	Cow's Milk (Unmodified)†	Conventional Milk-based Formula‡§	Proprietary Formulas "Humanized" Milk-based Formula‖	Soy-based Formula¶
Energy (kcal)	750**	660	700	700	700
Protein (g)	11**	35	15	15	18– 25
Fat (g)	45	37	37	36	30– 36
Minerals††					
Calcium (mg)	340	1170	536	445	700– 950
Phosphorus (mg)	140	920	454	300	500– 690
Sodium (mEq)	7	22	11	6	9– 24
Vitamins					
A (IU)	1898	1025	1650	2650	2100– 2500
Thiamine (μg)	160	440	510	710	400– 700
Riboflavin (μg)	360	1750	620	1060	600– 1060
Niacin (mg)	1.5	0.9	9	9	5.0– 8.4
Ascorbic acid (mg)	43	11	52	58	50– 55
Vitamin E (IU)	2	0.4	12	9	9– 11

* The composition of human milk may vary greatly

† Homogenized milk

‡ Milk-based formulas are similar and interchangeable

§ Enfamil, Similac

‖ SMA– SMA has a relatively low renal solute load

¶ Isomil, Neo-Mull-Soy, ProSobee, Nursoy—the soy-based formulas listed do not contain milk protein or lactose

** Values from Fomon S: Infant Nutrition. Philadelphia, WB Saunders, 1974

†† Levels of trace minerals would be difficult to interpret because of differences in bioavailability

(Adapted from Hambraeus L: Proprietary milk versus human breast milk. Ped Clin North Amer 24, No. 1:1736, 1977; Suitor CW, Hunter MF: Nutrition: Principles and Application in Health Promotion. Philadelphia, JB Lippincott, 1980)

Following are some of the procedures most often presented in a demonstration:

1. Picking up a young baby: Slide your arm under the baby up toward his head; with hand under head lift him up (Fig. 2– 23).
2. Bathing the baby: Until the cord stump falls off and the navel is healed, the baby should have sponge baths only, as the cord stump should be kept as dry as possible. Many parents like to give their baby a daily bath, but it is not really necessary. Every other day is adequate. On the nonbathing day wipe off the baby's face with water and a clean cloth and cleanse the diaper area at each change.

Sponge bath. Assemble the necessary articles for sponge bathing on the bathing table. Any sturdy table covered with a clean cloth can be used. Articles needed are the following:

Basin of warm water (100° F to 105° F), or warm to the elbow. It is preferable that the basin be used for this purpose only.

Cake of mild soap to be used only if needed.
Soft washcloth; towel for drying baby; large soft towel or cotton blanket on table on which to lay baby.
Small jar of clean cotton.
Paper bag for discarding cotton.
Small jar of mineral oil.
If needed, a jar or package of cornstarch to use instead of powder.
Clean clothes for baby.

Procedure. Have everything ready before picking up the baby. *Never* leave the baby on the table unattended: small infants can easily roll off the table. Place the baby on the blanket or towel and wash the face with clear water. If eyes have been draining, sponge them with a clean piece of cotton, wiping from the inner canthus outward and using clean cotton for each eye. Wash the outer folds of the ears and behind them, but do not poke in the infant's ear as serious harm can be done. Remember, "nothing smaller than your elbow in the ear." Next wash the baby's scalp with the washcloth. If soap is used, be sure to rinse thoroughly.

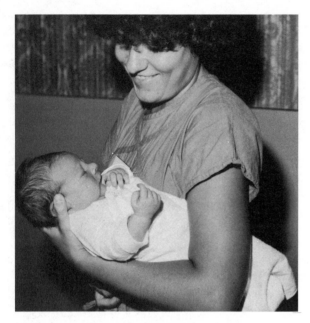

FIG. 2–23. The football hold is only one correct method of holding the newborn. (Reeder SJ, Mastroianni Jr L, Martin L: Maternity Nursing, 14th ed. Philadelphia, JB Lippincott, 1980)

Fill the tub about one-fourth full of water. If you have a thermometer, it should register about 100° F. A thermometer is not necessary; however, your elbow is a good indicator. The water should feel pleasantly warm, but not hot.

With the baby lying on the table, wash his face just as you would with a sponge bath. With either a sponge or tub bath, his scalp should be washed about every other day as cradle cap easily forms. The scalp can be washed quite vigorously with soap, taking care not to let any soapy water drip into the baby's eyes. If the scale on his scalp is difficult to remove, an application of mineral oil the night before is helpful. Be sure to wash carefully over the soft spots (fontanels) as well; you will not harm them. Now pick the baby up using the football hold and, with his head over the tub, rinse thoroughly, again taking care not to splash water into his eyes.

Lay the baby on the table, dry his head, and undress him. If he has had a bowel movement, cleanse the area before putting him into the tub. Hold him firmly in the tub, with back and head supported, and with your free hand wash him all over using soap if necessary. If soap is used, be sure to rinse thoroughly. Take him out of the tub; dry and dress him. Lotions and powders are not necessary; powder in particular may clog the pores of the skin and cause irritation. If his skin becomes irritated, especially in the creases, cornstarch applied to the areas is helpful.

When dressing the baby, it is helpful if the shirt unbuttons and does not have to be pulled over the head, as babies vigorously resist anything being pulled over their heads. If the shirt is the pullover type, stretch the neck of the shirt between your hands to help get it over the baby's head more easily. How much clothing you put on the baby depends mainly on the temperature of his room.

Many parents prefer to use diaper service at least for the first few weeks until mother regains her strength and has established a fairly regular schedule. If planning to use this service, be sure to notify the company in advance so that service can be started the first day home. Other parents find the use of disposable diapers acceptable. One precaution here needs to be mentioned: there is greater temptation to change the diaper less often than with a wet cloth diaper. Some babies develop diaper rash with these diapers, but this is minimized if they are changed before and after feedings, if needed; after a bowel movement, and if the baby seems uncomfortable or fretful.

The time of day for bathing the baby does not make any difference, although it is not practical to bathe him directly after feeding as he is likely to spit up.

After the demonstrations, which may include formula feedings (see Nutrition), time should be allowed for questions and discussion.

Following are some questions that mothers commonly ask:

1. How often should I weigh my baby? Should I weigh him before and after nursing to see how much milk he is getting?
   Answer: Weekly weighing is sufficient if the baby sleeps well and appears satisfied after feeding.

If he has a nasal discharge, wash the edge of his nostrils with cotton but do not poke in his nose. If you wish to dislodge dried mucus that is just inside the nostril, you may cleanse with a small piece of cotton dipped in water. This will usually make the infant sneeze and dislodge any mucus lodged further up in the nose.

Now undress the baby. If he has had a bowel movement you can cleanse the diaper area with clean cotton dipped in mineral oil before bathing the infant. Always clean from front to back to avoid contamination of the urinary system with fecal material. If necessary, use more than one piece of cotton, discarding after each use. Wash your hands before continuing the bath. (It is a good idea to have another small basin of water handy for handwashing.)

Now wash the baby's arms, trunk, and legs. Pay attention to skin folds, such as in the neck and underarms. Wash the genital area, getting into the creases. You can gently cleanse around the labia of girl babies, but do not try to retract the foreskin in uncircumcised males unless under the specific direction from the pediatrician.

Dry the baby, then turn him on his abdomen and wash the back of the neck, trunk, and lastly the buttocks cleansing around the rectum.

Discard the wet towel or blanket upon which the baby had been lying, and dress the baby.

Tub bath. After the cord stump has fallen off, babies can be given tub baths. You need the same utensils as for a sponge bath with the addition of an infant tub. Plastic tubs are available and inexpensive. Although it can be done, it is quite difficult and dangerous to bathe a very young baby in an adult tub. If you have a bathinet this can be used, although many parents do not think these are necessary.

If you don't have a scale, it seems unnecessary to buy one as long as the baby is taken to the well baby clinic or the pediatrician's office once a month. Most pediatricians do not feel it is necessary to weigh a baby before and after feeding, except perhaps in special circumstances.

Normal weight gain, after the initial newborn period of weight loss in the first week, is from 6 to 8 ounces. The baby should double his birth weight around the fifth or sixth month of life (see Table 6-1).

2. How warm should his room be, and how often should I take his temperature?

Answer: Newborn babies need little clothing, a shirt or gown and diaper are usually sufficient. The room temperature should be 70° F to 75° F during the daytime and may be 60° F to 65° F at night. A word of caution may be needed: Some mothers have heard so much against overdressing that they have erred in the opposite direction. Feel the baby's arms, legs, and body to determine if they are warm enough. Do not go by hands and feet, as they may feel cool although the body is comfortably warm. Use light blankets as needed.

It is well for a parent to know how to take a temperature and read a clinical thermometer, but there is no need to take an infant's temperature unless he appears ill or his body feels hot to the touch.

Note: The nurse may need to demonstrate how to take an infant's temperature (see p. 29 for explanation).

3. I do not have a crib for him yet. May I have him in the big bed during the day and beside me at night?

Answer: Even a new infant can roll around, and it is quite possible for him to roll off the bed. If you want to wait for a crib until he is older, you can take a regular clothes basket and line it with a padded lining. Secure the lining close to the basket so it cannot fall over the infant's face. You can use a folded blanket for a mattress, which is folded to size and stitched together. Do not use a pillow for the mattress as the baby can sink down into it and perhaps cover his face. A zippered plastic cover for the mattress can be used, but *never* a sheet of plastic that he can pull over his face.

Some parents wish to have the baby beside them in the bed at night so he can nurse when he wishes, but this is a dangerous practice. Babies have smothered when adults have rolled over in their sleep.

4. I have been told that a young baby sleeps much of the time. Just how much can I expect him to sleep? Should he sleep all night?

Answer: For the first weeks the baby wakes when he is hungry, otherwise sleeps most of the time. His sleep seems to be light; he may stretch and move his body, but external noises do not seem to disturb him. Toward the end of the first month he usually has longer periods of wakefulness.

As a rule, a very young infant cannot go all night without nourishment. Individual babies differ, but a young infant who is fretful and cries a great deal is not following a normal newborn pattern. If this happens, check with your pediatrician or public health nurse to attempt to find out what is troubling him. Most babies are able to sleep straight through the night by the fourth week of life, often before that.

5. I have been told that a newborn baby has immunity to common communicable diseases from his mother and, therefore, I do not need to worry if the older children are sick. Is this true?

Answer: For the first few weeks after birth some resistance to disease is provided by a passive transfer of antibodies to the child by the mother. This is only temporary and should not be relied upon to protect the infant if he comes in contact with an infectious disease.

Newborn infants should be protected from persons who are not in good health. Keep your baby away from the older child who has a cold or who is running a fever. Do not be afraid to tell visitors to stay away as well, even though they insist that "it is only an allergy." Don't take chances.

6. I have been careful to prepare my children for the new baby, even the 3-year-old is delighted to have a baby brother or sister. I see no reason why there should be any jealousy in our family over the new baby.

Answer: Things certainly should go well in your home. But even with the best preparation, a 3-year-old may have occasional feelings of displacement and perhaps feel some anger toward the person who has taken his place. It is well to be prepared for this and not be greatly disturbed. It is a good idea not to leave a very young child alone for any length of time with a young baby. It is possible that he may love him a little too hard, or, as children have been known to do, smile, pat the brother lovingly, and then pinch him. The conflict between love and jealousy is sometimes just a little too much.

the family adjusts to each other

Each new child reshapes the family into which he is born, because every member of that family is affected by the presence of this new person. By the same token, the family shapes the child. Couples who are parents for the first time probably have the greatest anxieties because they have totally new roles to learn. Early research on parent–infant attachment studied the "mothering" aspect of the relationship; very recent studies of neonatal behavior indicate that the infant has a definite role in the attachment process. Fathers are also the subject of more research than ever before, all of which has aided the understanding of how relationships are formed; the things that help or hinder; and how to avoid potential problems.

THE MOTHER'S ADJUSTMENT

Regardless of how much preparation the mother has had for her new role, it is still a totally new experience. She is prepared to love her child, and she does, but the fact remains that she has a new, live child who needs total care 24 hours a day. It looms as a terrific responsibility.

She perhaps has expected that a surge of motherly love instinctively will enable her to love and care for her baby without any doubt or trouble. When she feels inadequate, exhausted and discouraged, however—as many people do when confronted with a new and overwhelming responsibility—she is likely to feel resentment, followed by feelings of guilt over actually resenting the new baby. Even though she loves the baby, no one has prepared her for the purely normal resentment that the responsibility of total care for a helpless, demanding infant often brings.

Rather than trying to deny her resentment and what she considers as unworthy feelings, she needs help to admit them, and further, to understand that resentment is a normal reaction. She needs to understand that as she grows into her task, as she and her child begin to adjust to each other, resentment and feelings of inadequacy will fade away. Those who can learn to admit that they are normal women with a right to normal feelings have come a long way toward reaching equilibrium.

Another way to help is to find some way in which the mother can be relieved of some of the burden until her strength rises to the occasion. It might be helpful to have someone come in for an hour or so each day to take responsibility for the baby and let the mother rest or get out of the house for a short time.

THE FATHER'S ADJUSTMENT

Even a father who loves his new baby very much may feel left out and neglected when mother and baby come home and all her time and attention seem to be devoted to the baby. He may resent the fact that she seems exhausted, unless he understands just how much effort it takes to care for a helpless infant. Like the mother, he needs to be encouraged to admit his feelings because they are normal reactions to the situation.

THE INFANT'S ADJUSTMENT

Each infant reacts to his environment in his own way. As mentioned earlier, he needs to develop a sense of trust. After 9 months security he has been thrust into a world where he has to make known his needs, with no assurance that they will be met. He is in a strange country; he does not know the language, the customs, or the rules. Now he has moved again and he feels the difference. He is sensitive to attitudes that alter touch or to the tone of voice. He also needs reassurance.

summary

Knowledge about newborns and customs surrounding birth have altered dramatically during the last two decades. Though helpless and vulnerable, these infants are enormously complex and capable of responding to and eliciting responses from their caregivers. The trauma of birth and abrupt changes in environment make the first day of life a time of stabilization, demanding careful observation for any possible complications. Nurses and other health professionals are making it possible for babies and parents to be "introduced" in a more relaxed, less hurried atmosphere, hoping that a good beginning will result in a healthier infant and a stronger family relationship.

review questions

1. When do the following vessels close? Ductus arteriosus? Foramen ovale? Ductus venosus?
2. Explain the Apgar score.
3. Which organism causes ophthalmia neonatorum?
4. What nursing measure is taken to prevent ophthalmia neonatorum?
5. What are the four processes by which the newborn loses body heat?
6. Explain molding.
7. What are the shapes of the two fontanels? When do they close?
8. What is cradle cap (seborrheic dermatitis)?
9. What is the average respiratory rate in the newborn? What causes this rate to vary?
10. Differentiate between regurgitation and vomiting.
11. List and describe the reflexes of the neonate.
12. Discuss vascular nevus.
13. Define caput succedaneum.
14. Discuss physiologic jaundice (icterus neonatorum).
15. How does attachment take place between the mother and infant? The father and infant?
16. What is the reason for PKU testing?
17. What patient teaching should the nurse provide for the mother who is breastfeeding?

references

1. Klaus MH, Kennell JH: Parent—Infant Bonding, 2nd ed. St. Louis, CV Mosby, 1982
2. Greenberg M, Morris N: Engrossment: the newborn's impact upon the father. Am J Orthopsychiatr, 44, No. 4:520–531, 1974

bibliography

Bean M: Birth is a family affair. Am J Nurs 75:1659, 1975
Brazelton, T: Neonatal behavioral assessment scale. Clinics In Development Medicine, 50: England, Spastics International Publications, 1974.
Clark A, Affonso D: Infant behavior and maternal attachment: Two sides of the coin. Am J Mat Child Nurs 1, No. 2:94–99, 1976

Countryman BA: Alternative styles for childbirth, J Nurs Care 2, No. 8, 16–17, 1978

Endres JB, Rockwell RE: Food, Nutrition and the Young Child. St Louis, CV Mosby, 1980

Hervada A: et al: Drugs in breast milk. Perinatal Care 9, No. 2:19–25, 1978

Jensen MD, Benson R, Bobak IM: Maternity Care: The Nurse and the Family, 2nd ed. St Louis, CV Mosby, 1981

Klaus M, et al (eds): Maternal Attachment and Mothering Disorders, New Brunswick, Johnson & Johnson, 1974

Klaus M, Kennell JH: Parent–Infant Bonding, 2nd ed. St Louis, CV Mosby, 1982

Lipkin G: Parent–Child Nursing: Psychosocial Aspects, 2nd ed. St Louis, CV Mosby, 1978

Lum Sr B, Batzel RL, and Barnett E: Reappraising newborn eye care. Am J Nurs 80:1602–1603, 1980

McCall RB: Infants: The New Knowledge About the Years From Birth to Three. New York, Random House (Vintage), 1980

Oehler JM: Family-Centered Neonatal Nursing Care. Philadelphia, JB Lippincott, 1981

Phillips C, Anzalone J: Fathering: Participation in Labor and Birth. St Louis, The CV Mosby, 1978

Pipes PL: Nutrition in Infancy and Childhood, 2nd ed. St Louis, CV Mosby, 1981

Rubin R: Binding-in in the postpartum period. Mat Child Nurs 6:67–75, 1977

Waechter EH, Blake FG: Nursing Care of Children, 9th ed, Philadelphia, JB Lippincott, 1976

Whaley LF, Wong D: Nursing Care of Infants and Children. St Louis, CV Mosby, 1979

Wieczorek RR, Natapoff JN: A Conceptual Approach to the Nursing of Children. Philadelphia, JB Lippincott, 1981

the high-risk newborn

3

student objectives

The student successfully attaining the goals of this chapter will be able to

1 Define the following vocabulary terms:

apnea   hyaline membrane disease   hyperbilirubinemia   phototherapy
postmature   premature   retrolental fibroplasia   surfactant

2 Compare the appearance of the premature newborn with that of the normal term infant.

3 Discuss the possible emotional effects of a high-risk birth on the infant and family, and describe the nurse's role in providing emotional support.

4 Describe nursing measures to maintain adequate nutrition, hydration, and oxygenation for the premature infant.

5 Describe the appearance of the infant of a diabetic mother.

6 Describe the appearance of a newborn suffering from fetal alcohol syndrome.

Most infants readily adjust to life outside the uterus. Each year, however, about 5% of the babies born experience complications before, during, or immediately after birth. These infants (250,000 each year) are referred to as infants at risk or high-risk infants, because their survival and long-term well-being are seriously jeopardized. Only technologically advanced expert care by skilled health professionals and a controlled environment can offer them hope of realizing a normal life potential. A number of factors can place a fetus at risk (Table 3–1).

The largest number of high-risk newborns are small infants. About two-thirds of these are premature or preterm; the rest are term infants of low birth weight (SGA—small for gestational age). These tiny beings and their parents have multiple problems to deal with before they can be together as a family.

Immediate physical survival of the infant is not the only factor to be considered. Research indicates that nearly 40% of infants hospitalized at birth for a long time are later victims of neglect or abuse; several reasons are suggested for this tragic statistic. The infant's poor condition makes him even more unlike the "fantasy baby," and parents may feel guilty about this. His need to be in the intensive care nursery (ICN) means that the early bonding is interrupted, and the infant has little chance to be held, cuddled, and comforted, even though his emotional needs are probably more acute than those of a normal term baby. Unmet emotional needs can make the infant cross, unsta-

TABLE 3–1. FACTORS THAT PLACE A FETUS AT RISK

Factors	Ideal	At Risk	Potential Neonatal Problems of At-Risk Maternal Situations
Socioeconomic			
Age	20–29	Under 16	Low birth weight, fetopelvic disproportion
		Over 35	Congenital anomalies
Emotional stress	Minimal stress	Recent crisis event	
		History of emotional instability	? Prematurity
Smoking	None	Smokes	Low birth weight
			Abruptio placentae
Drug Use	None	Excessive use of alcohol	Fetal alcohol syndrome
		Use of addictive drugs	Withdrawal, growth retardation (heroin)
		Heavy use of tranquilizers	Withdrawal
Socioeconomic status	Middle to upper	Lower	Prematurity
			Increased incidence of neonatal complications
Marital status	Married	Single	Poor prenatal care
Prenatal care	First trimester	None or late in pregnancy	Multiple complications
Anatomical			
Cervix	Adequate	Incompetent	Prematurity
Uterus	Normal configuration	Abnormal	Prematurity, unusual placental implantation
Pelvis	Adequate for delivery	Small, questionable for vaginal delivery	Difficult labor and delivery; C section
Pregnancy history			
Parity	0–4	5 or more	Increased neonatal morbidity
History	Negative for catastrophic events during pregnancy	Previous abortion, stillbirth, neonatal death, or anomaly	Repeat neonatal disaster
Previous delivery	Uncomplicated vaginal	C section	C section
Maternal health–systems			
Endocrine	Normal	Disturbances—e.g., diabetes, thyroid dysfunction, etc.	Increased incidence of neonatal complications (see text)
Blood Pressure	Normal	Hypertension—i.e., 140/90 or increase of 30 mm systolic or 15 diastolic over initial pregnancy reading	Small for dates (SGA) infant; Abruptio placenta; Neonatal asphyxia
Renal	Normal	Repeated UTI; Chronic renal disease	Prematurity, neonatal asphyxia
Heart	Normal	Cardiac disease	Prematurity, neonatal asphyxia
Lungs	Normal	Pneumonia, asthma, cold	Prematurity, neonatal infection, asphyxia, SGA
Nutritional Status	Good	Malnourished	SGA infant
Weight	Normal for height	Underweight, obese	Macrosomia, fetopelvic disproportion
Other		Infection	Neonatal infection

TABLE 3–1. *(Continued)*

Factors	Ideal	At Risk	Potential Neonatal Problems of At-Risk Maternal Situations
Complications of pregnancy	None	Toxemia	SGA infant, asphyxia, hypoglycemia, hypocalcemia, aspiration syndrome, polycythemia
		Placental abnormalcy	Anemia, asphyxia, prematurity
		Multiple pregnancy	SGA, polycythemia, asphyxia (usually 2nd twin), prematurity
		Rh isommunization	Hyperbilirubinemia, anemia
		Failure to gain adequate weight	SGA
		Excessively large fetus	Trauma during delivery, asphyxia
		Premature rupture of membranes	Infection, prolapse of the cord
Labor and delivery			
Length	1st stage		
	3–12 hr primigravida	Over 12 hr, under 3 primigravida	
	2–8 hr multigravida	Over 8 hr, multigravida	Mechanical trauma
	2nd stage		
	30′ to 1 hr primigravida	Over 2 hr primigravida	Asphyxia, infection
	30′ or less multigravida	Over 30′ multigravida	
Forceps	Low or none	Mid	Mechanical trauma, asphyxia
Cord	No compression	Compression or prolapse	Asphyxia
Delivery mode	Vaginal	C section	Transient tachypnea, prematurity
Presentation	Vertex	Breech, face, shoulder, transverse	Bruising, brachial plexus damage or mechanical trauma, asphyxia
Meconium	None	Present before delivery	Meconium aspiration, pneumonia, asphyxia
Drugs	Local, regional or none	General	Neonatal depression
		Narcotics or CNS depressant	
		Less than 30′ before delivery	
		MgSO₄	

(Cranley MS: Fetal and maternal monitoring: Antepartal fetal assessment. Am J Nurs 78:2098 1978)

ble, and easily stressed, which is a source of great tension for the mother, who may feel exhausted and alone with an unfair responsibility. Health professionals who are aware of the potential problems can contribute much to the prevention of child abuse.

the premature infant

CONCEPT AND DEFINITION

At one time, prematurity was defined only on the basis of birth weight: any live infant weighing 2500 g (5 lb, 8 oz) or less at birth. Time proved this definition inadequate, because some infants born at full term weighed less than 2500 g and others weighed more than that even though delivered preterm.

The American Academy of Pediatrics has adopted the use of *premature* to mean any infant of less than 37 weeks gestation. A *term* infant is one born between the beginning of the thirty-eighth week and the end of the forty-second week of gestation, regardless of birth weight; and, a *postmature* (postterm) infant is one born after completion of the forty-second week of gestation, regardless of birth weight. In recent years new tests have been developed to determine gestational age, since calculating gestational age from the last menstrual period is not always reliable.

Generally the cause of prematurity is not known. Statistics show, however, that the incidence of prematurity is lowest in middle- to high-socioeconomic classes, where mothers are usually in good health, and have received adequate prenatal care.

The premature infant's untimely departure from the uterus may mean that various organs and systems are not sufficiently mature to adjust to extrauterine life. His chances for survival can be estimated in part by weight and gestational age. Infants who weigh 400 g to 1000 g at birth have only about a 10% chance of survival. Between 40% and 50% of those who weigh 1000 g to 1500 g can be expected to live with the benefit of intensive care. Those who weigh 1500 g to 2000 g have a much better prognosis—between 75% and 85%. The key factor in survival of premature infants is pulmonary function.

CHARACTERISTICS

Compared with the term infant, the premature infant (preemie) is tiny, scrawny, and red (Fig. 3–1). The extremities are thin with very little muscle or subcutaneous fat. Head and abdomen are disproportionately large, and the skin thin, relatively translucent and usually wrinkled. Veins of the abdomen and scalp are more visible. Lanugo is plentiful over the extremities, back, and shoulders. The ears have soft, minimal cartilage, and thus are very pliable. The soft bones of the skull have a tendency to flatten on the sides, and the ribs yield with each labored breath. Testes are undescended in the male; labia and clitoris are quite prominent in the female. The soles of the feet and palms of the hands have few creases. Many of the typical newborn reflexes are weak or absent (Fig. 3–2).

PROBLEMS OF THE PREMATURE INFANT

The premature infant's physiologic immaturity causes many difficulties (Table 3–2), the most critical of which is respiratory. Typically his respirations are shallow, rapid, and irregular, with periods of *apnea*, which is temporary interruption of the breathing impulse. Respirations may become so labored that the chest wall and perhaps even the sternum are retracted.

Pediatrician and nursery staff should be alerted to impending birth of a premature infant so that equipment for resuscitation and emergency care is made available.

Respiratory distress syndrome (RDS), also known as *hyaline membrane disease*, affects about one-half the preterm infants born each year. It occurs because the lungs are too immature to function properly. Normally the lungs remain partially expanded after each breath, owing to a substance called *surfactant*, a biochemical compound that reduces surface tension inside the air sacs. Premature infants' lungs are deficient in surfactant and thus collapse after each breath, greatly reducing the infant's vital supply of oxygen. This damages the lung cells, and these damaged cells combine with other substances present in the lungs to form a fibrous substance called *hyaline membrane*. This membrane fills the lungs and cuts off the supply of oxygen to the infant's bloodstream.

Infants with RDS now have a better prognosis if they can receive additional oxygen through *continuous positive airway pressure* (CPAP), using intubation or a plastic hood. This helps the lungs to remain partially expanded until they begin producing surfactant, usually within the first 5 days of life.

If premature delivery is expected, RDS can be prevented. Through amniocentesis, the amount of *lecithin*, the major component of surfactant, can be measured to determine lung maturity. If insufficient lecithin is present, the mother can be given steroid drugs that will cross the

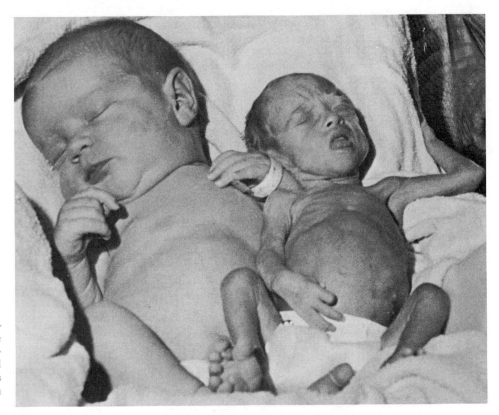

FIG. 3–1. The difference between full-term and premature infants is striking. The "preemie" has a relatively large head and loose skin. Sometimes loops of intestine are visible through the thin abdominal wall.

placenta and cause the infant's lungs to produce surfactant.

Cold stress is an even greater threat to the premature newborn than to the term infant. He cannot shiver and has no integration of reflex control of peripheral blood vessels.

Cold stress can result in hypoxia, metabolic acidosis, and hypoglycemia. Therefore, to prevent heat loss, and to control other aspects of the preemie's environment, he is placed in an isolette or incubator (Fig. 3–3). This unit has a clear plexiglas top that allows a full view of the infant

---

TABLE 3–2. SYSTEMS AND SITUATIONS THAT ARE MOST LIKELY TO CAUSE PROBLEMS IN THE PREMATURE INFANT

The premature infant has altered physiology due to immature and often poorly developed systems. The severity of any problem that occurs depends upon the gestational age of the infant.

Respiratory system
   Alveoli begin to form at 26–28 weeks' gestation; therefore, lungs are poorly developed.
   Respiratory muscles are poorly developed.
   Chest wall lacks stability.
   Production of surfactant is reduced.
   There is reduced compliance and low functional residual capacity.
   Breathing may be labored and irregular with periods of apnea and cyanosis.
   Infant is prone to atelectasis.
   Gag and cough reflexes are poor; thus, aspiration is a problem.

Digestive system
   Stomach is small, vomiting is likely to occur. It is difficult to provide caloric requirement in early days.
   Tolerance is decreased and there is impaired ability to absorb fat, vitamin D, and all fat-soluble vitamins.

Poor thermal stability
   Has very little subcutaneous fat; thus, there is no heat storage or insulation.
   Cannot shiver; has poor vasomotor control of blood flow to skin capillaries.
   There is a relatively large surface area in comparison to body weight.
   Sweat glands are decreased; infant cannot perspire.
   Has reduced muscle and fat deposits that restrict metabolic rate and heat production.
   Usually is less active.

Renal function
   Sodium excretion is probably increased, which may lead to hyponatremia; there is difficulty in excreting potassium.
   Ability to concentrate urine decreases; thus, when vomiting or diarrhea occur, dehydration is likely to follow.
   Ability to acidify urine decreases.
   Glomerular tubular imbalance accounts for sugar, protein, amino acids, and sodium present in urine.

Nervous system
   Response to stimulation is slow.
   Suck, swallow, and gag reflexes are poor; feeding and aspiration therefore are problems.
   Cough reflex is weak or absent.
   Centers that control respirations, temperature, and other vital functions are poorly developed.

Infection
   Actively formed antibodies are absent at birth (active immunity).
   No IgM is present at birth (passive immunity).
   Limited chemotaxis (reaction of cell to chemical stimuli).
   Decreased opsonization (preparation of cells for phagocytosis).
   Limited phagocytosis (digestion of bacteria by cells).

Liver function
   Does not have ability to handle and conjugate bilirubin.
   Does not store or release sugar well; thus, there is a tendency toward hypoglycemia.
   There is a steady decrease in hemoglobin after birth and in the production of blood; therefore, anemia may occur.
   Does not make or store vitamin K; thus, infant is susceptible to hemorrhagic disease.

Eyes
   Oxygen given beyond the point of infant need will cause retinal arteries to constrict, resulting in anoxic damage.
   The retinae detach from the surface of posterior chambers and a fibrous mass forms, resulting in an inability to receive visual stimulation. This is retrolental fibroplasia (RLF).
   There are many stages of RLF.
   The exact amount and level of oxygen needed to produce RLF is unknown.

(Brunner L, Suddarth D: Lippincott Manual of Nursing Practice, 2nd, Philadelphia, JB Lippincott, 1978)

---

from all aspects. The isolette maintains ideal temperature, humidity, and oxygen concentrations, and it isolates the infant from infection. Portholes at the side afford access to the infant with minimal temperature and oxygen loss.

The premature infant desperately needs nourishment, but his digestive system is often unprepared to receive and digest food. The stomach is small with a capacity of 1 or 2 ounces. The sphincters at either end of the stomach are immature, causing regurgitation or vomiting if feedings distend the stomach. The immature liver is unable to manage all the bilirubin produced by hemolysis, making the infant prone to jaundice and high blood bilirubin levels (*hyperbilirubinemia*) that can result in brain damage.

The infant is also immunologically immature because he does not receive enough antibodies from his mother and he cannot produce them himself. This makes him particularly vulnerable to infection.

Muscle weakness in the premature contributes to nutritional and respiratory problems, and to a posture distinct from that of the term infant (Fig. 3– 4). He may not be able to change positions, and will be prone to fatigue and exhaustion, even from eating and breathing. He needs gentle, but intensive care to survive and develop.

NURSING CARE

The physical handicaps of premature infants demand the finest nursing care, emphasizing cleanliness, continuous electronic monitoring, and frequent manual monitoring of vital signs, maintenance of adequate oxygenation, hydration, and nutrition; sensory stimulation for the infant and emotional support for the parents.

CLEANLINESS

Although the isolette provides a great deal of protection from infection, careful handwashing is still essential. Studies have shown that careful handwashing is more important in controlling nursery infections than caps and gowns and excluding important people such as parents and physicians from contact with the baby. Some nurseries are asking parents and staff to wear gowns only if they are going to hold the baby.

Another obvious line of protection is clean or sterile equipment. Modern incubators are designed to be as easy as possible to clean. Babies who are in these units for long periods should be transferred to fresh isolettes on a regular basis. Water in humidifiers should be changed frequently; every day is not too often, and every 8 hours is preferable.

MONITORING VITAL SIGNS

Close observation of the baby is a constant, primary responsibility of the nurse. Monitoring temperature, pulse, and respiration is one aspect of this responsibility. Blood pressure measurements are not routinely made on premature infants. Axillary temperatures are taken frequently and recorded; how often temperatures are taken will be determined by how unstable the baby's temperature is. The isolette thermostat is adjusted to maintain an axillary temperature of 96° F to 98° F. Maintaining the humidity level in the isolette will help the baby to stabilize his temperature.

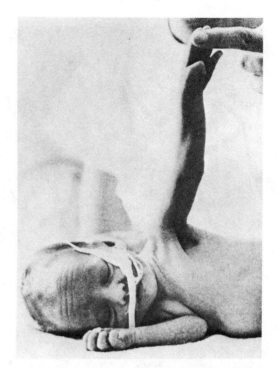

A

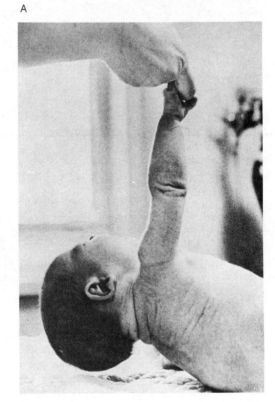

B

FIG. 3–2. (A) The grasp reflex present in the premature newborn is much weaker than that noted in the (B) full-term infant. (Courtesy Mead Johnson Laboratories, Evansville, Ind.)

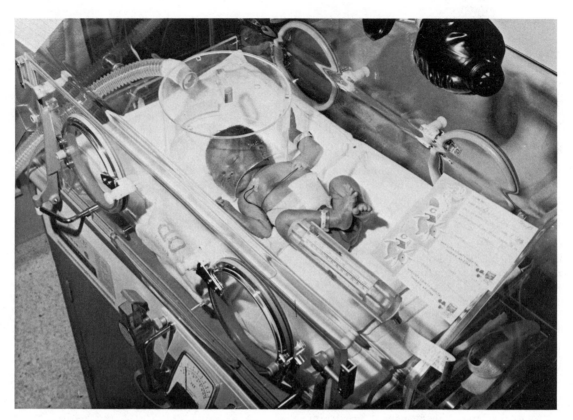

FIG. 3–3.   Isolette infant incubator. (Courtesy Air-Shields, Inc., Hatboro, Pa)

Most isolettes are equipped with a Servo Control system for temperature regulation. A temperature-sensitive electrode is attached to the baby's abdomen and connected to the isolette thermostat. The unit can then be set to turn the heater on and off according to the baby's skin temperature. It is still standard practice to take and record axillary temperatures when the baby is being monitored by Servo Control. In taking axillary temperatures the infant axilla should be dry, the arm held close to the body, and adequate time (5 to 10 minutes) allowed for the temperature to register. Rectal temperatures are not taken regularly after admission in order to prevent damage and overstimulation of the rectal sphincter.

Apical pulses are taken regularly, listening to the heart through the chest using a stethoscope for one full minute in order not to miss an irregularity in rhythm. Observations should include rate, rhythm, and strength. The pulse should be taken before rather than after such activities as feeding or taking the temperature, which may stimulate the baby. The pulse rate is normally rapid (120 to 140 per minute) and unstable. Preemies are subject to dangerous periods of bradycardia (down as low as 60 to 80 per minute) and tachycardia (up as high as 160 to 200 per minute). The nurse's observations of pulse rate, rhythm, and strength are essential to understanding how the baby is tolerating treatments, activity, feedings, and the temperature and oxygen concentration of the isolette.

Observation of the premature infant's respiration is obviously of utmost importance (Fig. 3–5). Measuring the rate of respiration and identifying retractions are essential to determining proper oxygen concentrations. One of the most hazardous characteristics of the premature infant is his tendency to stop breathing periodically (apnea). The hypoxia caused by this apnea and his general respiratory difficulty may cause mental retardation or other neurologic problems.

Frequently electronic apnea alarms are used. Electrodes are placed across the infant's chest with leads to the apnea monitor outside the isolette, giving a continuous reading of respiratory rate. Visual and audio alarms can be set to alert the nurse when the rate goes too high or low, or if the baby waits too long to take a breath.

In the fully equipped premature nursery, the apnea monitor is incorporated into a complete vital signs monitor. This monitor has temperature, pulse and respiration monitors. The pulse monitor gives a continuous rate reading and also has alarms to alert the nurse about extremes. The temperature monitor is similar.

It is a nursing responsibility to place, check and replace the leads from the baby. The electrodes should be removed and relocated slightly at least every day to protect the baby's sensitive skin from being damaged by the electrode paste and adhesive. The skin should be cleansed carefully between applications of the electrodes. Many false alarms are the result of leads coming loose. Some of these can be prevented by using a very small amount of electrode paste and being careful to keep the paste inside the circle of adhesive on the electrode.

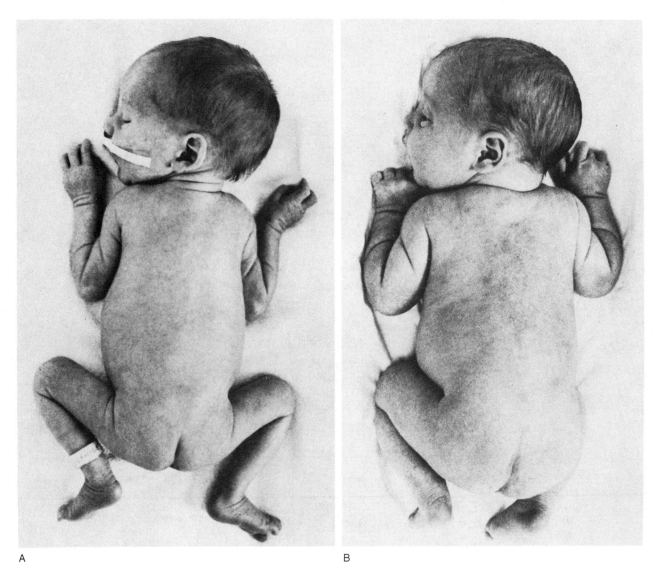

A   B

FIG. 3–4. It is easy to distinguish the premature newborn from the term infant when both are in the prone position. (A) the premature infant lies with pelvis flat and legs spread in a froglike position. (B) term infant lies with limbs flexed, pelvis raised, and knees drawn up under abdomen. (Courtesy Mead Johnson Laboratories, Evansville, Ind.)

Apical pulses, axillary temperatures and visual observations of the baby's respirations are still assessed at regular intervals by the nurse. The vital signs monitor serves as an extension of the nurse's eyes and ears, making her an even more constant, accurate and complete observer.

OXYGEN

Not all premature infants need extra oxygen, but many do. Isolettes are made with oxygen inlets and humidifiers for raising the oxygen concentration in the incubator from 20 to 21% (room air) to a higher percentage. This is the usual method of oxygen therapy. When the baby is cyanotic, breathing rapidly, and retracting, he needs more oxygen.

High blood concentrations of oxygen are dangerous. The immature retina is damaged, causing blindness. This condition is called *retrolental fibroplasia*. A baby with rela-

tively healthy lungs is likely to have his eyes damaged by concentrations of over 40% oxygen. A baby whose lungs are unable to transmit oxygen to his blood readily may be safe at 80% or 90% oxygen. Blood gas tests to determine the arterial blood oxygen are the most precise way to determine the proper oxygen concentration to prescribe for a baby. In the absence of a laboratory to do blood gas determination, the doctor and nurse must rely on careful, recorded, continual observations of the baby. Observations should be made of the pulse rate, the respiratory rate, retractions, skin color, muscle tone, alertness and activity. In the absence of lung pathology it is safer to keep the oxygen concentration below 40% unless hypoxia can be documented. For the baby's protection, incubators are constructed so that it is difficult to get over 40% concentrations without special maneuvers. It is part of the

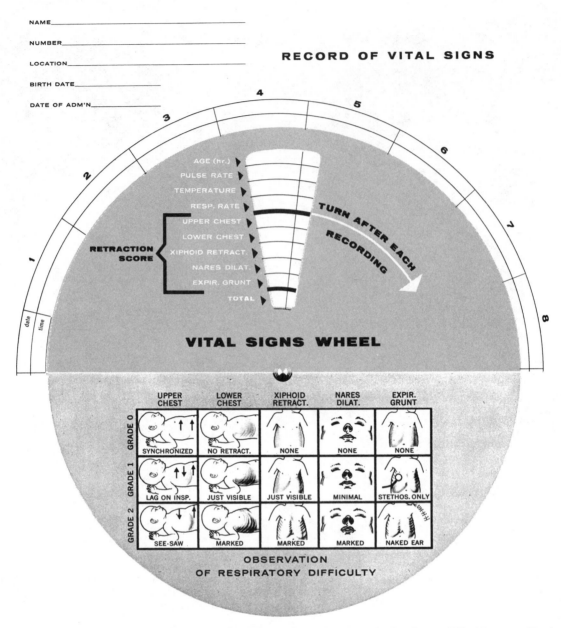

FIG. 3–5.   The vital signs wheel is used to follow up a baby's progress in the first hours of life. (Courtesy Mead Johnson Laboratories, Evansville, Ind.)

nurse's responsibility to measure the oxygen level in the isolette at regular intervals. This is done by means of an instrument called an oxygen analyzer.

Oxygen is also used in handling apnea. Usually a little gentle stimulation, such as wiggling a foot, is enough to remind the baby to breathe. There are times when respiration needs to be assisted by a bag and mask. Every nursery nurse should know how to "bag" a baby in order to be prepared for such times. The principles of this form of assisted respiration are very similar to those of mouth to mouth artificial respiration. The neck must be well extended to open the airway. The mask covers the baby's mouth and nose. A "tight seal" between the mask and the

baby's face must be maintained (see Fig. 2–3). The bag, filled with oxygen or air, is squeezed quickly. The quantity of air needed is relatively small and the pressure very gentle.

HYDRATION

When he is born, a preemie may be too weak to suck or not yet have adequate sucking and swallowing reflexes. For several hours or even a day he may be able to manage without fluids, but soon he will need intravenous fluids. In many cases an IV "life line" will be established right after delivery. Fluids are given through a catheter passed into the umbilical vein in the stub of the umbilical cord if it is still fresh. IV fluids can also be given through other veins. Very small amounts of fluid are needed; perhaps as little as 5 to 10 ml per hour or even less. They can be measured accurately and administered at a steady rate by using an infusion pump. Accurate and complete records of IV fluids are kept. All urinary output is measured and recorded by weighing the diapers before and after they are used. Normal range of urine volume is between 35 and 40 ml/kg per 24 hours during the first few days, increasing to between 50 and 100 ml. The nurse should also observe and record such observation as the number of urinations, color of the urine, and edema. Edema will change the loose wrinkled skin to tight, shiny skin. The open fontanels of the skull can also help in determining hydration. With a full-term child the fontanel will become soft and depressed in the case of dehydration.

FEEDING

At first some premature infants will get all their fluid, electrolyte, vitamin and caloric needs by IV routes. Others are able to start with a nipple and bottle (Fig. 3–6). Many will need gavage feedings. The frequency and quantity of the gavage feedings will be determined by the baby. Usually feedings are given every 2 hours. If the stomach is not being emptied by the next feeding, more time needs to be allowed between feedings or smaller feedings need to be given. Usually the quantity given is just as much as the baby can tolerate and is increased ml by ml as fast as tolerated. Starting a baby on 5 to 10 ml per feeding is not unusual. The feeding is not too large if the baby's stomach is not so distended that it causes respiratory difficulty, vomiting or regurgitation and if there is not much formula left in the stomach by the next feeding. The common preemie formula has 13 calories per ounce. A formula with 20 calories per ounce may also be used. If the formula is too rich the baby may have vomiting and diarrhea. If he is not gaining weight, after the usual postnatal weight loss, the calories may not be enough. Some infants are fed breast milk contributed by their mother or a wet nurse.

When a baby who is being gavage fed begins to suck on the gavage tube, his fingers or hands, he may be ready for nipple feeding. He is ready if he can take the same quantity of formula by nipple that he was tolerating by gavage and not become too tired. Some babies need alternating gavage and nipple feedings to see them through the transition period. The nipple for a premature infant is of softer rubber than the regular nipple. It is also smaller but no shorter than the regular nipple.

There are other methods by which preemies may be fed if neither gavage or nipple feeding is tolerated, and if IV fluids are not adequate. Some babies do better if fed with a rubber-tipped medicine dropper. For others it is necessary to provide gastrostomy feedings.

Premature infants need to be "bubbled" after feedings. Sometimes simply changing the baby's position is enough assistance. At other times it may be helpful to rub or pat the baby's back gently. After a feeding, the best position is probably on the left side with the head of the mattress slightly elevated.

The baby should be weighed daily at the same time in his feeding schedule. These daily weights will give an indication of the baby's overall health and indicate whether or not he is getting enough calories. The baby's doctor and parents probably will want to know the baby's current weight each day. Weighing the baby on the same scales in the same clothing at the same time will help ensure accurate, comparable data.

PHOTOTHERAPY

Jaundice is a common occurrence in prematurity. It is becoming quite common to expose the babies to "blue" fluorescent lights to prevent bilirubin levels from reaching the danger point (20 mg/100 ml). The lights are placed above and outside the isolette. The baby is nude and his

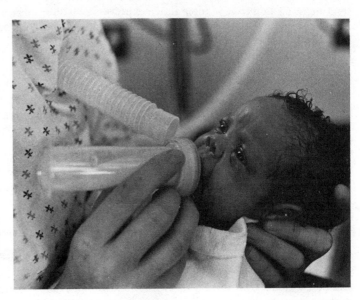

FIG. 3–6. This preterm infant with chronic lung disease still requires a small amount of supplementary oxygen but is able to be out of the isolette for short periods of time to be held for feedings. (Photo by Marcia Lieberman; Waechter EH, Blake FG: Nursing Care of Children, 9th ed. Philadelphia, JB Lippincott, 1976)

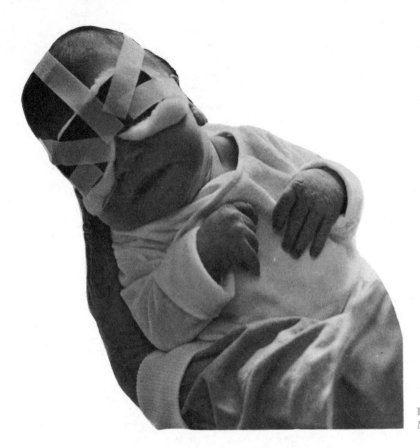

FIG. 3–7. Olympic Bili-Mask. (Courtesy Olympic Medical Corp., Seattle, Wash.)

eyes are shielded from the ultraviolet light (Fig. 3–7). Nurses can become creative in making miniature masks and eye patches to be taped over the baby's eyes with paper tape. The eye patches can promote infection if they are not clean, changed frequently, or applied so that they stay in place. Nurses should be aware that the light can cause skin rashes, "sunburn," or tanning, loose greenish stools, hyperthermia, increased metabolic rate, increased evaporative loss of water, and *priapism*, a perpetual abnormal erection of the penis. Infants undergoing phototherapy treatment need up to 25% more fluids to prevent dehydration. Protective measures for nurses working with these infants include wearing dark glasses, and a cap or scarf to prevent bulbs from scorching hair strands.

MEDICATIONS

The usual healthy premature needs very little medication. He probably will be given an injection of vitamin K at birth. Vitamins and/or iron may be added to feedings to improve nutrition. Some physicians will prescribe intramuscular antibiotics, such as penicillin, to prevent infections, and/or intramuscular phenobarbital to prevent hyperbilirubinemia. Dosage and quantities prescribed are minute, and must be calculated and measured with great care. Usually the best site for intramuscular injections is the anterior aspect of the upper thigh.

ENERGY CONSERVATION AND SENSORY STIMULATION

The premature newborn uses most of his energy to breathe and pump blood. The nurse should plan the baby's day so that he does not become exhausted from constant han-

dling and moving about. The baby's energy can be conserved by not bathing him regularly, but giving only "face and fanny" care as needed. Preemies usually wear only a diaper, if anything. This conserves energy, provides more freedom of movement and allows better opportunity to observe the baby. However, it should not mislead the nurse into ignoring or avoiding the baby, or discouraging parent–child contact essential to establishing a normal relationship.

Older premature babies have a special need for sensory stimulation. Visual stimulation can be provided by mobiles hung over the isolette and toys placed in or on the infant unit. Auditory stimulation can be provided by a radio turned low, a music box, or wind-up toy in the isolette. A very good form of auditory stimulation is the baby's parents, doctor, and nurse talking and singing to him. Being bathed, held, cuddled, and fondled provides needed tactile stimulation. Parent–infant contact is essential to baby and parents.

The nurse must position the premature infant carefully and change his position periodically. He can be positioned from side to side. If he is placed on his back or stomach, special care must be taken to see that he does not aspirate vomitus or bury his nose in sheets or diapers. Preemies have a knack of wriggling into corners and cracks from which they cannot extract themselves.

EMOTIONAL SUPPORT OF THE PARENTS

The premature infant creates a crisis for his parents. Their long-awaited baby is whisked away from them, sometimes to a remote neonatal center, and hooked up to a maze of machines. Parents feel anxiety, guilt, fear, depression, and perhaps anger. They cannot share the early sensitive attachment period. It may take weeks to establish touching and eye contact ordinarily achieved in 10 minutes with a normal term infant. Parents often leave the hospital empty-handed, without the perfect, healthy infant of their dreams. How can they learn to know and love the strange scrawny creature who now lives in that plastic box? These feelings are normal, but studies have shown that if these feelings are not expressed and resolved, they can damage the long-term relationship of parents and child, even resulting in child neglect or abuse.

It is important to consider the mother's condition too. If the infant was a cesarean birth, or if the labor was difficult or prolonged, she may feel abandoned and too weak to become involved with the baby.

Nurses who work with high-risk infants and parents can do much to help families cope with the crisis of prematurity and early separation. Explaining what is happening to their infant in the intensive care nursery, and reporting periodically on the infant's condition reassures parents that their child is receiving excellent care and that they are being kept informed. Listening to parents, and encouraging them to express their feelings can help them support one another. As soon as possible parents should see, touch, and help care for their infant (Fig. 3–8). Most intensive care nurseries do not restrict visiting hours for parents, and they encourage parents to visit their infants often, whenever it is convenient for the parents. Many hospitals offer 24-hour phone privileges to parents so that they are never out of touch with their infant's caregivers.

Before the mother is discharged from the hospital, plans can be made for both parents to visit the infant, and participate in his care. They need to feel that the infant belongs to them, not to the hospital. To help foster this feeling, and strengthen the attachment, nurses work closely with parents to help them progress toward successful parenthood (Fig. 3–9).

During the past few years, nurses have been instrumental in helping to form support groups of parents who have experienced the crisis that a premature infant causes. These parents visit new high-risk families in the hospital and at home. Early results indicate that these groups are quite successful in helping high-risk parents deal with their feelings and solve the problems that may arise when their infant is ready to come home, or if the infant dies. (See Stillbirth or the Death of a Newborn.)

Before the baby goes home, the mother must know how to hold, feed, bathe, dress, diaper, and protect him. This knowledge will give her confidence that she is capable of taking care of her infant. Some hospitals allow parents to stay overnight prior to the infant's discharge. Parents need to know that they can telephone their doctor and nurse at any time.

Premature infants are usually discharged when they weigh 4½ lb to 5 lb and are gaining weight steadily. They need to be able to nurse from a bottle and nipple or from the mother's breast. Through initial use of a breast pump, many mothers of high-risk infants are able to successfully provide this important nutrition for their hospitalized infant and gain the satisfying emotional rewards for themselves and their child.

Prior to discharge, the preemie will have successfully made the transition from isolette to open crib, thriving without artificial support systems. After the baby goes home, a nurse, usually a community health nurse, visits the family to check on the health of mother and baby. She provides additional teaching about the infant's care, if necessary, and answers any questions or concerns the parents might have.

other high-risk conditions

INFANTS OF DIABETIC MOTHERS

When diabetes is controlled in the mother, pregnancy usually does not threaten her health; however, the health of her infant is at great risk. With expert care, 75% to 85% of

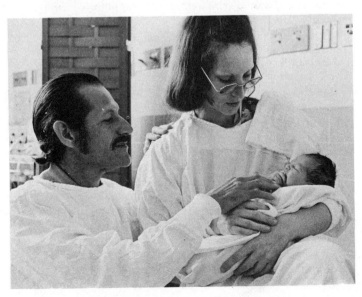

FIG. 3–8. Parents should be encouraged to visit and participate in the care of their high-risk newborn as soon and as often as possible. (Waechter EH, Blake FG: Nursing Care of Children, 9th ed. Philadelphia, JB Lippincott, 1976)

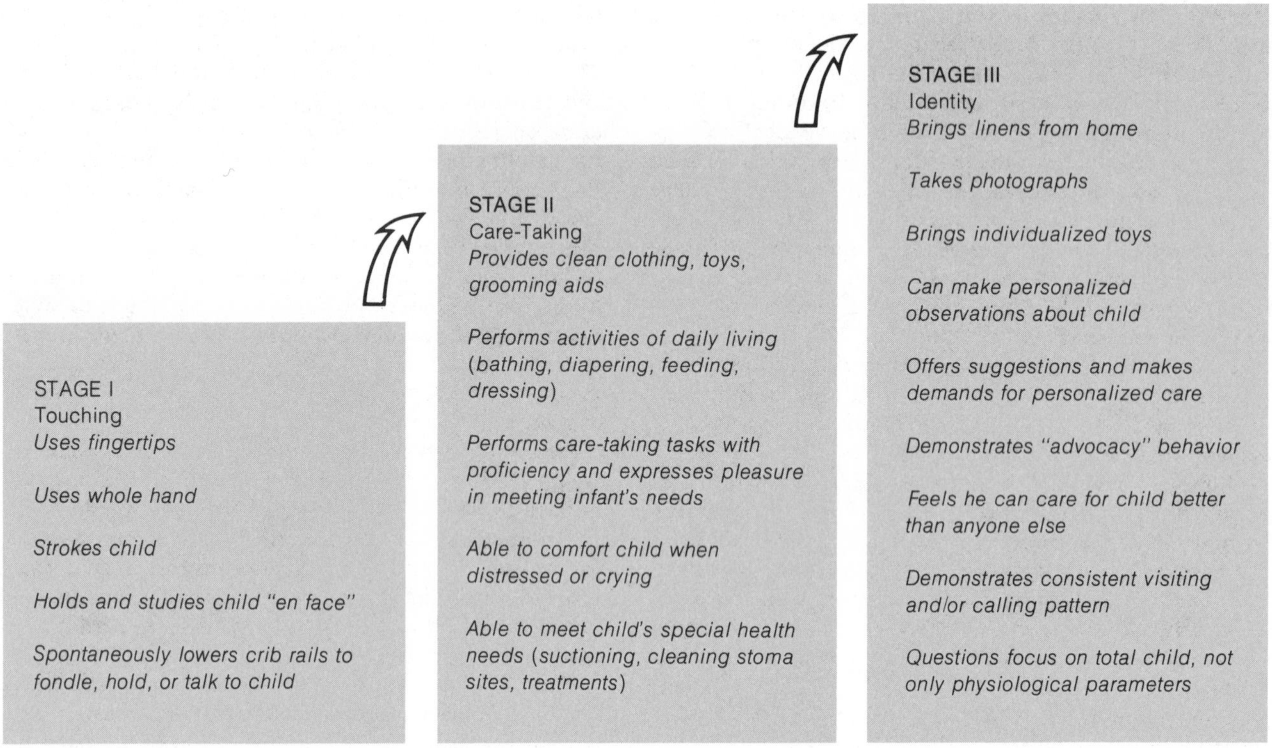

STAGE I
Touching
Uses fingertips

Uses whole hand

Strokes child

Holds and studies child "en face"

Spontaneously lowers crib rails to fondle, hold, or talk to child

STAGE II
Care-Taking
Provides clean clothing, toys, grooming aids

Performs activities of daily living (bathing, diapering, feeding, dressing)

Performs care-taking tasks with proficiency and expresses pleasure in meeting infant's needs

Able to comfort child when distressed or crying

Able to meet child's special health needs (suctioning, cleaning stoma sites, treatments)

STAGE III
Identity
Brings linens from home

Takes photographs

Brings individualized toys

Can make personalized observations about child

Offers suggestions and makes demands for personalized care

Demonstrates "advocacy" behavior

Feels he can care for child better than anyone else

Demonstrates consistent visiting and/or calling pattern

Questions focus on total child, not only physiological parameters

FIG. 3–9. Stages of parenting behaviors observed in parents of high-risk infants. (Adapted from the work of Reva Rubin, Susan Schaeffer Jay, Barbara Schraeder. In Schraeder BD. Attachment and parenting despite lengthy intensive care. Am J Mat Child Nurs 5:37–41, 1980)

these infants can survive; without it, only 50% of them will live.

Late in a diabetic pregnancy, the placenta ceases to function properly; therefore, the usual practice is to induce labor or schedule a cesarean delivery between 36 and 37 weeks gestation. Delivery prior to that time increases the risk of neonatal mortality; later delivery increases the risk of stillbirth.

Infants of diabetic mothers have a distinctive appearance (Fig. 3– 10). They are large for gestational age, plump and full-faced, coated with vernix caseosa. Both placenta and umbilical cord are oversized.

During their first 24 or more extrauterine hours, they lie on their backs, bloated and flushed, their legs flexed and abducted, their lightly closed hands on each side of their head, the abdomen prominent and their respiration sighing.[2]

These infants are subject to many hazards, including congenital anomalies, hypoglycemia, hypocalcemia, hyperbilirubinemia, and hyaline membrane disease. Hypoglycemia if left untreated can cause severe irreversible damage to the central nervous sytem. Although they are large, these infants are still premature and some of the complications may be related to this. These infants require careful observation and early feeding of 5% to 10% glucose followed by formula.

THE POSTMATURE INFANT

When pregnancy lasts longer than 42 weeks, the infant is considered to be *postmature* or *postterm*, regardless of birth weight. Approximately 12% of all infants are postmature, and the causes of delayed birth are not known. Some have an appearance similar to term infants, but others look like infants 1 week to 3 weeks old. Little lanugo or vernix remains, scalp hair is abundant, fingernails are long. Skin is dry, cracked, and wrinkled, and whiter than that of the normal newborn.

Like infants of diabetic mothers, these infants are threatened by failing placental function, and are at risk for intrauterine hypoxia during labor and delivery. It is customary, therefore, for the physician to induce labor or perform a cesarean delivery when the baby is markedly overdue.

The postmature infant has usually expelled meconium *in utero*. At birth, the meconium can be aspirated into the lungs. It obstructs the respiratory passages and irritates the lungs. Whenever meconium-stained amniotic fluid is detected, oral and nasopharyngeal suctioning should be performed as soon as the head is born. After delivery, gastric lavage may also be performed to remove any meconium swallowed and to prevent aspiration by way of vomiting.

INFANTS OF ADDICTED MOTHERS

As mentioned in Chapter 1, alcohol is one of the many teratogenic drugs that crosses the placenta to the infant. Fetal alcohol syndrome (FAS) is frequently apparent in infants of chronic alcoholic mothers, and sometimes, in infants of mothers who are moderate consumers of alcohol, the so-called "social drinkers." FAS is characterized by low birth weight, smaller height and head circumference, short palpebral fissures (eyelid folds), reduced ocular growth, and a flattened nasal bridge. These infants are prone to respiratory difficulties, hypoglycemia, hypocalcemia, and hyperbilirubinemia. Their growth continues to be slow and their mental development retarded, despite expert care and nutrition.

Infants of mothers addicted to heroin, methadone, or other narcotics, are born addicted, and many suffer withdrawal symptoms during the early neonatal period. These symptoms include tremors, restlessness, hyperactivity, disorganized reflexes, increased muscle tone, sneezing, tachypnea, and a shrill cry. Ineffective sucking and swallowing reflexes create feeding problems, and regurgitation and vomiting occur often after feeding. Typical treatment is administration of chlorpromazine or phenobarbital, intramuscularly, for 2 days to 4 days; then, orally for 7 days to 10 days. These babies respond favorably to movement and close body contact with their caregivers; therefore, some nurseries have instituted the practice of placing the babies in special carriers that hold them close to the nurse's chest as she moves about the nursery.

stillbirth or the death of a newborn

When a child dies, either before birth or in the first weeks after birth, parents are faced with the crisis of mourning someone they never really had a chance to know. They had expected a joyous event; they received a devastating loss. Nurses who work with these families need to understand the grieving process and their own feelings about death to help parents cope with this crisis.

Persons experiencing a loss or threat of a loss often react in a somewhat predictable way. Two pioneers in the study of grief have described the phases of mourning; the phases are comparable (Table 3–3).[3,4]

Mothers are sometimes aware that the fetus is dead long before any signs of labor appear; yet, many deny that something could be wrong until informed by their physicians. Parents, particularly the mothers, of a stillborn infant or one who dies immediately after birth, may need to see and touch the infant in order to accept the reality of the infant's death. This is something that each parent should decide *individually*, after discussing it with the nurse. Be-

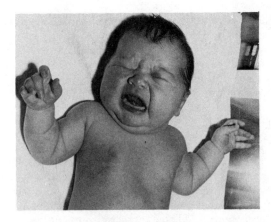

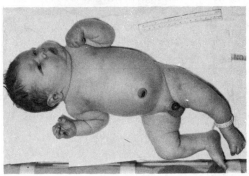

FIG. 3–10. Infant of diabetic mother (IDM). (Avery GB: Neonatology, 2nd ed. Philadelphia, JB Lippincott, 1981)

fore seeing the infant, parents need to be prepared for the infant's appearance—temperature, color, size, and any deformities or bruises. It is important that the mother be able to mourn this baby as a real person, without such well-meaning comments as, "you can have another baby;" comments that deny this baby as an individual.

Both parents need to feel that the nurse has the time and interest to listen, and that it is important for them to express their feelings. Attempts to cheer up the parents do not aid the grieving process, but strike a note of insincerity and insensitivity. Nurses need to know that it is all right for them to grieve with parents, to touch or hold them, and to cry with them.

TABLE 3–3. COMPARISON OF LINDEMANN PHASES OF MOURNING AND KUBLER-ROSS STAGES OF GRIEF

Lindemann (Three Phases)	Kubler-Ross (Five Stages)
1. Shock and disbelief	1. Denial and isolation: "No, not me."
	2. Anger: "Why me?"
	3. Bargaining: "If I . . . ."
2. Developing awareness and acute mourning	4. Depression and acute grief: "How can I . . . ."
3. Resolution and acceptance	5. Acceptance: "I can, I must."

The crisis of stillbirth or neonatal death is another instance where parent support groups can be remarkably effective. No one can better understand the feelings and problems of this tragic situation than parents who have lived through it and managed to rebuild their lives. They are proof that life can go on, even though it seems impossible at the time of crisis.

summary

The high risk infant often arrives unprepared for extrauterine life. Breathing, feeding, and regulating temperature are difficult, if not impossible, for him to manage on his own. Whether premature, postmature, or the infant of a diabetic or drug-addicted mother, this infant requires the finest, most advanced physical care available, plus sensitive response to his emotional needs. His parents need counseling and support to help them cope with this crisis. If the baby lives, they will need continued assistance in relating to and caring for him. If he dies, they will need understanding and guidance to help them mourn their loss. Nurses have been leaders among health professionals in recognizing and providing this critically important aspect of care.

review questions

1. Describe the appearance of the premature infant.
2. What specific treatment is given to a neonate with hyaline membrane disease?
3. Outline the nursing care required for a premature infant.
4. Describe the appearance of the fontanels in a dehydrated infant.
5. How are the infant's eyes protected during phototherapy?
6. How does the nurse conserve the energy of the premature infant?
7. In which ways can the nurse help the parents of a premature infant?
8. Describe the neonate whose mother has diabetes mellitus.
9. What are the characteristics of fetal alcohol syndrome?
10. What are the symptoms of narcotic withdrawal in the neonate?
11. How can the nurse help the parents after delivery of a stillborn or when an infant dies soon after birth?

references

1. Whaley L, Wong D: Nursing Care of Infants and Children. St Louis, CV Mosby, 1979
2. Farquhar JW: The child of the diabetic woman. Arch Dis Child 34:76, 1959
3. Lindemann E: Symptomatology and management of acute grief. Am J Psychol 101:141, 1944
4. Kubler-Ross E: On Death and Dying. New York, Macmillan, 1969

bibliography

Abbey BL, et al: Nursing responsibility in referring the convalescent newborn. Am J Mat Child Nurs 2:295–297, 1977

Babson SG, Pernoll ML, Benda GI, Simpson K: Diagnosis and Management of the Fetus and Neonate At Risk: A Guide for Team Care, 4th ed. St Louis, CV Mosby, 1979

Bock J: Closeup on fetal alcohol syndrome. Can Nurse 75, No. 11:35, 1979

Buerger EM: Developmental profile of the neonate. In McNall LK (ed): Contemporary Obstetric and Gynecologic Nursing. St Louis, CV Mosby, 1980

Christensen A: Coping with the crisis of a premature birth—one couple's story. Am J Mat Child Nurs 2:33–37, 1977

Crout TK: Caring for the mother of a stillborn baby. Nurs '80, 10, No. 4:70–73, 1980

Dingle RE, et al: Continuous transcutaneous O$_2$ monitoring in the neonate, Am J Nurs 80:890–893, 1980

Eager M: Long-distance nurturing of the family bond. Am J Mat Child Nurs 2:293–294, 1977

Eager M, Exoo R: Parents visiting parents for unequaled support. Am J Mat Child Nurs 5:35–36, 1980

Elmer E: Infant battery. In McNall LK (ed): Contemporary Obstetric and Gynecologic Nursing. St Louis, CV Mosby, 1980

Erdman D: Parent-to-parent support: The best for those with sick newborns. Am J Mat Child Nurs 2:291–292, 1977

Hawkins-Walsh E: Diminishing anxiety in parents of sick newborns. Am J Mat Child Nurs 5:30–34, 1980

Jensen MD, Bobak IM: Handbook of Maternity Care: A Guide for Nursing Practice. St Louis, CV Mosby, 1980

Johnson SH (ed): High-risk Parenting: Nursing Assessment and Strategies for the Family At Risk. Philadelphia, JB Lippincott, 1979

Klaus MH, Fanaroff AA: Care of the High-risk Neonate, 2nd ed. Philadelphia, WB Saunders, 1980

Korones S: High-risk Newborn Infants: The Basis for Intensive Nursing Care, 3rd ed. St Louis, CV Mosby, 1981

Kowalski K, Osborn MR: Helping mothers of stillborn infants to grieve. Am J Mat Child Nurs 2:29–32, 1977

Levin DL, Morriss FC, Moore GC: A Practical Guide to Pediatric Intensive Care. St Louis, CV Mosby, 1979

Metcalf SC: Getting to Know Your Premature Baby. Louisville, National Foundation March of Dimes.

Oehler J: Family-centered Neonatal Nursing Care. Philadelphia, JB Lippincott, 1981

Petrillo M: Emotional Care of Hospitalized Children, 2nd ed. Philadelphia, JB Lippincott, 1980

Pierog SH, Ferrara A: Medical Care of the Sick Newborn, 2nd ed. St Louis, CV Mosby, 1976

Rivard C: The fetal alcohol syndrome. J School Health 49, No. 2:96–98, 1979

Schraeder BD: Attachment and parenting despite lengthy intensive care. Am J Mat Child Nurs 5:37–41, 1980

Sheldon RE, Sellers P: The Expanding Role of the Nurse in Neonatal Intensive Care. New York, Grune & Stratton, 1980

Varner B, Ossenkop D, Lyon J: Prematures, too, need rooming-in and care-by-parent programs. Am J Mat Child Nurs 5:431–432, 1980

the newborn with special needs 4

student objectives

The student successfully attaining the goals of this chapter will be able to

1 Define the following vocabulary terms:

atresia   chordee   erythroblastosis fetalis   hydrocephalus   hypospadias
meningocele   myelomeningocele   omphalocele   talipes equinovarus

2 List four common birth injuries and describe the care of the infant with each.

3 Describe the nursing care of the infant following the surgical repair of a cleft lip.

4 List the two types of hydrocephalus and describe the differences between them.

5 List four common types of congenital heart disease and discuss the treatment for each.

6 Discuss the psychosocial needs of the hospitalized newborn and measures the nurse can take to help meet them.

Like other high-risk infants, the newborn with a defect creates a crisis for parents and caregivers. Depending on the nature of the defect, immediate or early surgery may be necessary. Rehabilitation of the infant and education of the parents in caring for him are essential, as are continuous observation and skilled nursing care. Attention to the infant's complex physical needs should not overlook his emotional needs for human contact and comforting.

Increased medical knowledge and advances in surgical techniques have improved the prognosis for many of these infants. Their ultimate well-being and their acceptance into the family, however, may well depend upon the quality of nursing care received during the first few days or weeks of life.

Whether their infant's defect is a result of injury at birth, or of abnormal intrauterine development, parents experience a grief response. They mourn the loss of the perfect child of their dreams; question why it happened; and wonder how they will show the infant to family and friends without shame or embarrassment. This grief is likely to interfere with parent–infant attachment. Parents need to understand that their response is normal, and that they are entitled to honest answers for their questions about the infant's condition. If there are other children in the family, parents must be careful to devote sufficient time and attention to these children to avoid jealousy toward the infant.

birth trauma

INTRACRANIAL HEMORRHAGE

Intracranial hemorrhage usually results from trauma during birth, and is particularly likely in difficult deliveries where the head is large in proportion to the size of the pelvic outlet (cephalopelvic disproportion). It is associated with precipitate delivery (rapid or sudden labor lasting less than 3 hours) or difficult breech delivery, because gradual molding of the head does not take place. Prolonged, hard

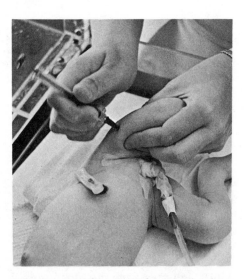

FIG. 4–1. An intramuscular injection into the anterolateral aspect of the thigh.

labors can also cause intracranial hemorrhage, and skilled, judicious use of forceps or a vacuum extractor may decrease the incidence of brain damage. Premature infants are at greater risk for this injury because of fragile intracranial vessel walls.

CLINICAL MANIFESTATIONS

The newborn may be difficult to arouse, the Moro reflex diminished or absent. Irregular and slow respirations, apnea, cyanosis, failure to suck well, high-pitched shrill cry, muscular twitchings, and convulsions are all symptomatic. Signs of mild hemorrhage may be limited to listlessness, poor appetite, and occasional vomiting. Diagnosis is based mainly on history of delivery and the clinical signs.

CARE

The infant should be handled gently and disturbed as little as possible. He should be placed in an incubator where temperature and oxygen can be regulated. Often the infant is positioned in a slightly reverse Trendelenburg position to reduce intracranial pressure and to aid lung expansion. Continuous observation is essential; therefore, he is best cared for in the intensive care nursery. An anticonvulsive drug, such as phenobarbital, may be ordered, and vitamin K may be given to minimize bleeding (Fig. 4–1). Sometimes cranial pressure is relieved by spinal or dural taps.

OUTCOME

The infant's future depends largely upon the severity of the condition. Death from respiratory failure may result within the first 3 days. Surviving infants may recover completely or may suffer cerebral palsy or mental retardation.

FRACTURES

The most common birth injury is fracture of the clavicle or collar bone. This injury occurs most often in breech or other difficult deliveries, particularly with large infants.

Clinical Manifestations. Though frequently undiagnosed at birth, fracture of the clavicle may be apparent at delivery. An audible click or snap, limited movement, and an absent Moro reflex on the affected side are signs of a fractured clavicle.

Care. When prescribed, treatment is immobilization of the shoulder and arm on the affected side, usually by means of a figure-of-eight bandage. Often nothing is prescribed other than proper body alignment and careful support of the affected side when handling the infant. Parents may be afraid of hurting these infants and must be taught how to handle them correctly in order to overcome this fear and avoid interruption of parent–infant attachment. Generally the fracture heals without complication.

FACIAL PALSY

Misapplication of forceps or prolonged compression in the birth canal can create damaging pressure on the facial nerve, resulting in temporary paralysis.

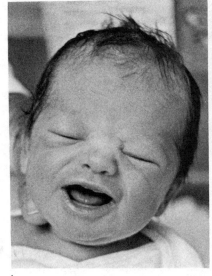 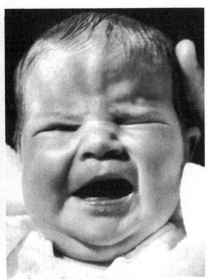

FIG. 4–2. (A) Normally the infant has a symmetrical facial expression and is able to close both eyes tightly. (B) Injury to the facial nerve produces paralysis on the affected side. (A photo by Marcia Lieberman; A, B from Waechter EH, Blake FG: Nursing Care of Children, 9th ed. Philadelphia, JB Lippincott, 1976)

A   B

Clinical Manifestations. Though temporary, facial palsy produces a rather grotesque expression on the infant, and is most apparent when he cries. The affected side of the face remains flattened, the forehead does not wrinkle, the eye remains partially open, and the mouth may droop at one corner (Fig. 4–2).

Care. Parents need reassurance that this condition is rarely permanent and recovery is usually complete within a few weeks. Particular care must be used during feeding, because of the infant's inability to close the mouth completely around the nipple. Breastfeeding is possible if the mother can aid the infant in holding onto and compressing the areola. If the infant is formula-fed, a soft rubber nipple with a large hole can be useful. Gavage feeding may be necessary to avoid aspiration.

Care must include protection of the eye that does not close completely. Daily instillation of artificial tears may be required to prevent drying of the cornea, conjunctiva, and sclera. Parents should be taught this procedure in case it is necessary after the infant goes home.

BRACHIAL PALSY

Also called *Erb's palsy* or *Erb-Duchenne paralysis,* this is a partial paralysis of one arm owing to excessive stretching of the nerve fibers that run from the neck through the shoulder. It occurs when traction is exerted on the head during delivery of the shoulder. It is seen more frequently with breech delivery but may result from a difficult vertex delivery.

Clinical Manifestations. The affected arm hangs limp, with the elbow extended, and the hand rotated inward (Fig. 4–3). Though the grasp reflex is present, the Moro reflex is weak and the deep tendon reflex absent.

Care. The main elements of treatment are peripheral immobilization, proper body alignment, and exercise to maintain joint range of motion and prevent contractures. Exercises are usually delayed until about the tenth day to prevent additional injury to the brachial plexus.

Outcome. In mild cases, spontaneous recovery occurs within a few weeks. Where injury to the nerve fibers is more severe, permanent damage may result. If recovery does not occur, neurosurgery may offer partial recovery.

PHRENIC NERVE INJURY (DIAPHRAGMATIC PALSY)

The phrenic nerve is the only one that activates the diaphragm and injury to it results in respiratory distress that, left untreated, causes pneumonia and death. Phrenic nerve injury is often associated with brachial palsy.

Clinical Manifestations. Irregular thoracic respirations with lack of abdominal movement on the affected side and cyanosis are characteristic of phrenic nerve palsy. The diagnosis can be confirmed by roentgenogram.

Care. Nursing care of the infant with phrenic nerve injury is directed at maintaining sufficient oxygen and nutrients (by the route most suitable for the infant—intravenous, gavage, nipple). Complete recovery usually occurs within 6 weeks to 1 year. Occasionally surgery is necessary to tighten and lower the diaphragm.

congenital anomalies

FACIAL DEFORMITIES

or hair lip

CLEFT LIP AND PALATE

The most common facial malformation, cleft lip and palate, occurs in about 1 in 1000 live births in whites; twice that in Japanese, less than half as many in American blacks.[1] Its cause is not entirely clear; it appears to be

Cleft lip is an opening of upper lip.

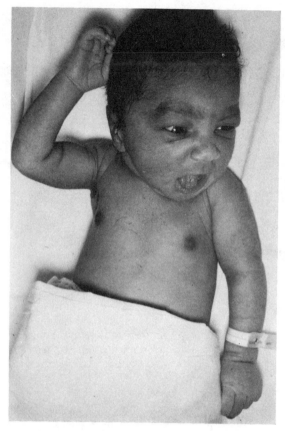

FIG. 4–3. Brachial-plexus injury. Note the position of the left arm, which is held close to the body and rotated inward. (Photo by Dr. R Platou; Waechter EH, Blake FG: Nursing Care of Children, 9th ed. Philadelphia, JB Lippincott, 1976).

other specialists, including a pediatrician, nurses, orthodontist, prosthodontist, otolaryngologist, speech therapist, and, occasionally, a psychiatrist. Even after long-term treatment, the child will likely have some defect in speech, facial appearance, or other problem related to the condition.

Plastic surgeons' opinions differ as to the best time for repair. Some are in favor of early repair, before the infant goes home; others prefer to wait until the infant is 1 or 2 months old.

If early surgery is contemplated, the baby should be healthy, of average or above average weight, and must be placed where he can be—and is—observed constantly. A newborn child has greater difficulty dealing with excess mucus than does an older infant. Good results are obtained when these infants are in the hands of competent plastic surgeons and experienced nurses.

Cheiloplasty cheiloplasty – lip repair

Nursing Care. There is little preoperative preparation for the infant who has surgery during the first few days of life. It would be well to accustom the older infant to elbow restraints, for he has to wear them for several days following surgery. It is also helpful if the nurse learns to feed the infant with an Asepto syringe. This special skill is difficult to acquire without practice.

Immediate postoperative care. Continuous, intelligent observation is essential. Swollen mouth tissues cause an excessive secretion of mucus that is poorly handled by a small infant. For the first few hours, he must *never* be left alone because he can quickly and easily aspirate the mucus. Cleanse c̄ sterile H₂O.

genetically influenced, but does occur in isolated instances.

This defect results from failure of the maxillary and premaxillary processes to fuse during the fifth to eighth week of intrauterine life. The cleft may be a simple notch in the vermilion line, or it may extend up into the floor of the nose (Fig. 4– 4). It may be either unilateral (one side of the lip) or bilateral (both sides). Cleft palate most often occurs with bilateral cleft lip. This defect is often accompanied by nasal deformity and dental disorders (deformed, missing, or supernumerary teeth).

Parents are naturally eager to see and hold their newborn infant, and must be prepared for the shock of seeing the disfigurement of a cleft lip. Their emotional reaction to such an obvious malformation is usually much greater than to a "hidden" defect such as congenital heart disease. They need encouragement and support as well as considerable instruction about the feeding and care of this infant until the defect can be repaired. More common in males.

Medical Treatment. Surgery, usually performed by a plastic surgeon, is a major part of the treatment of a child with a cleft lip and/or palate. Total care can involve many

palatoplasty – palate may need dental prosthesis,

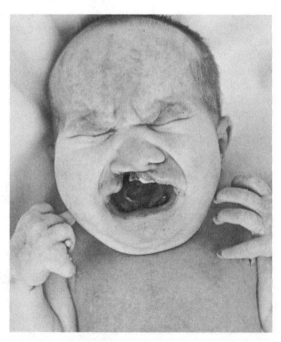

FIG. 4–4. Unilateral cleft lip extending into the floor of the nose.

Elbow restraints. A sore mouth calls for a comforting thumb, and this can quickly undo the difficult and costly repair. On this occasion the child's ultimate happiness and well-being must take precedence over his immediate satisfaction. Therefore, elbow restraints must be properly applied and checked frequently. Made with canvas and tongue blades, these are tied firmly around the arm, and pinned to the infant's shirt or gown to prevent them from sliding down below the elbow. The child can move his arm, but cannot bend his elbow to reach his face. The restraints must be applied snugly, but not allowed to hinder circulation.

Restraints need to be removed frequently, one at a time, controlling movements of the child's arm. A sufficient supply should be kept on hand to change soiled restraints.

The baby suffers emotional frustration because of the restraints, so satisfaction must be provided in other ways. He needs rocking and cuddling as any baby does, and probably more. Mother is the best person to supply this loving care, and no doubt the most willing. Nurses come next.

Care of suture line. The suture line is left uncovered after surgery and must be kept clean and dry to prevent infection with subsequent scarring. In many hospitals, a wire bow—called a Logan bar—is applied across the upper lip and attached to the cheeks with adhesive tape to prevent tension on the sutures (Fig. 4–5).

The sutures are carefully cleaned as often as necessary to prevent collection of dried serum. Frequent cleaning is essential for the first 2 or 3 days, as well as after every feeding as long as the sutures are in.

A *tray* containing the articles needed for suture care is kept at the bedside and changed daily. It should contain a covered jar of sterile cotton-tipped applicators, a sterile

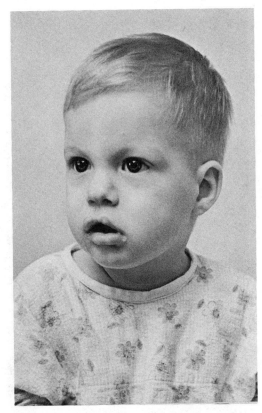

FIG. 4–6.   **This child has returned for slight revision of cleft lip repair.**

container of solution for cleansing and a paper bag for waste. Solutions used are commonly hydrogen peroxide, sterile saline, or water.

With clean hands, dip an applicator into the solution and gently clean each suture with a rolling motion. The sutures inside the lip also need cleaning. Application of an ointment after cleansing may be ordered.

The sutures are removed 7 to 10 days after surgery. The infant will probably be allowed to suck on a soft nipple at this time. Following effective surgery and intelligent, careful nursing care, the appearance of baby's face should be greatly improved.

The scar fades as time goes by. Parents need to know that the baby is probably going to need a slight adjustment of the vermilion line in later childhood. With today's surgery, they can expect that the child will not have the unsightly, thickened tissue seen in earlier days (Figs. 4–6 and 4–7).

Some infants who have a cleft lip also have a cleft palate. In such instances, the lip is repaired as described, but the palate repair is delayed until later.

Technique for feeding. Parents should be told that this baby can be fed and treated as any other. The baby is able to suck after the lip repair and should progress normally until ready for palate surgery. Some milk may seep through the cleft palate and out through the nose, but

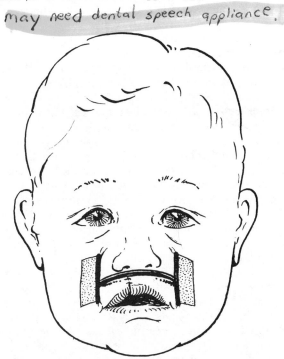

may need dental speech appliance.

FIG. 4–5.   Logan bar for easing strain on sutures.

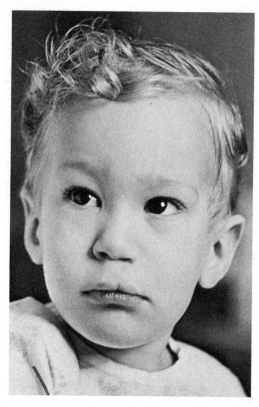

FIG. 4–7. This child may need a revision of the vermilion line.

most babies learn to handle this without too much difficulty.

Have ready a sterile Asepto syringe with the tip protected by a piece of sterile rubber tubing about 1 inch long. Plastic tubing is unsatisfactory as it may slide off and lodge in the infant's throat.

Place the syringe and warmed formula on the bedside stand within easy reach. Hold the infant in your arms in an upright position. Pour the formula into the syringe and place the rubber-covered tip in the child's mouth, away from the suture line. The formula usually drips quickly enough without squeezing the bulb. The nurse must regulate the drops to the infant's breathing and swallowing, something she and the baby soon learn. The baby swallows considerable amounts of air and needs burping frequently. About 30 minutes should be allowed for a feeding.

The baby is much safer when placed in his crib after his feeding if he is positioned on his side, in order to prevent aspiration if he vomits or regurgitates. If he cannot be satisfactorily restrained in this position but must instead be placed on his back, his head should be kept elevated and the child watched carefully.

DIGESTIVE TRACT DEFECTS

ESOPHAGEAL ATRESIA

Atresia is the absence of a normal body opening or the abnormal closure of a body passage. *Esophageal atresia,*

with or without fistula into the trachea, is a serious congenital anomaly, and among the most common anomalies causing respiratory distress. This condition occurs in about one in 2500 live births.

Though there are several types of esophageal atresia, more than 90% of them consist of the upper or proximal end of the esophagus ending in a blind pouch, with the lower, or distal segment from the stomach connected to the trachea by a fistulous tract (Fig. 4– 8).

Diagnosis. If the possible presence of this condition is recognized, diagnosis is not difficult. A rubber catheter passed through the infant's nose is blocked at the site of the atresia, and x-ray film shows the catheter coiled upon itself in the blind pouch.

Clinical Manifestations. Any mucus or fluid that an infant swallows goes into the blind pouch of the esophagus. This pouch soon fills and overflows, usually resulting in aspiration into the trachea.

Nursing Care. Few other conditions depend so greatly on careful nursing observation for early diagnosis, and therefore, improved chances of survival. The infant with this disorder has frothing and excessive drooling, periods of respiratory distress with choking and cyanosis. Many newborns have difficulty with mucus, but the nurse should be alert to the possibility of an anomaly and immediately report such difficulties to a supervisory person. The nurse should take responsibility for delaying the first feeding until the infant has been examined for the presence of this condition.

If early signs are overlooked, and feeding is attempted, the baby chokes, coughs, and regurgitates as the food enters the blind pouch. He becomes deeply cyanotic and appears to be in severe respiratory distress. During this process, he aspirates some of the formula with resultant pneumonitis, making necessary surgery an increased hazard to the child. In a very real sense, this infant's life may depend on the careful observation of the nurse.

Preoperative care. The infant needs to be placed in an incubator where highly saturated air, constant temperature, and oxygen are available. He should be positioned with head and chest elevated 30° to prevent reflux of gastric juice into the lung. A nurse should be in constant attendance. Frequent intermittent nasopharyngeal suction—as often as every 10 to 15 minutes—is needed to remove secretions. Care must be used to avoid injury to the blind pouch. Intravenous fluids are given by slow drip. Broad-spectrum antibiotics are used if pneumonitis or aspiration pneumonia is present.

Surgery may be delayed until the infant's condition is improved, and here again, the nurse must be constantly aware of his condition. She must watch for changes in color, temperature, pulse, and state of activity, keeping in mind the ever present danger of pneumonia or pneumonitis. The child must be turned frequently.

Not the least of the nurse's duties is to give adequate attention to the infant's family. It must be remembered

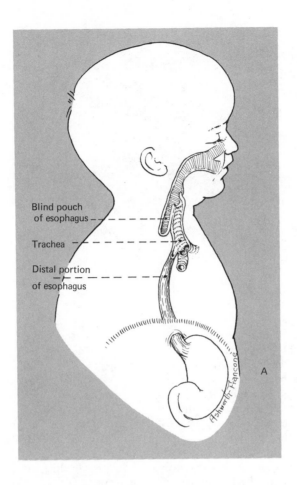

Blind pouch
of esophagus

Trachea

Distal portion
of esophagus

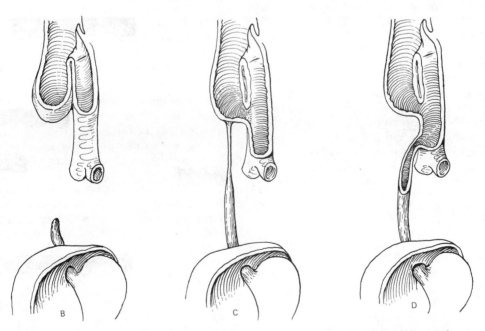

FIG. 4–8. (A) The most common form of esophageal atresia. (B) Both segments of the esophagus
are blind pouches. (C) Esophagus is continuous, but with narrowed segment. (D) Upper segment of
esophagus opens into trachea.

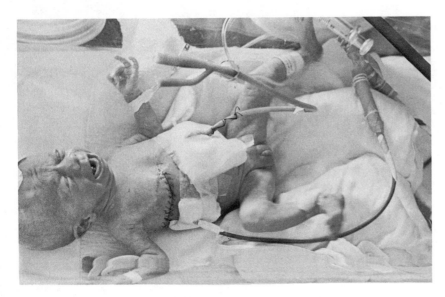

FIG. 4–9. Repair of tracheal esophageal atresia and fistula showing chest incision and drainage tube. Gastrostomy tube is also in place.

that this is a newborn infant who has never been home. Perhaps he is also premature, increasing the family's anxiety. Frequently, the infant has been removed from the place of his birth and taken to a center where more skilled care is available. This means that the mother does not get to see her child, and must rely on reports from her husband or from other members of the family.

It does not help the family for the nurse to say, "The baby is doing as well as can be expected." They certainly hope he is doing a little *better* than the picture allows them to expect. However, the nurse must guard against giving a false impression of well-being and optimism. A brush-off of, "You will have to ask the doctor" is not well accepted either. If the nurse does not know what is going on, or is not interested, the child is indeed in a sorry plight!

Time must be taken to listen to the family, and to give honest answers. The nurse refers them to the doctor as necessary, but she can give much supporting care herself. She can explain the various types of equipment, thus removing their mystery. She can explain the defect and its repair in simple, nonmedical terms. She can show a warm, human interest in the mother's progress and well-being. Above all, she does not show a feeling of irritation or hurriedness, but by her manner, convinces the family that their feelings and concerns are important.

Postoperative care.   While the infant is still in surgery, his nurse prepares for his return. The incubator must be clean, warm, and functioning properly. Ample supplies must be readied so there will be no interruption in her careful, constant observation when the infant returns.

Ordinarily complete chest expansion occurs in a few hours. The gastrostomy tube is sutured to the skin following surgery (Fig. 4–9). The dressing around the tube must be kept clean and changed as needed. An extra strip of adhesive around the tube at the site of insertion and attached to the skin will help prevent displacement of the tube. Following surgery, treatment is resumed much as

before. The child is placed in the warm, humidified incubator and kept free from excessive mucus by suctioning.

Feedings by gastrostomy tube are usually started on the second or third day. For this the nurse needs a sterile funnel or syringe barrel and a clamp. The funnel or syringe barrel is attached to the gastrostomy tube, and the solution placed in the funnel before the tube is unclamped. It is allowed to run in slowly, and the tube is again clamped when the feeding has reached the lower edge of the funnel or syringe barrel to avoid introduction of air.

For the first 2 or 3 days, glucose and water are used. In some hospitals, gastrostomy feedings are given by slow drip, using a special drip apparatus. After the physician is satisfied that the fluid is being well tolerated, warm formula is given according to the physician's directions.

Psychological needs.   The infant has psychological needs, one of which is the need to suck. Following an anastomosis, he can be given a sterile nipple stuffed with cotton or a pacifier to suck when he receives his gastrostomy feedings. After the feeding, he needs to be held and cuddled.

The infant who has not yet had an anastomosis cannot be permitted to suck, thus he has an even greater need for physical contact and warm acceptance. These infants continue to need gastrostomy feedings until further surgery.

Most of these infants, however, have had an anastomosis, and are ready for oral feedings after 8 to 10 days. A small-holed nipple should be used, and feedings given very slowly. Stenosis (narrowing of the passage) at the site of the anastomosis is not uncommon, so the nurse must be particularly watchful for choking or difficult swallowing.

When the mother is able, she should be encouraged to spend some time observing and helping with the care of her baby. She needs practice in the routine care of her newborn infant as well as in special procedures. She needs to develop confidence in bathing, weighing, and dressing a small infant.

Gastrostomy feeding. The mother should also learn how to give gastrostomy feedings. It is hoped that she will not have to give them, but many babies develop strictures at the site of the anastomosis, requiring temporary use of the gastrostomy tube for feeding. The wound itself should be well healed at the time of baby's discharge and require no special care or any dressing, so that baby can be put in the tube for bathing.

The mother also needs to practice oral feeding, and to learn what symptoms indicate impending trouble, such as a stenosis at the site of anastomosis. She should be told to call her doctor or the hospital resident if the baby chokes or regurgitates, and to stop feeding until the baby has been examined. With all of this, she must not be made too apprehensive.

The gastrostomy tube may be left in place for several months until the surgeon is satisfied that all need for its use is past. Frequently, several dilatations of the esophagus are necessary during the months following surgery.

Prognosis. is somewhat guarded, much depending on the infant's condition at time of surgery. Early diagnosis, especially before feedings are attempted, is an important factor in the infant's survival. For many infants, the condition is complicated by prematurity and by other congenital anomalies. However, through careful management, together with devoted nursing care, the mortality rate has been greatly reduced from the former prediction of "hopeless," and a normal life is now possible for many.

IMPERFORATE ANUS

In this condition, the rectal pouch ends blindly at a distance above the anus, and there is no anal orifice. There may be a fistula between the rectum and the vagina in females or between the rectum and the urinary tract in males.

Early in intrauterine life the membrane between the rectum and the anus should be absorbed, and a clear passage made from rectum to anus. If the membrane remains, blocking union between rectum and anus, an *imperforate anus* results.

Diagnosis. In some newborn infants, only a dimple indicates the site of the anus (Fig. 4–10A). When a rectal temperature is attempted, it is apparent that there is no anal opening. However, there may be a shallow opening in the anus, with the rectum ending in a blind pouch some distance higher (Figure 4–10B). For this reason it is imperative to understand that the ability to pass a rectal thermometer into the rectum is not a reliable indication of a normal rectal–anal canal. In fact, some newborn nursery personnel take axillary temperatures on infants from birth.

More reliable presumptive evidence is obtained by watching carefully for the first meconium stool. If the infant does not pass a stool within the first 24 hours, this should be reported to the physician. Abdominal distention also occurs. Definitive diagnosis is made by x-ray studies.

Surgical treatment. If the rectal pouch is separated from the anus by only a thin membrane, the surgeon can repair the defect from below. When a high defect is present, abdominal-perineal resection is indicated. In these infants a colostomy is performed, and extensive abdominal–perineal resection is delayed until the age of 3 to 5 months, or later. *Anoplasty*

Home Care. When the infant goes home with a colostomy, the parents will need to learn how to give colostomy care. The mother should be taught to keep the area around the colostomy clean with soap and water, and to diaper the baby in the usual way. Zinc oxide ointment is useful for protection of the skin around the colostomy.

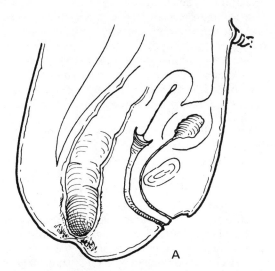 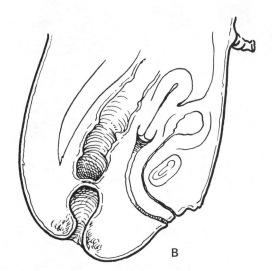

FIG. 4–10.   Imperforate anus (anal atresia). (*A*) Membrane between anus and rectum. (*B*) Rectum ending in a blind pouch at a distance above the perineum.

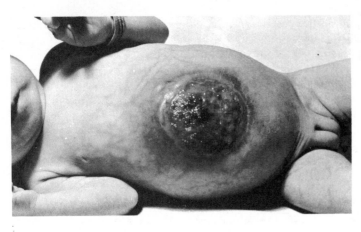

FIG. 4–11.   Omphalocele. (Waechter EH, Blake FG: Nursing Care of Children, 9th ed. Philadelphia, JB Lippincott, 1976)

HERNIAS

Diaphragmatic Hernia.   In this condition, some of the abdominal organs are displaced into the left chest through an opening in the diaphragm. The heart is pushed toward the right, and the left lung is compressed. Rapid, labored respirations and cyanosis are present on the first day of life, and breathing becomes increasingly difficult.

Surgery is essential and may be performed as an emergency procedure. During surgery the abdominal viscera are withdrawn from the chest, and the diaphragmatic defect is closed.

This defect may be minimal and easily repaired or so extensive that pulmonary tissue has failed to develop normally. The outcome of surgical repair depends on the degree of pulmonary development, and prognosis in severe cases is guarded.

Hiatal Hernia.   More common in adults than in newborns, this condition is caused when the cardiac portion of the stomach slides through the normal esophageal hiatus into the area above the diaphragm. This causes reflux of gastric contents into the esophagus and subsequent regurgitation. If upright posture and modified feeding techniques do not successfully correct the problem, surgery is necessary to repair the defect.

Omphalocele.   This is a rare anomaly existing at birth. Some of the abdominal contents protrude through into the root of the umbilical cord and form a sac lying on the abdomen (Fig. 4–11). This sac may be large and contain much of the intestines and the liver. The sac is covered with peritoneal membrane instead of skin. Surgical replacement of the organs into the abdomen may be difficult with a large omphalocele, as there may not be enough space in the abdominal cavity. Other congenital defects are present in many instances.

With large omphaloceles, surgery may be postponed and the surgeon will suture skin over the defect, creating a large hernia. The abdomen may enlarge enough as the child grows older so that replacement can be done.

Umbilical Hernia.   Normally the ring that encircled the fetal end of the umbilical cord closes gradually and spontaneously after birth. When this closure is incomplete, portions of omemtum and intestine protrude through the opening. More common in preterm and black infants, umbilical hernia is largely a cosmetic problem, which is upsetting to parents but with little or no morbidity (Fig. 4–12). In rare cases, the bowel can strangulate in the sac, requiring immediate surgery. Almost all of these hernias close spontaneously by age three. Those that do not should be surgically corrected before the child enters school.

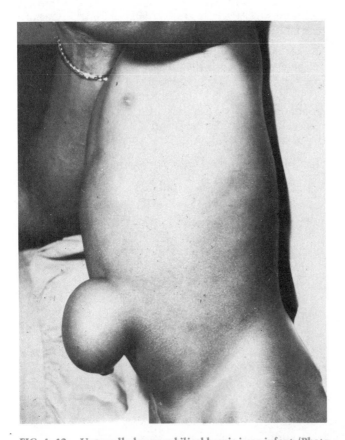

FIG. 4–12.   Unusually large umbilical hernia in an infant. (Photo courtesy of Dr. Mark Ravitch; Waechter EH, Blake FG: Nursing Care of Children, 9th ed. Philadelphia, JB Lippincott, 1976)

Inguinal Hernia. More common in males, inguinal hernias occur when the small sac of peritoneum surrounding the testes fails to close off after the testes descend from the abdominal sac into the scrotum. This allows intestine to slip into the inguinal canal, with resultant swelling. If the intestine becomes trapped (incarcerated) and the circulation to the trapped intestine is impaired (strangulated), surgery is necessary to prevent intestinal obstruction and gangrene of the bowel. As a preventive measure, inguinal hernias normally are repaired as soon as diagnosed.

CENTRAL NERVOUS SYSTEM DEFECTS

SPINA BIFIDA

Caused by a defect in the neural arch, generally in the lumbosacral region, *spina bifida* is a failure of the posterior laminae of the vertebrae to close, leaving an opening through which the spinal meninges and spinal cord may protrude.

Clinical Manifestations. The occurrence of a bony defect without soft tissue involvement is called *spina bifida occulta.* In most cases it is asymptomatic and presents no problems. A dimple in the skin or a tuft of hair over the site may cause one to suspect its presence or it may be entirely overlooked.

When a portion of the spinal meninges protrudes through the bony defect and forms a cystic sac, the condition is termed *spina bifida with meningocele.* No nerve roots are involved; therefore, no paralysis or sensory loss below the lesion appears. The sac may, however, rupture or perforate, thus introducing infection into the spinal fluid and causing meningitis. For this reason, as well as for cosmetic purposes, surgical removal of the sac, with closure of the skin, is indicated.

Spina bifida with myelomeningocele signifies a protrusion of the spinal cord and the meninges, with nerve roots embedded in the wall of the cyst (Fig. 4–13). The effects of this defect vary in severity from sensory loss or partial paralysis below the lesion, to complete flaccid paralysis of all muscles below the lesion. Complete paralysis involves the lower trunk and legs as well as bowel and bladder sphincters. It is not always possible however to make a clear-cut differentiation in diagnosis between a meningocele and a myelomeningocele on the basis of symptoms alone.

The condition myelomeningocele may also be termed *meningomyelocele.* The associated spina bifida is always implied, but not necessarily named. *Spina bifida cystica* is the term used to designate either of these protrusions.

Outcome. It is difficult to predict the future for these infants. Many of those with hydrocephalus and myelomeningocele appear to have a hopeless prognosis at birth. Many who do survive in spite of severe handicaps, succumb to infection during early life. Some, however, live through the hazardous early years. These children, with skillful help and favorable circumstances, may be able to achieve useful, satisfactory lives.

The majority of neurosurgeons and orthopedists prefer

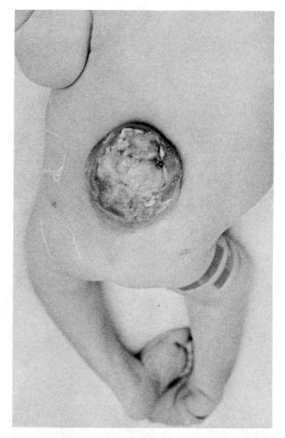

FIG. 4–13. A myelomeningocele showing an additional defect of clubfeet.

to give the child every possible assistance, even if the prospect does not appear particularly favorable. Shunting devices and repair of spinal defects are instituted early. If satisfactory results have been attained, orthopedic procedures should be carried out in anticipation of the possibility of future ambulation. These may include casting for talipes equinovarus and hip dysplasia, as well as intensive physical therapy to prevent progression of deformities.

As the child grows older, he can progress from a stroller to a wheelchair, with the prospect for many of learning to walk with the help of braces and crutches. Increasingly, as medical knowledge advances, more such handicapped children are helped to a relatively normal way of life.

The courage and persistence demanded from these children and their parents is nearly more than the unaffected person can grasp. They deserve a great deal of emotional support and encouragement. Considerable physical and financial help is necessary for most families.

The child who does achieve ambulation through use of braces and crutches, and is able to take his place as a well adjusted member of society, rewards all those who gave so much time, effort and unending patience. The child in Figure 4–14 is such an example. A myelomeningocele was successfully repaired in infancy. He learned to walk with crutches and braces; at the age of five he re-entered the hospital for new braces, an Achilles tenotomy, and

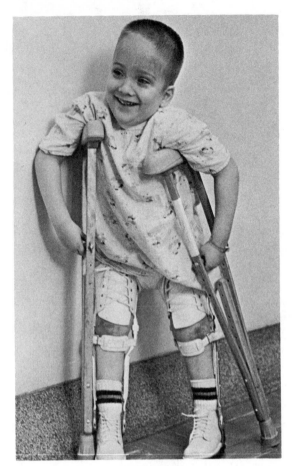

FIG. 4–14. Learning to use new braces, this boy underwent successful surgery for repair of a myelomeningocele during infancy.

urinary tract evaluation. He was a friendly, outgoing child with a sunny disposition, a lively imagination and quick mental ability. The picture shows him ready to leave the hospital with his new braces. Giving such a child hope for a relatively normal life seems well worth the effort put forth by so many—not the least of whom was the child himself.

Surgical Treatment. Surgical repair of a myelomeningocele cannot be expected to decrease the neurological disability, although many surgeons believe that future function is improved to some extent in those carefully repaired. It has been observed that some newborn infants show a limited motor ability that rapidly decreases after birth. Many neurosurgeons advocate immediate repair.

A leaking sac calls for immediate repair to prevent meningitis. Some infants with a thin membrane over the sac, through which spinal fluid is leaking, show signs of meningitis at birth.

The primary objective of surgical repair is closure of the defect, with replacement of neural elements within the vertebral canal whenever possible. Nerve roots that can be freed are replaced in the canal, the sac amputated at its base or turned inward, and plastic surgery employed for covering the site of the defect.

Nursing care. In some hospitals the baby is placed on a Bradford frame to facilitate handling. The canvas frame must be covered with soft sheets to prevent skin irritation, and the edges of the open section below the perineal region protected with sheets of plastic that drape down into the receptacle placed on the bed below the frame.

The child is positioned on his abdomen with flannel restraints to hold him in place. A rolled towel under his ankles or a rolled blanket under his legs is needed to prevent pressure on his toes. It is possible to position a small infant on his side while on a Bradford frame, with the use of a rolled blanket against his back above the lesion, and restraints to hold him in place.

Nurses and parents are encouraged to hold the child at intervals, particularly for feedings. Of course he must be held in such a manner as to avoid pressure on the sac, but the child can be fitted comfortably into one's arm. Parents may be frightened and need encouragement as well as help in correctly positioning the child.

Preoperative care. The infant with a spinal lesion cannot be allowed to lie on his back, but must be positioned on his side or abdomen. His position must be frequently changed.

It is most important that the sac be kept clean and dry, with all pressure avoided. Any leakage of spinal fluid must be reported immediately. Avoidance of contamination from urine or fecal material is of particular importance. A sheet of plastic may be taped between the defect and the anus, and folded back on itself to form a barrier, and taped into place. If the sac covering is thin, a sterile dressing, either dry or medicated, may be ordered to be placed over it.

Perhaps the greatest nursing challenge is in keeping the perineum clean and in preventing excoriation when paralysis of the sphincter muscles is present, because the lack of sphincter control results in constant dribbling of urine and feces. Because the infant cannot be placed on his back, fecal material runs down over the perineum. The constant dribbling of urine and feces causes severe skin irritation. To help prevent excoriation, scrupulous cleanliness must be maintained. The perineum should be cleansed frequently with an unmedicated oil and left exposed to the air at all times.

Postoperative care. Following repair of a meningocele or myelomeningocele, the infant is placed in a prone or knee-chest position and not moved unnecessarily until the operative site is completely healed. This means that all procedures must be carried out with the infant in this position, including feeding and bathing.

Usual postoperative observations are followed. Perineal care must be continued, and special precautions for keeping the operative site clean and dry strictly observed. When feedings are begun, the nurse turns the baby's head to one side and holds the bottle, at the same time keeping the baby in the prone position. The surgeon decides when he can be moved or turned.

Continuing care. A number of methods have been devised to achieve urinary continence for the child, none of which has proved to be entirely satisfactory. A very few children have achieved successful control after long-term, rigorous training. Control of fluid intake, with strict regularity of mechanical bladder emptying by the Credé method, combined with unlimited patience, has produced good results. Few parents or children are able to carry out these long-term programs. Even if control is achieved in this manner, the bladder may not be completely emptied.

Indwelling catheters may be useful for short periods, especially when an infection is being treated. Transplant of the ureters into the sigmoid is a procedure that has been widely used, but the ascending infection that usually results has been discouraging.

The most encouraging procedure employed at present is an ileal loop, or cutaneous ileoureterostomy. A small segment of the ileum is isolated, its distal end closed, and the proximal end brought to the skin surface of the abdomen. The remaining bowel is anastomosed for continuity of function. The ends of the ureters are inserted into the sides of the ileal segment, which then acts as a conduit for the urine to the surface of the body. An ileostomy bag fitted over the stoma receives the urine. The parents and child need careful instruction and practice in learning to apply the bag correctly to prevent leakage.

Bowel control is not so difficult to achieve. A slightly constipating diet may be necessary at first. The parent places the child on the toilet at the time he usually has a bowel movement, perhaps using a suppository until habit is established. Accidents may happen at first, but intelligent regulation is usually effective.

Associated Conditions. Hydrocephalus of the obstructive type is frequently associated with these two defects.

Bypass procedures may arrest the hydrocephaly, but cannot affect or restore the neural function involved in a myelomeningocele. It was formerly thought that surgical repair of the spinal defect would frequently cause hydrocephaly not previously present, and parents were so advised. This has not been proved, however. The concept accepted by many neurosurgeons today is that hydrocephaly is already present, the surgical repair of the sac accelerating its development. Other defects are frequently present, the most common being talipes equinovarus. Hip dysplasia may also be present.

HYDROCEPHALUS

Hydrocephalus is a condition characterized by an excess of cerebrospinal fluid witin the ventricular and subarachnoid spaces of the cranial cavity. Normally there is a delicate balance between the rate of formation and the absorption of cerebrospinal fluid. The entire volume is absorbed and replaced every 12 to 24 hours. In hydrocephalus this balance is disturbed.

Cerebrospinal fluid is formed by the choroid plexus, mainly in the lateral ventricles. It is absorbed into the venous system through the arachnoid villi. Cerebrospinal fluid circulates within the ventricles and the subarachnoid space. It is a colorless fluid, consisting of water with traces of protein, glucose and lymphocytes.

The *noncommunicating* type of congenital hydrocephalus occurs when there is an obstruction in the free circulation of cerebrospinal fluid. This blockage causes increased pressure on the brain or spinal cord. The site of obstruction may be at the foramen of Monro, the aqueduct of Sylvius, the foramen of Lushka, or the foramen of Magendie (Fig. 4–15).

In the *communicating* type of hydrocephalus, there is no obstruction of the free flow of cerebrospinal fluid between the ventricles and the spinal theca. The condition is caused by defective absorption of the cerebrospinal fluid, this causing pressure on the brain or spinal cord to build

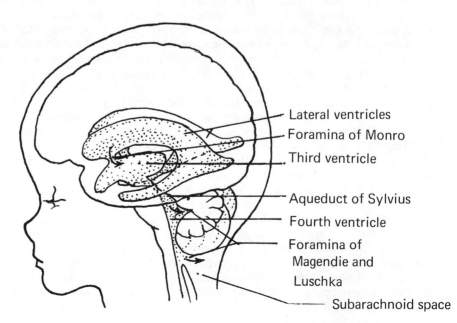

FIG. 4–15. Ventricles of the brain and channels for the normal flow of cerebrospinal fluid. (Courtesy of Dr. AJ Raimondi; Raffensberger J, Primrose R (eds): Pediatric Surgery for Nurses. Boston, Little, Brown, 1968)

Lateral ventricles
Foramina of Monro
Third ventricle
Aqueduct of Sylvius
Fourth ventricle
Foramina of Magendie and Luschka
Subarachnoid space

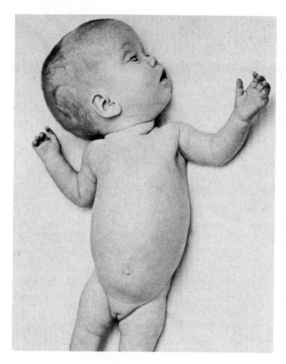

FIG. 4–16. A child with hydrocephalus. Note the pull on the eyes giving the "setting sun" appearance. Note also the site of incision for a ventriculo-auricular shunt.

up. Congenital hydrocephalus is most frequently of the obstructive or noncommunicating type.

Hydrocephalus may be recognized at birth, or it may not be evident until after a few weeks or months of life. Occasionally, the condition may not be congenital, but may instead occur during later infancy or during childhood as the result of a head injury, or an infection such as meningitis.

When hydrocephalus occurs early in life before the skull sutures close, the soft pliable bones separate to allow head expansion. This is manifested by a rapid growth in head circumference. The fact that the soft bones are capable of yielding to pressure in this manner may partially explain why many of these infants fail to show the usual symptoms of brain pressure, and may exhibit little or no damage to mental function until later in life. Other infants show severe brain damage, often occurring before birth.

Clinical Manifestations. An excessively large head at birth is suggestive of hydrocephalus. Rapid head growth with widening cranial sutures is also strongly suggestive. Positive diagnosis is made through the use of pneumoencephalograms and ventriculograms.

A rapidly enlarging head may be the first manifestation of this condition. An apparently large head in itself is not necessarily significant. Normally, every infant's head is measured at birth, and the rate of growth is checked at subsequent examinations. Any infant's head that appears to be abnormally large at birth, or appears to be enlarging, should be measured frequently.

As the head enlarges, the suture lines separate, and the spaces can be felt through the scalp. The anterior fontanel becomes tense and bulging; the skull enlarges in all diameters; the scalp becomes shiny, and its veins dilate. The eyes appear to be pushed downward slightly, with the sclera visible above the iris, giving the so-called "setting sun" sign (Fig. 4–16).

As the condition progresses, the head becomes increasingly heavy, the neck muscles fail to develop sufficiently, and the infant has difficulty raising or turning his head. Unless the hydrocephalus is arrested, the infant becomes increasingly helpless, and symptoms of brain pressure eventually develop. These may include irritability, vomiting, failure to thrive, and arrested development.

Outcome. Prognosis is guarded in all cases. Many affected infants show severe brain damage at birth. Surgical intervention is the only effective means for relieving brain pressure and preventing further damage. Some children who have suffered only minimal brain damage are able to function within a normal mental range. Motor function is usually retarded.

Surgical Treatment. For the majority of cases the only available procedure is a shunting device that bypasses the point of obstruction, draining the excess cerebrospinal fluid into a body cavity. This procedure arrests excessive head growth and prevents further brain damage. Installation of a shunting device is considered to be indicated for any hydrocephalic infant whose condition permits, most surgeons being unwilling to wait for a possible spontaneous arrest.

Shunting procedures. A number of types of surgery have been devised over the years for this condition with varying success. The most successful kind of surgery has consisted of a shunting procedure, using rubber, polyethylene, or silicone tubing to bypass the point of obstruction and to drain the excess into a body cavity.

Among the shunting procedures developed are, ventriculo-ureteral, ventriculo-peritoneal, and ventriculo-atrial shunts. Each has advantages and disadvantages and all are subject to mechanical difficulties such as obstruction, kinking, or separation of the tubing, and to infection, usually staphylococcal, which is the most common complication.

Ventriculo-ureteral shunting drains cerebrospinal fluid from the lateral ventricle into a ureter. This procedure necessitates the removal of one kidney, and requires the addition of measured amounts of salt to the diet, to be continued indefinitely. The amount of salt excreted from the body owing to the loss of cerebrospinal fluid seriously upsets the electrolyte balance, unless it is replaced.

Ventriculo-peritoneal shunting (Fig. 4–17) has become the preferred procedure for treating hydrocephalus since development of silicone catheters in the mid-1960s.[2] Though this procedure is not without potential complications, the rate of serious complications is much lower than with ventriculo-atrial shunting.

Ventriculo-atrial shunting is still an accepted procedure. Because it drains cerebrospinal fluid into the right atrium of the heart, complications are often life-threatening. Frequent revisions are necessary due to children's growth and resultant displacement of the catheter.

Nursing Care. *Postoperative care.* Following a shunting procedure, the infant is kept with his head turned away from the operative site until the incision is healed. If the child is able to turn his head, sandbags may be needed to keep it turned to one side. Vital signs are taken routinely as they would be after any surgical procedure. He should be watched carefully for change of color, excessive irritability or lethargy, and for abnormal vital signs. The fontanel is frequently depressed after shunting; this is to be expected. A suction machine for removal of excessive mucus from the nose and the mouth should be readily available.

The side of the head on which the baby lies should be examined for pressure sores, particularly if the head is large and heavy. Sponge rubber under his head may be useful. Tincture of benzoin applied to irritated places may prevent such breakdown. Any broken area should be reported at once.

The child may receive intravenous fluids immediately following surgery, with oral feedings started when he is able to tolerate them.

Psychosocial aspects of care. Every infant has the need and the right to be picked up and held, cuddled, and comforted. An uncomfortable or painful experience increases the need for emotional support. An infant perceives such support principally through physical contact made in a soothing, loving manner. When a nurse must cause discomfort to a child, such as giving an intramuscular injection, she must immediately follow with emotional support, which is an integral part of treatment. Preferably this support is given by the person who has caused the pain.

The nurse should never feel that she does not have time for emotional care, any more than she would feel that she did not have time to wash her hands or put on sterile gloves when indicated. Occasionally physical reasons prohibit taking a child out of his crib. Then the nurse must convey her concern by her touch and her soothing voice (Fig. 4–18).

The infant needs social interaction, to be talked to, played with, and given the opportunity for activity. Toys appropriate for his physical and mental capacity must be provided. If the child has difficulty moving about his crib, toys must be within his reach and vision, such as a cradle gym tied close enough for him to maneuver its parts. If he cannot turn his head in pursuit of an elusive toy, he will be unnecessarily frustrated.

Unless the infant's nervous system is so impaired that all activity increases his irritability, he needs stimulation as much as any child. If turning an infant from side to side means turning him away from the sight of activity, the crib can be turned around so that he is not facing the wall or unit divider.

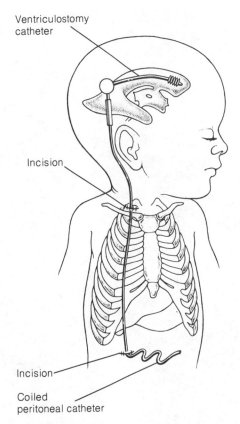

FIG. 4–17. Ventriculo-peritoneal shunt. (Jackson PL: Ventriculo-peritoneal shunts, Am J Nurs 80:1104, 1980)

Attention and stimulation are essential to the well-being of every infant. The infant that lies in his crib day after day, receiving all necessary physical care but no emotional stimulation; is never played with, talked to, or picked up, does not fit the definition of a normal child; is not treated as one; and therefore does not act as one. Because of his limitations, he cannot provide self-stimulation.

An infant with the same handicap who is given all the contact and support that any infant requires, develops a personality because he is nourished by emotional stimulation. The nurse's time for physical care is also a time for social interaction. She talks, laughs, and plays with him, and visits him at times between the necessary occasions for giving physical care.

Comparing the two infants, one would note the personality development and mental alertness of the second child, finding the first child dull and apathetic. Both may have had the same capacity for development, but are products of differing environments, re-emphasizing that nursing care is much more than the meeting of physical needs.

Bathing. Sponge baths may be necessary if the hydrocephalic infant has poor head control. Special care to the areas behind the ears and in the creases of the neck is important. As in everything done for these infants, special

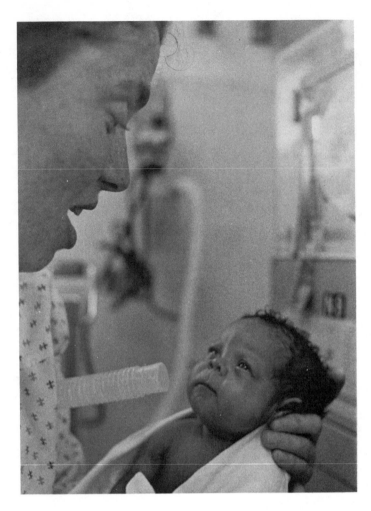

FIG. 4–18. Because they undergo many painful treatments, infants with a defect need to be soothed with a loving touch even more than normal newborns. (Waechter EH, Blake FG: Nursing Care of Children, 9th ed. Philadelphia, JB Lippincott, 1976)

attention can be a means of alleviating some of the inherent frustrations.

Comfortably warm bath water is soothing. Too often, one finds only a few inches of cool or lukewarm water in the bath basin, especially when the nurse has prepared the water before collecting other bath equipment.

A few minutes spent in giving a gentle back rub is likely to be appreciated by an infant who must lie in his crib for long intervals. A soft, gentle voice helps soothe and comfort the infant during the backrub or any other part of the bathing process.

Feeding.   Feeding techniques also assume importance for this child. These babies have a need to be held, if permitted, when they are fed, even more than healthy babies; often this need is not met. The nurse may need to select a chair with an arm on which to rest her elbow while supporting the heavy head. When these children have difficulty holding their heads erect, bubbling them becomes more difficult. Bottle feeding should be given carefully and slowly, with special attention to the absence of air in the nipple. Smaller, more frequent feedings may prove more comfortable for both infant and nurse.

When the baby cannot be held for feeding, there may be a temptation to prop the bottle. However, this is an unacceptable practice in the care of any hospitalized infant.

Head measurement.   The baby's head circumference should be measured daily, or at intervals ordered by the doctor. The tape measure is placed around the largest portion of the child's head, over the forehead, and around the occipital region. In the interest of accuracy, it is better if the same person does the measurement each time, using the same tape measure.

Emotional Support for Parents.   A nurse does not find it difficult to understand the anxiety and apprehension of parents whose child is hydrocephalic, but she may feel quite helpless in trying to give support. Her own acceptance of the child with her tender care and concern for his welfare helps convey her warmth of feeling. Her matter-of-fact acceptance of his handicap, as well as her treatment of him as a baby with normal needs, helps put the situation on a more realistic basis.

Arrangements should be made to give much of the normal, daily care at times when parents can be present. They need to learn how to hold and handle the baby in as normal a manner as possible. Undoubtedly, they need much encouragement. Can they harm him by the way they care for him? Should he be kept quietly by himself to avoid too much stimulation? Many other questions may be asked of the nurse, who has an opportunity to clear up many misunderstandings.

A mother should be encouraged to help with her child's care when there are others present to give her support. She can be encouraged to feel the valve in the shunting device, and to develop an understanding of its function. Both parents need to understand the importance of careful observation for any abnormal developments, and at the same time, attempt to create as normal a life as possible for their child.

CIRCULATORY SYSTEM DEFECTS

CONGENITAL HEART DISEASE

Parents are greatly alarmed when their child is discovered to have a heart abnormality. The heart is *the* vital organ; one can live without a number of other organs and appendages, but life itself depends on the heart. To know that an infant is starting life with an imperfect heart is a matter of great concern. Natural questions are, "How serious is it? Is there a chance that the child can outgrow the condition? Can it be fixed?"

These are difficult questions for a doctor or nurse to try to answer. First, a definite answer may not be known. Second, answers that encourage optimism and hope may give false assurances and encourage unfounded hope. For example, a mother was upset because her child was about to have a cardiac catheterization. She was sure he would not survive this procedure and was not helped at all by the assurance that children don't die from cardiac catheterization. Her child *did* die during the procedure, however. The mother was understandably bitter, and the nurse learned an unforgettable lesson.

A brief discussion of the development and function of the embryonic heart is useful to understanding malformations that occur.

Pathophysiology.   The heart begins beating early in the first month of intrauterine life. When first formed, the heart is a simple tube receiving blood from the placenta and pumping it out into its developing body. During this period it rapidly develops into the normal, but complex, four-chambered heart.

Adjustments in circulation must be made at birth. During fetal life, the lungs are inactive, requiring only a small amount of blood to nourish their tissues. Blood is circulated through the umbilical arteries to the placenta, where waste products and carbon dioxide are exchanged for oxygen and nutrients. The blood is then returned to the fetus through the umbilical vein.

At birth, the umbilical cord is cut, and the infant establishes his own independent system. Certain circulatory bypasses, such as the *ductus arteriosus*, the *foramen ovale*, and the *ductus venosus* are no longer necessary. They close and atrophy after birth, although probably more gradually than had formerly been supposed (Figs. 2–4 and 4–19).

During this period of complex development, any error in formation can cause serious circulatory difficulty. The incidence of cardiovascular malformations is about 6 per 1000 live births.

Etiology.   Rubella in the expectant mother during the first trimester is a common cause of cardiac malformation. Irradiation or ingestion of certain drugs during pregnancy may also be a cause. The drug *thalidomide* has had a high association with congenital heart disease. Maternal malnutrition and heredity are assumed to play a role also.

The newborn with a severe abnormality, such as a transposition of the great vessels, is cyanotic from birth, requiring oxygen and special treatment. A less seriously affected child, whose heart is able to compensate to some degree for the impaired circulation, may not have symptoms severe enough to call attention to the difficulty until he starts to walk. Others may live a fairly normal life and not be aware of any heart trouble until a murmur or an enlarged heart is discovered on physical examination in later childhood. Some abnormalities are slight, and allow the person to lead a normal life without correction. Others cause little apparent difficulty but need correction to improve the chance for a longer life and for optimum health. Some severe anomalies are incompatible with life for more than a very short time, and others may be helped but not cured by surgery.

Clinical Manifestations.   A cardiac murmur discovered early in life necessitates frequent physical examinations. This may be a functional, "innocent" murmur that may disappear as the child grows older, or it may be the chief manifestation of an abnormal heart or an abnormal circulatory system. The most frequent parental complaint is of feeding difficulties. Infants with cardiac anomalies severe enough to cause circulatory difficulties have a history of being poor eaters, tiring easily from the effort to suck, and fail to grow or to thrive normally.

Manifestations of congestive heart failure may appear the first year of life in infants with such conditions as transposition of the great vessels, large ventricular septal defects, and with other serious defects. One indication of congestive heart failure in infancy is easy fatigability, manifested by feeding problems. The baby tires, breathes hard, refuses a bottle after one or two ounces but soon becomes hungry again. He has difficulty lying flat, and appears to be more comfortable if held upright over an adult's shoulder.

Other signs are failure to gain weight, a pale, mottled or cyanotic color, a hoarse or weak cry, and tachycardia. Rapid respiration (with an expiratory grunt), flaring of the alae nasi, and the use of accessory respiratory muscles with retractions at the diaphragmatic and the suprasternal level are other clinical manifestations of congestive heart failure. Edema is a factor, and the heart generally shows enlargement. Anoxic attacks (fainting spells) are common.

Treatment.   Treatment for congestive failure includes digitalization, diuretics to reduce any edema, oxygen, and the use of small doses of morphine for relaxation if neces-

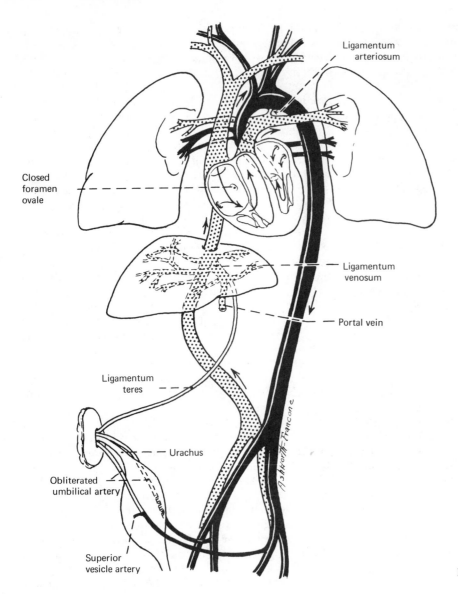

Ligamentum
arteriosum

Closed
foramen
ovale

Ligamentum
venosum

Portal vein

Ligamentum
teres

Urachus

Obliterated
umbilical artery

Superior
vesicle artery

FIG. 4–19. Normal blood circulation.

sary. The infant should be placed in a slanting position with the head elevated.

Because surgery carries less danger for an older child than for an infant, whenever possible, affected children should be maintained on medical treatment until the optimal time for surgical procedure.

Advances in medical technology are making it possible to repair even the hearts of infants less than 1 day old and other very young children. Miniaturization of instruments, earlier diagnosis, better intensive care facilities staffed with skilled nurse specialists, and more sophisticated monitoring techniques have all contributed to these advances.

Many physicians now think it is important to operate as early as possible to repair defective hearts. Inadequate circulation can prevent adequate growth and development, and may cause permanent, irreparable physical damage.

Care at home before surgery.   A child with congenital heart disease may show easy fatigability and retarded growth. If he has a cyanotic type of heart disease with clubbing of his fingers or toes, periods of cyanosis and reduced exercise tolerance are evident. This young child assumes a squatting position when he is tired from play.

Such a child should be allowed to lead as normal a life as possible. Parents are naturally apprehensive and find it difficult not to overprotect the child. They frequently increase their child's anxiety and make him fearful about participating in normal activities. Children are rather sensible about finding their own limitations, and will usually limit their activities to their capacity if they are not made unduly apprehensive.

Some parents are able to adjust well and provide guidance and security for their sick child. Others may become confused and frightened, and show hostility, disinterest or neglect, needing guidance and counseling.

Routine visits to a clinic or to a doctor's office become a way of life, and the child may come to see himself set apart from others. Doctors and nurses have a responsibility to both the parents and the child to give clear explanations of the defect, using readily understandable terms and illustrating their explanations with appropriate diagrams, pictures or models. A child can accept much and can continue with the business of living if he understands what it is all about.

Cardiac catheterization. Cardiac catheterization may be performed before heart surgery for more accurate information of the child's condition. The child or infant will be sedated or anesthetized for this process, during which a radiopaque tube is inserted through a vein into the right atrium of the heart.

Preoperative preparation. When a child enters the hospital for cardiac surgery, it seldom is his first admission. Generally, it has been preceded by cardiac catheterization or perhaps by other hospitalizations. Admission is scheduled to precede surgery by a few days, in order to give time for adequate preparation. Parents should understand that blood may be drawn for typing and cross-matching and for other determinations as ordered. Possibly additional roentgenograms may be made, and the child may be photographed.

Apparatus to be used after surgery should be described with drawings and pictures. If possible, the parents and their child should be taken to a cardiac recovery room and should be shown chest tubes, an oxygen tent, and the general appearance of the unit. Judgment should be shown about the timing and the extent of such preparation, because nothing is gained by arousing additional anxiety with premature or excessively graphic descriptions. A young child can become familiar with the surgical dress worn by personnel, with the oxygen tent, and perhaps listen to his own heart beat. He should practice coughing, and should understand that he will be asked to cough after surgery, even though it will hurt a little.

Cardiac surgery. Open heart surgery, using the heart–lung machine, has made extensive heart correction possible for many children who would have been otherwise hopelessly doomed to invalidism and a short life span not many years ago. Machines are now available for infants and small children.

Hypothermia is a useful technique that helps make early surgery possible. By gradually lowering the baby's body temperature, physicians increase the time that the circulation can be stopped without causing brain damage. The baby is packed in ice, and the temperature of the blood further reduced by the use of cooling agents in the heart–lung machine. This provides a dry, bloodless, motionless field for the surgeon.

Postoperative care. At the end of surgery, the child is taken to the intensive care unit to be skillfully nursed by specially trained personnel for as long as necessary. Children who have had closed chest surgery need the same careful nursing.

By the time the child returns to the ward, his chest drainage tubes have been removed, he has started taking oral fluids and is ready to sit up in bed or in a chair. He probably feels rather weak and helpless after his experience, and needs encouragement and reassurance. As he recovers, however, a child is usually quite ready for activity. His improved health provides the incentive. Mothers usually need to reorient themselves and to accept their child's new status—an attitude that is not easy to acquire after years of anxious watching.

The surgeon and his staff evaluate the results of the surgery and make any necessary recommendations regarding the resumption of the child's activities. Plans should be made for both follow-up and supervision, as well as for counseling and guidance, as the parents need it.

Common Types of Congenital Heart Disease. Congenital heart defects are commonly described as cyanotic or acyanotic conditions. Cyanotic heart disease implies an oxygen saturation of the peripheral arterial blood of 85% or less. This condition occurs when a heart defect allows any appreciable amount of oxygen-poor blood in the right side of the heart to mix with the oxygenated blood in the left side of the heart. Defects that permit right-to-left shunting can occur at the atrial, ventricular, or aortic level.

Many defects occur in combination, giving rise to complex situations. Many of the complex defects, and most of the rare, isolated defects may never be seen by the average nurse. The conditions discussed here are common enough that the pediatric nurse needs to be familiar with their diagnosis and treatment.

Ventricular septal defect. This is the most common intracardiac defect. It consists of an abnormal opening in the septum between the two ventricles, allowing blood to pass directly from the left to the right ventricle. There is no leakage of unoxygenated blood into the left ventricle, and thus no cyanosis (Fig. 4–20).

Small, isolated defects are usually without symptoms, and are frequently discovered during a routine physical examination. A characteristic loud, harsh murmur, associated with a systolic thrill, is occasionally heard on examination. There may be a history of frequent respiratory infections during infancy, but growth and development are not affected. The child leads a normal life.

Corrective surgery should be postponed, if at all possible, until the age of three years, when the surgical risk is less than that for infants. A very ill infant may be cared for medically with the use of digitalis, diuretics and antibiotics. A banding procedure has frequently brought about a marked improvement in those infants with large ventricular septal defects who have a large pulmonary blood flow and heart failure. This is accomplished by the application of a nylon cloth band around the root of the pulmonary arterial trunk, causing a reduction in the pulmonary flow and a drop in pulmonary artery pressure. At subsequent corrective surgery, the band is removed.

Atrial septal defects. In general, left-to-right shunting occurs in all true atrial septal defects. A patent foramen ovale, which is situated in the atrial septum, however, is present in a large number of healthy persons, and normally

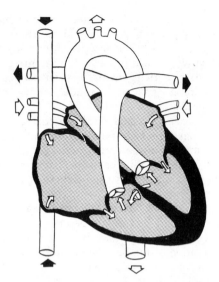

FIG. 4–20. A ventricular septal defect is an abnormal opening between the right and left ventricle. Ventricular septal defects vary in size and may occur in either the membranous or muscular portion of the ventricular septum. Owing to higher pressure in the left ventricle, a shunting of blood from the left to the right ventricle occurs during systole. If pulmonary vascular resistance produces pulmonary hypertension, the shunt of blood is then reversed from the right to the left ventricle, with cyanosis resulting. (Courtesy of Drs. Moller and Anderson and Ross Laboratories, Columbus, Ohio)

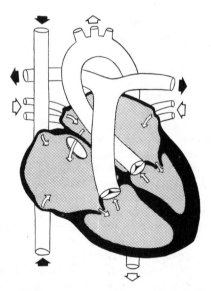

FIG. 4–21. An atrial septal defect is an abnormal opening between the right and left atria. Basically, three types of abnormalities result from incorrect development of the atrial septum. An incompetent foramen ovale is the most common defect. The high ostium secundum defect results from abnormal development of the septum secundum. Improper development of the septum primum produces a basal opening known as an ostium primum defect, frequently involving the atrioventricular valves. In general, left to right shunting of blood occurs in all atrial septal defects. (Courtesy of Drs. Moller and Anderson and Ross Laboratories, Columbus, Ohio)

causes no problems. This is because the valve of the foramen ovale is anatomically structured to withstand left chamber pressure, and makes the patent foramen ovale functionally closed (Fig. 4–21).

True atrial septal defects are common heart anomalies and may occur as isolated defects or in combination with other heart anomalies.

Treatment.   The ostium secundum defect is amenable to surgery, with a low surgical mortality risk. Since the advent of the heart-lung bypass machine, this repair can be performed in a dry field, replacing the older "blind" technique. The opening is either sutured or is closed with a nylon patch.

Patent ductus arteriosus.   The ductus arteriosus is a vascular channel between the left main pulmonary artery and the descending aorta. In fetal life, this allows blood to bypass the nonfunctioning lungs and go directly into the systemic circuit. After birth, the duct normally closes, eventually becoming obliterated and forming the ligamentum arteriosum. If the ductus remains patent, however, blood continues to be shunted from the aorta into the pulmonary artery. This overfloods the lungs and overloads the left-heart chambers (Fig. 4–22).

Normally the ductus arteriosus is nonpatent after the first or second week of life, and should be obliterated by the fourth month. Why it fails to close is not known at the present time. Patent ductus arteriosus is common in infants who exhibit the rubella syndrome, but most of the infants with this anomaly give no history of exposure to rubella during fetal life.

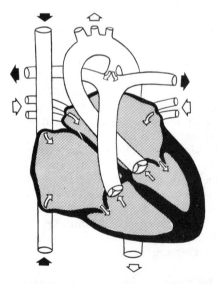

FIG. 4–22. The patent ductus arteriosus is a vascular connection that, during fetal life, short-circuits the pulmonary vascular bed and directs blood from the pulmonary artery to the aorta. Functional closure of the ductus normally occurs soon after birth. If the ductus remains patent after birth, the direction of blood flow in the ductus is reversed by the higher pressure in the aorta. (Courtesy of Drs. Moller and Anderson and Ross Laboratories, Columbus, Ohio)

Clinical manifestations. Symptoms are frequently absent during childhood. Growth and development may be retarded in some children, with an easy fatigability and dyspnea on exertion.

Diagnosis. This can be based on a characteristic, machinery-like murmur over the pulmonary area, a wide pulse pressure, and a bounding pulse. Cardiac catheterization is diagnostic but is not required in the presence of classical clinical features.

Treatment. Surgery is indicated in all diagnosed cases, even if they are asymptomatic. Some persons may possibly live a normal life span without correction, but the risks involved far outweigh the surgical ones.

Surgical procedures. Surgical correction consists of closure of the defect by ligation or by division of the ductus. Division is the method of choice if the child's condition permits, because the ductus occasionally reopens after ligation. Optimal age for surgery is between two and five years, with earlier surgery for severely affected infants. Prognosis is excellent following a successful repair.

Coarctation of the aorta. This is a congenital cardiovascular anomaly consisting of a constriction or narrowing of the aortic arch, or of the descending aorta, usually adjacent to the ligamentum arteriosum (Fig. 4—23 and Fig. 4—24).

A majority of children with this condition are asymptomatic until later childhood or young adulthood. A few infants have severe symptoms in their first year of life showing dyspnea, tachycardia, and cyanosis, all signs of developing congestive heart failure.

Diagnosis. The condition is easily diagnosed from hypertension present in the upper extremities, and from hypotension in the lower extremities. The radial pulse is readily palpable but the femoral pulses are weak or even impalpable. Blood pressure is normal or elevated in the arms and is low or undetectable in the legs. A high-pitched systolic murmur is usually present, heard over the base of the heart and over the interscapular area of the back. Diagnosis can be confirmed by aortography.

Obstruction to blood flow caused by the constricted portion of the aorta does not cause early difficulty in an average child because the blood bypasses the obstruction by way of the collateral circulation. The bypass is chiefly from the branches of the subclavian and the carotid arteries which arise from the arch of the aorta. Eventually, the enlarged collateral arteries erode the rib margins, and the rib notching can be visualized by x-ray examination.

The uncorrected coarctation may cause hypertension and cardiac failure later in life. The optimal age for surgery is probably between the ages of five to ten or twelve years. Early surgery may be necessary for a gravely ill infant if medical measures fail, but the mortality rate is high.

Treatment. Surgery consists of resection of the coarcted area with an end-to-end anastomosis of the proximal and the distal ends of the aorta. Occasionally a long defect may necessitate an end-to-end graft, using tubes of dacron or similar material. Prognosis is excellent for the restoration of normal functions after surgery.

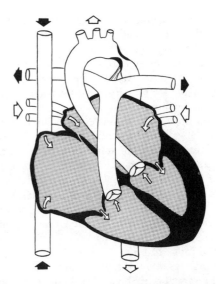

FIG. 4—23. Coarctation of the aorta is characterized by a narrowed aortic lumen. It exists as a preductal or postductal obstruction, depending on the position of the obstruction in relation to the ductus arteriosus. Coarctations exist with great variation in anatomic features. The lesion produces an obstruction to the flow of blood through the aorta causing an increased left ventricular pressure and work load. (Courtesy of Drs. Moller and Anderson and Ross Laboratories, Columbus, Ohio)

Tetralogy of Fallot. This is a fairly common congenital heart defect, involving 50% to 70% of all cyanotic congenital heart diseases. It consists of a grouping of heart defects, the term "tetralogy" denoting four abnormal condi-

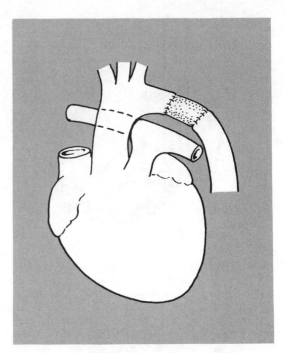

FIG. 4—24. A coarctation of the aorta is shown resected and a graft applied.

tions. These are *pulmonary stenosis, ventricular septal defect, overriding aorta,* and *right ventricular hypertrophy.*

The pulmonary stenosis is usually of the infundibular type, in which there is a narrowing of the upper portion of the right ventricle. It may include, however, stenosis of the valve cusps. Pulmonary stenosis results, in turn, in right ventricular hypertrophy.

The aorta appears to straddle the ventricular septum, overriding the ventricular septal defect. This defect allows a shunt of unsaturated blood from the right ventricle into the aorta, or into the left ventricle (Fig. 4–25).

Clinical manifestations.   The child may be precyanotic in early infancy with the cyanotic phase starting at from 4 to 6 months. Some severely affected infants, however, may show cyanosis earlier. It is believed that as long as the ductus arteriosus remains open, enough blood passes through the lungs to prevent cyanosis.

The infant presents feeding difficulties and poor weight gain with retarded growth and development. Dyspnea and easy fatigability become evident, especially when the child begins to walk. Cyanosis becomes grossly severe after the first year, even when the child is at rest.

Exercise tolerance depends somewhat on the severity of the disease, some children becoming fatigued after very little exertion. As the child experiences fatigue, breathlessness and increased cyanosis, he usually assumes a squatting posture for relief. Squatting apparently increases the systemic oxygen saturation.

Attacks of paroxysmal dyspnea are common during infancy and early childhood. An anoxic spell is heralded by sudden restlessness, gasping respiration, and increased cyanosis, leading into a loss of consciousness and possibly into convulsions. These attacks last from a few minutes in length to several hours and appear to be unpredictable, although stress does seem to trigger some episodes.

Iron-deficiency anemia is a common complication caused by the poor food intake. Cardiac catheterization, using angiocardiography helps present a clear picture of the anomalies involved.

Treatment.   Treatment is aimed at medical management until the child can tolerate surgery. The constant aim, of course, is to keep the child in the best possible physical condition.

An infant suffering an anoxic spell should be placed in a knee–chest position for the greatest possible relief. Oxygen is administered, and morphine is given to relax any child suffering an anoxic episode. Intravenous sodium bicarbonate has also been proved useful in severe spells. As the child grows older, however, he learns his physical limitations, and the anoxic episodes become fewer.

Anemia, if present, is treated with iron therapy. Surgery on the nose, the throat or on the ears carries the danger of subacute bacterial endocarditis. Therefore, antibiotic therapy is utilized if such surgery is necessary. Fevers, vomiting, and diarrhea diminish the fluid component of the blood, aggravating the existing polycythemia.

Surgical relief is imperative for these children as early as possible. The average age span for uncorrected cases is not over ten years. Heart surgery does carry a risk, and thus it is necessary for the child to be in the best possible physical condition.

1. Blalock-Taussig procedure. This is an end-to-end anastomosis of a vessel arising from the aorta, usually the subclavian, to the corresponding right or left pulmonary artery (Fig. 4–26A).
2. Potts procedure. This is a side-to-side anastomosis between the aorta and the left pulmonary artery (Fig. 4–26B).

Total surgical correction.   This procedure can only be carried out in a dry field, necessitating the use of a cardiopulmonary bypass machine. The heart is opened, and extensive resection is done. The septal defect is closed by use of an Ivalon patch and the valvular stenosis and infundibular chamber are resected.

Total correction is delayed, if possible, until after the age of 3 to 5 years. Palliative surgery carries the young child along and does not interfere with later correction. Because of the high surgical risk involved if correction is attempted in infancy, most surgeons prefer the sequence of palliative surgery at an early age, followed by total correction. Some surgeons have attempted total correction on selected infants with reported good results, but the risk for an average infant is still high.

Successful total correction transforms a grossly abnormal heart into a functionally normal one, as far as we can tell from present knowledge. Most of these children are left without a pulmonary valve, however. Whether this will prove harmful with age we cannot tell as yet.

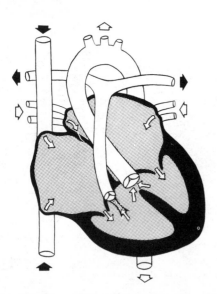

FIG. 4–25. Tetralogy of Fallot is characterized by the combination of four defects: (1) pulmonary stenosis, (2) ventricular septal defect, (3) overriding aorta, and (4) hypertrophy of the right ventricle. It is the most common defect causing cyanosis in patients surviving beyond 2 years of age. The severity of symptoms depends upon the degree of pulmonary stenosis, the size of the ventricular septal defect, and the degree to which the aorta overrides the septal defect. (Courtesy of Drs. Moller and Anderson and Ross Laboratories, Columbus, Ohio)

HEMOLYTIC DISEASE OF THE NEWBORN

Hemolytic disease is another name for *erythroblastosis fetalis*, a condition in which the infant's red blood cells are broken down (hemolyzed) and destroyed, producing severe anemia and hyperbilirubinemia. This rapid destruction of red blood cells can produce heart failure, brain damage, and death.

Prior to the mid-1960s, hemolytic disease was largely the result of Rh incompatibility between the blood of mother and fetus. The introduction of Rho immune globulin (RhoGAM*) in the mid-1960s has markedly reduced the incidence of this disorder. Hemolytic disease occurring today is principally the result of ABO incompatibility, and is generally much less severe than Rh-induced disorder.

Rh Incompatability. The Rh factor is a protein substance that is called an *antigen*, and is found on the surface of red blood cells. It is called Rh because it was first identified in the blood of rhesus monkeys. Those persons who possess the factor are referred to as Rh positive (D), and those lacking it as Rh negative (d).

The blood type of an individual is inherited, following the same hereditary rules regarding dominant and recessive traits. Rh positive is dominant. If both members of a couple are Rh negative, there will be no hemolytic disorder with their children. However, if the mother is Rh negative, the father is Rh positive, and the child inherits Rh positive blood, then the disorder can occur.

If the father is homozygous positive, then both of his genes carry the D (dominant) trait, but if he is heterozygous positive, one of the genes is a D and the other a d. Thus, if the father is heterozygous positive and the mother Rh negative, there is a 50–50 chance of their having a baby who is Rh negative (without hemolytic disease). Because of the mechanism by which the mother is sensitized to the Rh factor, there is little chance of the first baby being affected.

The incidence of hemolytic disease is directly related to occurrence of certain blood groups in our population. About 85% of the white population is Rh positive and 15% is Rh negative. This percentage varies among different racial groups. Thus, only a small percentage of marriages (about 13% in the U.S.) hold the potential for development of this complication.

Pathophysiology. The mechanism is based on the principles of the *antigen–antibody response*. Although fetal and maternal circulations are completely separated, a break in the placental barrier may allow some of the fetal red blood cells to escape into the maternal circulation. Often the break occurs at the time the placenta separates during delivery; or, it may take place after an abortion. The Rh positive fetal cells entering the maternal circulation act as a "mini-transfusion" causing the mother to form protective antibodies. It may take some time, however, for the antibodies to form so that the first baby is rarely affected.

With the next pregnancy, if any of the baby's red blood

*Orthodiagnostics, Raritan, NJ

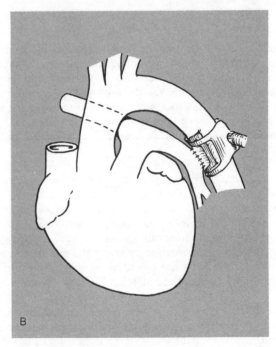

FIG. 4–26. (*A*) The Blalock-Taussig procedure is an end-to-end anastomosis of a vessel arising from the aorta to the corresponding right or left pulmonary artery. (*B*) The Potts procedure is a side-to-side anastomosis between the aorta and the left pulmonary artery.

cells enter the maternal circulation, antibodies form rapidly. Consequently, the maternal antibodies enter the fetal circulation and begin to hemolyze the baby's red blood cells (Fig. 4–27).

The rapid destruction of red blood cells causes excretion of bilirubin into the amniotic fluid. The baby's body

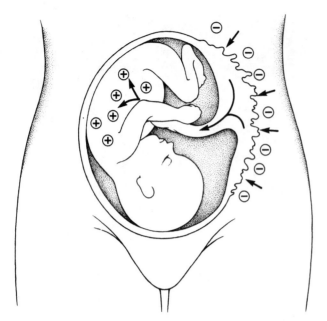

FIG. 4–27. Antibodies from mother enter the child and begin destroying its blood cells.

makes a valiant attempt to replace the red blood cells being destroyed by sending out large amounts of immature red blood cells called "erythroblasts" into his blood stream. For this reason, the disease is called *erythroblastosis fetalis*. As the process of rapid destruction of the red blood cells continues the baby develops anemia which, if severe enough, can result in heart failure and death of the baby *in utero*.

Treatment.   All expectant mothers should have their blood tested for blood group and Rh type at the initial prenatal visit. If the woman is found to be Rh negative then she should be followed closely throughout her pregnancy.* At periodic intervals she should have blood titers done as a screening method to detect the presence of antibodies. This allows the attending physician to evaluate the health of the fetus and plan for the baby's delivery and care.

When titers show the presence of antibodies the doctor then tries to determine how much the fetus is affected. Since there is no direct way to sample the infant's blood to find out the degree of anemia, indirect means must be used. A recent advance in diagnosing fetal diseases has been through the use of a procedure called *amniocentesis*. By inserting a needle into the amniotic sac, 10 to 15 ml of amniotic fluid is removed. The fluid is sent to the laboratory for spectophotometric analysis which shows the amount of bile pigments (bilirubin) in the amniotic fluid. Thus it can be determined if the fetus is mildly, moderately, or severely affected.

* Her husband's blood should also be typed and if he is Rh positive, a genotype may be done to determine if he is homozygous or heterozygous.

If analysis of the amniotic fluid shows that the fetus is severely affected, the physician will either perform an intrauterine transfusion of Rh negative blood, or, if the mother is beyond 32 weeks gestation, induce labor or perform cesarean delivery. After delivery, the baby is turned over to a pediatrician who will arrange for exchange transfusions.

Prevention.   The dramatic reduction in *erythroblastosis fetalis* is due largely to the introduction of Rho immune globulin (RhoGAM). It is effective only in mothers who do not have Rh antibodies, and must be injected into the mother within 72 hours after delivery of an Rh positive infant, or after abortion of an Rh positive fetus. It is *never* given to an infant or to a father.

The use of RhoGAM on all patients who are candidates for it offers the hope of eliminating hemolytic disease caused by Rh incompatability. The criteria for giving RhoGAM are

- The mother must be Rh negative.
- The infant must be Rh positive.
- The direct Coombs' test, a test for antibodies done on cord blood at delivery, is weakly reactive or negative.

ABO Incompatibility.   The major blood groups are A, B, AB, and O, and each has antigens that may be incompatible with those of another group. The most common incompatibility in the newborn occurs between an infant with type A or B blood and a mother with type AOB. Although the reactions are usually less severe than in Rh incompatibility, the clinical manifestations are similar, including jaundice, enlarged liver and spleen, but usually without severe anemia. Treatment is also similar; no preventive measures exist, however.

Care of the Infant with Erythroblastosis Fetalis.   Infants with known incompatibility to the mother's blood are examined carefully at birth for pallor, edema, jaundice, enlarged spleen and liver. A severely affected infant may be stillborn or have *hydrops fetalis*, with extensive edema, marked anemia and jaundice, and enlargement of the liver and spleen. These babies are in critical condition and will need exchange transfusions at the earliest possible moment.

The severely affected infants who survive without treatment run the risk of severe brain damage, called *kernicterus*. Symptoms appear after about the third day of life. At first, these include lethargy, poor muscle tone and poor sucking, often followed by spasticity and convulsions. Death occurs in about 75% of infants with kernicterus; those who survive may be mentally retarded or develop spastic paralysis or nerve deafness. Exchange transfusions are given at once to those infants who have signs of neurologic damage when first seen, although there is no proof that the damage can be reversed. Fortunately, present day ability to detect and treat hemolytic disease has reduced the number of infants who become permanently damaged.

A severely affected newborn will usually be transfused

without waiting for laboratory confirmation. All other suspected infants will have a sample of cord blood sent to the laboratory for a Coombs' test for the presence of damaging antibodies, Rh and ABO typing, hemoglobin and red cell level, and measurement of plasma bilirubin. A positive direct Coombs' test indicates the presence of antibodies on the surface of the infant's red blood cells. A negative direct Coombs' test indicates that there are no antibodies on the infant's red blood cells.

Treatment. A positive Coombs' test indicates presence of the disease but not the degree of severity. If bilirubin and hemoglobin are within normal limits, the infant will be watched carefully; frequent laboratory blood tests will be done. Phototherapy may also be ordered. (See Chapter 3.) Hemoglobin below the level of 10.5 mg/100 ml., or a rising bilirubin will be an indication for an exchange transfusion.

Exchange transfusions. Exchange transfusions require elaborate preparations and are time-consuming. The infant may be cared for in the intensive care unit, and will receive his transfusions there. It is important that the infant be kept in a warm environment at about 75° F to 80° F. A Servocontrolled isolette may be used for this purpose. Resuscitative equipment must be readily available: intubation equipment, laryngoscope, means for providing endotracheal suction, oxygen and resuscitative drugs.

Nursing care. After an exchange transfusion the infant is carefully observed for signs of shock or other reactions. Temperature, pulse and respirations are recorded routinely. He may be fed about 1 hour after the transfusion, or 6 hours after birth. If he is not too severely ill, he may be breastfed by his mother, then returned to his incubator. These babies need to be kept well hydrated. Intravenous feedings may be needed if the baby is premature.

These infants are lethargic and weak and need frequent changes of position. A careful watch must be kept for signs of impending kernicterus, such as loss of Moro reflex and decreased responsiveness.

Any infant admitted to the newborn nursery should be examined for jaundice during the first 36 hours. The nurse must keep in mind that early development of jaundice is a probable indication of erythroblastosis.

Infants whose bilirubin has been restored to normal levels, may be removed from their isolettes and returned to the regular nursery. They are discharged to routine home care, just as any well newborn.

SKELETAL DEFECTS

Infants with congenital skeletal defects usually receive primary treatment on the general pediatric ward, and thus the nurse needs to understand the nature and treatment of these abnormalities. Children with these conditions and their parents often face long periods of exhausting, costly treatment, and therefore need continuing support, encouragement, and education.

The two most common and important skeletal deformities are *clubfoot* (talipes equinovarus) and *dislocation of the hip.*

CONGENITAL TALIPES EQUINOVARUS

Congenital clubfoot is a deformity in which the entire foot is inverted, the heel is drawn up, and the forefoot is adducted. The Latin *talus,* meaning ankle, and *pes,* meaning foot, make up the word talipes, and is used in connection with many foot deformities. Equinus, or plantar flexion, and varus, or inversion, denote the kind of foot deformity present in this condition. The equinovarus foot has a clublike appearance, hence the term clubfoot (Fig. 4–28).

Congenital talipes equinovarus is the most common congenital foot deformity, appearing as a single anomaly, or in connection with other defects, such as myelomeningocele. It may be bilateral or unilateral. Etiology is not clear; an hereditary factor is occasionally observed. A theory that receives some acceptance postulates an ar-

clubfoot - one which is turned in or outward,

cause: abnormal pressure on feet in utero + inproper position in utero.

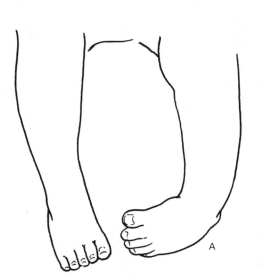

FIG. 4–28. Unilateral clubfoot. (A) front view, (B) back view.

rested growth of the germ plasm of the foot during the first trimester of pregnancy.

Diagnosis.   Talipes equinovarus is easily detected in a newborn infant but must be differentiated from a persisting fetal "position of comfort" assumed in utero. The positional deformity can be easily corrected by the use of passive exercise, but the true clubfoot deformity is fixed. The positional deformity should be explained to the parents at once to prevent anxiety.

Nonsurgical Treatment.   If treatment is started during the neonatal period, correction can usually be accomplished by manipulation and bandaging, or by application of a cast. While the cast is being applied, the foot is first gently moved into as near normal position as possible. Force should not be used. If the infant's mother can be present to help hold him while the cast is being applied, she will have the opportunity to understand what is being done. The very young infant gets his satisfaction from sucking, therefore a bottle of glucose water or formula will engage his attention and help prevent squirming while the cast is being applied.

The cast is applied over the foot and ankle (and usually to mid-thigh) to hold the knee in right-angle flexion (Fig. 4–29). Casts are changed frequently to provide gradual, nontraumatic correction. Treatment is continued until complete correction is confirmed by x-ray and clinical observation, usually in a matter of months.

Any cast applied to a child's body should have some type of waterproof material protecting the skin from the sharp plaster edges of the cast. One method is to apply strips of adhesive vertically around the edges of the cast in a manner called *petaling*. This is done by cutting strips of adhesive 2 to 3 inches long and 1 inch wide. One end is notched and the other end cut pointed to aid smooth application.

An alternative method involves the use of a Denis Browne splint. The splint is composed of a flexible, horizontal metal bar attached to two foot plates. The child's foot is attached to the foot plate with adhesive tape, and the attachment of the horizontal bar permits changing the relationship of the bar to the plate as necessary. This splint must be used for a period of time, as long as seven or eight months, until a wide overcorrection is attained (Fig. 4–30).

Following correction from a cast or a splint, a Denis Browne splint with shoes attached is used to maintain correction for another 6 months or so. After overcorrection has been attained, a special clubfoot shoe should be worn—a laced shoe with a turning out of the shoe and the outer wedge of the sole. The Denis Browne splint may still be worn at night, and passive exercises of the foot should be carried out by the child's parent.

Surgical Treatment.   Children who do not respond to nonsurgical measures, especially older children, need surgical correction. This involves several procedures depending on the age of the child and upon the degree of the deformity. It may involve lengthening of the Achilles tendon, capsulotomy of the ankle joint, release of medial strictures, and, for the child over ten years of age, an operation on the bony structure. Prolonged observation, after correction by either means, should be carried out at least until adolescence; any recurrence is treated promptly.

Nursing Care.

Postoperative care.

Check vital signs until they are stable.
Observe the cast for signs of bleeding.
Elevate the affected leg.
Observe circulation and temperature of the toes.
Be alert for any signs of infection.

Continuing care.   The infant or small child in a cast cannot explain to his nurses that his cast is too tight, im-

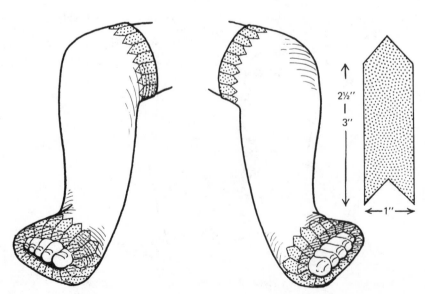

FIG. 4–29. Casting for clubfoot showing petalling of cast.

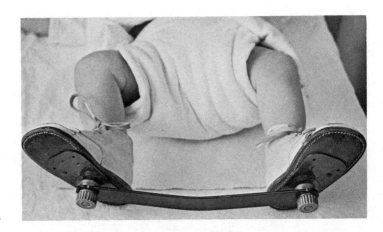

FIG. 4–30. A Denis Browne splint with shoes attached.

pairing circulation, or is irritating his skin. Nursing observation should include the following:

Check the color and the temperature of the toes at frequent intervals. Check excessive irritability—indicating acute discomfort—with the attending physician.

Prevent the child from banging and denting his cast before it is dry. A clovehitch restraint may be necessary.

Petal edges of the cast, when dry, with adhesive to prevent skin irritation.

Hold and comfort the child when possible. Better still, if his mother or father are present they can do this.

If a Denis Browne splint is used instead of a cast, check the foot for irritation from adhesive tape, for swelling or for any other indication of circulation impairment from the tight strapping. Check frequently the position of the foot on the foot plate. These splints are uncomfortable until the infant becomes accustomed to them. He cannot kick the way he is accustomed to; in fact there is less freedom of movement than when casts are used. These babies have a special need to be held and comforted.

Home Care.   If the mother has helped with the hospital care, her infant's needs will be better met when he goes home. The mother must continue to watch for skin irritation and for signs of pressure from a cast that has become too tight. She must be prompt for appointments, and understand the importance of notifying the physician or the clinic whenever the cast needs attention or if the splint appears to have slipped. The family must also be prepared to give additional emotional support until the infant becomes accustomed to the splint or cast.

CONGENITAL DISLOCATION OF THE HIP

A defective development of the acetabulum, with or without dislocation, may be present in the newborn infant. The malformed acetabulum permits dislocation, the head of the femur becoming displaced upward and backward. The condition is difficult to recognize during early infancy. When there is family history of the defect, increased observation of the young infant is indicated. The condition is approximately seven times more common in girls than in boys and is frequently bilateral.

due to malformed hip socket.

Diagnosis.   Early recognition and treatment, before an infant starts to stand or walk, is extremely important for successful correction. Early signs include the following.

Asymmetry of the gluteal skin folds (they are higher on the affected side) (Fig. 4–31).

Limitation of abduction of affected hip. This is tested by placing infant on his back with his knees flexed and then abducting both knees passively until they reach the examination table without resistance. If dislocation is present, the affected side cannot be abducted beyond 45°. Sometimes a clicking sound may be elicited as the head of the femur slips over the rim of the acetabulum.

Later signs, after the child has started walking, include: lordosis, sway-back, protruding abdomen, shortened extremity, duck-waddle gait, positive Trendelenburg sign. To elicit the sign, the child stands on his affected leg and raises his normal leg. The pelvis tilts downward rather than upward toward the unaffected side.

Roentgen studies are usually made to confirm the diagnosis. Uncorrected dislocation causes limping, easy fatigue, hip and low back discomfort, and postural deformities.

Treatment.   When the dislocation is discovered during the first few months, treatment consists of manipulation of the femur into position and application of a spica cast or brace. If treatment is delayed until after the child has commenced to walk, open reduction followed by a spica cast is usually needed. After the cast is removed, a metal or plastic brace is applied to keep the legs in wide abduction. *in frog leg position.*

It is important that the legs be kept in the proper position. The Frejka splint (Fig. 4–32) is a kind of harness attached to a pillow that holds the legs wide apart. It is applied over the diaper, so much care is needed to keep the baby's legs in position while diapers are being changed.

A metal or plastic splint is applied after the cast has been removed. A newer product made of lightweight nontoxic polyethylene plastic has foam padded edges and laced cuffs.* The splint is moisture-proof, sanitary, well-

2 0 3 diapers applied.

* Camp Plastic Abduction Splint.

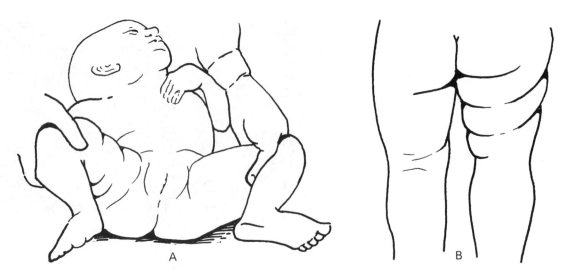

FIG. 4–31.   Congenital hip dislocation. (*A*) Limitation of abduction in the affected leg; (*B*) asymmetry of skin folds of the thighs.

ventilated, and can be fitted over or under the diaper (Fig. 4–33).

Nursing Care.   The child in a cast needs careful observation of circulation, attention to his skin, and comfortable positioning. A hard mattress is needed, with pillows for positioning while the cast is drying. Complaints of pain should be heeded and reported. The cast, which extends from the upper abdomen to the toes, should be petaled with adhesive around the waist and the toes with a plastic sheet tucked under the cut-out pubic area and taped over the cast for protection from soiling and wetting.

If open reduction has been performed, the child should be watched for signs of shock and bleeding; fluids and diet are resumed as usual. The edges of the cast should be petaled with adhesive or otherwise covered to avoid irritation to the skin.

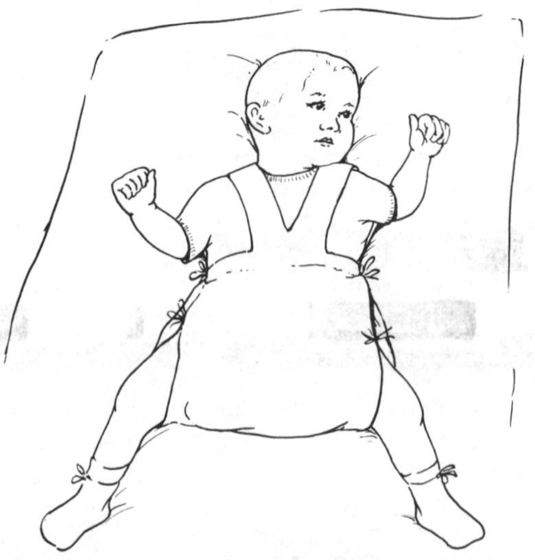

The skin around and under the edges of the cast should be watched for irritation, particularly for crumbs of plaster or food that may fall under the cast. The child may stuff a small toy or some food that he is supposed to have eaten, into the cast. The cast around the perineal area should be inspected daily for dampness or soiling, and the waterproof material washed, dried and reapplied as needed.

The child may be held after the cast is dry; with a frog-leg cast he can sit on the nurse's lap, particularly for his meals. In bed he must be turned frequently and should be taken to the playroom or perhaps on rides about the hospital on a stretcher for diversion. Parents need to learn the proper home care—learning most easily acquired through participation in the child's care before discharge.

GENITOURINARY TRACT DEFECTS

Most congenital anomalies of the genitourinary tract are not life-threatening in a physical sense, but can present social problems with life-long implications for the child and his family. Thus, early recognition and supportive, understanding care of these problems are essential.

HYPOSPADIAS AND EPISPADIAS

Hypospadias is a congenital condition of a male child in which the urethra terminates on the underside (ventral) of the penis, instead of at the tip. A cordlike anomaly (called a *chordee*) extends from the scrotum to the penis, pulling the penis downward in an arc. Urination is not interfered with, but the boy is unable to void while standing in the normal male fashion. Surgical repair is recommended before the child starts to attend school to avoid the psychological damage he will suffer through ridicule from his male classmates.

Surgical repair is performed in two stages. The primary surgery is for the purpose of releasing the chordee. Later, during the preschool period, plastic surgery is used to ex-

FIG. 4–32.   The Frejka splint is used to correct congenital dislocation of the hip.

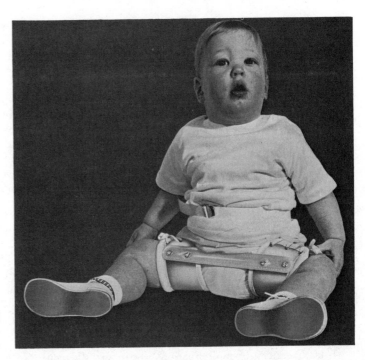

FIG. 4–33. The Camp plastic abduction splint may be used with the child who has congenital hip dislocation. (Courtesy SH Camp and Co.)

tend the urethra to the tip of the penis and to close the ventral opening. These infants should not be circumcised, as the foreskin is used in the repair.

In *epispadias* the opening is on the dorsal (top) surface of the penis. This condition frequently occurs with exstrophy of the bladder. Surgical repair is indicated.

EXSTROPHY OF THE BLADDER

This urinary tract malformation occurs in one out of every 30,000 live births in the U.S. and is usually accompanied by other anomalies such as epispadias, cleft scrotum, cryptorchidism (undescended testes), a shortened penis in males, and cleft clitoris in females. It is also associated with malformed pelvic musculature, resulting in prolapsed rectum and inguinal hernias. Children with this defect have a widely split symphysis pubis and posterolaterally rotated hip sockets, causing a waddling gait.

In this condition, the anterior surface of the urinary bladder lies open on the lower abdomen (Fig. 4–34). The exposed mucosa is red and sensitive to touch, and allows direct passage of urine to the outside. This makes the area very vulnerable to infection and trauma. Surgical correction of this condition is thought to be most effective between 12 and 18 months of age. Thus, parents need to be taught how to care for this condition, and how to deal with their own feelings toward this less-than-perfect child. Their emotional reaction may be further complicated if the malformation is so severe that the sex of the child can only be determined by a chromosome test. (See Sexual Ambiguity.)

Nursing care of the infant with exstrophy of the bladder should be directed toward prevention of infection, prevention of skin irritation around the seeping mucosa, meeting the infant's need for touch and cuddling, and educating and supporting the parents during this crisis.

May need iliostomy or urostomy.

SEXUAL AMBIGUITY

The birth of an infant with ambiguous genitalia presents a highly charged emotional climate, and possible long-range social implications. Regardless of the cause, it is important to establish the genetic sex and the sex of rearing as early

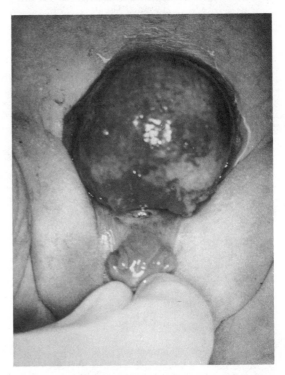

FIG. 4–34. Exstrophy of bladder. (Avery GB: Neonatology, 2nd ed. Philadelphia, JB Lippincott, 1981)

as possible, so that surgical correction of anomalies can take place before the child begins to function in a sex-related social role. Authorities believe that the infant's anatomy, rather than the genetic sex, should determine the sex of rearing. It is possible to surgically construct a functional vagina and to administer hormones to offer an anatomically incomplete female a somewhat normal life. To date it is not possible to offer comparable surgical reconstruction to males with an inadequate penis. Parents may feel guilt, anxiety, and confusion about their child's condition, and will need empathetic understanding and support to help them cope with this emergency.

OTHER CONGENITAL DISORDERS

CONGENITAL RUBELLA

It is now apparent that the rubella virus infection acquired by the fetus *in utero* generally persists throughout fetal life, and for as long as 18 months after delivery. Persons coming into intimate contact with these babies may develop the disease; therefore, all women of childbearing age who are not immune to rubella should avoid contact with an infected infant.

A large variety of malformations constitute the congenital rubella syndrome, including, cataracts and other eye defects such as glaucoma; also deafness, cardiac anomalies, especially patent ductus arteriosus, and septal defects; intrauterine growth retardation, subnormal head circumference, and retarded functional development.

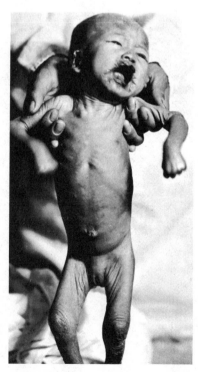

FIG. 4-35. Some of the skin manifestations of congenital syphilis. (Waechter EH, Blake FG: Nursing Care of Children, 9th ed. Philadelphia, JB Lippincott, 1976)

Reliance on immunization by presumed attacks of rubella during the individual's childhood is generally not dependable because many rashes resemble that of rubella, and symptoms of childhood rubella are mild. Testing for the presence of rubella serum antibody is desirable in areas where adequate laboratory facilities are available. A positive reaction shows the person to be immune either as a result of the disease itself, or from immunization. Parents of infected infants should understand the dangers presented to pregnant women.

Care of the infant is concerned with treating concomitant conditions and giving routine care accorded any newborn infant. Some infants are extremely ill from complications present at birth, and rates of permanent damage are high.

Prevention. A rubella vaccine is now available that produces long lasting immunity. This is a live virus vaccine administered in a single subcutaneous injection. In the United States, mass vaccination for children between the ages of 1 and 12 years is being attempted as vaccine becomes available. Priority is given to kindergarten and early school age children, as this is the age group most likely to disseminate the disease. History of rubella in a child is usually not reliable enough to omit vaccination.

Women of childbearing age in the United States are not given the vaccine unless there is no possibility of pregnancy within 2 months following vaccination. Each case is considered individually. Medically acceptable methods of contraception should be followed to insure against pregnancy. Vaccination with live rubella virus is contraindicated during pregnancy.

Rubella in a woman in the first trimester of pregnancy is now legally recognized as an indication for abortion in many states of the United States, and in many other countries.

CONGENITAL SYPHILIS

Syphilis, whether congenital or acquired, is caused by the spirochete *Treponema pallidum.* Fetal infection does not occur much before the fourth month of fetal life after the fetal organs are formed, therefore, anomalies rarely occur. The infection is contracted through the mother by placental transfer. About one fourth of infected infants are stillborn. Infants born live may not show any clinical symptoms for months or years.

Diagnosis. A Wasserman test on cord blood at delivery is done when congenital syphilis is suspected. Passively acquired antibodies may give a false positive, therefore other serological tests will be given later. If results are doubtful, treatment will usually be instituted to avoid a full blown infection.

In *early* congenital syphilis, symptoms may appear before the sixth week of life. Rhinitis, with a profuse, mucopurulent nasal discharge is usually the first symptom. A maculopapular skin rash next appears, heaviest over the back, buttocks and backs of the thighs. Bleeding ulcerations and mucous membrane lesions appear around the mouth, anus, and the genital areas (Fig. 4-35). Anemia is present, pseudoparalysis and pathological fractures may occur. These symptoms usually subside without treatment while the infectious organism lies latent in the child's tissues.

Late symptoms, appearing after infancy, involve the skeletal framework, the eyes and the central nervous system. The child may acquire a flat bridge of the nose, known as "saddle nose." His permanent teeth are affected, the incisors are peg-shaped (Hutchinson's teeth). A condition of the eyes called *interstitial keratitis* frequently occurs later in the disease with lacrimation, photophobia, and opacity of the lens which may lead to blindness.

Treatment. Ideally, treatment is preventive, consisting of treatment of the affected mother early in pregnancy. Treatment for the affected infant consists of a course of penicillin therapy.

Early congenital syphilis usually responds to vigorous treatment; and growth and development will not be affected. Late congenital syphilis responds well to treatment, but pathological changes in the bones, eyes, and nervous sytem are permanent.

GONORRHEAL OPHTHALMIA NEONATORUM

Gonorrheal eye infection in the newborn is a serious condition usually resulting in blindness when prophylactic treatment at birth is omitted. The infectious agent is *Neisseria gonorrhoeae*, the gonococcus. The infant becomes infected as he passes through the birth canal of an infected mother.

Symptoms are acute redness and swelling of the conjunctiva with a purulent discharge from the eyes, occurring within 36 to 48 hours after birth. The condition is communicable for 24 hours after specific therapy is instituted, or when no therapy is used, until discharge from the eyes has ceased.

Prevention. In the United States, all states have laws requiring the use of specific preparations instilled into the eyes at birth. A number of states require instillation of 1% silver nitrate. In other states antibiotic drops or ophthalmic ointments such as tetracycline or erythromycin are used.

Treatment. Penicillin is a specific for the treatment of gonorrheal infections, including gonorrheal ophthalmia.

HERPESVIRUS HOMINIS, TYPE 2 INFECTION

Infants of mothers infected with this virus must be delivered by cesarean method before rupture of membranes, if they are to survive. Even then the prognosis is grave, and the probability high for ocular or neurologic damage. This condition is highly contagious and can be transmitted from infected lesions through breaks in the skin of caregiver's ungloved hands.

summary

The infant who sustains damage during intrauterine life or at birth has a better chance for survival today than ever before. The more serious the damage, the greater the ten-dency to concentrate on meeting the infant's physical needs, sometimes ignoring his acute need for tender loving care and social interaction. Meeting these needs is a very real part of nursing care. So are the comfort and understanding support that parents of these special infants require as they mourn the loss of their hoped-for perfect child, and begin learning how to make life as normal as possible for their real child and for the family.

review questions

1. What is the most common birth injury?
2. Discuss how to feed an infant following the repair of a cleft lip. How is aspiration prevented after feeding?
3. Describe esophageal atresia.
4. What is spina bifida?
5. What are the two types of hydrocephalus?
6. What is the "setting sun" sign?
7. Describe the surgical treatments of hydrocephalus.
8. How does the nurse help meet the psychosocial needs of an infant?
9. What are the two most common skeletal deformities? How are these deformities treated?
10. What drug is responsible for reducing the incidence of erythroblastosis fetalis?
11. Identify the distinctive characteristics for each of the following congenital heart defects: (a) ventricular septal defect, (b) atrial septal defect, (c) patent ductus arteriosus, (d) coarctation of the aorta, (e) tetralogy of Fallot.
12. Explain ABO incompatibility.
13. What organism causes syphilis? Gonorrhea?
14. What is the drug of choice used to treat syphilis and gonorrhea?

references

1. Whaley L, Wong D: Nursing Care of Infants and Children. St Louis, CV Mosby, 1979
2. Jackson PL: Ventriculo-peritoneal shunts. Am Nurs 80:1104–1109, 1980

bibliography

Bishop WS, Head JJ: Care of the infant with a stoma, Am J Mat Child Nurs 1:315–319, 1976

Clay C: There is something wrong with your baby. In McNall LK, Galeener JT (eds): Current Practice in Obstetric and Gynecologic Nursing, vol 1. St Louis, CV Mosby, 1976

Conway BL: Carini and Owens' Neurological and Neurosurgical Nursing, 7th ed. St Louis, CV Mosby, 1978

Conway, BL: Pediatric Neurologic Nursing. St Louis, CV Mosby, 1977

Featherstone H: A Difference in the Family. New York, Basic Books, 1980

Hill S: The child with ambiguous genitalia. Am Nurs 77:810–814, 1977

Hilt NE, Cogburn S: Manual of Orthopedics. St Louis, CV Mosby, 1979

Hilt NE, Schmitt W: Pediatric Orthopedic Nursing. St Louis, CV Mosby, 1975

Jensen MD, Benson R, Bobak IM: Maternity Care: The Nurse and the Family, 2nd ed. St Louis, CV Mosby, 1981

Korones SB: High-risk Newborn Infants: The Basis for Intensive Nursing Care, 3rd ed. St Louis, CV Mosby, 1981

Mercer RT: Crisis: a baby is born with a defect. Nurs '77 7, No. 11:45– 47, 1977

Mills GC: Supporting parental needs after birth of a defective infant. In Brandt PA, Chinn PL, Smith ME (eds): Current Practice in Pediatric Nursing, vol 1. St Louis, CV Mosby, 1976

Moller JH: Essentials of Pediatric Cardiology, 2nd ed. Philadelphia, FA Davis, 1978

Passo SD: Positioning infants with myelomeningocele. Am J Nurs 74:1658– 1660, 1974

Rankin H: Handicap: a parent's perspective. Can Nurse 11:38– 39, 1979

Shirkey HC: Pediatric Therapy, 5th ed. St Louis, CV Mosby, 1975

Stevens MS, Reinitz M: Nursing a child through exstrophic bladder reconstruction surgery. Am J Mat Child Nurs 5:265– 270, 1980

Uzark K: A child's cardiac catheterization: Avoiding the potential risks. Am J Mat Child Nurs 3:158– 161, 1978

Whaley L, Wong D: Nursing Care of Infants and Children. St Louis, CV Mosby, 1979

Wieczorek RR, Natapoff JN: A Conceptual Approach to the Nursing of Children. Philadelphia, JB Lippincott, 1981

Young RK: Chronic sorrow: parent's response to the birth of a child with a defect. Am J Mat Child Nurs 2:38– 42, 1977

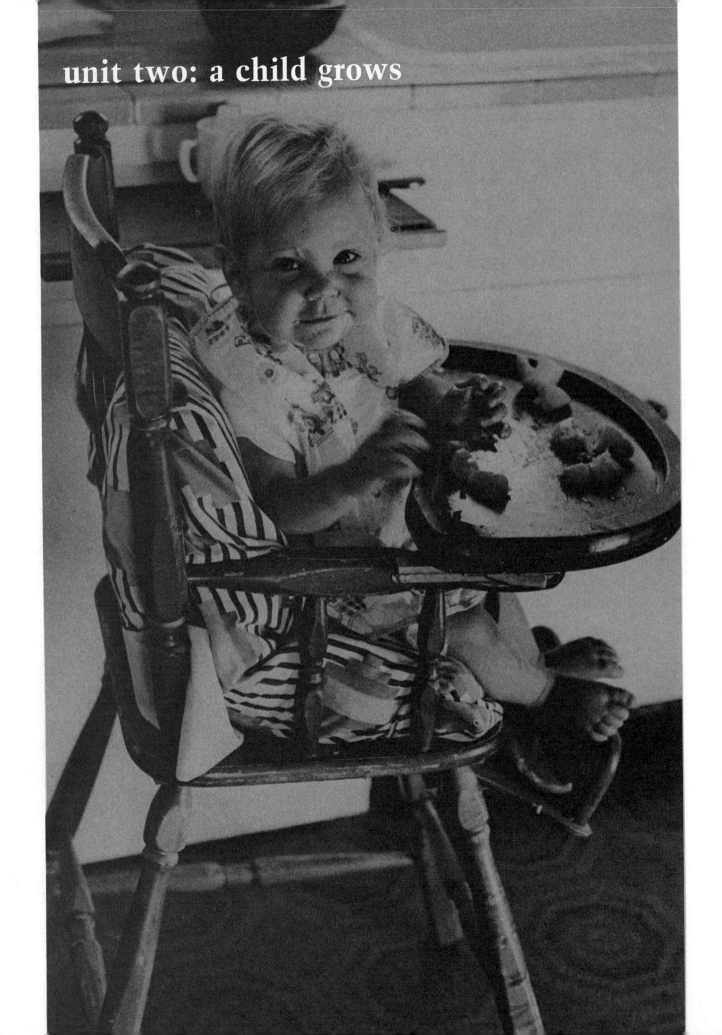

the child and the family

student objectives

The student successfully attaining the goals of this chapter will be able to

1 Define the following vocabulary terms:

archetypes   circadian rhythms   egocentric   extended family
individuation   nuclear family   Oedipal stage   socialization   superego

2 Describe three primary functions of the family.

3 Explain how circadian rhythms may affect the relationship of a newborn with his family.

4 Describe the six stages of Freud's psychosexual theory of development.

5 Describe the seven developmental tasks of Erikson's psychosocial theory of development.

6 List the four principal stages of intellectual development as described by Piaget.

The birth of a baby alters forever the relationship of his parents and establishes a new social unit—a family—in which all members influence and are influenced by each other. Each subsequent child born into that family continues the process of reshaping the individual members and the family unit. In addition, family members are individually and collectively affected by the larger community around them.

Nursing care of children demands a solid understanding of normal patterns of growth and development—physical, psychological, social, and intellectual (cognitive)—and an awareness of the many factors that influence those patterns. It also demands an appreciation for the uniqueness of each child and each family. To be complete and therefore as effective as possible, a child must be considered as a member of a family and a larger community.

Today's American child enters a family that may resemble only faintly the traditional nuclear family of 20 or 30 years ago, in which the father worked outside the home and the mother cared for the children. Family structure is changing in response to turbulent social and economic conditions, and its very meaning is being redefined based on the functions it performs for its members.

Continuing research studies of children and family behavior are changing and increasing the knowledge of how children and families affect each other. This new knowledge can point the way toward more stable, healthful family relationships and thereby better health for children and other family members.

family function

The family is mankind's oldest and most basic social unit, and its primary purpose is to continue the society and its knowledge, customs, values, and beliefs. It establishes the individual's primary connection with a group responsible for him until he becomes an independent person. Although family structure varies among different cultures, its functions related to children are similar: providing physical care, educating and training children, and protecting children's psychological and emotional health.

PHYSICAL CARE

The family is responsible for meeting each child's basic needs for food, clothing, shelter, and protection from harm, including illness. The work necessary to meet these needs was once clearly divided between mother and father, with the mother providing total care for the child and the father providing the resources that made it possible. These attitudes have changed in many areas of today's society, so that each parent has an opportunity to share in the joys and trials of child care and other aspects of family living.

EDUCATION AND TRAINING

Within the family unit, a child learns the rules of the society and the culture in which he lives: its language, values, ethics, and acceptable behaviors. This process is called *socialization* and is accomplished by training and education. Children are trained by teaching them acceptable ways of meeting physical needs such as eating and elimination, and certain skills such as dressing oneself. Children are educated by teaching them about relationships to other persons within and outside the family. They learn what is permitted and approved within their society and what is forbidden.

PSYCHOLOGICAL AND EMOTIONAL HEALTH

Research studies continue to support the importance of early parent–child relationships to emotional adjustment of the individual in later life. As mentioned earlier in the discussion of attachment, even a few hours can constitute a critical period in the emotional bond between parents and child. Though results of these recent studies are controversial, it is generally agreed that young children are highly sensitive to psychological influences, and those influences may have long-range effects, either positive or negative.

With the family, the child learns who he is and how his behavior affects other family members. He observes and imitates their behavior, learning quickly which behaviors are rewarded and which are punished.

Participation in a family is a child's only rehearsal for parenthood. How he is treated by each parent has a powerful influence on how he will treat his own children. Studies have shown that often parents who abuse their children were abused by their parents as children.

family structure

Two principal kinds of family structure occur in many cultures; they are the nuclear family and the extended family. Other variations include the single-parent family, the communal family, the polygamous family, and the homosexual family. To be considered a family does not require legal sanction, but for societal and economic reasons, a legalized union is most often preferred.

NUCLEAR (CONJUGAL) FAMILY

This structure is composed of a man, a woman, and their children (either biologic or adopted) who share a common household (Fig. 5–1). This was once the typical American family structure; now less than one-third of U.S. families fit this pattern. It is a more mobile and independent unit than an extended family, but is often part of a network of related nuclear families within close geographic proximity.

EXTENDED FAMILY

Typical of agricultural societies, the extended family consists of one or more nuclear families plus other kinsmen. The needs of individual members are subordinate to the needs of the group, and children are considered an economic asset. Grandparents aid in childrearing, and children learn respect for their elders by observation of their parents' behavior toward the older generation.

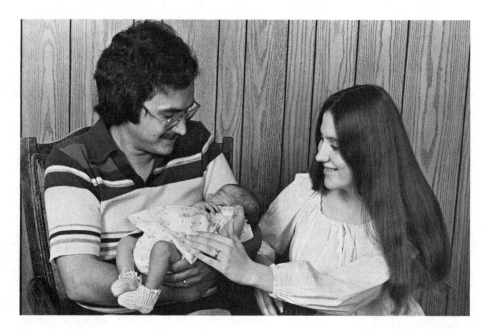

FIG. 5–1. The nuclear family: mother, father, and child. (Wolff L, Weitzel MH, Fuerst EV: Fundamentals of Nursing, 6th ed. Philadelphia, JB Lippincott, 1979)

NON-TRADITIONAL FAMILIES

Rising divorce rates, the women's movement, increasing acceptance of illegitimacy, and a more liberal attitude toward adoption have combined to produce a growing number of *single-parent families.* More than 7% of U.S. households fall in this category (a 40% increase between 1970 and 1980) and most are headed by women. Though this family situation places a heavy burden on the parent, no conclusive evidence is available to show its effects on children.

During the early 1960s, increasing numbers of young adults began to challenge the values and traditions of the American social system. One of the results of that challenge was the establishing of communal groups and collectives, or *communal families.* This alternative structure occurs in many settings and may favor either a primitive or modern lifestyle. Members of a communal family share responsibility for homemaking and childrearing; all children are the collective responsibility of adult members. Not actually a new family structure, the communal family is a variation of the extended family.

Although *polygamy* (having more than one spouse at a single time) is illegal in the U.S., it is practiced illegally in certain parts of the country. In this situation, a husband usually has more than one wife and assumes responsibility for his wives and all their children. Generally this creates economic as well as emotional difficulties.

Another type of family that has only recently begun to be openly acknowledged is the *homosexual family.* In this circumstance, two persons of the same sex, bound by formal or informal commitment, raise children. These children may be the result of a prior heterosexual mating, adoption, or artificial insemination. Studies are not available to evaluate the effects of this family structure on its members.

family factors that influence children

FAMILY SIZE

The number of children in the family makes a decided difference in parents and children. The smaller the family, the more time there is for individual attention to each child. Children in small families, particularly "only" children, often spend more time with adults and therefore relate better with them than with their peers. Only children tend to be more advanced in language development and intellectual achievement.

A large family understandably emphasizes the group more than the individual child. There is greater interdependence among these children, and less dependence on the parents (Fig. 5–2). Less time is available for parental attention to individual children.

SIBLING ORDER AND SEX

Whether a child is the firstborn, the middle child, or the youngest also makes a difference in his relationships and behavior. Firstborn children command a great deal of attention from parents and grandparents, and are also affected by their parents' inexperience, anxieties, and uncertainties. Many times parents' expectations for the oldest child are greater than for subsequent children. Generally firstborn children are greater achievers than their siblings.

With second and subsequent children, parents tend to be more relaxed and permissive. These children are likely to be more relaxed and slower to develop language skills. They identify more with peers than with parents.

Sexual identity in relation to siblings also affects a child's development. Girls raised with boys tend to have more masculine characteristics than girls raised with girls. Boys raised with older brothers are more aggressive than boys who have older sisters.

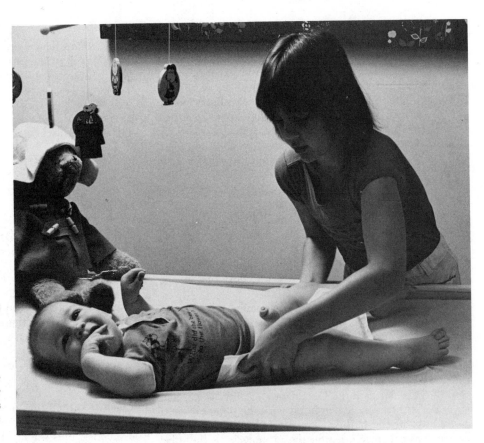

FIG. 5–2. Children from larger families learn to care for each other and are not as dependent on parents as only children. (Photo by Bruce Grindle)

PARENTAL BEHAVIOR

Many factors have conspired to change the traditional mother-at-home, father-at-work image of the American family (Fig. 5–3). More than half of U.S. mothers work outside the home, some because they are the family's only source of income, others because the family's economic goals demand a second income. This means that probably more than half of all children between the ages of 3 and 5 spend part of their day being cared for by someone other than their parent. Mothers are concerned with more than childcare responsibilities, often affecting the quality of the time that they have at home with the children.

Many fathers are away from home for most of their children's day; some fathers have jobs that require travel and thus are away for days or weeks at a time. This "absent" father, when at home, is often too tired to participate in family activities, thus creating feelings of resentment and neglect on the part of children and perhaps the mother.

Families spend less time together because of many factors. Separate jobs for mother and father, school activities for children, absorption in television rather than family conversation at mealtime, emphasis on acquisition of material goods rather than development of relationships—all contribute to a breakdown in family communication, which is typical of many families, and unmeasured in impact on today's children, the parents of tomorrow.

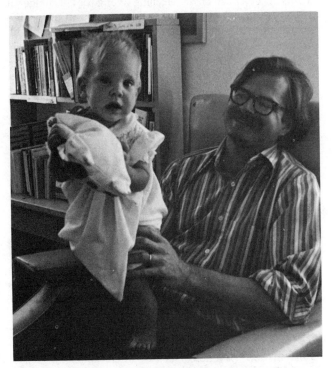

FIG. 5–3. Father's increased participation in childcare is a welcome change in many American families.

DIVORCE

During the decade of 1970 to 1980, the number of divorces granted increased 65%. This fact holds nothing good for the children involved, but to determine the exact extent of the damage is difficult. Children whose lives were seriously disrupted before a divorce may feel relieved when the situation is resolved. Others who felt that their lives were happy may feel frightened and abandoned. All these feelings depend upon the individuals involved, their ages, and the kind of care and relationships they experience with their parents following the divorce.

CIRCADIAN RHYTHMS

Scientists now know that all our biologic functions vary throughout the day according to innate mechanisms called *circadian rhythms* (from the Latin, meaning, "about one day"). The most obvious of these is sleep, but research has shown that blood pressure, hormone levels, and pulse all follow their own pattern.[1]

Studies have shown that newborn infants have innate but undeveloped circadian rhythms that, over varying periods of time, take on the regularity of an adult's rhythms.

While these rhythms are developing, every member of the newborn's family may experience considerable disruption of their life pattern. The infant's feeding, wake, and sleep cycles are not synchronized with the older children and adults in the family. Normally the sleep and wake pattern has begun to resemble the adult cycle by the third week of life and by the end of the 18th week the baby begins to do most of his sleeping at night. The longer it takes the infant's rhythms to adjust to adultlike regularity, the more likely that the infant will be considered "difficult," possibly interfering with parent–child relationships. Much remains to be learned about mankind's circadian rhythms, but even limited knowledge indicates that they are a very real factor in the development of family relationships.

concepts of child development

How a helpless infant grows and develops into a fully functioning independent adult has fascinated scientists for years. Three pioneering researchers in this area whose theories are widely accepted are Sigmund Freud, Erik Erikson, and Jean Piaget (Table 5–1). Their theories present human development as a series of overlapping stages that occur in somewhat predictable patterns in an individual's life. It is important to remember that these stages are only approximations of what is likely to happen at various ages in a child's life, and that each child's development may differ from these in varying degrees.

SIGMUND FREUD

Most modern psychologists base their understanding of children at least partly on the work of Sigmund Freud. His theories are concerned primarily with the child's sexual development and appreciation of his own body, and his relationships to others.

ORAL STAGE (AGE 0 TO 2 YEARS)

The newborn first relates almost entirely to its mother (or someone taking a motherly role), and the first experiences with body satisfaction come through the mouth. This is true not only of sucking, but also of making noises, crying, and, often, breathing. It is through the mouth that the baby expresses its needs and finds satisfaction, and thus first begins to make sense of the world.

ANAL STAGE (AGE 2 TO 3 YEARS)

This is the child's first encounter with the serious need to learn self-control and to take responsibility. Toilet training looms large in the minds of many people as a very important phase in childhood. Because elimination is one of the child's first experiences of creativity, it represents the beginnings of the desire to mold and control the environment—the mudpie period in a person's life.

Cleanliness and a child's natural pride in what he has created do not always go together, so that it is necessary to help direct his pride and interest into more acceptable behaviors. This is an important part of learning to take part in society. Playing with such materials as modeling clay, crayons, and dough helps put the child's natural interests to good use, a process called *sublimation*.

PHALLIC (INFANT GENITAL) STAGE (AGE 3 TO 5 YEARS)

It is only natural that interest moves to the genital area as a source of pride and curiosity. To the child's mind, this area constitutes the big difference between boys and girls, a difference that he is beginning to be aware of socially.

Until this time, girls and boys enjoy the same toys and games, and are treated somewhat alike. Now, the boy begins to take pride in being a male and the girl in being a female. In many families a new brother or sister arrives at about this time, arousing the child's natural interest in human origins. A hospital setting can prompt questions that might be delayed or avoided at home, and can also provide answers the child might not get at home.

This is the age when the child begins to understand what it means to be a boy or a girl. Parents' reaction to the child's genital exploration can determine whether the child learns to feel satisfied with himself as a sexual being, or is laden with feelings of guilt and dissatisfaction all his life.

For most children of this age, boys as well as girls, playing with dolls is a way of working out family relationships and expressing feelings that naturally build up, without fear of punishment.

OEDIPAL STAGE (AGE 5 TO 6 YEARS)

This is a time of conflict in the child's emotional relationships with his parents. The conflict occurs between attachment to and imitation of the parent of the same sex, and the appeal of the other parent. The boy who for years has depended on his mother for all his emotional and physical needs is now confronted by his desire to be a man. The girl, who has imitated her mother, now finds her father a real attraction. This is not only social, but sexual; it is through contact with parents that the child learns to relate to the opposite sex. This is not just a physical interest but

TABLE 5–1. COMPARATIVE SUMMARY OF FREUD, ERIKSON, AND PIAGET THEORIES

Age	Stage	Erikson (Psychosocial Development)	Freud (Psychosexual Development)	Piaget (Intellectual Development)
1	Infancy	Trust vs mistrust	Oral stage	Sensorimotor phase
2	Toddlerhood	Autonomy vs shame	Anal stage	Preoperational phase
3		Initiative vs guilt		
4	Preschool age (early childhood)		Infant genital stage	
5			Oedipal stage	
6			Latency stage	
7	School age (middle childhood)	Industry vs inferiority		Concrete operational phase
8				
9				
10				
11			Genital stage (puberty)	Formal operational phase
12				
13	Adolescence	Identity vs identity confusion		
14				
15				
16				
17				
18				
	Early adulthood	Intimacy vs isolation		
	Young and middle adulthood	Generativity vs self-absorption		
	Later adulthood (Senescence)	Ego integrity vs despair		

a need to learn the interests, attitudes, concerns, and wishes of the opposite sex.

A child usually feels rather ambivalent at this age, sometimes wanting the comfort and support of his own sex, at other times disdaining it. It is also the time when embarrassment begins, when a boy may be acutely embarrassed by having a female nurse insert a rectal thermometer, but would be less uncomfortable having a man do it.

LATENCY STAGE (AGE 6 TO 10 YEARS)

This is the time of primary schooling, when the child is preparing for adult life but must await maturity to exercise his own initiative in adult living. It is the time when the child's sense of moral responsibility (the *superego*) is built, based on what he has been taught through words and actions by his parents.

When placed in an unfamiliar setting, children in this stage may become confused because they do not know what is expected of them. They need the sense of security that comes from approval and praise, and usually respond favorably to a brief explanation of "how we do things here."

GENITAL STAGE (AGE 11 TO 13 YEARS)

Physical puberty continues to occur at an increasingly early age, and social puberty occurs even earlier, due largely to the influence of sexual frankness on television, in movies, and in print media. At puberty, all the child's earlier learning is concentrated on the powerful biologic drive, finding and relating to a mate. In earlier societies, mating and forming a family took place at a young age. Our society delays mating for many years after puberty, creating a time of confusion and turmoil during which biologic readiness must take second place to educational and economic goals. This is a sensitive period when privacy is very important, and great uncertainty exists about relating to any members of the opposite sex.

ERIK ERIKSON

Building on Freud's theories, Erikson describes human psychosocial development as a series of tasks or crises. This development depends on a self-healing process within the individual that helps counterbalance the stresses created by natural and accidental crises. The self-healing process is delayed by any major crisis, such as hospitalization, which interrupts normal development. Interruptions may cause regression to an earlier stage, such as the older child who begins to wet the bed when hospitalized. Erikson comments that "children 'fall apart' repeatedly, and unlike Humpty Dumpty, grow together again," if they are given time and sympathy, and are not interfered with.[2]

Erikson formulated a series of eight developmental tasks or crises, the first five of which pertain to children and youth. In each, the individual must master the central problem before moving on to the next one. Each holds positive and negative counterparts, and each implies new developmental tasks for parents (Table 5–2).

TRUST VERSUS MISTRUST (AGE 0 TO 1 YEAR)

The infant has no way to control his world other than crying for help and hoping for rescue. During the first year, the child learns whether the world can be trusted to give love and concern, or only frustration, fear, and despair. The infant who is fed on demand learns to trust that his cries will be answered. The baby fed according to the schedule of hospital or mother does not understand the importance of routine but only that his cries may go unanswered.

AUTONOMY VERSUS DOUBT AND SHAME (AGE 1 TO 3 YEARS)

Even the smallest child wants to feel like an individual, and needs to learn to "do it himself," even when this takes a long time or makes a mess. The toddler gains reassurance from feeding himself, from crawling or walking alone where it is safe, and being free to handle and learn about things in his environment.

Just as the toddler explores his environment, he begins to explore and learn about his body. If parents react appropriately to this very normal behavior, the child will gain self-respect and pride. If, however, they shame him for responding to this natural curiosity, he will sustain the feeling that somehow he is "dirty, nasty, and bad."

INITIATIVE VERSUS GUILT (AGE 3 TO 6 YEARS)

During this period, the child engages in active, assertive play. His steadily improving physical coordination and expanding social skills encourage "showing off" to gain adult attention, and, he hopes, approval. Still very self-centered, he plays by himself, though in the company of other children. Interaction comes later. These children want to know what the rules are, and enjoy "being good" and the adult approval that action gains. During this time, the child develops a conscience, and accepts punishment for doing wrong because it relieves his feelings of guilt.

Children in this phase of development generally do not have a concept of time and the changes it imposes on nursing shifts. Explaining that it is time for a nurse to go

---

TABLE 5–2.   CHILD AND PARENT DEVELOPMENT

Stage of Child Development (Erikson)	Stage of Parent Development	Parental Task
I. Infant—trust	Learning the cues	To interpret infant needs
II. Toddler —autonomy	Learning to accept growth and development	To accept some loss of control while maintaining necessary limits
III. Preschooler —initiative	Learning to separate	To allow independent development while modeling necessary standards
IV. School-age —industry	Learning to accept rejection without deserting	To be there when needed without intruding unnecessarily
V. Teenager —identity	Learning to build a new life, having been thoroughly discredited by one's teenager	To adjust to changing family roles and relationships during and after the teenager's struggle to establish an identity

(Wieczorek R, Natapoff J: A Conceptual Approach to the Nursing of Children: Health Care From Birth Through Adolescence. Philadelphia, JB Lippincott, 1981)

home to her family can help an unhappy child realize that the nurse is not deserting him because he was naughty.

INDUSTRY VERSUS INFERIORITY (AGE 6 TO 12 YEARS)

Children begin to seek achievement in this phase. They learn to interact with others, and sometimes to compete with them. They like activities they can follow through to completion and tangible results.

Competition is healthy as long as the standards are not so high that the child feels he has no chance of winning. Praise, not criticism, helps the child to build his self-esteem and avoid feelings of inferiority. It is important to emphasize that everyone is a unique person and deserves to be appreciated for his or her own special qualities.

IDENTITY VERSUS IDENTITY CONFUSION (AGE 12 TO 18 YEARS)

The adolescent is confronted by marked physical and emotional changes, and the knowledge that soon he will be responsible for his own life. He develops a sense of being an independent individual with his own ideals and goals, and may feel that the adults in his world refuse to grant that independence. He may break rules just to prove that he can. Stress, anxiety, and mood swings are typical of this phase. Relationships with peers are more important than ever.

INTIMACY VERSUS ISOLATION (EARLY ADULTHOOD)

This is the period during which the individual tries to establish intimate personal relationships with friends and an intimate love relationship with one person. Difficulty in establishing intimacy results in feelings of isolation.

GENERATIVITY VERSUS SELF-ABSORPTION (YOUNG AND MIDDLE ADULTHOOD)

For many people, this phase means marriage and family, but for others it may mean fulfillment in some other way—a professional or business career, or a religious vocation. The person who does not find this fulfillment becomes self-absorbed, and ceases to develop socially.

EGO INTEGRITY VERSUS DESPAIR (OLD AGE)

This final phase is the least understood of all, for it means finding satisfaction with oneself, one's achievements, and present condition, without regret for the past or fear for the future.

JEAN PIAGET

Freud and Erikson studied psychosexual and psychosocial development of humans; Piaget brought new insight into intellectual (cognitive) development—how a child learns and develops that quality called intelligence. He describes intellectual development as a sequence of four principal stages, each made up of several substages.[3] All children move through these stages in the same order, but each at his or her own individual pace.

SENSORIMOTOR (AGE 0 TO 2 YEARS)

The newborn behaves at a sensorimotor level linked entirely to his desires for physical satisfaction. He feels, hears, sees, tastes, and smells countless new things, and moves his body in an apparently random way. His purposeful activities are controlled by reflexive responses to the environment. For example, while nursing, he gazes intently at his mother's face, grasps her finger, smells the nipple and tastes the milk, thus involving all his senses.

As the infant grows, he gains an understanding of cause and effect. When random arm motions strike the string of bells stretched across his crib, he hears the sound that is made, and eventually is able to manipulate his arms to deliberately make the bells ring.

In the same way, a newborn cannot understand words or even the tone of voice, but only through hearing conversation directed to him can he pick out sounds and begin to understand. As he produces noises with his own mouth, the response of those near him encourage him, and eventually help him learn to talk.

PREOPERATIONAL (AGE 2 TO 7 YEARS)

The child in this phase of development is *egocentric*; that is, he cannot put himself in another's place. He interprets the world from his own point of view and in terms of what he can see, hear, or otherwise experience directly.

This child has no conception of quantity; if it looks like more, it *is* more. Four ounces of juice poured into two glasses looks like more than four ounces in one glass. His sense of time is not developed, and thus he cannot always tell whether something happened a day ago, a week ago, or a year ago.

CONCRETE OPERATIONS (AGE 7 TO 11 YEARS)

During this stage, children develop the ability to begin problem solving in a concrete, systematic way. They can classify and organize information about their environment, and they begin to understand that volume or weight can remain the same even though the appearance changes, unlike in the preoperational stage. These children can consider another's point of view, and can deal simultaneously with more than one aspect of a situation.

FORMAL OPERATIONS (AGE 12 TO 15 YEARS)

The adolescent is capable of dealing with ideas, abstract concepts described only in words or symbols. He begins to understand jokes based on double meanings, and enjoys reading and discussing theories and philosophies. He can observe and then draw logical conclusions from his observations.

OTHER THEORISTS

Freud, Erikson, and Piaget are only three of the many researchers who have studied the development of children and families. During the 1940s and 1950s, Arnold Gesell studied many infants and talked with their parents concerning children's behavior. From his studies emerged a series of developmental landmarks that are still considered valid and the observation that children progress through a series of "easy" and "difficult" phases as they develop. For example, he labeled one period the "terrible twos," the time when a toddler begins to assert his new mobility and coordination to gain parental attention, even if the attention is unfavorable. Knowing that these cycles are normal makes it easier for parents to cope.

Carl Jung's contribution to the study of child growth and development focused on the inner sequence of events that shape personality. He emphasized that human development follows predetermined patterns called *archetypes*. These archetypes replace the instinctive behavior present in other animal life. Interaction of the archetypes with the outside environment is evident throughout human life. For example, a normal child learns to suck, crawl, walk, talk, without any instruction, but the details of how he does these things come from observation and imitation of others.

The interaction of inner development and environment is particularly clear in studies of young children who have been deprived in some way. Bowlby's studies of children who were not held or loved, and Bettelheim's studies of children given good physical care but little or no emotional satisfaction, indicate how vital psychological interaction is.

Jung believes that the first 3 years of a child's life are spent in coordinating experiences and learning to make a conscious personality, a distinct person who is separate from the rest of the environment. In the following years, the child learns to make sense of his environment by associating new discoveries to his general approach to the world. Dreams and nightmares help to express developments of the personality, which for some reason do not find a conscious outlet.

According to Jung, the principal psychological task of the first half of life (up to age 40) is one of learning to adapt to the environment and to society. This is the first half of the process of *individuation*, of becoming a real individual.

During the second half of life, the main task is to come to grips with the many areas of personality development that had been put aside in the interests of a career or marriage. This involves the formation of new attitudes, new values, and a discovery that the center of life is within the spirit of the individual and not in the material world or in other people.

Jung points out that what happens to a child is not so critical to the child's development as the responses to these happenings. A hospital experience can permanently scar a child's personality if the child's natural feeling of terror is overlooked. It may be accepted and even become a point of pride, however, if carried out in an atmosphere of assurance and support of the child's emotional concern, and need for love and acceptance.

summary

Research studies continue to explore how children and parents develop together, and what specific skills and abilities children acquire at various ages. It is now recognized that infants respond to parents from birth, and parents, in turn, respond to infants' behavior. Nurses and other health professionals must understand those patterns of response to contribute to the healthy growth and development of children and families.

review questions

1. What is the primary purpose of the family?
2. How does the child learn who he is?
3. What have studies shown about parents who abuse their children?
4. What are the developmental tasks formulated by Erikson?
5. What is meant by the term cognitive?
6. What are the four principal stages of intellectual development formulated by Piaget?

references

1. Deters GE: Circadian rhythm phenomenon. Am J Mat Child Nurs 5:249–251, 1980
2. Erikson EH, Senn MJE: Symposium on the Healthy Personality. New York, Macy Foundation, 1958
3. Piaget J: The Language and Thought of the Child. Cleveland, World Publishing, 1967

bibliography

Austin J: Family-centered discharge planning classes. Am J Mat Child Nurs 5:96–97, 1980

The American family: Bent but not broken. U.S. News and World Report 88:48–50, 1980

Bee HL: The Developing Child. New York, Harper & Row, 1978

Bettleheim B: Love Is Not Enough. New York, Macmillan, 1970

Bowlby J: Attachment. New York, Basic Books, 1969

Brazelton TB: On Becoming a Family. New York, Delacorte, 1981

Cameron JR: Parental treatment, children's temperament and the risk of childhood behavioral problems, II, Am J Orthopsychiatr 48, No. 1:41–43, 1978

Duvall EM: Family Development, 4th ed. Philadelphia, JB Lippincott, 1971

Erikson EH: Childhood and Society, 2nd ed. New York, Norton, 1963

Fong B, Resnick M: The Child: Development Through Adolescence. Palo Alto, Addison-Wesley, 1980

Friedman S, Hoekelman R: Behavioral Pediatrics. New York, McGraw-Hill, 1980

Hymovich D, Bernard M: Family Health Care: General Perspectives, Vol 1. 2nd ed. New York, McGraw-Hill, 1979

Lowry GH: Growth and Development of Children. Chicago, Year Book Publishers, 1978

Marano HE: Biology is one key to the bonding of mothers and babies. Smithsonian 12, No. 2:60–69, 1981

Miner R: The story of a father who tried to be a mother. Family Health 12, No. 2:36–42, 1980

Palmer JD: An Introduction to Biological Rhythms. New York, Academic Press, 1976

Petrillo M, Sanger S: Emotional Care of Hospitalized Children, 2nd ed. Philadelphia, JB Lippincott, 1980

Schuster C, Ashburn S: The Process of Human Development. Boston, Little, Brown & Co, 1980

Smith DD, Burman E, Robinson E: The Biologic Ages of Man from Conception Through Old Age. Philadelphia, WB Saunders, 1978

growth and development of the infant: 28 days to 1 year

6

student objectives

The student successfully attaining the goals of this chapter will be able to

1 Define the following vocabulary terms:

"bottle mouth" caries   deciduous teeth   fontanel   immunization
ossification   pedodontist   weaning

2 Describe the growth and development of the infant in the following areas: personal–social development, fine motor skills, gross motor skills, language development, and cognition.

3 Identify the age at which the average infant can be expected to, 1) double his birth weight, 2) experience eruption of the first deciduous teeth, and 3) begin eating solid foods.

4 Describe the recommended immunization schedule for infants, listing each immunization and the approximate age at which it should be administered.

5 Describe the infant's nutritional need for iron and explain how it may be added to his diet.

6 Describe the problems that long-term hospitalization may cause in the development of the infant and discuss two ways that the nurse can help to solve these problems.

The infant who has lived through the first month of life has a busy year ahead. During this year he grows and develops skills at a faster rate than he ever will again. In the short span of a single year, this tiny, helpless bit of humanity becomes an individual with strong emotions of fear, jealousy, anger, and love, and the ability to rise from a supine to an upright position and move about purposefully.

Both weight and height increase very rapidly. During the first 6 months the infant doubles his birth weight and adds about 6 inches to his height. Growth slows slightly during the second 6 months, but is still rapid. By 1 year of age, the infant triples his birth weight, and adds 10 to 12 inches to his height.

It is misleading to think in terms of the "average" child. To determine whether an infant is reaching acceptable levels of development, he must be evaluated in relation to his own birth weight and height. A baby weighing 6 pounds at birth cannot be expected to weigh as much at 5 or 6 months as the baby who weighed 9 pounds at birth, but each is expected to double his own birth weight at about this time. A growth graph is helpful to the nurse or pediatrician for assessing a child's progress.

Table 6–1 gives the average heights and weights of children from birth to age 11 years. This table is based on the average heights and weights of a sampling of white, North American children whose growth ranges from the 5th to the 95th percentile for their ages.

physical development

HEAD AND SKULL

At birth an infant's head circumference is usually slightly larger than his chest circumference. At about 1 year of age, both become approximately equal. The head of the newborn averages about 13¾ inches or 35 cm in circumference. Chest circumference measures approximately the same as the abdomen and less than that of the head.

The head increases in circumference to approximately 18 inches or 47 cm at 1 year of age. The chest also grows rapidly, catching up to the head circumference at about 5 to 7 months of age. From then on it can be expected to exceed the head in circumference.

FONTANELES AND CRANIAL SUTURES

The posterior fontanel is usually closed by the second or third month of life. The anterior fontanel may increase slightly in size during the first few months of life. After the sixth month it begins to decrease in size, becoming closed between the 12th and 18th months. The sutures between the cranial bones do not ossify until later childhood.

SKELETAL GROWTH AND MATURATION

During fetal life the skeletal system is completely formed in cartilage at the end of 3 months gestation. Ossification and growth of bones occur during the remainder of fetal life and throughout childhood. The pattern of maturation is so regular that the "bone age" can be determined by radiologic examination. When the bone age matches the child's chronological age, the skeletal structure is maturing at a normal rate. Radiologic examination is performed *only* if a problem is suspected, to avoid unnecessary exposure to radiation.

ERUPTION OF DECIDUOUS TEETH

Calcification of the primary, or deciduous, teeth starts early in fetal life. Shortly before birth, calcification begins in those permanent teeth that will be the first to erupt in later childhood. On the average the first deciduous teeth erupt between 6 and 8 months of age. The first to erupt are usually the lower central incisors.

Babies in good health and showing normal development may differ in timing of tooth eruption. Some families show a tendency toward very early or very late eruption, without other signs of early or late development. Figure 6–1 shows the eruption pattern of the deciduous teeth.

Nutritional deficiency or prolonged illness in infancy may interfere with calcification of both the deciduous and the permanent teeth. The role of fluoride in strengthening calcification of teeth has been well documented. In areas where the fluoride content of drinking water is inadequate or absent, its administration to infants and children is recommended by the American Dental Association.

CIRCULATORY SYSTEM

During the first year of life the circulatory system undergoes several changes. During fetal life a high level of hemoglobin and of red blood cells was necessary for adequate oxygenation. After birth when oxygen is supplied through the respiratory system, hemoglobin decreases in volume and red blood cells gradually decrease in number until the third month of life. Thereafter the count gradually increases until adult levels are reached.

Blood pressure is extremely difficult to obtain with accuracy in an infant. The flush method is sometimes used when a reading of the systolic blood pressure is desired. Average blood pressure during the first year of life is 85/60. However, variability can be expected to exist among children of the same age and body build (Table 6–2).

An accurate count of the infant's heartbeat requires an apical pulse count. Place a stethoscope over the left chest in a position where the heartbeat can be clearly heard, and count for 1 full minute (Fig. 6–2). During the first year of life an average apical beat ranges from 70 (asleep) to 150 (awake), and up to 180 while crying.

BODY TEMPERATURE AND RESPIRATION RATE

Body temperature follows the average normal range after the initial adjustment to postnatal living. Respirations average 30 per minute, with a wide range according to the infant's activity.

MATURATION AND DEVELOPMENT

As the infant grows, his nerve cells mature, his fine muscles learn to coordinate, and he follows an orderly pattern of development. Naturally his parents are full of pride if he learns to sit or stand before the neighbor's baby, but actu-

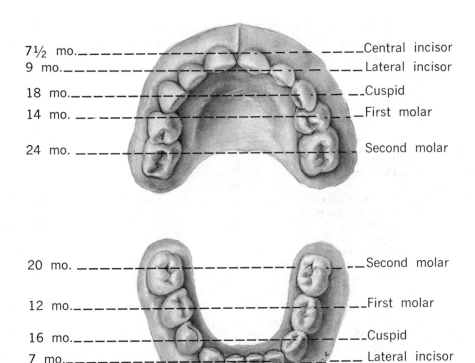

7½ mo. _Central incisor
9 mo. _ _ _ _ _ _ _ _ _ _ _ _ _ _ _ _ _ _ _Lateral incisor
18 mo. _ _ _ _ _ _ _ _ _ _ _ _ _ _ _ _ _ _Cuspid
14 mo. _ _ _ _ _ _ _ _ _ _ _ _ _ _ _ _ _First molar
24 mo. _ _ _ _ _ _ _ _ _ _ _ _ _ _ _ Second molar

20 mo. _ _ _ _ _ _ _ _ _ _ _ _ _ _ _ _ _Second molar
12 mo. _ _ _ _ _ _ _ _ _ _ _ _ _ _ _ _ _First molar
16 mo. _ _ _ _ _ _ _ _ _ _ _ _ _ _ _ _ _Cuspid
7 mo. _ _ _ _ _ _ _ _ _ _ _ _ _ _ _ _ _Lateral incisor
6 mo. _ _ _ _ _ _ _ _ _ _ _ _ _ _ _ _ _ _Central incisor

FIG. 6–1. Approximate ages for the eruption of deciduous teeth.

TABLE 6–1. AVERAGE BOY–GIRL HEIGHTS AND WEIGHTS OF CHILDREN 0–11 YEARS

Age	Height (in inches)		Weight (in lbs)	
	5th p	95th p	5th p	95th p
Birth	18.4	20.9	5.6	9.0
1 mo	19.7	22.7	7.0	10.5
3 mo	22.4	25.2	10.0	15.2
6 mo	24.9	28.0	14.1	20.6
9 mo	26.8	29.9	16.1	24.6
1 yr	28.0	31.6	18.1	26.9
2 yr	31.9	36.6	22.8	32.6
3 yr	35.3	40.0	26.7	38.1
4 yr	38.2	43.3	29.4	42.8
5 yr	40.5	46.3	32.6	48.6
6 yr	42.8	49.0	35.8	54.7
7 yr	44.7	51.3	39.3	62.6
8 yr	46.7	53.9	43.2	71.4
9 yr	48.5	56.5	46.6	81.3
10 yr	50.3	59.2	49.8	93.2
11 yr	51.9	61.5	54.4	105.6

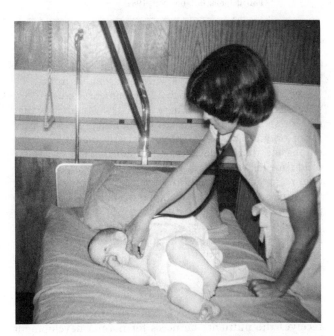

FIG. 6–2. Listening to heart sounds in an infant. (Courtesy of Wieczorek R, Natapoff J: A Conceptual approach to the Nursing of Children: Health Care From Birth Through Adolescence. Philadelphia, JB Lippincott, 1981)

TABLE 6-2.   SELECTED VALUES OF BLOOD PRESSURE, BLOOD COUNT, AND SPINAL FLUID DURING INFANCY

	Age			
	Birth	**2 Weeks**	**3 Months**	**1 Year**
Pulse	70-170/min	120-140/min		80-140/min
Blood pressure	60-90 systolic			60-120 systolic
	20-60 diastolic			50-70 diastolic
Red blood cells (millions/cu mm)	4.9-5.5	4.5-5.5	3.9-4.8	4.5-5.0
Hemoglobin (g/100 ml)	16-20	14-17	10.5-11.5	12-13
Hematocrit (%)	44-64		35-49	30-40
White blood cells (thousands/cu mm)	10-20	8-12	5-9	6-10
Lymphocytes (%)	30-45	45-55	50-60	50-60
Platelets (thousands/cu mm)	200-300	350	200-300	250-350
Spinal fluid Pressure				70-200 mm H_2O
Cell count				0-10 (lymphocytes)
Protein (mg/100 ml)	20-120			15-40
Sugar (mg/100 ml)				50-90
Chlorides (mg/100 ml)				650-750

(Wieczorek R, Natapoff J: A Conceptual Approach to the Nursing of Children: Health Care From Birth Through Adolescense. Philadelphia, JB Lippincott, 1981)

ally such precocity means very little. Each child follows his own rhythm of progress within reasonable limits.

Average rates of growth and development are useful for purposes of evaluation. There are a few landmarks that call for special attention, even though their absence may mean only a lack of environmental stimulation. Do not emphasize routine developmental tables with parents; a mild time lag will probably mean nothing. A large lag may require greater stimulation from the environment or a watchful attitude to discover how overall development is proceeding.

Table 6-3 summarizes accepted norms for development in personal-social, motor, language, and cognitive behavior for the first year of life.

nutrition

Except for vitamins C and D, and iron, the young infant receives the nutrients he needs for normal development from milk, either breast milk or modified cow's milk formula. A healthy, full-term infant will have stored enough iron in his tissues to supply him for about the first 4 months. The American Academy of Pediatrics Committee on Nutrition recommends that, not later than 4 months of age in a term infant, iron supplements be added to all infants' diets. These supplements can come from iron-fortified cereal or formula, or medicinal iron. Premature infants will need iron supplements by 2 months of age since their stores were inadequate at birth.

Vitamins C and D need to be added to the infant's milk in the form of vitamin drops. Daily amounts required for nutritional health remain constant during the first year, and these are 30 mg of vitamin C and 400 units of vitamin D.

Fluoride is needed in minute quantities for strengthening calcification of the teeth and preventing tooth decay. In areas where the water supply is deficient in fluoride, a solution of sodium fluoride can be given by mouth, or vitamin-fluoride drops can be used.

ADDITION OF SOLID FOODS

There is no exact time or order for starting solid foods. About 4 to 6 months of age, however, the infant's iron supply becomes low and he needs supplements of iron-rich foods. Guidelines for introducing new foods into an infant's diet are provided in Table 6-4.

INFANT FEEDING

The baby knows only one way to take food, and that is to thrust his tongue forward as if to suck, which has the effect of pushing the solid food right out of his mouth (Fig. 6–3). The process of transferring food from the front of the mouth to the throat for swallowing is a complicated skill that must be learned. The eager, hungry baby is quite puzzled over this new turn of events, and is apt to become frustrated and annoyed, protesting loudly and clearly. It is best, therefore, to let the very hungry baby take the edge off his appetite with part of his formula before proceeding with this new experience. If a mother understands that pushing food out with the tongue does not mean rejection, she can be patient.

The baby's clothing (and his mother's too) needs protection when he is sitting in his mother's arms. A small spoon fits his mouth better than a large one, and makes it easier to put food further back on the tongue, but not far enough to make the baby gag. The mother needs to catch the food if it is pushed out and offer it again, but her baby soon learns how to manipulate his tongue, and comes to enjoy this novel way of eating.

Foods are started in small amounts, one or two teaspoonsful daily. Babies like their food smooth, thin, lukewarm, and bland. The choice of mealtime does not matter. It works best, at first, to offer one food for several days until the baby becomes accustomed to it before introducing another.

When the teeth commence to erupt, the infant appreciates a piece of zwieback or toast to practice chewing on. About this time chopped foods can be substituted for pureed foods. The formula will probably be changed to whole milk or reconstituted evaporated milk around 4 to 6 months of age. The infant will soon commence to learn to drink from a cup, although he doubtless will derive comfort from sucking at breast or bottle for some time to come.

PREPARATION OF FOODS

A great variety of pureed baby foods, chopped junior foods and prepared milk formulas, are on the market, and they certainly relieve the mother of much preparation time. It should be remembered, however, that prepared foods involve a considerable expense that many families can ill afford.

The nurse can point out that vegetables and fruits can be cooked and strained at home, and are just as well accepted by the baby. Cereals can be cooked, and formulas prepared at home as well. Some families prefer to spend more for convenience and economize elsewhere, but no one should be made to feel that a baby's health or well-being depends on commercially prepared foods.

The well baby's appetite is the best index of the proper amount of food. Healthy babies enjoy eating and accept most foods, but not strong-flavored or bitter foods. If the baby shows a definite dislike for any particular food, there is no point in forcing it, because this is one of the best ways to make certain that he sees feeding time as an occasion for a battle of will power. However, a dislike for a certain food does not need to be permanent, and the re-

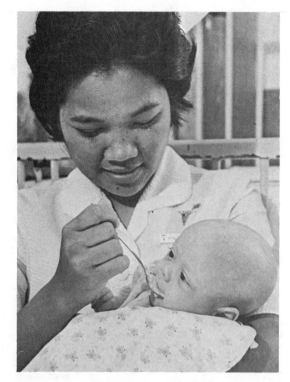

FIG. 6–3.   A baby tends to push his first solids out of his mouth with his tongue.

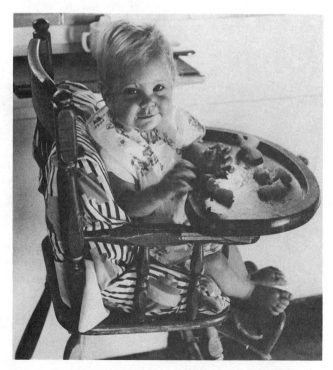

FIG. 6–4.   This child is feeding herself. (Photo by Carol Baldwin)

TABLE 6–3.   GROWTH AND DEVELOPMENT CHART: THE INFANT

Age	Personal–Social	Fine Motor
Birth– 4 weeks	Some smiling Begins Erikson's stage of "trust vs mistrust"	Grasp reflex very strong Hands flexed
6 weeks	Smiling in response to familiar stimuli	Hands open Less flexion noted
10– 12 weeks	Aware of new environment Less crying Smiles at significant others	No longer has grasp reflex Pulls on clothes, blanket, but does not reach for them
16 weeks	Responses to stimulus Sees bottle, squeals, laughs Aware of new environment and shows interest	Grasps objects with two hands Grasps objects in crib voluntarily and brings them to mouth Eye– hand coordination beginning
20 weeks	Smiles at self in the mirror Cries when limits are set or when objects are taken away	Holds one object while looking at another one Grasps objects wanted
24 weeks	Likes to be picked up Knows family from strangers Plays "peek-a-boo" Knows what he likes and dislikes	Holds bottle fairly well Tries to retrieve a dropped article
28 weeks	Fear of strangers Imitates simple acts Responds to "no" Shows preferences and dislikes for food	Holds cup Transfers objects from one hand to the other
32 weeks	Dislikes diaper and clothing change Afraid of strangers Fear of separating from mother	Adjusts body position to be able to reach for an object May stand up holding on
36 weeks	Imitates waving "bye-bye" Repeats facial expressions; cries when yelled at	Releases objects with flexed wrist Good finger and thumb grasp
40 weeks– 1 year	Does things to attract attention Tries to follow when being read to Imitates parents Looks for objects not in sight	Holds tool with one hand and works on it with another Puts toy in box after demonstration Stacks blocks Holds crayon to scribble on paper

jected food may be offered again at a later date. The important point is to avoid making an issue of likes or dislikes.

SELF-FEEDING

The infant has an overpowering urge to investigate and to learn. He early grabs the spoon from his mother, examines and mouths it. He also sticks his fingers in his food to feel the texture and to bring it to his mouth for tasting (Fig. 6– 4). All this is an essential, although messy, part of his learning experience. After preliminary testing, his next task is to try feeding himself. He soon finds the motions involved in getting a spoon right side up into his mouth are too complex for him, and he drops the spoon in favor of his fingers. But he returns to the spoon again and again until he eventually succeeds in getting some food from spoon to mouth at least part of the time. The nurse can

TABLE 6–3.   (*Continued*)

Gross Motor	Language	Cognition
Catches and holds objects in sight which cross visual field Can turn head from side to side when lying in a prone position When prone, body in a flexed position When prone, moves extremities in a crawling fashion	Cries when upset Makes enjoyment sounds during mealtimes	At 1 month sucking activity associated with pleasureful sensations
Tries to raise shoulders and arms when stimulated Holds head up when prone Less flexion of entire body when prone	Cooing is predominant Smiles to familiar voices Babbling	***Primary Circular Reactions*** Begins to repeat actions
No longer has Moro reflex Symmetrical body positioning Pumps arms, shoulders, head from prone position	Makes noises when spoken to	Beginning of coordinated responses to different kinds of stimuli
Plays with hands Brings objects to mouth Balances head and body for a short period in sitting position	Laughing aloud Sounds "n," "k," "g," "p," "b"	Likes social situations Defiant, bored if unattended
Able to sit up Can roll over Can bear weight on legs when held in a standing position	Cooing noises Squeals with delight	Visually looks for an object that has fallen
Able to control head movements Tonic neck reflex disappears Sits alone in high chair, back erect Rolls over and back to abdomen	Makes sounds "guh, bah" Sounds "p," "m," "b," "t" are pronounced Bubbling sounds Babbling decreases Duplicates "ma-ma" "pa-pa" sounds	***Secondary Circular Reactions*** Repeats actions that affect an object Beginning of object permanence
Reaches without visual guidance Can lift head up when in a supine position		
Crawls around Pulls toy toward self	Combines syllables but has trouble attributing meaning to them	
Creeping around; stands when holding onto furniture Pulls self to stand Sits up Recovers balance when falls over	Imitates sounds Knows what "no" means	Now aware that objects are separate from self ***Secondary Circular Reactions*** Actions memorized
Stands alone; begins to walk alone Can change self from prone to sitting to standing position	Words emerge Says "da-da" "ma-ma" with meaning	Coordination of secondary schemes; masters barrier to reach goal; symbolic meaning

help mothers understand that all this is not messing, to be forbidden, but rather it is a very necessary part of the infant's learning.

WEANING THE INFANT

Weaning, either from breast or bottle, needs to be attempted gradually without fuss or strain. The infant is still testing his environment, and an abrupt removal of his main source of satisfaction—sucking—before he has conquered his basic distrust of his environment may prove detrimental to his normal development. The speed with which weaning is accomplished should be suited to the individual infant's readiness to give up this form of pleasure for a more mature way of life.

At the age of 5 or 6 months, the infant who has watched others drink from a cup will usually be ready to try a sip

TABLE 6–4. INTRODUCING NEW FOODS INTO AN INFANT'S DIET

When to Introduce	Approximate Total Daily Intake of Solids*	Description of Foods and Hints about Giving Them
4–5 mo (6–7 mo if infant is breastfed)	Dry cereal: Start with ½ tsp (dry measurement), gradually increase to 2–3 Tbsp Vegetables: Start with 1 tsp, gradually increase to 2 Tbsp Fruit: Start with 1 tsp, gradually increase to 2 Tbsp Divide food among 4 feedings per day (if possible)	Cereal: Offer iron-enriched baby cereal or plain Cream of Rice first. Begin with single grains (rice, barley, corn). Mix cereal with an equal amount of breast milk, formula, or water Vegetables: Try a mild-tasting vegetable first (carrots, squash, peas, green beans). Stronger-flavored vegetables (spinach, sweet potatoes) may be tried after the infant accepts some mild-tasting ones Fruits: Mashed ripe banana and unsweetened, cooked, bland fruits (apples, peaches, pears) are usually well-liked. Apple juice and grape juice (unsweetened) may be introduced. Initially, dilute juice with an equal amount of water Introduce one new food at a time and offer it several times before trying another new food Give a new food once a day for a day or two; Increase to twice a day as the infant begins to enjoy the food. Watch for signs of intolerance Include some foods that are good sources of Vitamin C (other than orange juice)
5–6 mo (6–7 mo if infant is breastfed)	Dry cereal: Gradually increase up to 4 Tbsp Fruits and vegetables: gradually increase up to 3 Tbsp of each Meat: Start with 1 tsp and gradually increase to 2 Tbsp Divide food among 4 feedings per day (if possible)	Meat: Offer pureed or milled poultry (chicken or turkey) followed by lean meat (veal, beef); lamb has a stronger flavor and may not be as well-liked initially. Liver is a good source of iron: it may be accepted at the beginning of a meal with a familiar vegetable Continue introducing new cereals, fruits, and vegetables as the infant indicates he is ready to accept them, but always one at a time
6–8 mo (7–9 mo if infant is breastfed)	Dry cereal: Up to ½ c Fruits and vegetables: Up to ¼ to ½ c of each Meats: Up to 3 Tbsp Divide food among 4 feedings per day (if possible)	Soft table foods may be introduced; e.g., mashed potatoes and squash and small pieces of soft, peeled fruits Toasted whole grain or enriched bread may be added when the infant begins chewing If introduction of solids is delayed until now, it is not necessary to use strained fruits and vegetables Continue using *iron-fortified* baby cereals
8–12 mo	Dry cereal: Up to ½ c Bread: About 1 slice Fruits and vegetables: Up to ½ c of each Meat: Up to ¼ c Divide food among 4 feedings per day (if possible)	Table foods may be added gradually. Cut table foods into small pieces. Start with ones that do not require too much chewing (cooked, cut green beans and carrots, noodles, ground meats, tuna fish, soft cheese, plain yogurt). If fish is offered, check closely to be sure there are no bones in the serving Mashed, cooked egg yolk and orange juice may be added at about 9 mo of age Sometimes offer peanut butter or thoroughly cooked dried peas and beans in place of meat

* Some infants do not need or want these amounts of food; some may need a little more food. (Suitor CW, Hunter MF: Nutrition: Principles and Application in Health Promotion, Philadelphia, JB Lippincott, 1980)

for himself when it is offered. He seldom is ready at this point, however, to give up the pleasures of sucking altogether. Forcing the child to give up sucking creates resistance and suspicion. It is better to let the infant follow his own timetable. An infant who takes his food from a dish and his milk from a cup during the day may be reluctant to give up his bedtime bottle. However, many *pedodontists* (dentists who specialize in care and treatment of children's teeth) discourage the bedtime bottle as such intermittant sucking can cause erosion of the enamel on the deciduous teeth, often resulting in a condition known as "bottle mouth" caries.

A few babies, although accepting food from a spoon, resist drinking from a cup. Fruit-flavored yogurt, custards, and other milk dishes will help fill their milk needs until they become accustomed to drinking from a cup.

During the second half of the first year, the infant's milk consumption is not likely to be sufficient to meet his caloric, protein, mineral, and vitamin needs (Table 6–5).

health maintenance

Every infant is entitled to the best possible protection against disease, and because he cannot take the proper precautions himself, parents and health professionals must do it for him. This care extends beyond his daily needs for food, sleep, cleanliness, love, and security, to a concern for his future health and well-being (Table 6–6).

Within a short time, medical science has discovered measures providing immunity against a number of serious or crippling diseases. Means now exist to assure protection against conditions such as diphtheria, smallpox, tetanus, polio, mumps, measles, and German measles (rubella), making it unnecessary to take chances with children's health owing to inadequate immunization.

The chronically ill child may not need to forego this protection, depending on his condition and our present knowledge; but whether he is given immunization, or protected from contact from these diseases, is a matter to be discussed in connection with the condition itself.

IMMUNIZATION SCHEDULE

The Academy of Pediatrics, through its committee on the control of infectious diseases, has recommended a schedule of immunization for healthy children living under normal conditions (Table 6–7). Children with certain chronic or acute conditions, or children who can be expected to be exposed to certain infectious conditions such as typhoid, need a modification of this schedule.

psychosocial development

The very young infant experiences the give-and-take of life when his need for food induces him to seek it actively. Being fed on demand builds his sense of trust in his world. Eventually he becomes aware that every felt need is not always met immediately on demand. Dimly he begins to sense that something outside himself supplies relief. Gradually he learns that through his own efforts and signals, he influences his environment to respond to his de-

TABLE 6–5. RECOMMENDED DIETARY ALLOWANCES FOR INFANTS DURING THE FIRST YEAR

	0–6 Months 6 kg–60 cm	6–12 Months 9 kg–71 cm
Energy (kcal)	115 kcal/kg (690)	105 kcal/kg (945)
Protein (g)	2.2 g/kg (13.2)	2.0 g/kg (18)
Vitamin A (RE)	420* (1400 IU)	400 (2000 IU)
Vitamin D (mcg)	10 (400 IU)	10 (400 IU)
Vitamin E (mg α-TE)	3	4
Ascorbic Acid (mg)	35	35
Folacin (mcg)	30	45
Niacin (mg NE)	6	8
Riboflavin (mg)	0.4	0.6
Thiamin (mg)	0.3	0.5
Vitamin B_6 (mg)	0.3	0.6
Vitamin B_{12} (mcg)	0.5	1.5
Calcium (mg)	360	540
Phosphorus (mg)	240	360
Iodine (mcg)	40	50
Iron (mg)	10	15
Magnesium (mg)	50	70
Zinc (mg)	3	5

* Assumed to be all as retinol in milk during the first 6 months of life. All subsequent intakes are assumed to be half as retinol and half as beta-carotene when calculated from international units. As retinol equivalents, three-fourths are as retinol and one-fourth as beta-carotene. (Anderson L, Dibble MV, Turkki PR, et al: Nutrition in Health and Disease, 17th ed. Philadelphia, JB Lippincott, 1982, adapted from Food and Nutrition Board: Recommended Dietary Allowances. Washington, DC, National Academy of Sciences/National Research Council, 1980)

sires. He is now aware that he and his environment exist separately.

The mother who expects too much too soon from her infant is not encouraging his optimal development. Rather than teaching him the rules of life before he has learned to trust his environment, she is actually teaching him that he gains nothing by his own activity and that the world will not respond to his needs.

Conversely, the mother who rushes to anticipate the infant's every need gives him no opportunity to test his environment. He has difficulty developing the understanding that his own actions have manipulated the environment to suit his desires. Table 6–8 summarizes healthy childrearing patterns during infancy.

No mother is perfect and every ordinary mother is certainly going to misinterpret her infant's signals at times. She may be tired, preoccupied, responding momentarily to her own needs. She may not be able to ease his pain or restlessness, but this too is learning for the baby.

As mentioned earlier, the infant's development depends on a reciprocal relationship between him and his environment, of which parents play the most important role. Table 6–9 summarizes significant parent–infant interactions.

During the first few weeks of life, actions such as kicking or sucking are simple reflex activities. In the next sequential stage, reflexes are coordinated and elaborated. For example, the child's eyes follow his random hand movements (Fig. 6– 5). The infant finds that repetition of chance movements brings interesting changes, and in the latter part of the first year his acts become clearly intentional (Fig. 6– 6). He expects that certain results follow certain actions.

An infant soon learns to connect the smiling face looking down at him with pleasure—being picked up, fed, or bathed. His face lights up and he squirms with anticipation toward anyone who smiles and talks softly with him. In only a few weeks, however, he learns that one particular person is the main source of his comfort and pleasure.

An infant cannot apply abstract reasoning, but understands only through his five senses. As he matures enough to recognize his mother or mother-figure, he becomes fearful when she disappears. Out of sight has always meant, to him, out of existence, and he cannot tolerate this. So he sets about the task of assuring himself that objects and people do not cease to exist when out of sight. This is a very real learning experience upon which his entire attitude toward life depends.

The ancient game of "peek-a-boo" is a universal example of this learning technique. It is also one of the joys of infancy, as the child affirms his ability to control his own disappearance and reappearance. In the same manner by

---

TABLE 6–6.   RECOMMENDED HEALTH MAINTENANCE FOR INFANTS FROM 2 WEEKS TO 1 YEAR OF AGE

Procedure	2 Weeks	2 Months	4 Months	6 Months	9 Months	12 Months
Health history	Take the prenatal and birth history and family and social history; discuss events in first 2 weeks and family concerns.	Update history, including eating, sleeping, and elimination patterns. Discuss family concerns.	Update history; discuss family concerns and infant's reactions to immunizations.	Update history and discuss family concerns.	Same as at 6 months	Same as at 6 months
Physical examination*	Measure height, weight, and head circumference; take infant's temperature; perform a complete physical examination and vision evaluation.	Same as for 2 weeks, except include hearing and vision evaluation	Same as at 2 weeks, with vision evaluation	Same as at 2 weeks, except include hearing and vision evaluation	Same as at 2 weeks, except add dental examination and vision evaluation	Same as at 2 weeks, except include dental examination
Laboratory procedures	PKU check				Hematocrit, hemoglobin, and blood count; sickle cell screening	Urinalysis
Immunizations	None	DPT,† TOP‡	DPT, second TOP	DPT, third TOP		Tuberculin test
Feeding	100– 110 cal/kg/day; discuss feeding method and answer family's questions.	Water is added to feeding; there is now a need for iron in formula if infant is bottle-fed.	May begin adding solids depending on family preference and infant response	Milk, either breast or bottle (24 oz/24 hr); continue or begin solid foods, including finger foods and foods that alleviate sore gums.	May begin to follow family eating patterns. Some infants are ready for cup. Continue use of finger foods.	Infant should follow family eating patterns. Provide foods equal to recommended daily allowances from four food groups. Appetite may begin to decrease. Self-feeding activities may begin (earlier in some, later in others).

TABLE 6–6. (*Continued*)

Procedure	2 Weeks	2 Months	4 Months	6 Months	9 Months	12 Months
Teaching and Counseling§	Discuss normal variations of newborn (*e.g.,* skin color, head shape); need for tactile and visual stimulation; prevention of infection; hygiene; differences in infant temperament; attachment behaviors; and need for consistency (basic trust).	Discuss immunizations and possible reactions; sleep patterns; accident prevention; differences in temperament; visual, tactile, and auditory stimulation; repetition of infant sounds and vocal stimulation; family needs for rest, privacy, and break from routine; need for consistency; and attachment behaviors.	Discuss immunizations and possible reactions; sleep and wake patterns; need for activities to strengthen head (*e.g.,* infant swing); stimulation of all senses; moving baby around in home; and opportunity for movement on floor.	Discuss immunizations and possible reactions; accident prevention; care of minor infections such as colds, diarrhea, and vomiting; teething; family interactions; continued need for stimulation including roughhouse play; need for room to crawl, scoot, and roll over; and fear of strangers.	Discuss accident prevention, including possibility of walking; care of teeth; separation anxiety; surprise toys like jack-in-the-box and separation games like "peek-a-boo"; sound and language stimulation; and child-rearing practices.	Discuss accident prevention (the toddler years are here!); dental care and care of minor accidents (falls, cuts); developing sense of autonomy; satisfaction of curiosity needs; language stimulation; putting-in and taking-out activities; and developing independence and start of temper tantrums.

* Include developmental screening tests of proven reliability and validity such as the Denver Developmental Screening Test or Bayley Scales of Infant Development.

† Diphtheria, pertussis, tetanus

‡ Trivalent oral polio

§ Only highlights of teaching and counseling are given here. Much discussion with the family will center on individual concerns. (Wieczorek R, Natapoff J: A Conceptual Approach to the Nursing of Children: Health Care From Birth Through Adolescence. Philadelphia, JB Lippincott, 1981; data from Chow M, Durand B, Feldman M, et al: Handbook of Pediatric Primary Care. New York, Wiley, 1979; and Kempe CH, Silver HK, O'Brien D: Current Pediatric Diagnosis and Treatment. Los Altos, CA, Lange Medical Publications, 1978)

which he affirms his own existence, he confirms that of others, even when temporarily out of sight.

implications for hospital care

Hospitalization, however brief, hampers the infant's normal pattern of living. As long as he is given sufficient affection and loving care, and is promptly restored to his family, the infant is not likely to suffer any grave psychological problems. Long-term hospitalization, however, can present serious problems, even with the best of care.

Illness in itself is frustrating, causing pain and discomfort, and limits normal activity, none of which the infant can understand. Add to these problems the cold, sterile, unfamiliar atmosphere, and possible lack of cuddling or rocking, and an infant may fail to respond to treatment, despite cleanliness and proper hygiene. When this happens, it becomes readily apparent that touching, rocking, and cuddling a child are essential elements of nursing care (Fig. 6– 7).

Hospitalization can have other adverse effects. The small infant matures largely as a result of his physical development. Hindered from reaching out and responding to his environment, he becomes apathetic and ceases to learn. This is particularly apparent when restraints are necessary to keep the child from undoing surgical procedures or from harming himself. The child in restraints needs an extra measure of love and attention from nurses and parents, and every possible method available to relieve his discomfort.

PARENT–NURSE RELATIONSHIP

The nurse's relationship with parents is most important. Mothers and fathers should be allowed and encouraged to feed their baby, change his diaper, hold him, and participate in his total care as fully as they feel capable of doing. Many parents are timid or frightened, and think that they are not allowed to do this. The nurse should ask the parent if she or he would like to hold or feed the child, being careful not to make the parents feel guilty if they do not feel adequate to the situation.

In the hospital, the infant must cope with discomfort,

TABLE 6–7.   IMMUNIZATION SCHEDULES

Recommended Schedule for Active Immunization of Normal Infants and Children

2 mo	DTP*	TOPV†
4 mo	DTP	TOPV
6 mo	DTP	‡
1 yr		Tuberculin Test§
15 mo	Measles,‖ Rubella‖	Mumps‖
1½ yr	DTP	TOPV
4–6 yr	DTP	TOPV
14–16 yr	Td# —repeat every 10 years	

* DTP—diphtheria and tetanus toxoids combined with pertussis vaccine.

† TOPV—trivalent oral poliovirus vaccine. This recommendation is suitable for breast-fed as well as bottle-fed infants.

‡ A third dose of TOPV is optional but may be given in areas of high endemicity of poliomyelitis.

§ Frequency of repeated tuberculin tests depends on risk of exposure of the child and on the prevalence of tuberculosis in the population group. For the pediatrician's office or outpatient clinic, an annual or biennial tuberculin test, unless local circumstances clearly indicate otherwise, is appropriate. The initial test should be done at the time of, or preceding, the measles immunization.

‖ May be given at 15 months as measles-rubella or measles-mumps-rubella combined vaccines.

#Td—combined tetanus and diphtheria toxoids (adult type) for those more than 6 years of age, in contrast to diphtheria and tetanus (DT) toxoids, which contain a larger amount of diphtheria antigen. *Tetanus toxoid at time of injury:* For clean, minor wounds, no booster dose is needed by a fully immunized child unless more than 10 years have elapsed since the last dose. For contaminated wounds, a booster dose should be given if more than 5 years have elapsed since the last dose.

Concentration and Storage of Vaccines

Because the concentration of antigen varies in different products, the manufacturer's package insert should be consulted regarding the volume of individual doses of immunizing agents.

Because biologics are of varying stability, the manufacturer's recommendations for optimal storage conditions (e.g., temperature, light) should be carefully followed. Failure to observe these precautions may significantly reduce the potency and effectiveness of the vaccines.

(Report of the Committee on Infectious Diseases. Evanston, IL, American Academy of Pediatrics)

pain, and strangeness. Some hospitals permit a parent to live-in with the infant to avoid the additional burden of infant–parent separation. Separation is a very real problem in hospitals where parents are limited to visiting hours with their infants.

PHYSICAL CARE

A child enters the hospital for one purpose only, and that is, to become physically well. It has been demonstrated that a child cannot thrive physically if he is emotionally disturbed or if he is allowed to stagnate mentally. All of his needs must be met as completely as possible.

In meeting the child's emotional needs, one must not neglect physical care. The basic goal remains the same: to restore the child to physical health and return him to his parents.

BATHING

A daily bath is desirable if the infant's condition permits. The hospitalized infant should have his own bath basin, soap, and bathing table. Placing him in the bath rather than giving him a sponge bath, can have a soothing and comforting effect, as long as there are no contraindications to this.

Tub Bath.   Gather together the following equipment before starting:

- large basin or small tub
- mild soap
- clean cotton balls
- soft washcloth
- large, soft towel or small, cotton blanket
- clean diaper and shirt

Water in the basin should be about 95° F to 100° F, measured with a bath thermometer or tested with the elbow. Water should feel comfortably warm to the elbow. Small babies squirm and move about much more than an inexperienced person might expect. (A basic rule is *never* to turn one's back on an infant when the crib side is down.) A sensible precaution when bathing a baby is to put the bath basin into the crib and thus eliminate the need for turning from the baby. Crib mattresses are plastic-covered and sheets can be changed, so that splashed water is no problem (Fig. 6–8).

Before undressing a baby, wash his face with clean water, using either the washcloth or cotton balls. This includes washing eyes and ears. Cotton balls are useful if any discharge is present, as a clean one can be used each time and then discarded.

If dried mucus is present in the anterior nares, a wisp of cotton may be twisted, dipped in clear water, and used for cleaning the nose. This may cause the baby to sneeze and bring down more mucus, which can be wiped away. Applicators should *not* be used in the ordinary cleaning of a baby's eyes, ears, or nose. Injury to the mucous membrane can easily occur as the baby squirms. Any material in the ears or nose that is too deep to remove without probing should only be removed, if necessary, by the use of appropriate instruments in the hands of a trained person.

Next, the baby's scalp may be soaped, then the baby picked up by sliding the hand and arm under him, grasping his head firmly while holding him over the basin to rinse the soap away (Fig. 6–9).

After drying the head, undress the baby and examine him for rashes or excoriations. If the baby's diaper is soiled, the feces should be wiped from his buttocks before placing him into the basin. Then soap the infant's body all over and lift him into the basin, supporting the head and shoulders on your arm. Some nurses prefer to soap the infant with their free hand while he is in the tub because a soapy baby is slippery and difficult to pick up.

If the baby is enjoying this experience, make it a leisurely one, and let him stay in the water for a few minutes

TABLE 6-8. HEALTHY CHILDREARING PATTERNS DURING THE INFANT'S FIRST YEAR OF LIFE

Age of Child	Recommended Childrearing Practices
Birth– 6 wk	Practices include holding the infant frequently, giving the infant a feeling of being loved and cared for, and rocking and soothing the infant.
6 wk– 3½ mo	Giving the infant a feeling of being loved and cared for; giving the infant more things to look at in his environment
3½ – 5 mo	Playing regularly with the child; continuing to give the infant a variety of things to look at; talking to the infant; responding to the infant's cries
5½ – 8 mo	Continuing to give the infant a feeling of being loved and cared for; talking to the infant; putting the infant on the floor more so he can roll and move about
8– 12 mo	Accident-proofing the house; giving the infant maximum access to a living area; supplying the infant with playthings; being available to the infant so he can use the parents in situations he cannot yet handle well; talking to the infant to help develop language

(Adapted from White B: The First Years of Life. Englewood Cliffs, Prentice Hall, 1975)

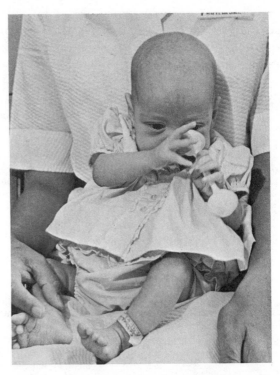

FIG. 6–5. Eye–hand coordination is good at 4 months.

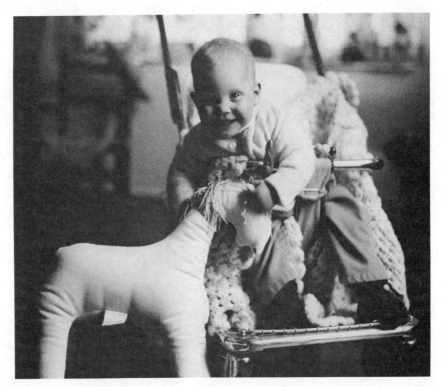

FIG. 6–6. This 5-month-old infant is able to grasp and hold on to the toy of her choice.

TABLE 6–9. PARENT–INFANT ADAPTIVE AND MALADAPTIVE INTERACTIONS

Critical Period	Adaptive	Maladaptive
Feeding behaviors	Offers appropriate amounts and/or types of food to infant Holds infant in comfortable position during feeding Burps baby during and/or after feeding Prepares food appropriately Offers food at a comfortable pace for infant	Provides inadequate types or amounts of food for infant Does not hold infant, or holds in uncomfortable position during feeding Does not burp infant Prepares food inappropriately Offers food at pace too rapid for infant's comfort
Infant stimulation	Provides appropriate verbal stimulation for infant during visit Provides tactile stimulation for infant at times other than during feeding or moving infant away from danger Provides age-appropriate toys Interacts with infant in a way that provides for infant's satisfaction	Provides none or only aggressive verbal stimulation for infant during visit Does not provide tactile stimulation, or only that of aggressive handling of infant No evidence of age-appropriate toys Frustrates infant during interactions
Infant rest	Provides quiet or relaxed environment for infant's rest, including scheduled rest periods Ensures that the infant's needs for food, warmth, and/or dryness are met before sleep	Does not provide quiet environment or consistent schedule for rest periods Does not attend to infant's needs for food, warmth, and/or dryness before sleep
Perception	Demonstrates realistic perception of infant's condition in accordance with medical and/or nursing diagnoses Has realistic expectations of infant Recognizes infant's unfolding skills or behavior Shows realistic perception of own mothering behavior	Shows unrealistic perception of infant's condition Demonstrates unrealistic expectations of infant Has no awareness of infant's development Shows unrealistic perception of own mothering
Initiative	Shows initiative in attempts to manage infant's problems, including actively seeking information about infant	Shows no initiative in attempts to meet infant's needs or to manage problems; does not follow through with plans
Recreation	Provides positive outlets for own recreation or relaxation	Does not provide positive outlets for own recreation or relaxation
Interaction with other children	Demonstrates positive interaction with other children in the home	Demonstrates hostile and aggressive interactions with other children in the home
Mothering role	Expresses satisfaction with mothering	Expresses dissatisfaction with mothering

(Adapted from Harrison L: Nursing intervention with the failure-to-thrive family. Reproduced with the permission of The Am J Mat Child Nurs 1, Vol. 2: 112, March/April 1976)

while you talk to and play with him. When finished, lift him out and pat him dry, paying attention to creases.

After the bath, the labia of female infants should be separated and cleansed with cotton and clean water. Wipe from front to back to avoid introducing any bacteria from the anal region into the vagina or urethra. Male infants who have been circumcised only need to be inspected for cleanliness. An uncircumcised male infant may have the foreskin gently retracted and any accumulation of smegma or debris washed off. If the foreskin does not easily retract, do not force it, but report this to the pediatrician.

For the baby with healthy skin, powders, lotions, and ointments are unnecessary and sometimes harmful. Powder tends to cake in the creases and cause irritation; also, it is sometimes inhaled by the infant, causing respiratory

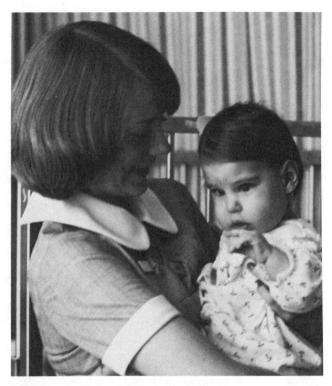

FIG. 6–7. Holding and cuddling can ease the discomfort and fear of a hospital experience. (Courtesy J Nurs Care)

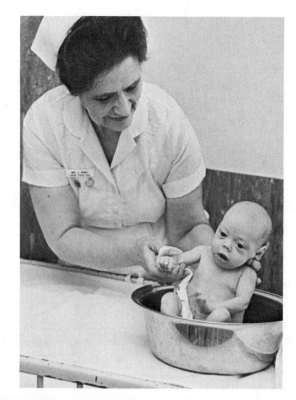

FIG. 6–8. The bath basin should be set inside the crib for safety.

problems. A baby may have an allergy to the ingredients in baby lotion; in any case, a clean baby smells sweet enough without any extras.

Excessively dry skin may benefit from the application of mineral oil or a neutral lubricant. If powder is needed, cornstarch is nonirritating. Various medicated ointments are available for excoriated skin areas.

A baby's fingernails need to be inspected and cut if they are long, because he can scratch his face during random arm movements. The nails should be cut straight across, using care to hold the arm and the hand firmly while cutting.

The bathing procedure is essentially the same for the older infant. When old enough to sit and move about freely, the infant may enjoy the regular bathtub, but usually this is frightening to him. Splashing about in a small tub may be more fun, especially with the addition of a floating toy. Try to schedule your time so that this can be a leisurely process, a time for nurse and baby to enjoy together.

Sponge Bath. See procedure in Chapter 2, The Normal Newborn, page 29.

DRESSING THE INFANT

Hospitalized infants wear cotton shirts or gowns and diapers except in hot weather when a diaper alone is sufficient. The easiest way to dress a small infant is to grasp his hand and pull his arm through the sleeve. If gowns are used that

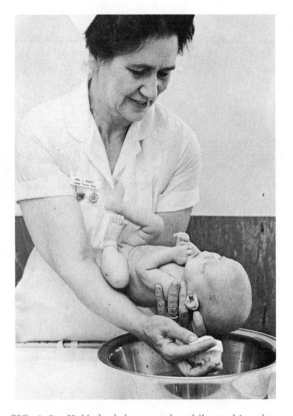

FIG. 6–9. Hold the baby securely while washing the head.

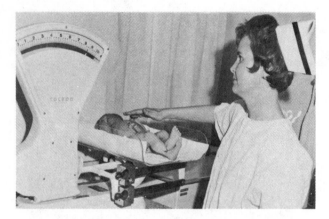

FIG. 6–10. While weighing the infant, the nurse keeps one hand ready to take hold if the infant becomes active. Note the paper on the scale to prevent the infant from directly contacting with the scale. (Bethea DC: Introductory Maternity Nursing, 3rd ed. Philadelphia, JB Lippincott, 1979)

WEIGHING THE INFANT

A baby should be weighed daily, semiweekly, or weekly, as ordered. He should be weighed at the same time each day, preferably before breakfast, using a regular baby scale. The procedure for weighing is as follows:

1. Ascertain the baby's previous weight from the record of the last weighing.
2. Place a clean diaper, sheet, or paper liner on the scoop of the scale in which the baby is to lie.
3. Balance the scale.
4. Place the baby, completely undressed, on the scale and weigh (Fig. 6– 10). Use a small piece of clean paper to manipulate the scales if this is the practice in the nursery.
5. In case of a significant discrepancy from the previous recorded weight, check the scale balance and have your findings checked by a second person.
6. Remove the infant from the scale, discarding the scoop liner.
7. Enter weight in the appropriate space on the chart with weight recording countersigned by a second person if necessary.

TAKING THE INFANT'S TEMPERATURE

In most sick baby nurseries, rectal temperatures are routine, although some favor axillary temperature taking. Unless an electronic thermometer with disposable shields is used, each baby should have his own thermometer which should be cleaned after each use. The thermometer should be kept in a special container in the bedside stand, or in a container attached to the wall of his cubicle.

Before taking the temperature, inspect the thermometer for breakage, especially at the bulb. If the thermometer has been kept in a solution, rinse it and shake it to below 98°.

If the baby has his temperature taken rectally, hold his

tie in back, care must be taken to see that they fit properly, are not too tight around the neck, or too loose, or the baby might get tangled up in his clothing.

Diapers come in various sizes and shapes. Whatever size and folding method used, the important point to remember is that there should not be bunched material between the thighs. Two popular diaper styles are either the oblong strip pinned at the sides or the square diaper folded "kite" fashion. The latter kind has the advantage of being useful for different ages and sizes.

The older infant needs his diaper pinned snugly at hips and legs to prevent feces from running out at the open spaces. Cleaning a soiled crib and smeared baby once or twice serves as an effective reminder for the nurse.

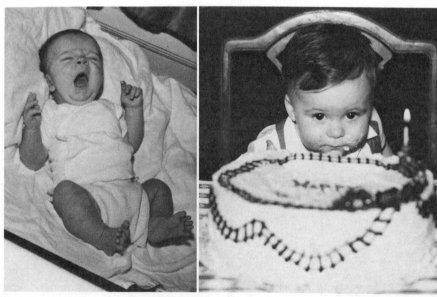

A   B

FIG. 6–11. (A) Infant at 28 days. (B) The same child at age one. (Photos by Don Evans)

ankles firmly as you raise his legs to expose the rectum, and insert the thermometer into the rectum just past the bulb of the thermometer. Both the thermometer and the baby should be held firmly, and the nurse should keep her mind on the business at hand, because thermometers have been broken by kicking and squirming babies. Three or four minutes is considered a sufficiently long insertion to get an accurate temperature.

After use, clean the thermometer with a soapy cotton ball, rinse it with water, and soak it in an antiseptic solution for the designated time, then dry it, and replace it in its container.

summary

From entry into the world until the first birthday, the child undergoes astounding changes in size, appearance, personality, abilities, and understanding. (Fig. 6–11). He view his world from an upright position and knows how to make things happen in that world as he moves through it. Parents, grandparents, siblings, and friends are important to his expanding social network and the shaping of his attitudes and behavior. He recognizes himself as separate from his environment, and becomes increasingly assertive in his need to explore and understand that environment.

review questions

1. When does the infant double his birth weight? Triple it?
2. What is meant by ossification?
3. At what age do the first deciduous teeth erupt? Name the first teeth to erupt.
4. How many deciduous teeth are there in a complete set?
5. At what age should iron supplements be added to the infant's diet?
6. Should infants be forced to give up sucking? Why?
7. At what age is weaning gradually begun?
8. What can the game of "peek-a-boo" teach the child?
9. Why are cotton-tipped applicators not recommended in the ordinary cleaning of a baby's eyes, nose, and ears?

bibliography

Begley S, Carey J: The wisdom of babies. Newsweek 97, Vol. 5:71–72, 1981

Bishop B: A guide to assessing parenting capabilities. Am J Nurs 76:1784–1787, 1976

Bower TGR: A Primer of Infant Development. San Francisco, Freeman, 1977

Endres JB, Rockwell RE: Food, nutrition and the Young Child. St Louis, CV Mosby, 1980

Kempe CH, Silver H, Obrien D (eds): Current Pediatric Diagnosis and Treatment. Los Altos, Lange, 1978

Lowrey GH: The Growth and Development of Children. Chicago, Year Book Publishers, 1978

Pipes PL: Nutrition in Infancy and Childhood, 2nd ed. St Louis, CV Mosby, 1981

Robeck MC: Infants and Children: Their Development and Learning. New York, McGraw-Hill, 1978

Selekman J: Immunization: What's it all about? Am J Nurs 80:1440–1443, 1980

Slattery JS: Nutrition for the normal healthy infant. Am J Mat Child Nurs 2:105–112, 1977

Stone LJ, Smith HT, Murphy LB: The Social Infant. New York, Basic Books, 1978

Suitor CW, Hunter MF: Nutrition: Principles and Application in Health Promotion. Philadelphia, JB Lippincott, 1980

Vaughan VC, McKay, RJ, Behrman RE: Nelson's Textbook of Pediatrics, 11th ed. Philadelphia, Saunders, 1979

Webster-Stratton C, Kogan K: Helping parents parent. Am J Nurs 80:240–244, 1980

health problems of the infant

psychological problems
failure to thrive
gastrointestinal disorders
malnutrition
diarrhea
colic
vomiting and regurgitation
cleft palate
congenital hypertrophic pyloric stenosis
congenital aganglionic megacolon
prolapse of the rectum
intussusception
circulatory system disorders
blood dyscrasias
respiratory system disorders
acute nasopharyngitis (common cold)
acute otitis media
acute bronchiolitis
pneumococcal pneumonia
hemophilus influenzae and other pneumonias
sudden infant death syndrome

genitourinary system disorders
acute pyelonephritis
Wilms' tumor
nervous system disorders
acute or nonrecurrent convulsions
febrile convulsions
hemophilus influenzae meningitis
skin disorders
miliaria rubra (prickly heat)
diaper rash
acute infantile eczema
impetigo
seborrheic dermatitis (cradle cap)
summary
review questions
references
bibliography

student objectives

The student successfully attaining the goals of this chapter will be able to

1 Define the following vocabulary terms:

failure to thrive   Hirschsprung's disease   intussusception   meningitis
miliaria rubra   pellagra   pyelonephritis   pyloric stenosis   rickets
scurvy   SIDS   Wilms' tumor

2 List four disorders that are caused by malnutrition.

3 Describe the appearance of the failure-to-thrive infant and explain the most common cause for this problem.

4 List three good sources for each of the following nutrients: protein, vitamin A, vitamin B, vitamin C, vitamin D, calcium, iron, and iodine.

5 List three nursing actions that help prevent excoriation of the skin that can accompany diarrhea.

6 List five items that should be included on the patient's record when the child has had a convulsion.

Infancy is a period of continuing adjustment for the child and his family. The child is adjusting to physical life outside the uterus and social life within a family. Family members are adjusting to their new roles as parents or siblings, and to the presence of this new person in their midst. Although the adjustment is more gradual than the abrupt transition required at birth, it can still involve sufficient physiologic and psychosocial stress to create health problems during the first year of life.

Wieczorek and Natapoff have identified three factors that determine how health problems are manifested in the infant:[1]

1. The pathogenic agent—how virulent the organism or stress is.
2. The environment—how favorable or unfavorable the setting is, including nutrition and hygiene.
3. The individual child—his resistance and ability to adapt to stress, his bodily responses to biologic, chemical, or physical injury.

All three factors need to be considered when planning nursing care for the infant and his family, remembering that even a minor health problem can create great anxiety for concerned parents.

Infants can rapidly become very ill, often with a high fever (102° F to 103° F). Fortunately, with proper treatment, they can recover with equal speed. Diagnosis of an infant's health problem is no simple matter, partly because the infant cannot "tell you where it hurts," and partly because the clinical manifestations are similar for many different disorders; some minor, some quite serious.

Most acute health problems result from a respiratory or gastrointestinal infection, or from an uncorrected, and perhaps even undetected, congenital deviation. Respiratory problems occur more often and with greater severity in infants because of their immature body defenses and tiny anatomic structures (Fig. 7–1). Sometimes these problems require hospitalization, interrupting development of the infant–family relationship and the infant's patterns of sleeping, eating, and stimulation. If the illness is acute, but the recovery rapid and hospitalization brief, the infant probably will experience few if any long-term effects. If, however, the condition is chronic or so serious that it requires lengthy hospitalization, both infant and family may suffer serious consequences.

psychological problems

FAILURE TO THRIVE

Infants who fail to gain weight and show signs of delayed development with no apparent physical cause are de-

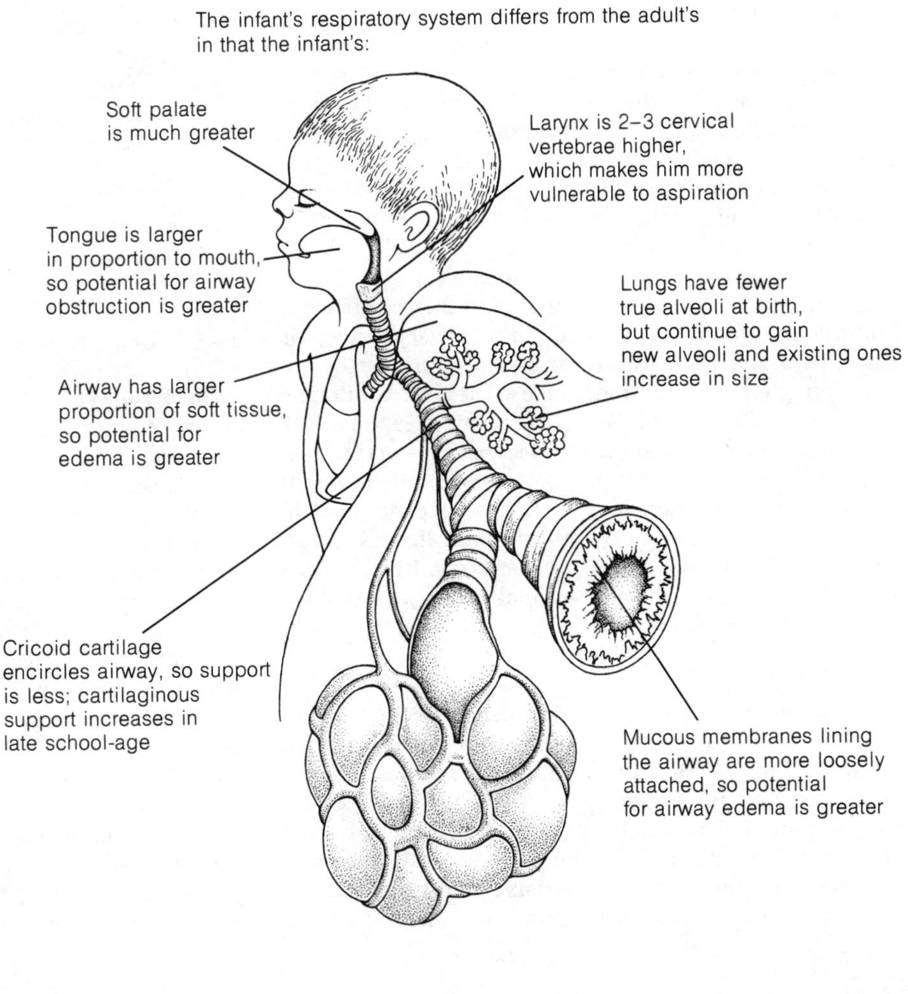

The infant's respiratory system differs from the adult's in that the infant's:

Soft palate is much greater

Larynx is 2–3 cervical vertebrae higher, which makes him more vulnerable to aspiration

Tongue is larger in proportion to mouth, so potential for airway obstruction is greater

Lungs have fewer true alveoli at birth, but continue to gain new alveoli and existing ones increase in size

Airway has larger proportion of soft tissue, so potential for edema is greater

Cricoid cartilage encircles airway, so support is less; cartilaginous support increases in late school-age

Mucous membranes lining the airway are more loosely attached, so potential for airway edema is greater

FIG. 7–1. The infant or young child is at greater risk for airway obstruction due to anatomical differences in the respiratory tract. Alveolar damage in infancy is often not permanent, but airway damage remains throughout life. (Redrawn from Simkims, R. The crises of bronchiolitis, American Journal of Nursing 81:514–516, 1981)

scribed as failure-to-thrive (FTT) infants. Early studies of these children were done by Rene Spitz and John Bowlby, who studied children raised in institutions.[2,3] Later researchers studied children with the same problem who lived in a home with one or both parents. Often when these babies were hospitalized, they began to show rapid weight gain.

Four principal factors are necessary for human growth: food, rest and activity, adequate secretion of hormones, and a satisfactory relationship with a parent (or parent substitute), who provides loving, human contact and stimulation. When any of these four factors are missing, or when the infant has a major birth defect such as congenital heart disease or kidney disorders, growth is disturbed and development delayed.

CLINICAL MANIFESTATIONS

Infants with failure to thrive (FTT) are listless, seriously below normal in weight and height, immobile for long periods of time, and seem unresponsive to cuddling and vocalization. Examination of the infant is likely to reveal no organic cause for this condition. Examination of the family relationship, particularly the mother–infant relationship, however, can often provide important insight into the problem.

The family relationship of this unfortunate infant is often so disrupted that there is no warm, close relationship with the mother. For some reason or reasons, attachment has not occurred. Often the father is immature or absent, making the mother feel isolated and perhaps inadequate, leading to stress and marital conflict.

It is important that the nurse understand that the problem is not with the mother alone, nor with the infant, but instead with their interaction and mutual lack of responsiveness. They are not in harmony. The mother does not stimulate the infant; therefore, he has no one to whom he can respond, and so he fails to do the "cute baby" things that would gain him attention and stimulation.

A frequent characteristic of failure-to-thrive infants is *rumination* (voluntary regurgitation). Fleisher suggests that this problem may occur because the mother or primary caregiver does not understand what gives comfort or satisfaction to the infant.[4] When the infant tries to evoke a response, and fails, rumination occurs. This activates a series of events that further strains the mother–infant relationship. The infant loses weight, sometimes becoming severely emaciated, grows increasingly listless and irritable, and because of the frequent vomiting, smells strongly of vomitus. None of this makes him an attractive baby to love and cuddle.

NURSING CARE

When failure-to-thrive infants are hospitalized, the nurse can play a critical role in reversing the infant's growth failure and improving mother–infant interaction. By providing sensory stimulation, adequate food (140 cal/kg) for weight gain, and tender loving care, the nurse can help change the infant's behavior for the better. As the baby becomes less fretful, more responsive, and gains weight, he is much more appealing to the mother, and the attach-

ment process that has been delayed for several months now has a chance to begin.

As with every hospitalized infant, the mother's participation in his care is important. The nurse can point out the infant's development and responsiveness, and praise the mother's positive parenting behaviors. If the mother has felt the absence of a close, warm childhood relationship with her mother, she may not understand the infant's needs for cuddling and stimulation. Teaching about these needs must be done carefully, so as not to further damage the mother's self-esteem. Long-term care of these infants and their families may require counseling that involves several members of the health care team—family therapist, clergy, social worker, and public health nurse.

gastrointestinal disorders

MALNUTRITION

The World Health Organization has abundantly publicized the malnutrition and outright hunger that affect more than half the world's population. Even within the affluent United States of America, cases of kwashiorkor, marasmus, rickets, scurvy, vitamin A deficiency, and anemia affect poor children.

Malnutrition is a term used to indicate a condition in which one or more nutrients essential for health is lacking (Fig. 7–2). Malnutrition accompanies many chronic diseases, but the greatest number of cases of malnutrition are due to insufficient intake of essential nutrients. A deficient diet may have other than economic causes. Lack of understanding of the nutritional needs of children is one. Another is ignorance of inexpensive ways of supplying the child's needs.

PROTEIN MALNUTRITION

Protein malnutrition results from an insufficient intake of good quality protein or from a condition in which there is an impaired absorption of protein. Clinical evidence of protein malnutrition may not be striking until the condition is well-advanced.

Kwashiorkor. This syndrome, a protein–calorie malnutrition, results from severe deficiency of protein, and is a condition accounting for most of the malnutrition among the world's children today. Its highest incidence is among children age 4 months to 5 years.

An affected child develops a swollen abdomen, retarded growth with muscle wasting, edema, gastrointestinal changes, apathy, and irritability. In untreated cases, mortality rates are 30% or higher. Even when children are brought for treatment, the condition has often advanced sufficiently to keep mortality rates as high as 15 to 20% at some treatment centers. Although strenuous efforts are being made around the world to prevent this condition, its causes are complex.

Traditionally, these babies have been breast-fed up to the age of 2 or 3 years. The child is weaned abruptly and is then given the regular family diet, which contains mostly starch foods with very little meat or vegetable protein. Cow's milk is not generally available, and in many places where goats are kept their milk is not considered fit for human consumption.

In fact, the name kwashiorkor means in African dialect, "the sickness the older baby gets when the new baby comes."

VITAMIN DEFICIENCY DISEASES

Rickets. This disorder is caused by a lack of vitamin D. Children who live in the sunshine and wear little clothing may absorb sufficient vitamin D from the sun's ultraviolet rays, but the infant or small child in a temperate or an arctic climate rarely has opportunity to receive his antirachitic vitamin in this manner.

Rickets is a disease affecting the growth and calcification of bones. The absorption of calcium and phosphorus is diminished due to the lack of vitamin D, the function of which is to regulate the utilization of these minerals. Early manifestations include craniotabes (a softening of the occipital bones) and delayed closure of the fontanels. There is delayed dentition, with defects of tooth enamel and a tendency to develop caries. As the disease advances, thoracic deformities, softening of the shafts of long bones and spinal and pelvic bone deformities develop. The muscles are poorly developed and lacking in tone, thus delaying standing and walking.

These deformities occur during the periods of rapid growth, and although rickets in itself is not a fatal disease, complications such as tetany, pneumonia and enteritis are more likely to cause death in rachitic children than in healthy children.

Infants and children require an estimated 400 units of vitamin D daily for the prevention of rickets. Because of the uncertainty of a small child receiving sufficient exposure to ultraviolet light in temperate climates, it is administered orally in the form of fish liver oil or synthetic vitamin. Whole milk and evaporated milk, fortified with 400 units of vitamin D per quart, are available throughout the United States. *sunlight*

Scurvy. Inadequate vitamin C in the diet causes scurvy. Early inclusion of vitamin C (ascorbic acid) in the form of orange or tomato juice, or a vitamin preparation, is insurance against the development of this disease. Febrile diseases seem to increase the need for vitamin C. A variety of fresh vegetables and fruits supply vitamin C for the older infant and child, although a considerable proportion of vitamin C content is destroyed by boiling, or by exposure to air for long periods of time.

Early clinical manifestations of scurvy are irritability, loss of appetite and digestive disturbances. A general tenderness in the legs, severe enough to cause a "pseudoparalysis" develops. The infant is apprehensive about being handled, and assumes a "frog" position, with hips and knees semi-flexed and the feet rotated outward. The gums become red and swollen, and hemorrhages occur in various tissues. Characteristic hemorrhages in the long bones are subperiosteal, especially at the ends of the femur and tibia.

Recovery is rapid with adequate treatment, but death may occur from malnutrition or exhaustion in untreated

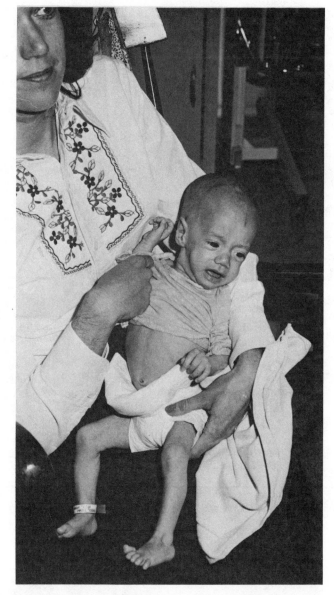

FIG. 7–2. Five-month-old infant with malnutrition due to unknown causes, admitted for observation and diagnosis.

cases. Treatment consists in therapeutic daily doses of ascorbic acid. *raw leafy veg.*

Thiamin Insufficiency. The major vitamin B complex components are thiamin, riboflavin and niacin. Children whose diets are poor in thiamin exhibit irritability, listlessness, loss of appetite and vomiting. A severe lack of thiamin in the diet causes the disease called *beriberi,* characterized by cardiac and neurological symptoms. Beriberi does not occur where balanced diets are eaten which include whole grains.

Riboflavin Insufficiency. This deficiency usually occurs in association with thiamin and niacin deficiencies. It is manifested mainly by skin lesions.

Niacin Insufficiency. Lack of niacin in the diet causes a disease known as *pellagra*, which has gastrointestinal and neurologic symptoms. Children whose intake of whole milk is adequate do not get pellagra; nor do those whose diet is well balanced.

MINERAL INSUFFICIENCY

Anemia. Iron deficiency results in anemia. The condition is not uncommon among children over the ages of 4 to 6 months whose diets lack iron-rich foods. Anemia is frequently found in poor children under age 6 in the U.S.

Hypocalcemia. Calcium is necessary for bone and tooth formation. It is also needed for proper nerve and muscle functioning. Insufficient calcium causes neurologic damage including mental retardation.

OTHER CAUSES OF MALNUTRITION

Allergic reactions to foods may limit the child's diet to the point that he is not getting the proper nutrients, and parents usually need a dietician's help in working out substitutes for the foods he cannot tolerate.

HOSPITAL CARE OF THE MALNOURISHED INFANT

The malnourished infant admitted to the hospital presents problems that are not easily resolved. The underlying cause must be found and eliminated or treated. If the difficulty lies in the parents' inability to give proper care, whether owing to ignorance, financial difficulty, or indifference, these causes need consideration, with perhaps the help of several health and social services.

The nurse responsible for the daily care of the infant has her own problems when attempting to meet his needs.

One problem may be persuading the infant to take more nourishment than he wants. Inexperienced nurses find it very difficult to persuade an uninterested infant to take his formula, and it can become frustrating. Perhaps the nurse's insecurity and uncertainty communicate themselves to the child in the way she handles him. Frequently an experienced nurse is successful in feeding an infant 3 or 4 ounces in a short time, while the inexperienced nurse who seems to be going through the same motions, persuades the infant to take only 1 ounce or less. As nurse and infant become accustomed to each other, however, they both relax, and feeding becomes easier.

In addition to a lack of interest, the infant is weak and debilitated, with little strength to suck. Intravenous or gavage feeding may be employed, but it is important for the infant to develop an interest in food and in the process of sucking. A hard, or small-holed nipple may completely discourage him. The nipple should be soft, with holes large enough to allow the formula to drip without pressure, but not so soft that it offers no resistance and collapses when it is sucked on, or with holes so large that milk pours out, causing him to choke. These experiences easily frustrate a weak infant, who soon gives up any attempt to nurse.

The baby who is held snugly in the nurse's arms, wrapped closely and rocked gently, will find it easier to relax and take a little more. An impatient, hurried nurse nearly always communicates her tension to the child. If the nurse is tense because of other feedings she must attend to, she should ask for help. And she should never prop the bottle in the crib.

Some of the babies may be on a 2- or a 3-hour feeding schedule, because most weak babies are able to handle frequent small feedings better than the every 4-hour feedings. In this case, it is more important than ever that the

---

GOOD SOURCES OF ESSENTIAL NUTRIENTS

Protein

Meat, poultry, fish, milk products and eggs. Whole wheat grains, nuts, peanut butter, legumes are also good sources of protein, but need to be supplemented by some animal protein, such as meat, eggs, milk, cheese, cottage cheese or yogurt.

Vitamin A

Green leafy vegetables, deep yellow vegetables and fruits, whole milk or whole milk products, egg yolk.

Vitamin B

Thiamin. Meat, fish, poultry, eggs, whole grain, legumes, potatoes, green leafy vegetables.

Riboflavin. Milk (best source), meat, egg yolk, green vegetables.

Niacin. Meat, fish, poultry, peanut butter, wheat germ, brewer's yeast. Although the amount in milk is small, children whose intake of milk is adequate do not develop pellagra.

Vitamin C

Citrus fruits and tomatoes, fresh or frozen citrus fruit juices, strawberries, cantaloupe. Breast milk is an adequate source of vitamin C for young infants only if the mother's diet contains sufficient vitamin C.

Vitamin D

Sunlight, fish liver oils, fortified milk and synthetic vitamin D.

Minerals

Calcium. Milk and milk products, squash, sweet potatoes, raisins, rhubarb, well-cooked dried beans, turnip greens, Swiss chard, mustard greens.

Iron. Green leafy vegetables, liver, meats and eggs, dried fruits, whole grain or enriched bread and cereals.

Iodine. Seafoods, plants grown on soil near the sea, iodized salt.

feedings be given on time. Also, as sucking takes considerable energy, the weak infant tires easily. It is not good practice to take more than 20 or 30 minutes for feeding such an infant. If the baby does not take at least two-thirds of his formula, this should be reported. Accurate intake recording is essential, because these babies may need help in the form of small transfusions or parenteral fluids to furnish them with enough energy to take more oral nourishment.

Self-demand feedings, if used at all with these infants, must be used cautiously. A normal, healthy baby promptly makes his needs known if he is hungry, and will quickly fall into a routine, following the rhythmic filling and emptying of his stomach. If such a child sleeps through his feeding time only to waken an hour later in a near-famished state, he usually is the best gauge of his own needs. But the malnourished baby probably has lost the power to regulate his own supply and demand schedule.

DIARRHEA

Diarrhea in infants is a fairly common symptom of a variety of conditions. It may be mild with a small amount of dehydration, or may be extremely severe, calling for prompt and effective treatment (Fig. 7–3).

ETIOLOGY

Chronically malnourished infants with diarrheal symptoms constitute a common problem in many areas of the world. This condition is prevalent in areas where clean water and sanitary facilities are lacking or inadequate.

Allergic reactions to food are not uncommon, and can be controlled by avoidance of the offending food. Overfeeding as well as underfeeding, or an unbalanced diet may be the cause of diarrhea in an infant. Adjustment of the infant's diet, cutting down on the sugar added to formula, or reducing bulk or fat in the diet may be necessary. Certain metabolic diseases, such as cystic fibrosis have diarrhea as a symptom.

Many diarrheal disturbances in infants may be caused by contaminated food. The infectious organisms may be salmonella, *E. coli*, dysentery bacilli, and various viruses. It is difficult to determine the causative factor in the majority of cases. Because of the seriousness of infectious diarrhea among infants, most hospitals isolate the child with moderate or severe diarrhea until it can be definitely proved that there is no infectious agent involved.

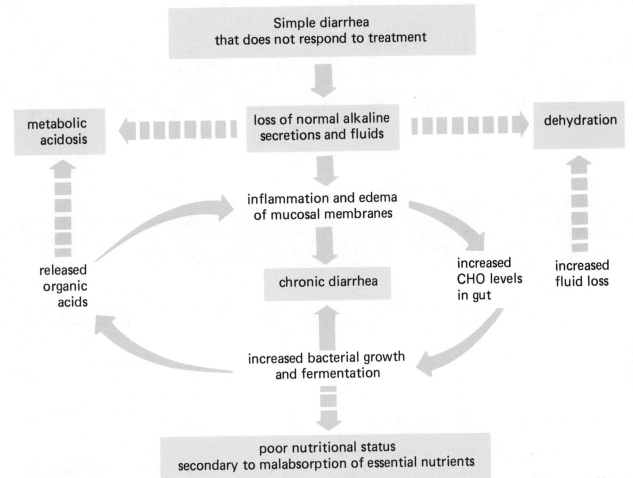

FIG. 7–3. The vicious cycle of infant diarrhea. (Redrawn from Copeland L: Chronic diarrhea in infancy. Am J Nurs 77:461–463, 1977. Copyright © 1977, American Journal of Nursing Company. Reproduced with permission)

CLINICAL MANIFESTATIONS

Mild diarrhea may show little more than loose stools, which may number from two to four to as many as ten or 12 per day. There may be irritability and loss of appetite. Vomiting and gastric distention are not significant factors and dehydration is minimal.

Severe diarrhea may develop gradually with the condition becoming progressively more serious, with marked dehydration. The skin becomes very dry and loses its turgor. The fontanel becomes sunken, the pulse is weak and rapid. The stools become greenish liquid and may be blood-tinged.

TREATMENT

The important factor in treatment is to establish normal fluid and electrolyte balance.

The physician may treat the mild dehydration by giving oral feedings of five per cent glucose in saline solution, or a commercial preparation in place of milk or food. Sometimes a period of complete omission of oral feedings is ordered for a period of a few hours before commencing the oral electrolyte solution. As the diarrhea clears, skim milk may be offered followed by gradual additions of infant formula and food.

Mild or moderate diarrhea can convert rather quickly to severe diarrhea in an infant. Vomiting usually accompanies the diarrhea; together they cause large losses of body water and electrolytes. The infant becomes severely dehydrated, and is gravely ill. Oral feedings are discontinued completely. Fluids to be given intravenously must be carefully calculated to replace the lost electrolytes. Frequent laboratory determinations of the infant's blood chemistries will be necessary for guidance in this replacement therapy.

NURSING CARE

In addition to maintaining the intravenous fluid at a correct speed and keeping accurate records of fluids, the nurse also needs to keep strict account of the number and character of the infant's stools and the amount and character of vomitus and urine. A record is kept of skin condition, the child's temperature and state of activity. Strict isolation techniques must be observed unless otherwise ordered. If high fever is present, tepid sponge baths or a cooling water mattress will be ordered.

Excoriation of the skin in the genital area must be prevented as much as possible. This area should be cleansed frequently with mineral oil or vaseline and a mild ointment applied. Leaving the diaper off, exposing the buttocks and genital area to the air is helpful. Disposable pads under the infant will facilitate easy and frequent changing. Cold cream may be applied to the child's dry lips to help prevent cracking and sores.

Meeting the infant's emotional needs will be difficult but of great importance. His mother is the one who can best fulfill the infant's needs, if she can be taught the principles of strict aseptic technique and can be relied on to maintain them.

If the infant can be picked up and rocked, this will be helpful. However, if there is a possibility that the intravenous needle may be displaced, this will not be permitted. Getting a needle into the small veins of an infant is difficult and replacement may be nearly impossible, but the infant's life may depend on the proper parenteral therapy.

Soothing the baby by gentle head stroking and soft speech helps him bear the frustrations imposed on him by his illness as well as by the treatment. His sucking needs may be met by means of a pacifier. When the child's mother cannot be with him, the nurse has an obligation to take her place in filling his emotional needs as much as possible.

COLIC

The recurrent paroxysmal bouts of abdominal pain that are not uncommon among young infants have earned for the condition the name of 3-month colic. The fact that the condition disappears around the age of 3 months gives small comfort to the parent vainly trying to sooth a colicky baby.

ETIOLOGY

Exact cause is unknown. Air swallowing and hunger have been suggested. A state of tension in the family, communicating itself to the infant may be a factor.

CLINICAL MANIFESTATIONS

Attacks occur quite suddenly, usually late in the day or evening. The infant cries loudly and continuously. His abdomen is tense and distended, his legs drawn up and the hands clenched. He appears to be in considerable pain. The baby may only momentarily be soothed by rocking or holding. Eventually he cries himself to sleep from exhaustion.

Differentiation from other conditions will need to be made. Allergic reaction to certain foods and intestinal obstruction or infection should be ruled out.

TREATMENT

No single treatment is consistently successful. A *warm* water bottle or heating pad on low setting with the infant lying prone across it is sometimes helpful. Great care must be taken to ensure that the bottle or pad are not too warm for the baby's tender skin. The pad or water bottle should be placed *outside* his clothing, not next to his skin. The doctor may order a rectal glycerine suppository to help the infant expel flatus. Sedation such as phenobarbital for attacks that persist is sometimes useful. Attacks rarely persist after the age of 3 months.

Methods of feeding and of burping the infant should be examined for possible cause. However, the mother should not be made to feel guilty or inefficient in her child's care. Frequently no mismanagement in the feeding practices can be found.

VOMITING AND REGURGITATION

Vomiting is one of the commonest disturbances of infancy and childhood. It can be a symptom of a wide variety of conditions. Attention must be given toward discovering the cause and correcting it. It may be simply a matter of overfeeding or swallowing too much air.

More serious conditions can be pyloric stenosis, allergic reaction to cow's milk, infections or organic obstructions in any body system.

Some well-nourished, active infants tend to spit up (regurgitate) small amounts of feeding rather frequently. These infants seem to regurgitate easily, especially when excited. There appears to be no particular causative factor, and change of formula seldom helps. This type of regurgitation tends to disappear as the infant grows older.

Thorazine or phenagar

CLEFT PALATE

The child born with a cleft palate (but with an intact lip) does not have the external disfigurement that may be so distressing to the new mother—but his problems are more serious. Although a cleft lip and a cleft palate frequently appear together, either defect may appear alone. In embryonic development, the palate closes at a later time than does the lip, and the failure to close is for somewhat different reasons. The manner in which the palate normally closes is interesting.

ETIOLOGY

When the embryo is about 8 weeks old, there is still no roof to the mouth: the tissues that are to become the palate are two shelves running from the front to the back of the mouth, and projecting vertically downward on either side of the tongue. The shelves move from a vertical position to a horizontal position, their free edges meeting and fusing in midline. Later, bone forms within this tissue to form the hard palate.

Normally the palate is intact by the tenth week of fetal life. Exactly what happens to prevent this closure is not known with certainty. It occurs more frequently in near relatives of persons with the defect than in the general population, and there appears to be some evidence that environmental and hereditary factors may each play a part in this defect.

A cleft palate may involve the soft palate alone, or it may extend into the nose and into the hard palate. It may be unilateral or bilateral, an isolated defect, or in conjunction with cleft lip.

TREATMENT

The goal is to give the child a union of the cleft parts that would allow intelligible and pleasant speech, and to avoid injury to the maxillary growth. Timing of surgery is individualized, according to the size, the placement and the degree of deformity. The optimal time for surgery is considered to be between the ages of 6 months and 5 years. Because the child is not able to make certain sounds when he starts to talk, undesirable speech habits are formed which are difficult to correct. If surgery must be delayed beyond the third year, a dental speech appliance may help the child develop intelligible speech.

Cleft lip and cleft palate centers provide teams of specialists who can give the professional services that these children need through their infancy, preschool and school years. Members of the professional team include a pediatrician, a plastic surgeon, an orthodontist, a speech therapist, a social worker and a public health nurse. The services of a child nutritionist are also available. Explanations and counseling concerning the child's diet, his speech training, his immunizations and his general health supervision can be given. Questions can be answered and misconceptions can be cleared up.

It may sound strange to speak about preparation for speech training for an infant only a few weeks of age. The babbling and cooing of a young infant is an important precursor of speech activity, and the stimulation that the parents normally give when they repeat the sounds back to him is essential. Parents normally do this, but they may be too disturbed and tense to behave in a natural manner before an infant with a palate defect. This child, however, needs to hear these sounds as a pattern for learning, even more than an infant who does not have to overcome a physical impediment.

Dental care for the deciduous teeth is of more than usual importance. The incidence of dental caries is high in children with a cleft palate, but the preservation of the deciduous teeth is important for the best results in speech as well as for appearance.

Home Care before Surgery. The infant with a cleft palate (but with an intact lip) can learn to suck without much difficulty. A rather large nipple, with holes that allow the milk to drip freely, makes sucking easier for this child, who does not get quite as much suction as a child with an intact palate. The activity of sucking is an important one for the development of speech muscles. Special cleft palate nipples, with a flange to cover the cleft, are commercially available. They are expensive and unnecessary for the average infant with cleft palate. An occasional infant, with a wide cleft, may be able to suck more easily with one of these. It may be necessary to feed such an infant with a medicine dropper. Most of these infants can learn to take milk from a spoon, slowly, at an early age.

Strained foods are introduced at the usual time and in the routine manner, within the framework of a normal diet. A little food or milk may seep through the cleft and out through the nose, and the mothers should be informed of this possibility.

NURSING CARE

For preoperative and immediate postoperative care, see Chapter 4.

The operating surgeon will have a routine for postoperative repair that he finds most successful. Generally, the patient is allowed clear liquids after nausea has ceased. Spoons and straws are usually forbidden, only drinking from a cup or a glass being allowed. Clear liquids that are usually accepted are Jello water, apple juice, and the synthetic, fruit-flavored drinks. Broth may be offered, but is not a popular drink with this age group. Clear liquids are allowed for a period of from three to five days, followed by full liquids for approximately 10 days, after which semiliquids such as cereal, ice cream or Jello may be fed with a spoon. Some variations from this schedule may be desired by different plastic surgeons.

The sutures are not cleansed or manipulated in any way. Water, or a clear liquid after a milk drink is helpful to keep the sutures clean if the child will cooperate. In addition to vigilance in keeping toys or any objects out of the mouth, considerable care must be exercised to keep anyone with a suspicion of a cold or a cough away from the patient, whether it is a staff nurse, a family member, or some other patient. A cough or a nasal infection may well damage the best repair.

If all goes well, the child can probably be discharged about the tenth day, returning to the clinic or to his doctor's office for suture removal about the third week.

OUTCOME

Orthodontic treatment is necessary for the majority of these children. There may be a distortion of the maxillary arch causing malocclusion, and interference with optimal growth and development of the upper jaw. Orthodontic observation and treatment are continued until the permanent teeth are in good occlusion.

Speech therapy is continued after surgery to aid the child in correcting faulty sounds learned before the defect was corrected. Parents and therapists work together with the child to help him achieve clear speech without disagreeable nasal tones.

Occasionally it is necessary to delay surgery until the fourth or fifth year of life in order to take advantage of the palatal changes that occur with growth. If surgery is delayed beyond the third year, a prosthesis will be needed to help the child develop intelligible speech. The formation of teeth is usually delayed in the area of the defect. These missing teeth can be replaced by a denture to which is attached, posteriorly, a contoured speech bulb.

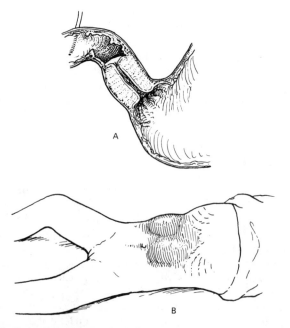

FIG. 7–4. Pyloric stenosis. (A) Narrowed lumen of the pylorus. (B) Visible peristalsis.

CONGENITAL HYPERTROPHIC PYLORIC STENOSIS

Pyloric stenosis is rarely symptomatic during the first days of life. It has on occasion been recognized shortly after birth, but the average affected infant does not show symptoms until about the third week of life. Symptoms rarely appear after the second month.

Although symptoms appear late, pyloric stenosis is classified as a congenital defect. Its cause is not known.

narrowing of exit of stomach

PATHOPHYSIOLOGY

The condition is characterized by hypertrophy of the circular muscle fibers of the pylorus, with a severe narrowing of its lumen. The pylorus is thickened to as much as twice its size, is elongated and has a consistency resembling cartilage. As a result of this obstruction at the distal end of the stomach, the stomach becomes dilated (Fig. 7–4A).

CLINICAL MANIFESTATIONS

During the first weeks of life, the infant with pyloric stenosis probably eats well and gains weight. Then he starts vomiting occasionally after meals. Within a few days the vomiting episodes increase in frequency and force, becoming projectile. The vomited material may contain mucus, but never bile, because it has not progressed beyond the stomach.

Because the obstruction is a mechanical one, the baby does not feel ill, is ravenously hungry, and is eager to try again and again, but the food invariably comes back.

As the condition progresses the baby becomes irritable, loses weight rapidly and becomes dehydrated. A condition of alkalosis develops from the loss of potassium and hydrochloric acid, and he becomes very ill.

Constipation becomes progressive because little food gets into the intestines, and the urine is scanty. Gastric peristaltic waves passing from left to right across the abdomen can usually be seen during or after feedings.

DIAGNOSIS

Diagnosis usually can be made on the clinical evidence. The nature, type and times of vomiting, observation of gastric peristaltic waves, (Fig. 7–4B) and a history of weight loss with hunger and irritability point in this direction. The olive-size pyloric tumor can often be felt through deep palpation by an experienced physician. Roentgenographic examination with barium swallow shows an abnormal retention of barium in the stomach and increased peristaltic waves.

TREATMENT

The condition is well-known and is suspected if a previously well infant commences to vomit his feedings. When under a pediatrician's care, either in a private office or in a clinic, these infants are carefully watched to prevent the critical degree of dehydration that was formerly so frequent. However, all too frequently infants do not come into the hospital until dehydration and malnutrition are obvious, thus presenting an infant in very poor condition for surgical correction.

Treatment to correct pyloric stenosis is routinely surgical in the United States. The procedure commonly used is the Fredet-Remstedt operation. This procedure simply splits the hypertrophic pyloric muscle down to the submucosa, allowing the pylorus to expand so that food may pass. If performed by a competent surgeon on an infant in good condition, the operation is simple, and it gives excellent results.

In the United States, the older method of medical treatment is rarely used. This treatment consists of feedings of cereal-thickened formula, antispasmodic drugs and sedation. This treatment must of necessity be of long duration, is frequently unsatisfactory, and serves to increase the hazards to the child who is already malnourished and in poor condition. It may on occasion be used for a short time while a diagnosis is being established, but not for the child with pyloric stenosis who has lost much weight or who is already in alkalosis. *Atropine - rapid pulse + flush skin*

NURSING CARE

Preoperative Care. The infant who comes into the hospital after unsuccessful attempts at home treatment is not, as a rule, in a condition for immediate surgery. He needs laboratory tests to determine his metabolic deficits and state of chemical imbalance. Intravenous fluids are given to restore proper hydration and to correct the hypokalemic alkalosis.

The nurse should follow directions exactly as to the amount and type of fluid to be given. Mixing fluids, if this is required to meet the child's needs, is a very exact procedure, and should be done only by a nurse familiar with this procedure.

When the baby is in the hospital awaiting surgery, it will be very helpful if the mother is allowed to participate in his care. Both the mother and the baby are going to be happier if nurses can recognize their mutual needs. The nurse also needs a better opportunity to explain the purpose of waiting for surgery and the function of the intravenous fluids. *IV in to scalp for newborn*

Feedings. If the baby does need a period of hospitalization before surgery, a smooth-muscle relaxant such as atropine may be ordered prior to oral feedings. Feedings may be thickened by mixing cooked cereal with the formula, and the child fed through a large-holed nipple, in the hope that some nutrients may be retained.

Documentation. The nurse needs to record accurately the amount of feeding given, and the approximate amount retained, as well as the frequency and type of emesis. Urinary output is estimated or measured; the skin turgor is noted as well as the general physical appearance, state of irritability, lethargy, or any change in response to external stimulation.

Oral fluids are omitted for a specified time before surgery. Some surgeons order a stomach lavage shortly before surgery, with the nasogastric tube left in place. Preoperative medication such as atropine intramuscularly is usually ordered.

While the baby is in surgery, some attention is paid to the mother's needs, including a comfortable place to wait, and something to do. If she waits in the general waiting room, some member of the staff can seek her out for an occasional friendly word. Recovery room delay should be explained because many parents become alarmed at a wait of several hours after the doctor has assured them that surgery is simple and of short duration.

Postoperative Care. Postoperatively, the child should be positioned on his side and watched carefully to prevent aspiration of mucus or vomitus, particularly during the anesthesia recovery period. When fully awake, but restless, he may relax if his mother holds him. If so, she should be given a gown to protect her clothing.

The first feeding is usually given about 6 hours postoperatively, and generally is glucose water. If well tolerated, this feeding can be alternated with small amounts of dilute formula at frequent intervals, gradually increasing in amount and in frequency. The baby may vomit a time or two, but should progress quite rapidly toward complete recovery. Intravenous feedings may be needed until the child can tolerate sufficient oral feedings.

With early diagnosis, and surgery before dehydration and malnutrition have become severe, the child has an excellent chance for returning to a satisfactory condition in a period of weeks, and of progressing steadily on to complete recovery. Operative fatality rate under these conditions has become less than 1%. *fed up right*

CONGENITAL AGANGLIONIC MEGACOLON

Also called Hirschsprung's disease, this condition is characterized by obstinate constipation resulting from partial or complete intestinal obstruction of mechanical origin. The condition may be severe enough to be recognized during the neonatal period. In other cases, it may not be diagnosed until later infancy or early childhood.

PATHOPHYSIOLOGY

Parasympathetic nerve cells regulate peristalsis in the intestines. In Hirschsprung's disease there is a congenital absence of parasympathetic ganglion cells within the muscular wall of the distal colon and the rectum. In their absence, the affected segment narrows, and the portion of the colon directly *above* the affected area becomes greatly dilated, filled with feces and gas (Fig. 7–5).

CLINICAL MANIFESTATIONS

The *newborn* may pass no meconium during the first 24 hours. This may be symptomatic of other conditions such as imperforate anus. In any case, it is of extreme importance that accurate records be kept of the first stool, its timing and character. Failure to pass a stool within the first 24 hours should always be reported.

Other neonatal symptoms are of complete or partial intestinal obstruction, such as bile-stained emesis and generalized abdominal distention. Gastroenteritis with diarrheal stools may be present, and ulceration of the colon may occur.

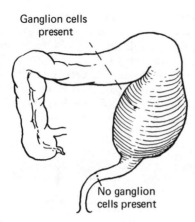

Ganglion cells present

No ganglion cells present

FIG. 7–5. Dilated colon in Hirschsprung's disease.

Symptoms in the *older infant* or *young child* are obstinate, severe constipation dating back to early infancy. Stools are ribbonlike or consist of hard pellets. Formed bowel movements do not occur except with the use of enemas, and soiling does not occur. The rectum is usually empty, as the impaction occurs above the aganglionic segment.

As the child grows older the abdomen becomes progressively enlarged and hard (Fig. 7–6). General debilitation and chronic anemia are usually present. Differentiation must be made between this condition and psychogenic megacolon due to coercive toilet training or other emotional problems. In aganglionic megacolon there is no withholding of stool or defecating in inappropriate places, and no soiling.

Encopresis – incont. of B.M. ₃ any apparent reason.

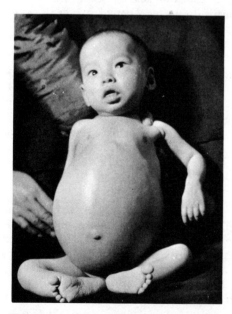

FIG. 7–6.   A baby with Hirschsprung's disease. (Waechter EH, Blake FG: Nursing Care of Children, 9th ed. Philadelphia, JB Lippincott, 1976)

DIAGNOSIS

Definitive diagnosis requires radiologic examination following barium enema and, frequently, rectal biopsy.

TREATMENT

Treatment requires abdominal resection. In early infancy, a colostomy is usually performed to relieve the obstruction. Resection is deferred until later infancy.

Best results have been obtained through the Swenson pull-through procedure. In this procedure the narrowed section is pulled through and sutured to the anal opening. Modifications of the Duhamel side-to-side anastomosis are also being evaluated.

NURSING CARE

Preoperative Care.   The colon must be emptied of fecal material prior to diagnostic procedures, and also prior to surgery. Oil retention enemas, followed by colonic irrigation are necessary daily or at frequent intervals to empty the colon. Oil retention enemas consisting of three or four ounces of mineral or olive oil may be used.

Colonic irrigations or enemas must always consist of *isotonic saline solution*. Due to the lack of peristaltic action, the water in plain tap water enemas or soap suds enemas is retained and absorbed into the tissues, causing water intoxication. Syncope, shock, and frequently death result even after only one or two tap-water irrigations. Enemas of magnesium sulfate have caused magnesium poisoning. Isotonic saline solutions should be used routinely.

Postoperative Care.   If a colostomy only has been performed, routine colostomy care is given.

Children generally tolerate this long, difficult surgery very well. The child should be closely observed until he is thoroughly awake. Vital signs are observed and recorded as in any major abdominal operation. A nasogastric tube will be left in and intravenous feedings given until bowel function is established. Temperatures should not be taken rectally. For the infant and young child, axillary temperatures can be taken. The nurse needs to be alert for rectal bleeding, abdominal distention, a rise in pulse or temperature. Any of these signs should be reported promptly. Successful surgery allows these children to grow and develop normally.

PROLAPSE OF THE RECTUM

Rectal prolapse is a descent of the mucous membrane of the rectum into the anus, with or without protrusion through the anal opening. The term *procidentia* of the rectum is used when all of the coats of the rectum descend.

CLINICAL MANIFESTATIONS

Infants and children who suffer from severe malnutrition disturbances are prone to rectal prolapse when straining at stool in constipation, or during diarrheal episodes. Prolapse of the rectum is common in children with cystic fibrosis. The protruding mass is bright or dark red and may be several inches in length (Fig. 7–7).

NURSING CARE

The protrusion may recede spontaneously, but generally needs to be replaced manually. A gloved finger, covered with a piece of toilet tissue, is gently introduced into the lumen of the mass, and the mass is pushed gently back into the rectum. The toilet tissue will adhere to the mucous membrane, permitting the withdrawal of the gloved finger. The tissue will later be expelled spontaneously.

During defecation, the child's buttocks should be held firmly together. Whenever a prolapse occurs, the rectal tissue should be replaced.

TREATMENT

Treatment should be directed toward relieving the cause. For intractable cases, perineal surgery may become necessary.

INTUSSUSCEPTION

Intussusception is the invagination or telescoping of one portion of the bowel into a distal portion. It occurs most frequently at the juncture of the ileum and the colon, although it can appear elsewhere in the intestinal tract. The invagination is from above downward; the upper portion, the intussusceptum, slipping into the lower, the intussuscipiens, pulling the mesentery along with it (Fig. 7–8).

The condition occurs more often in boys than in girls, and is the most frequent cause of intestinal obstruction in childhood. The greatest incidence occurs in infants between the ages of 4 months to 10 months.

ETIOLOGY

The condition usually appears in healthy babies without any demonstrable cause. Its production is supposed to be favored by the hyperperistalsis and the unusual mobility of the cecum and ileum normally present in early life. Occasionally, a lesion such as a Meckel's diverticulum or a polyp may be present.

CLINICAL MANIFESTATIONS

The infant who has previously appeared healthy and happy suddenly becomes pale, cries out sharply, and draws up his legs in a severe colicky spasm of pain. This spasm may last for several minutes, after which the infant relaxes and appears well until the next episode, which may be 5, 10, or 20 minutes later.

Most of these infants start vomiting early, a vomiting that becomes progressively more severe and eventually is bile stained. The infant strains with each paroxysm, emptying his bowels of fecal contents, after which the stools consist of blood and mucus, earning the name of "currant jelly" stools.

Symptoms of shock appear quickly. Rapid pulse, paleness, and marked sweating are characteristic. Shock, vomiting and currant jelly stools are the cardinal symptoms of this condition. Fortunately, these symptoms, coupled with the paroxysmal pain, are severe enough to bring the child into the hospital early.

Because the nurse is often consulted by neighbors, friends and relatives if things go wrong, she needs to be informed and alert. Therefore, a word of caution is needed.

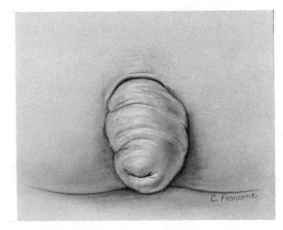

FIG. 7–7. Drawing showing prolapse of the rectum.

On rare occasions a more chronic form appears, particularly during an episode of severe diarrheal disturbance. The onset is more gradual and may not show all of the classic symptoms, but the danger of a sudden, complete strangulation is present. Presumably, such an infant is already under a doctor's care.

DIAGNOSIS

Diagnosis can usually be made by the physician from the clinical symptoms, rectal examination, and palpation of the abdomen during the calm interval when it is soft. A baby is often not willing to tolerate this palpation, and sedation may be ordered. In many cases, a sausage-shaped mass along the colon can be felt through the abdominal wall.

TREATMENT

Unlike pyloric stenosis, this condition is a true emergency in the sense that prolonged delay is dangerous. The telescoped bowel rapidly becomes gangrenous, thus markedly reducing the possibility of a simple reduction. Adequate treatment during the first 12 to 24 hours should have a

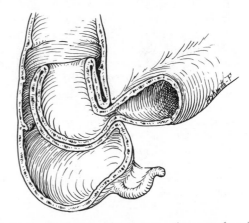

FIG. 7–8. In this drawing of intussusception note the telescoping of a portion of the bowel into the distal portion.

good outcome, with complete recovery. The outcome becomes more uncertain as the bowel deteriorates, making resection necessary.

Emergency Treatment. The baby is, of course, given nothing by mouth, and intravenous fluids are started. A cut-down or catheter into the vein will probably be used.

Surgical Treatment. Traditionally, surgery has been preceded by a diagnostic barium enema, and it has been observed in some cases that the reduction has been accomplished by the hydrostatic pressure itself. Most surgeons prefer to follow the enema with surgery to assure themselves of complete reduction and absence of other lesions.

Surgery consists of a gentle milking of the intussusceptum back into place. This is a simple procedure, requiring a small incision, and affords an opportunity for visual assurance of complete reduction as well as identification of any possible lesion that might be present. Should the bowel be found to be gangrenous or the intussusception irreducible, resection will be necessary.

NURSING CARE

Preoperative Care. The infant needs very careful watching because his condition can deteriorate rapidly. Vital signs need to be checked frequently, warmth applied if symptoms of shock are present, and general condition noted. Aspiration of vomited material is a very real danger, especially as the child becomes weaker. The baby will probably not tolerate being held to any extent.

Support of the Parents. Every parent is entitled to as complete and accurate an explanation as she or he can understand. The parents need to understand the condition, and its severity. Medical and nursing procedures are frequently complicated and extremely frightening to the uninformed person.

The baby, lying in his crib, has a tubing extending from his nose and connected to a continuous suction apparatus. Another tube extends from a bottle of fluid into a vein in his scalp. He may have still another tubing coming from his bladder into a drainage bottle. None of these may have great significance, but even the most informed nurse might have a few qualms if this child was her own.

An explanation of the whys and wherefores can help relieve parental anxiety. The nurse who listens attentively can show sympathy and understanding, help correct misunderstandings, and give assurance that the child's welfare is of the greatest concern to all.

The nurse should try to make the parents comfortable, and make them feel that they are part of the group and not hindrances or unavoidable nuisances.

It is unwise and unfair to offer parents false hope or to be unrealistically optimistic. Their child is sick and no one can predict a recovery with certainty.

Postoperative Care. Following a simple reduction of the intussusception, treatment is symptomatic. Intravenous feeding is necessary until normal bowel sounds are present, at which time feedings are cautiously resumed. The surgical area must be kept clean, dry, and uncontaminated by urine or fecal material.

If resection has been necessary, this assumes the gravity of any major abdominal surgery. Constant gastric suction is necessary to keep the stomach and upper intestinal tract empty. Drainage must be measured, and may be analyzed for electrolyte losses that must be replaced in the intravenous fluids.

These patients must be turned frequently because they cannot learn to cough or breathe deeply to keep the lungs clear. A nasal suction machine must be on hand to keep the airways clear of mucus, and activity should be stimulated by frequent turning and, if necessary, by making the infant cry. This must be explained to the parents, who may resent measures that make the child temporarily uncomfortable.

circulatory system disorders

BLOOD DYSCRASIAS

Anemia is a common childhood blood disorder. It may be the result of an inadequate production of red blood cells or of hemoglobin, or from an excessive loss of either red cells or of hemoglobin. The following are examples of the more common types of anemia found in childhood; there are many others.

1. Inadequate production of erythrocytes or of hemoglobin, as in iron deficiency anemia and in anemia of chronic infection.
2. Excessive loss of red cells, as in hemorrhage.
3. Hemolytic anemia associated with congenital abnormalities of erythrocytes or hemoglobin, as in thalassemia or sickle cell disease.
4. Hemolytic anemia associated with acquired abnormalities of erythrocytes or hemoglobin, from drugs, chemicals, or bacterial reaction.

IRON DEFICIENCY ANEMIA

Iron deficiency anemia is a common nutritional deficiency among young children. It is a hypochromatic, microcytic anemia, i.e., the blood cells are smaller than normal, and deficient in hemoglobin, common between the ages of 9 and 24 months. The full-term newborn has a high hemoglobin that decreases during the first 2 to 3 months of life. However, considerable iron is reclaimed and stored, usually in sufficient quantity to last for 4 to 9 months of life.

A child needs to absorb 0.8 mg to 1.5 mg of iron per day. As only 10% of dietary iron is absorbed, a diet containing 8 mg to 10 mg of iron is needed for good health. During the first years of life it is often difficult for a child to obtain this quantity of iron from his food. If the diet is inadequate, anemia quickly results.

Babies with an inordinate fondness for milk, sometimes taking an astonishing amount, have their appetites satisfied, and show little interest in solid foods. Infants and toddlers have come into the hospital with a history of taking 2 to 3 quarts of milk daily and accepting no other foods, or at best, only foods with a high carbohydrate content. Many parents believe, incorrectly, that milk is a perfect food, so why not let him have all he wants?

Many of these children, however, are undernourished strictly because of the family's economic problem. Much work is needed to help provide necessary nutrients for the nation's children. It is not an economic problem alone but also a need for proper nutritional knowledge and a need to learn ways to use money for food to the best nutritional advantage.

A few children have a hemoglobin so low, or their anorexia so acute, that they need additional therapy. An iron dextran mixture for intramuscular use (Imferon) is available, which is markedly efficient in bringing the hemoglobin to normal levels. A special technique for administering this medication, called the Z-track method, is necessary to avoid leakage into the subcutaneous tissues.

Home Care. The most important aspect of treatment for this condition is education for the parents. They need to understand the importance of iron in their child's diet, and the foods that are best for meeting this need. One mother was quite severely criticized in the pediatric outpatient clinic because of her child's anemic condition. "Mrs. Black," said the pediatrician, "you simply have to give your child more foods that contain iron." Mrs. Black looked at him in bewilderment and exclaimed, "But doctor, after liver—what?"

A nurse has a splendid opportunity to teach good nutritional habits in such a situation—habits that may improve the health of the entire family. She can guide the mother to use green and yellow vegetables, egg yolk, and iron-rich fruits such as peaches, in addition, of course, to liver. Some of the pamphlets published by commercial food companies are excellent for teaching parents, and perhaps can refresh the nurse's memory as well. These give the iron and the vitamin content of foods, and list the requirements for various age levels.

Prognosis is excellent for restored health in iron deficiency caused by poor iron intake with dietary correction. If untreated, anemia becomes progressive, with possible resultant cardiac failure.

SICKLE CELL DISEASE

Sickle cell disease is an hereditary trait occurring primarily but not exclusively in the Negro race. It appears as an asymptomatic trait when the sickling trait is inherited from one parent alone (heterozygous state). When inherited from both parents (homozygous state) anemia develops. A rapid breakdown of red cells carrying hemoglobin S, an abnormal hemoglobin, causes a severe hemolytic anemia. The sickling trait occurs in about 10% of American blacks: there is a much higher incidence in parts of Africa. The disease itself has an incidence of 0.3% to 1.3%. The tendency to sickle can be demonstrated by laboratory tests. In those who carry one gene for the *sickle cell trait*, hemoglobin level and red cell count is normal, and the child is asymptomatic.

Clinical symptoms of the disease itself do not usually appear before the latter half of the first year of life. Sickle cell disease causes a chronic anemia with hemoglobin levels of 6 g/ml to 9 g/100 ml, or lower. Easy fatigability and anorexia are the usual manifestations of any form of anemia. The frequent sickle cell crises, however, make the disease a serious one.

Sickle Cell Crisis. This may be the first clinical manifestation of the disease, and may recur frequently during early childhood. This disturbance presents a variety of symptoms. The most common symptom is severe, acute abdominal pain, together with muscle spasm, fever, severe leg pain that may be muscular, osseous, or localized in the joints, which become hot and swollen. The abdomen becomes boardlike, with an absence of bowel sounds, making it extremely difficult to distinguish the condition from an abdominal condition requiring surgery. The crisis may have a fatal outcome caused by cerebral, cardiac, or hemolytic difficulties.

Treatment. The child should be kept in optimum health between crises. Adequate hydration is vital; intake of fluids should be between 1500 ml and 2000 ml daily, and under stressful situations as much as 3000 ml daily. Small blood transfusions help to bring the hemoglobin level near normal, but the increase is only temporary. Treatment for crises is supportive and symptomatic, and bedrest is indicated. Analgesics are given for pain and dehydration and acidosis is vigorously treated. Oral intake of iron has no effect on the disease. The spleen becomes greatly enlarged, but in later childhood may become small and fibrotic and is rarely palpable in childhood.

Outcome. Prognosis is guarded, depending on the severity of the disease. *avoid high altitudes.*

respiratory system disorders

ACUTE NASOPHARYNGITIS (COMMON COLD)

The common cold is one of the most common infectious conditions of childhood. The young infant is as susceptible as the older child but is not generally as frequently exposed.

ETIOLOGY

The illness is of viral origin, rhinoviruses being the principal agents. Bacterial invasion of the tissues may cause complications such as ear, mastoid and lung infections. The young child appears to be more susceptible to complications than an older person.

CLINICAL MANIFESTATIONS

The infant over the age of 3 months usually develops fever early in the course of the infection, often as high as 102° F to 104° F, that is, 38.9° C to 40° C. (Younger infants usually are afebrile.) He sneezes frequently, becomes irritable and restless. The congested nasal passages interfere with nursing, increasing the infant's irritability. The infant may have accompanying vomiting or diarrhea. This nasopharyngeal condition also appears as the first symptom of many childhood contagious diseases, such as measles. The common cold also needs to be differentiated from allergic rhinitis.

PREVENTION

Because complications can be very serious for the infant, efforts should be made to keep him away from persons suffering from colds.

TREATMENT

Nose drops of normal saline will help relieve the nasal congestion. Oily nose drops should *never* be used because of the danger of lipoid pneumonia if aspirated.

NURSING CARE

Nursing care of the irritable, uncomfortable infant includes holding, rocking and soothing him.

Administering Nose Drops. The infant is placed across the nurse's lap with his head lowered, or placed on his back in his crib with a folded blanket under his shoulders to allow his head to drop back. A plastic dropper with a rounded tip should be used to avoid injury to the child's nasal membrane. He should be kept in this position for a minute or two to allow the medication to shrink the nasal mucosa.

Nose drops should be administered 10 to 15 minutes before feedings and at bedtime. A bottle of nose drops should be used by only one person and discarded after its use is discontinued, as the solution easily becomes contaminated.

ACUTE OTITIS MEDIA

The eustachian tube in an infant is shorter and wider than in the older child. It is also straighter, thereby allowing nasopharyngeal infections to enter the middle ear more easily. *Hemophilus influenzae* is an important causative agent of otitis media in infants.

CLINICAL MANIFESTATIONS

roll or   *pain*

A restless infant who repeatedly shakes his head or rubs his ear should be checked for ear infection. Symptoms include fever and irritability. There may be vomiting or diarrhea. Examination of the ear with an otoscope reveals a bulging eardrum. Spontaneous rupture of the eardrum may occur, in which case there will be purulent drainage and pain will be relieved.

according to weight

TREATMENT *, IM vastus lateralus*

Antibiotics are used during the period of infection and for several days following, to prevent chronic infection and mastoiditis. Myringotomy may be necessary if improvement does not follow the use of antibiotics.

Recurrences of otitis media are common in infancy.[1] Myringotomy (incision of the eardrum) to establish drainage and to obtain pus for culture is necessary in persistently recurring otitis media. Antibiotics are used as with acute otitis media. Selective antibiotics, most effective in destroying the specific organism, are used as soon as cultures have shown the causative bacterium.

Complications: mastoiditis + deafness

Treatment of chronic otitis media also includes surgical insertion of tiny polyethylene tubes into the tympanic membrane to act as drains. Eventually the tubes will fall out spontaneously.

NURSING CARE

Emotional and physical support necessary for any ill infant should be freely given. If there is drainage from a ruptured eardrum or following myringotomy, the outer ear must be kept scrupulously clean. If ear wicks are to be inserted, the ear lobe is pulled down and back to straighten the ear canal in an infant. Ear wicks made of sterile gauze should be inserted carefully and loosely, and changed frequently. Placing the infant on the affected side helps promote drainage.

ACUTE BRONCHIOLITIS

Acute bronchiolitis (acute interstitial pneumonia) occurs with the greatest frequency during the first 6 months of life, and is rarely seen after the age of 2 years. The majority of cases occur in infants who have been in contact with older children or adults suffering from upper respiratory viral infections.

ETIOLOGY

Acute bronchiolitis is caused by a viral infection. The causative agent in over 50% of cases has been shown to be the respiratory syncytial virus. Other viruses associated with the disease are the parainfluenza, adenoviruses, and other viruses not always identified.

PATHOLOGY

The bronchi and bronchioles become plugged with a thick, viscid mucus, causing air to be trapped in the lungs. The infant can breathe air in, but has difficulty expelling it. This hinders the exchange of gases, and cyanosis appears.

CLINICAL MANIFESTATIONS

Onset of dyspnea is abrupt, sometimes preceded by a cough or a nasal discharge. There is a dry, persistent cough, extremely shallow respiration, air hunger, and cyanosis, which is frequently marked. Suprasternal and subcostal retractions are present. The chest becomes barrel-shaped from the trapped air. Respirations are 60 to 80 per minute.

Body temperature elevation is not great, seldom rising above 101° F to 102° F (38.3° C to 38.9° C). Dehydration may become a serious factor if competent care is not given. The infant appears apprehensive, irritable and restless.

NURSING CARE

Elevation of the child's head and chest aids his breathing. He should be turned at least every hour, and needs frequent changes of clothing because of the moist atmosphere.

If he is to be fed, clean his nares as much as possible before offering a bottle. Use a relatively small-holed nipple so that he does not choke, but do not make him work hard enough to tire him. If he can be removed from his

Croupette, he no doubt will fare better when he is held for feeding. If he needs to stay in his humidified atmosphere continually, be certain that his head is elevated, and hold his bottle, watching for choking or signs of exhaustion.

The nurse must remember that the baby is working hard in an effort to breathe, and can become exhausted very easily. Handling should be at a minimum consistent with intelligent nursing care. Intravenous fluids may be substituted for oral feedings until the infant is breathing more easily.

Medication is usually minimal because antihistamines, expectorants and sedatives do not appear to be useful. Antibiotics may be given to control secondary bacterial infections. Tracheostomy is not indicated in this condition.

OUTCOME

With careful nursing care and intelligent treatment, the condition can be expected to improve within a few days. Mortality rate is low if adequate supportive care is given. Complications, however, can include cardiac failure, respiratory failure from exhaustion, severe dehydration from loss of fluid because of hyperventilation, and bacterial bronchopneumonia.

PNEUMOCOCCAL PNEUMONIA

Pneumococcal pneumonia is the most common form of pneumonia found among infants and children. Its incidence has decreased over the last several years. This disease occurs mainly during the late winter and early spring months, principally in children under 4 years of age.

PATHOPHYSIOLOGY *X-ray, C+S of sputum, lab tests WBC ↑ urine S.G. ↑*

In infants, pneumococcal pneumonia is generally of the bronchial rather than the lobar type seen in older children. It is generally of the secondary type, following an upper respiratory viral infection.

The most common finding in infants is a patchy infiltration of one or several lobes of the lung. Lobar consolidation is unusual in infants and young children. Pleural effusion is frequently present.

CLINICAL MANIFESTATIONS

The onset of the pneumonic process is usually abrupt, following a mild upper respiratory illness. Temperature rises rapidly to 103° F to 105° F (39.4° C to 40.6° C). Respiratory distress is marked, with obvious air hunger, flaring of the nostrils, circumoral cyanosis and chest retractions. Tachycardia and tachypnea are present, with a pulse rate frequently as high as 140–180 per minute, and respirations as high as 80.

Generalized convulsions may occur during the period of high fever. Cough may not be noticeable at the onset but may appear later. Abdominal distention due to swallowed air or paralytic ileus is common.

TREATMENT

The use of antibiotics early in the disease gives prompt and favorable response. Penicillin has proved to be the most effective and is generally used unless the infant has a penicillin allergy. Oxygen started early in the disease process is important. Infants do best when placed in a Croupette.

Intravenous fluids are often necessary to supply the needed amount of fluids.

NURSING CARE

The infant needs considerable emotional support in his obvious distress. Having his mother at his bedside to reach into the Croupette and stroke his head gently and talk to him soothingly is the preferable method of support. If his mother cannot be present, this will be a nursing function.

The temperature and oxygen flow rate in the Croupette need frequent checking. The infant is usually more comfortable and finds breathing easier when his head is elevated. Suction apparatus should be at the cribside or

---

PROCEDURE FOR USE OF AN ICE-COOLED MIST TENT (CROUPETTE*) *makes easier to breath by liquifying secretions*

1. Make up the crib in the usual manner. Place a cotton blanket over the sheet to absorb the increased moisture caused by humidity in the croupette (optional).
2. Unfold the frame, and set it in the crib. Open the plastic canopy and fit it over the frame, with the apron of the canopy extending toward the foot of the crib. The zippered side openings permit nursing care.
3. Fill the ice chamber at the back of the tent with ice for cooling the tent. (The croupette is occasionally operated without ice if the child's temperature is below normal.)
4. Fill with distilled water the jar through which oxygen or air passes.
5. Connect the designated tubing to an oxygen wall outlet or a tank, or to the air compressor motor.
6. Allow humidified oxygen or air to flow into the tent for a few minutes before placing the child in the tent.
7. Set the liter gauge at the prescribed pressure.
8. Place the child in the tent, explaining the procedure if he can understand it. Position the child on his side, with his head slightly elevated. This usually helps to alleviate respiratory distress.
9. Keep the distilled water jar filled. Clean it thoroughly when refilling.
10. When ice in the chamber has melted, the drainage tubing should be allowed to drain into a basin, and the chamber should be refilled.
11. After the child is removed from the croupette, wash all apparatus, and send the canopy to be autoclaved.

* Air-Shields, Inc. Hatboro, Pa.

within ready access for use to remove excess secretions if necessary.

OUTCOME

With present day prompt and effective treatment, prognosis for recovery is excellent. Mortality rates have dropped to less than 1% in infants. The most common complication in infants is empyema, but this seldom occurs when adequate treatment has been started early in the disease.

HEMOPHILUS INFLUENZAE AND OTHER PNEUMONIAS

Hemophilus influenzae pneumonia also occurs in infants and young children. Its clinical manifestations are similar to those of pneumococcal pneumonia. However, its onset is more insidious, its clinical course longer and less acute. It is usually lobar in distribution.

Complications are frequent in the young infant. Most commonly seen are empyema and bacteremia.

Treatment consists of the same measures used in other pneumonias, with emphasis on the adequate use of antibiotics.

Staphylococcal pneumonia is still a menace to the newborn and very young infant. Streptococcal pneumonia is rarely seen in the infant.

SUDDEN INFANT DEATH SYNDROME

Sudden infant death syndrome (SIDS) has caused much grief and anxiety among many families for centuries. One of the leading causes of infant mortality, it claims an estimated 10,000 lives annually in the United States alone.

Throughout history this syndrome has presented a most vexing problem. Commonly known as "crib death," it is defined as "the sudden and unexpected death of an infant who was either well or almost well prior to death, and whose death remains unexplained after the performance of an adequate autopsy."[5]

Varying theories have been suggested about the cause of SIDS. In ancient writings, it was attributed to "overlaying" by the infant's mother or nurse. The adult supposedly rolled over onto the infant during sleep. This was eventually ruled out, particularly as many affected infants were alone in their cribs when they ceased breathing.

Later, an enlarged thymus was believed to be the cause. Other possible causes were also tested, but none could be definitely implicated.

Recent research suggests the possibility that SIDS results from respiratory failure followed by cardiac arrest. It is believed that respiratory failure is caused either by laryngeal spasm, or by a partial nasal obstruction that causes a sucking back of the tongue over the larynx.

The National Institute of Child Health and Human Development has sponsored a research program, which supports a variety of SIDS research projects. Several of these are still in progress in the U.S. and other countries, investigating respiratory, cardiac, and laryngeal factors as well as genetic and environmental responses. Psychological stress experiences of the families of SIDS victims are also considered.

Infants affected are most frequently between the ages of 2 months to 3 months, although some deaths have occurred during the first and second weeks of life. Few infants over 6 months of age die of SIDS. SIDS is a greater threat to low-birth-weight infants than to term infants. It occurs more often in winter, and affects more male infants than female infants, those who have had slight cold symptoms, and infants from minority and lower socioeconomic groups.

SIDS is rapid and silent, occurring most frequently in the early morning hours while the infant is sleeping. The infant has been put to bed in apparent good health and later when checked is found dead. No outcry is said to have been heard, nor is there any evidence of a struggle. Persons who have been sleeping nearby claim to have heard nothing unusual before the death was discovered. It is not uncommon for the infant to have been recently examined by a physician and found to be in excellent health. Autopsies frequently reveal a mild respiratory disorder but nothing considered serious enough to have caused death.

EMOTIONAL SUPPORT FOR PARENTS AND FAMILIES

The effects of SIDS on parents and families are devastating. Grief is coupled with guilt, even though it is known that SIDS cannot be predicted or prevented. For this reason, it is recommended that an autopsy be done and the results promptly made known to the family. Even though parents are told that they are not to blame for the infant's death, it is difficult for most parents not to keep searching for evidence of some possible neglect on their part. Prolonged depression usually follows the initial shock and anguish over the infant's death.

Probably the most helpful resource available for these parents is a local chapter of the Sudden Infant Death Syndrome Foundation. This organization and other similar ones can put parents of SIDS victims in touch with other parents who have gone through the same experience.

Other children in the family need truthful, compassionate information concerning the infant's death. An article by C. Hardgrove and L. Warrick, "How shall we tell the children?" provides sound advice.[6]

Eventually some parents may want to have another baby. When that subsequent child is born, parents will be understandably anxious and are likely to need counseling. The following comments are from Carolyn Szybist, a nurse, and a mother of a SIDS baby. She offers important insight into the feelings of SIDS parents.[7]

- Two important facts are that 1) SIDS is a disease entity that cannot be predicted or prevented, and 2) SIDS is not hereditary.
- Everyone who has lost a child to SIDS has encountered someone who did not understand.
- When you hold your new baby for the first time, you may find that old memories come flooding back.
- Will you spend 24 hours a day by the crib? The answer is no. Even if you try, eventually you will get tired. That is when you learn to trust—in living, in yourself.
- You will probably check on your sleeping baby more frequently. Parents of subsequent children admit that in

the past they used to check their babies to see if they were covered, now they check respiration.

- Even the youngest child (sibling) reacts in some way to the death of the previous child.
- Panic can be caused by too much time alone, too much time to think, and perhaps the terrible burden of believing that your presence alone is keeping the baby alive, that you are a round-the-clock human respirator.
- Parents of subsequent children are inclined to view the common cold with more alarm than open-heart surgery.
- The most uncomfortable period will be the point when your subsequent child reaches the age of the child who died.

genitourinary system disorders

ACUTE PYELONEPHRITIS

Infections of the urinary tract are fairly common in the "diaper age," particularly between the ages of 2 months and 2 years. Pyelonephritis (pyuria, pyelitis) is the most common urinary tract infection and the most common renal disorder of infants and children.

PATHOPHYSIOLOGY

The condition occurs more commonly in girls than in boys. Although many different bacteria may infect the urinary tract, intestinal bacilli account for the infection in about 80% of acute episodes. The female urethra is shorter and straighter than that in the male, thus being more easily contaminated with feces. Inflammation may extend into the bladder, ureters, and the kidney.

CLINICAL MANIFESTATIONS

In acute pyelonephritis the onset is abrupt with high fever for a day or two. Occasionally there is little or no fever.

Vomiting is common; diarrhea may occur. The infant is irritable; convulsions may occur during the period of high fever.

DIAGNOSIS

Diagnosis is based on finding of pus in the urine under microscopic examination. It is important that the urine specimen be fresh and uncontaminated. A "clean catch" voided urine, properly performed, is essential for microscopic examination. If a culture is needed, the infant must be catheterized. *IVP - intravenous pylegram*

TREATMENT

Fluids should be given freely. The symptoms usually subside within a few days, but this is not an indication that the infection is completely cleared. Medication is usually continued after symptoms disappear.

NURSING CARE

The nurse will give the infant supportive care as needed. She will need to use ingenuity in persuading the infant or young child to take the necessary amount of fluids. Glucose water or liquid gelatin dessert, is usually well accepted. The nurse should not be discouraged if only a few swallows at a time are taken. Persistence is the answer.

OUTCOME

Chronic and recurring urinary infections are frequently associated with obstructions in the urinary tract. The urinary system should be carefully studied through the use of x-ray visualization procedures.

WILMS' TUMOR *a highly malignant tumor - embryotal tumor*

Wilms' tumor is an adenosarcoma in the kidney region and is one of the most common of the abdominal neo-

Hydrocele is common in newborns + usually corrects itself.

OBTAINING A CLEAN URINE SPECIMEN

In Infants

Equipment

1. A sterile basin containing cotton balls saturated with aqueous Zephiran 1 : 1000 or a soap solution.
2. A plastic urine collector (Fig. 7 – 9).
3. A sterile specimen bottle. (Alternatively, the plastic collector may also be used as the specimen bottle.)

Procedure

1. Wash genitalia with soaked cotton balls using downward strokes. For girls, first separate the labia, washing away from the urethral meatus. Wash the outer surface of the perineum and the anal region. Discard cotton ball after each stroke.
2. Dry the skin. While one person holds the infant with legs abducted, the nurse firmly presses the adhesive surface of the bag down around the urethra (Fig. 7 – 10A). In girls, care should be taken to ensure the adhesive adheres to the strip of skin between the vagina and the rectum.

3. Observe the infant frequently for voiding. After the specimen is obtained, remove collector, press sides of adhesive around opening together to make a sterile container (Fig. 7 – 10B).
4. Label and send to laboratory.
5. Record the time and other pertinent data.

In Older Children

1. Clean genitalia as outlined.
2. A small child may sit on a potty chair and void into a sterile basin or into a sterilized potty. An older child may void into a sterile bedpan, a sterile urinal, or directly into a specimen bottle.
3. A midstream specimen is desirable, but difficult to obtain from small children. To obtain a midstream specimen, the child should start to void into an unsterile receptacle, stop the stream, and void into a sterile receptacle.

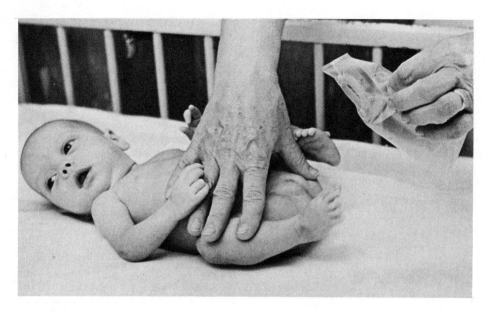

FIG. 7–9.   One method of applying a plastic urine collector.

plasms found in early childhood. The tumor arises from bits of embryonic tissue remaining after birth. This tissue has the capacity to begin rapid cancerous growth in the area of the kidney.

The tumor is rarely discovered until it has reached a size large enough to be palpated through the abdominal wall. As the tumor grows it invades the kidney or the renal vein

IVP - diagnosis   don't palpate or rub abd.

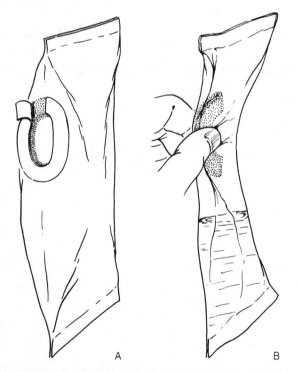

FIG. 7–10.   The plastic urine collector has a soft sponge around the opening (A), and the sides of the opening are pressed together to make the collector into a specimen container (B).

and disseminates to other parts of the body. Treatment consists of surgical removal as soon as possible after the growth is discovered. The medication now being used is actinomycin D given before and after surgery. Irradiation is also used postoperatively.

Prognosis is generally good for children under the age of 2 years. The use of actinomycin D has brought about a significant decrease in the mortality rate from this disorder. If the child appears well and no metastasis is evident after the age of 2, he is considered cured.

nervous system disorders

ACUTE OR NONRECURRENT CONVULSIONS

A convulsion may be a symptom of a wide variety of disorders. In infants and children under the age of 2 or 3 years, febrile convulsions are the most common. These convulsions occur in association with a high fever, frequently one of the initial symptoms of an acute infection somewhere in the body. Less frequent causes of convulsions are intracranial infections such as meningitis, toxic reactions to certain drugs or minerals such as lead, metabolic disorders, and a variety of brain disorders.

CLINICAL MANIFESTATIONS

A convulsion may appear suddenly without warning; however, frequently, restlessness and irritability may precede an attack. The infant's body stiffens and he loses consciousness. In a few seconds clonic movements occur. These are quick, jerking movements of the arms, legs, and facial muscles. Breathing is irregular and there is an inability to swallow saliva.

TREATMENT

Phenobarbital sodium is usually ordered by the physician, and given intramuscularly.

NURSING CARE

A child whose fever or other symptoms indicate that a convulsion may be anticipated should be placed where he can be easily watched. Crib sides should be padded to prevent injury, but some space should be left at the foot of the crib so that the infant is not entirely isolated from his environment. An airway or a padded tongue blade should be kept at the bedside.

When an infant starts to convulse, the nurse should turn his head to one side to prevent aspiration of saliva or vomitus. However, the child's movements should not be restrained. Mouth suctioning, using a soft catheter, removes excess saliva. A padded tongue blade placed between the jaws of an older infant or young child prevents him from biting his tongue.

Documentation should be detailed and complete. The record should include

1. Any symptoms observed previous to the convulsion.
2. Kind of movements: rigidity, jerking, twitching, whether generalized or localized in one part of the body.
3. Duration of seizure.
4. Child's color, pulse and respiration rates and quality.
5. Any deviant eye movements or other abnormal signs.

OUTCOME

An isolated convulsion may cause no harm, but repeated convulsions may result in brain damage. Most physicians will give the child a thorough physical and neurological examination following a single convulsion, and will carefully check the child's history concerning all phases of his health and of his level of development.

FEBRILE CONVULSIONS

Febrile convulsions are usually in the form of a generalized seizure, occurring early in the course of a fever. Although usually associated with high fever, 102° F to 106° F (38.9° C to 41.1° C), some children appear to have a low seizure threshold and convulse when a fever of 100° F to 102° F (37.8° C to 38.9° C) is present.

Prompt reporting of elevated temperatures is essential for all sick children. Aspirin and tepid sponges or a cooling mattress are usually ordered for reduction of fever.

A convulsion is a frightening occurrence to parents. Explanations are needed to reassure them that febrile convulsions are not uncommon in small children. Parents also need to understand that the thorough examination given a child after he has had a convulsion does not mean the physician suspects some serious condition. He is seeking to *rule out* any possible cause other than the nervous system irritation caused by high fever.

HEMOPHILUS INFLUENZAE MENINGITIS

Purulent meningitis in infancy and childhood is caused by a variety of agents. Among these are the meningococcus, tubercle bacillus and the *Hemophilus influenzae*. The most common form is the influenza bacillus meningitis.

Peak occurrence of influenza bacillus meningitis is between the ages of 6 and 12 months. It is rare during the first 2 months of life and seldom seen after the fourth year. Purulent meningitis is an infectious disease. Strict isolation techniques should be carried out for 24 hours after the start of effective antimicrobial therapy, or until pathogens can no longer be cultured out from the nasopharynx.

CLINICAL MANIFESTATIONS

The onset may be either gradual or abrupt following an upper respiratory infection. Young infants with meningitis may have a characteristic high pitched cry, fever and irritability. Other symptoms include headache and stiffness of the neck and spine. Projectile vomiting may be present. Generalized convulsions are common in infants. Coma may occur early, particularly in the older child.

DIAGNOSIS

Early diagnosis and treatment are essential for uncomplicated recovery. A spinal tap should be done promptly whenever symptoms raise a suspicion that the disease may be present.

The spinal fluid will be found to be under increased pressure. Laboratory examination of the fluid will reveal

---

PROCEDURE FOR TEPID BATH TO REDUCE FEVER

Equipment
A basin containing tepid water.
A bath blanket (two for an older child).
A wash cloth.

Technique
1. Take the child's temperature and record it.
2. Wash your hands, and assemble the equipment.
3. Undress the child, and place a bath blanket under the child (to absorb moisture and to prevent undue chilling).
4. Cover an older child with a second bath blanket.
5. Expose his arms and his chest. Wring washcloth lightly from tepid water, sponge gently, making long, even strokes. Apply gentle friction with your

hands, following the sponge. Repeat 2 or 3 times, giving attention to the axillary area.
6. Sponge the abdomen, the legs and the feet in the same manner.
7. Turn the child on his abdomen and sponge his back.
8. Sponge the inner surface of the groin and the perineal region. (Sponge the anal region last.)
9. Do not continue longer than 15 or 20 minutes.
10. Take the child's temperature every ½-hour until it is reduced to an acceptable level. Note: The child's temperature may continue to fall after sponging. Wait for 30 minutes before resuming the sponge bath. The child may be left uncovered following the sponge bath if his temperature remains elevated.

increased protein and decreased glucose content. Very early in the disease the spinal fluid may be clear, but it rapidly becomes purulent. The causative organism can usually be determined from stained smears of the spinal fluid. It enables specific medication to be started very early, without waiting for growths of organisms on culture media.

TREATMENT

Treatment consists primarily in administration of medication in effective dosage. At present, ampicillin or chloramphenicol is the treatment of choice. Initially these medications are usually given by the intravenous route for rapid assimilation or by intramuscular injection. Later in the disease, they may be given orally. Treatment is continued for at least 7 days, and longer if there is persistent fever, subdural effusion or otitis media.

COMPLICATIONS

Subdural effusion may complicate the condition among infants during the course of the disease. Fluid accumulates in the subdural space between the dura and the brain. Needle aspirations through the infant's open suture lines or burr holes (in the skull of the older child) are used to remove the fluid. Repeated aspiration may be required.

Other complications of influenzal meningitis are hydrocephalus, nerve deafness, mental retardation and paralysis. The risk of complications is lessened when appropriate medication is started early in the disease.

NURSING CARE

Because of the irritability associated with meningitis, noises and bright lighting should be kept at a minimum. The child should be handled as little as possible during the stage of irritability. However, frequent turning is necessary to avoid skin breakdown and upper respiratory infection. All turning and handling must be done as gently as possible. The mother or nurse may help calm the child by sitting at his bedside within his range of vision and speaking to him softly.

Nursing care includes attention to such manifestations as vomiting, convulsions, urinary retention, food and fluid intake. Prompt reporting and accurate recording are essential. When the fever is high, a cold water mattress, or tepid sponges are usually indicated. Mouth and skin care are given as needed. During convalescence, careful record should be kept of an unusual behavior, or signs of deafness, enlarging head or any abnormality.

OUTCOME

Since the advent of the use of sulfa drugs and antibiotics, the recovery rate has been about 95%. However, serious and permanent complications do occur, in spite of optimal treatment.

skin disorders

MILIARIA RUBRA (PRICKLY HEAT)

This condition, often called *prickly heat,* is common in infants who are exposed to summer heat or are over-dressed. It may also appear in febrile illnesses and may be mistaken for the rash of one of the communicable diseases. The rash appears as pinhead-sized erythematous (reddened) papules. It is most noticeable in areas where sweat glands are concentrated, as in folds of the skin, the chest and about the neck. It usually causes itching, making the infant uncomfortable and fretful.

Treatment should first be preventive. Mothers should be taught to avoid bundling their infants in layers of clothing in hot weather. A diaper may be all the child needs. Tepid baths without soap will help control the itching. A sprinkling of cornstarch at diaper changes will help relieve the infant's discomfort.

DIAPER RASH

Diaper rash is a common occurrence in infancy. Bacterial decomposition of urine produces ammonia which is very irritating to an infant's tender skin. Diarrheal stools also produce a burning erythematous area in the anal region. Infants who become easily irritated in the diaper area may have inherited a sensitive skin. Other causes may be: prolonged exposure to wet or soiled diapers, (aggravated by the use of rubber or plastic covers, or disposable diapers); incomplete cleansing of the diaper area, especially after a bowel movement; sensitivity to certain soaps or to plastic pants; and use of strong detergents with incomplete rinsing for washing diapers and crib bedding.

TREATMENT

Exposure of the diaper area to the air helps to clear up the dermatitis. When the area is excoriated and sore, the physician may prescribe an antibiotic or other ointment.

PREVENTION

Diapers washed at a commercial diaper service are sterilized, preventing the growth of ammonia-forming bacteria. Diapers washed at home should be rinsed thoroughly, and an antiseptic such as Diaper Sweet added to the final rinse. Drying diapers in the sun, or in a heated dryer, also helps destroy the bacteria.

Mothers should be cautioned to change diapers each time the infant urinates, and to check diapers frequently if infant is wearing plastic pants or disposable diapers, which prevent moisture from becoming apparent.

ACUTE INFANTILE ECZEMA inflammation of skin

Infantile eczema is an atopic dermatitis considered to be at least in part an allergic reaction to some irritant or irritants. It is fairly common during the first year of life after the age of 3 months. It is uncommon in breastfed babies before they are given additional foods.

ETIOLOGY

Infantile eczema is characterized by

1. A hereditary predisposition. Also, those infants who have eczema tend to have hay fever or asthma later in life.
2. Hypersensitivity of the deeper layers of the skin to protein or proteinlike allergens.

3. Allergens to which the child is sensitive may be inhaled, ingested, or absorbed through direct contact. Examples are house dust, egg white, and wool.

CLINICAL MANIFESTATIONS

Eczema usually starts on the cheeks and spreads to the extensor surfaces of the arms and legs. Eventually the entire trunk may become involved. The initial reddening of the skin is quickly followed by papule and vesicle formation. Itching is intense, and the scratching the infant does makes the skin weep and crust. The areas easily become infected by hemolytic streptococci or by staphylococci.

DIAGNOSIS

The most common allergens concerned in the manifestation of eczema are:

Foods: egg white, cow's milk, wheat products, and orange and tomato juice.
Inhalants: house dust, pollens, and animal dander.
Materials: wool, nylon, and plastic.

However, diagnosis is not simple. The infant may show skin-test sensitivity to one or many allergens but still show no improvement when they are eliminated. Factors other than allergy appear to be involved. These may include the sensitive nature of the skin of an infant, which reacts more quickly to marked changes in temperature and to other environmental factors.

Diagnostic Diet. An elimination diet may be helpful in ruling out offending foods. A basic diet, consisting of only hypoallergenic foods, is started. Some form of milk or milk substitute should be included, as well as vitamin supplements. If the child's skin condition shows improvement, other foods are added one at a time, and the effects are carefully noted.

Great care must be taken not to foster undernourishment. One child with severe eczema was kept on such a strict regimen that he was in an extremely poor nutritional state and became susceptible to infection. The infection cleared when someone with common sense placed the emphasis on building up the child's nutritional status; and the emotional satisfaction this gave the child enabled him to express his needs in other than physical symptoms. Needless to say, an elimination program must always be under the strict supervision of a competent physician.

Hyperallergenic Foods. The protein in egg white is such a common offender that most pediatricians advise against feeding whole eggs to any infant until late into the first year of life.

Cow's milk seems to cause or aggravate eczema in some infants. Because of this fact, evaporated milk may be tolerated when regular bottled milk is not. Some babies tolerate goat's milk well, but many do best on feedings of hypoallergenic milk substitutes. These are prepared from soya (soy bean) or hydrolized casein. However, it should be kept in mind that *breast* milk rarely causes allergic reactions.

Hypoallergenic milk substitutes are prepared by commercial firms and appear to be nutritionally satisfactory.

Inhalant and Contact Allergens. These substances should be avoided as far as possible. In the infant's sleeping room window drapes, dresser scarfs and rugs should be removed, and furniture washed off frequently. He should not come in contact with feather pillows; stuffed toys should be carefully chosen. Sadly, it may be necessary to provide new homes for household pets.

TREATMENT

Smallpox vaccination is definitely contraindicated for the child with eczema. In fact, he must be kept away from anyone who has recently been vaccinated. A serious condition called *eczema vaccinatum* results when an infant with eczema is vaccinated or is exposed to the vaccination of another person. The infant becomes seriously ill and mortality rates have been high.

In the presence of infection, antibiotics will be ordered, preferably by mouth. Sedatives and antihistamines help control the itching and calm the infant. Antihistamine ointments and local anesthetics *should not* be used.

Bulky, cool wet packs help alleviate the itching. These packs should not be wrapped in plastic or bandages, but may be pinned together loosely or tied with straps.

Ointments should be applied with long, smooth strokes for the soothing effect. After an ointment has been applied, the area should be bandaged with strips of soft cotton cloth and held in place with 2-inch Ace bandages.

A face mask may be needed to hold wet dressings in place or to ensure retention of ointments applied to the face. A mask is made by cutting holes in a piece of cotton material to correspond in location to eyes, nose and mouth. The holes should be hemmed to avoid fraying. The mask is made to go around the head and is held in place with tapes or drawstrings. Care should be taken to avoid friction or binding (Fig. 7–11).

Colloid Baths. Tub baths using tepid water, cornstarch, and baking soda are soothing. For a small infant tub, use about one fourth cup of baking soda and one fourth cup of cornstarch mixed together. Oatmeal baths are also used. Cooked oatmeal is put in a cheesecloth bag and squeezed through the bath water. A commercial preparation called Aveeno may be used in place of the homecooked oatmeal. Use according to directions.

The child is bathed in one of these colloid baths for about 15 minutes. Soap should not be used. He should be dried by light dabs, not by rubbing.

NURSING AND HOME CARE

Coping with the care of an infant with eczema is an exhausting task. The mother can be assured that most cases of infant eczema clear up by the age of 2, but this assurance does little to relieve the present situation. Whenever possible, hospitalization should be avoided because these infants pick up infections in the hospital very easily. There are times when hospitalization seems to be

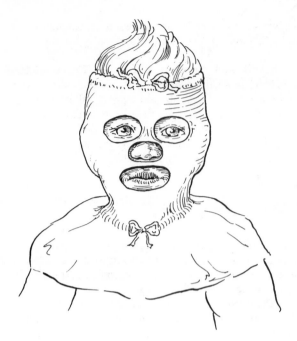

FIG. 7–11. To prevent his scratching eczema of the face, the child is protected with a facial mask.

indicated, either to give the child more intensive care or to relieve an exhausted parent. Great care must be taken to shield the child from infection while giving him the comfort and emotional support he desperately needs.

Physical Care.   The infant is apt to express his discomfort through scratching and rubbing the itching areas. He must be prevented from scratching and making his condition worse, but restraints should be used only when no alternative will work. He does not need any more frustration than he is already experiencing.

Use of Restraints.   When restraints must be used, elbow restraints are probably the most effective. Fingernails and toenails should be kept short. Mitts put on the child's hands will help prevent scratching.

Emotional Support.   The infant with eczema needs at least as much cuddling and affection as the healthy child. Deprived of normal avenues of sensory stimulation, he needs opportunity to develop his mental and physical abilities, as well as to achieve emotional satisfaction.

His frustration may be relieved by use of a pacifier to provide additional sucking pleasure. Soft, smooth toys can occupy his hands and divert his attention from his discomfort. If old enough to creep or walk, he needs opportunities to do so. Some mothers may be fearful or repulsed by the child's unattractive appearance. They will need help to view their child as a normal child with a distressing, but temporary, skin condition.

IMPETIGO

This infection of the skin occasionally appears in newborn or infant nurseries when strict aseptic technique is not carried out, or in home situations that are not sanitary. Impetigo may be either a staphylococcal or streptococcal skin infection, but in newborns or infants it is usually due to staphylococci. Lesions appear anywhere on the body.

CLINICAL MANIFESTATIONS

The lesions are vesicular, becoming rapidly seropurulent with an area of erythema surrounding each lesion. Rupture of the pustules causes spread to other areas.

Susceptibility among newborns seems to be general. The infecting organism may be carried by attending personnel with minor staphylococcal lesions. The condition can spread quickly through a nursery unless strict isolation of the infected infant is carried out.

TREATMENT

The lesions should be washed with an antiseptic detergent solution. If crusts have formed, they should be carefully removed after softening with 1 : 20 Burow's solution compresses. Antibiotic ointment may be applied locally. Systemic antibiotic therapy may also be used if condition is not controlled topically.

OUTCOME

The disease is generally mild with complete recovery if the infant is cared for properly. In the past, sepsis has occurred primarily in sick and premature babies.

SEBORRHEIC DERMATITIS (CRADLE CAP)

Generally this condition can be prevented by daily washing of the infant's hair and scalp. Characterized by yellowish, scaly or crusted patches on the scalp, it occurs in newborns and in older infants who are beginning to feed themselves with their fingers and periodically run their fingers through their hair.

Parents may be afraid to wash vigorously over the "soft spot." They need to understand that this is where cradle cap often begins, and that careful but vigorous washing of the area with a washcloth can prevent this disorder. Using a fine baby comb after shampooing is also a helpful preventive measure.

Once the condition exists, daily application of mineral oil will help loosen the crust. No attempt should be made to loosen it all at once; otherwise, the delicate skin on the scalp may break or bleed, and easily become infected.

summary

The remarkable growth and development that occurs during the first year of an infant's life affects all the years that follow. Even with ideal nutrition and a warm family relationship, a few minor health problems are inevitable, usually with no serious long-term effects. Infants who live in less than an ideal environment are vulnerable to major health problems. Owing to immature body systems and defenses, and small anatomical structures, even minor problems can become serious, and major problems life-threatening, if not promptly diagnosed and treated. Depending on the pathogenic agent, the family environment, the individual child, and the care received from health professionals, health problems can be a source of growth or a source of crisis for the infant and family.

review questions

1. Describe the mother–infant relationship of infants with failure-to-thrive.
2. What is the nurse's role when a failure-to-thrive infant is hospitalized?
3. What is the cause of the following disorders: Rickets? Scurvey? Beriberi? Pellagra?
4. Name three sources of vitamin C, calcium, iron, and iodine.
5. What nursing measures must be taken to prevent the excoriation of the skin that accompanies diarrhea?
6. Describe projectile vomiting.
7. Prior to the surgical correction of pyloric stenosis, what type of feedings are given?
8. How does the nurse prevent hypostatic pneumonia in an infant who has had surgery?
9. What behaviors by the infant would suggest otitis media?
10. What nursing measure will facilitate breathing in an infant with acute bronchiolitis?
11. What is the most helpful community resource the nurse can suggest to parents who have experienced SIDS?
12. What nursing measures are necessary when an infant experiences a febrile convulsion?
13. Differentiate between sickle cell disease and sickle cell trait.
14. Explain sickle cell crisis and its treatment.

references

1. Wieczorek RR, Natapoff JN: A Conceptual Approach to the Nursing of Children: Health Care From Birth Through Adolescence. Philadelphia, JB Lippincott, 1981
2. Spitz R: The First Year of Life. New York, International Universities Press, 1965
3. Bowlby J: Child Care and the Growth of Love. Baltimore, Penguin, 1953
4. Fleisher DR: Infant rumination syndrome. Am J Dis child 133:266–269, 1979
5. Bergman AB, et al: Studies of SIDS in Kings County, Washington, Part 3, Epidemiology. J Pediatr 49:860, 1972
6. Hardgrove C, Warrick L: How Shall We Tell the Children? Am J Nurs 74:448–450, 1974
7. Szybist C: The subsequent child. DHEW No. (HSA) 76-545. Rockville, U.S. Public Health Service, 1976

bibliography

Barnard MU, et al: Handbook for Comprehensive Pediatric Nursing. New York, McGraw-Hill, 1981

Bishop WS, Head J: Care of the infant with a stoma. Am J Mat Child Nurs 1:315–319, 1976

Chinn PL: Child Health Maintenance: Concepts in Family-centered Care, 2nd ed. St Louis, CV Mosby, 1979

Ein SH, Stephens CA: Intussusception: 354 cases in 10 years. J Pediatr Surg 6:16, 1971

Fochman D, Raffensperger JG: Principles of Nursing Care for the Pediatric Surgery Patient, 2nd ed. Boston, Little, Brown & Co., 1976

Fox JA: Primary Health Care of the Young. New York, McGraw-Hill, 1980

Harrison L: Nursing intervention with the failure-to-thrive family. Am J Mat Child Nurs 1:112, 1976

Howry LB, Bindler RM, Tso Y: Pediatric Medications. Philadelphia, JB Lippincott, 1981

Johnson SH (ed): High-risk Parenting: Nursing Assessment and Strategies for the Family At Risk. Philadelphia, JB Lippincott, 1979

McGrath BJ: Fluids, electrolytes and replacement therapy in pediatric nursing. Am J Mat Child Nurs 5:58–62, 1980

Miller JR, Janosik EH: Family-focused Care. New York, McGraw-Hill, 1980

Nutrition: World Health Magazine. World Health Organization (WHO), May 6, 1977

Pinney M: Pneumonia. Am J Nurs 81:517–518, 1981

Rutter M: Maternal deprivation, 1972–1978: New findings, new concepts, new approaches. Child Development 50:283–285, 1977

Simkins R: Bronchiolitis. Am J Nurs 81:514–516, 1981

Simkins R: Croup and epiglottis. Am J Nurs 81:519–520, 1981

Spenner D: When the baby is sick and the mother's concern is ignored. Am J Nurs 80:2223–2224, 1980

Sudden Infant Death Syndrome Research Program of National Institute of Child Health and Human Development, DHEW No. (NIH) 77-1436, Rockville, U.S. Public Health Service, 1977

normal growth and development of the toddler: 1 to 3 years 8

physical development
nutrition
health maintenance
accident prevention
teaching oral hygiene
toilet training
psychosocial development
discipline
sharing with a sibling
implications for hospital care
toilet training
discipline problems
eating problems
summary
review questions
references
bibliography

student objectives

The student successfully attaining the goals of this chapter will be able to

1 Define the following vocabulary terms:

caries   dawdling   discipline   ipecac   negativism   plaque   ritualism

2 Describe the growth and development of the toddler in the following areas: personal–social development, fine motor skills, gross motor skills, language development, and cognition.

3 Discuss how the eating pattern of the toddler may change and list six suggestions that may be helpful in solving the eating problems of the toddler.

4 Identify the four leading causes of accidental death during childhood and describe safety measures that can be used to prevent each of them.

5 List six suggestions the nurse can give parents about toilet training their child.

6 Describe the terms negativism, ritualism, and dawdling as they pertain to the psychosocial development of the toddler.

Soon after a child's first birthday, important, sometimes dramatic changes take place. Physical growth slows considerably, mobility and communication skills improve rapidly, and a determined, often defiant little person begins to create a whole new set of problems for his parents. "No" and "want" are favorite words. Temper tantrums appear.

During this transition from infancy to early childhood, the child learns many new physical and social skills. Additional teeth and better motor skills make it possible for him to feed himself a whole new array of foods, and also, if unsupervised, to taste many nonfood items that may be harmful, even fatal.

This transition is a time of unpredictability: one moment, the toddler insists on "doing it himself;" the next moment, he reverts to dependence on mother or other caregiver. As he seeks to assert his independence and achieve autonomy, he experiences fear of separation. Curiosity about the world around him increases as does his ability to explore (Fig. 8–1). Parents soon discover that this exploration can wreak havoc on orderly routine and a well-kept house, and that the toddler requires close supervision to prevent injury to himself and objects in the environment.

Toddlerhood is a difficult time for parents. Just as they are beginning to feel confident in their ability to care for and understand their infant, he changes into a walking, talking stranger whose attitudes and behaviors disrupt the entire family. Accident-proofing safety measures and firm but gentle discipline are paramount tasks for parents of toddlers. Learning to discipline with patience and understanding is difficult, but eventually rewarding. At the end of the "terrible twos," children's behavior generally becomes more acceptable and predictable.

physical development

Toddlerhood is a time of slowed growth and rapid development. Each year the toddler adds 5 to 10 pounds to his weight and about 3 inches to his height. Continued erup-

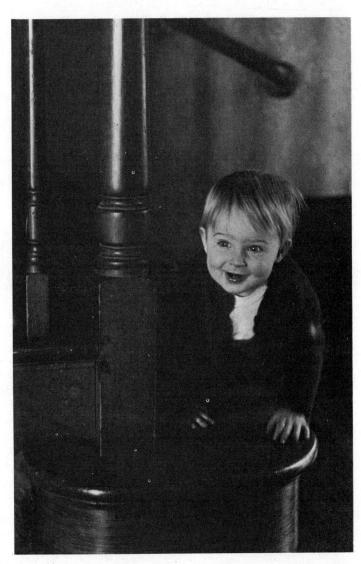

FIG. 8–1.   The toddler explores the stairs on his own. (Photo by Carol Baldwin)

tion of teeth, particularly the molars, help him learn to chew food. He has learned to stand alone (Fig. 8–2), and perhaps, to walk, between the ages of 1 and 2 years. During this time, most children say their first words, and continue to improve and refine their language skills. By the end of this period, they may have learned partial or total toilet training.

The rate of development varies with each individual child, depending on his personality and the opportunities he has to test, explore, and learn. Significant landmarks in growth and development of the toddler are summarized in Table 8–1.

nutrition

Between the ages of 1 and 3, eating problems frequently appear. These occur for a number of reasons such as the following:

1. The child's growth rate has slowed; therefore, he may want and need less food than before. Parents need to know that this is normal.
2. The child has a strong drive for independence and autonomy. This compels him to assert his will, to prove

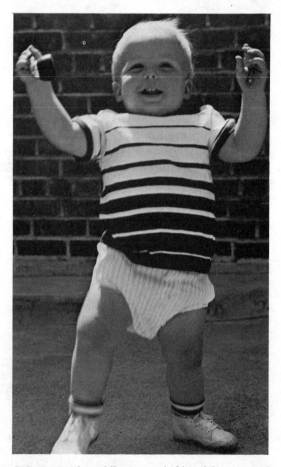

FIG. 8–2. The toddler is proud of his ability to stand alone. (Photo by Carol Baldwin)

to himself and others that he is an individual in his own right.
3. A child's appetite varies according to the kind of foods offered, and he is likely to go on "food jags," desiring only one kind of food for periods of time.

To minimize these eating problems and assure that the child gets a balanced diet with all the proteins, carbohydrates, minerals, and vitamins essential for health and well-being (Table 8–2), meals should be planned with an understanding of the toddler's developing feeding skills (Table 8–3). The following suggestions also may be helpful to parents and to caregivers in the hospital:

1. Serve small portions, and let the child ask for seconds. This will foster his growing autonomy and remove the need to rebel.
2. Remember that there is no *one* food positively essential to health. Allow substitution for a disliked food.
3. Toddlers like simply prepared foods, served warm or cool, *not* hot or cold.
4. Most children eat better when they eat with the family. They learn by imitating the acceptance or rejection of foods by other family members.
5. Children prefer foods they can pick up with their fingers; however, they should be allowed to use a spoon or fork when they want to try.
6. Parents should let a child eat, not force him to eat. When he has eaten all he wishes, he should be allowed to leave the table. If he has refused most of his food, it is better to make no comment, but to withhold additional food until the next meal or snack period.
7. Dawdling at mealtime is common with this age group and can be ignored unless it stretches on to unreasonable lengths or becomes a play for power. Then the food can be calmly removed without comment.
8. Making desserts a reward for good eating habits is not appropriate. It gives unfair value to the dessert and makes vegetables or other foods seem less desirable.
9. Offer regularly planned nutritious snacks, such as milk, crackers and peanut butter, cheese cubes, pieces of fruit.

A sample daily food plan is provided in Table 8–4.

health maintenance

Activities that protect the health of the toddler and help ensure continuing growth and development include prevention of accidents and infection, formation of good oral health habits, toilet training, and providing a stimulating environment and the opportunity to explore it. Nurses assist families with toddlers in these activities by health teaching, support of positive parenting behaviors, and reinforcement of the toddler's achievements (Table 8–5).

ACCIDENT PREVENTION

Toddlers are explorers who demand constant supervision in a controlled environment to prevent injury. When supervision is inadequate, or the environment unsafe, tragedy often results, making accidents the leading cause

TABLE 8–1. GROWTH AND DEVELOPMENT CHART: THE TODDLER

Age (months)	Personal–Social	Fine Motor	Gross Motor	Language	Cognition
12–15	Begins Erikson's stage of "autonomy vs shame and doubt" Seeks novel ways to pursue new experiences Imitations of people are more advanced	Builds with blocks, finger paints Able to reach out with the hands and bring food to the mouth Holds a spoon Drinks from a cup	Movements become more voluntary Postural control improves; able to stand and may take few independent steps	First words are not generally classified as true language. They are generally associated with the concrete and are usually activity-oriented	Begins to accommodate to the environment, and the adaptive process evolves
18	Extremely curious Becomes a communicative social being Parallel play Fleeting contacts with other children "Make-believe" play begins	Better control of spoon; good control when drinking from cup Turns pages of a book Places objects in holes or slots	Walks alone; gait may still be a bit unsteady Begins to walk sideward and backward	Begins to use language in a symbolic form to represent images or ideas that reflect the thinking process Uses some meaningful words such as "hi," "bye-bye," "all gone" Comprehension is significantly greater	Demonstrates foresight and can discover solutions to problems without excessive trial-and-error procedures Is able to imitate without the presence of a model (deferred imitation)
24	Language facilitates autonomy. Sense of power from saying "no" and "mine" Increased independence from mother	Turns pages of a book singly Adept at building a tower of 6–7 cubes When drawing, attempts are made to enclose a space	Runs well with little falling Throws and kicks a ball Walks up and down stairs	Begins to use words to explain past events or to discuss objects not observably present Rapidly expands vocabulary to approximately 300 words; uses plurals	Enters preconceptual phase of cognitive development State of continuous investigation Primary focus is egocentric
36	Basic concepts of sexuality are established. Separates from mother more easily Attends to toilet needs	Copies a circle and a straight line Grasps spoon between thumb and index finger Holds cup by handle	Balances on one foot; jumps in place; pedals tricycle	Quest for information furthered by questions like "why," "when," "where," and "how" Has acquired the language that will be used in the course of simple conversation during the adult years	Preconceptual phase continues; can only think of one idea at a time; unable to think of all parts in terms of the whole

(Wieczorek RR, Natapoff JN: A Conceptual Approach to the Nursing of Children: Health Care From Birth Through Adolescence. Philadelphia, JB Lippincott, 1981)

TABLE 8–2.   RDA FOR TODDLER COMPARED TO INFANT

	Infant 6–12 Months 9 kg–71 cm	Toddler 1–3 Years (13 kg)
Energy (kcal)	105 kcal/kg (945)	1300
Protein (g)	2.0 g/kg (18)	23
Vitamin A (RE)	400 (2000 IU)	400
Vitamin D (meg)	10 (400 IU)	10
Vitamin E (mg α-TE)	4	5
Ascorbic acid (mg)	35	45
Folacin (mcg)	45	100
Niacin (mg)	8	9
Riboflavin (mg)	0.6	0.8
Thiamin (mg)	0.5	0.7
Vitamin B$_6$ (mg)	0.6	0.9
Vitamin B$_{12}$ (mcg)	1.5	2.0
Calcium (mg)	540	800
Phosphorus (mg)	360	800
Iodine (mcg)	50	70
Iron (mg)	15	15
Magnesium (mg)	70	150
Zinc (mg)	5	10

(Adapted from Anderson L, Dibble MV, Turkki PR, et al: Nutrition in Health and Disease, 17th ed. Philadelphia, JB Lippincott, 1982; from Food and Nutrition Board Recommended Dietary Allowances. Washington, DC, National Academy of Sciences/National Research Council, 1980)

of death for children between the ages of 1 and 4 years.[1] Accidents involving motor vehicles, drowning, burns, and poisoning are the most frequent killers (Table 8–6).

MOTOR VEHICLE ACCIDENTS

Many childhood deaths or injuries resulting from motor vehicle accidents could be prevented by proper use of re-straints when toddlers are passengers in moving vehicles. Harnesses, car seats, or seat belts could save many young lives if used consistently. Many other toddlers are killed or injured by moving vehicles while playing in their own yards, driveways, or garages. Parents need to be aware that these tragedies can occur and take proper precautions at all times.

DROWNING

Although drowning of young children is often associated with bathtubs, the increased number of home-owned swimming pools has added significantly to the number of accidental drownings. Often these pools are fenced on three sides to keep out nonresidents, but are bordered on one side by the family home, making the pool accessible to infants and toddlers. These and small plastic wading pools hold enough water to drown an unsupervised toddler. Any family living near even a small body of water must be cautioned not to leave a mobile infant or toddler unattended, even for a moment, to avoid potential tragedy.

BURNS

The third most significant cause of accidental death during childhood is burn accidents, which occur most often as scalds from immersions and spills, and from exposure to uninsulated electrical wires or live extension cord plugs. Children are also burned while playing with matches, or while left unattended in a home where a fire breaks out. Whether the fire results from a child's mischief, an adult's carelessness, or some unforeseeable event, the injuries, even if not fatal, can have long-term or permanent effects. Many burns can be prevented by being sure that:

1. Electrical cords do not dangle within the reach of toddlers and are repaired if frayed.
2. Electrical wall outlets are covered by safety caps (Fig. 8–3).
3. Pans of hot liquid on the stove are turned toward the back of the stove, and if possible are placed on back burners out of the toddler's reach (Fig. 8–4).
4. Cups of hot liquid are placed out of reach.
5. Small children are supervised at all times while in the bathtub, so they cannot turn on the hot water tap.
6. Matches are placed in metal containers, out of reach of small children.
7. Small children are not left unattended by an adult or responsible teenager.

INGESTION OF TOXIC SUBSTANCES

The curious toddler wants to touch and taste everything. Left to his own devices, he may sample household cleaners, parents' prescriptions, children's or regular aspirin, kerosene, gasoline, or peeling paint from the wall. Poisoning is still the most common medical emergency in children, with the highest incidence occurring between the ages of 1 and 4 years.

Parents need continual cautioning about the possibility of childhood poisoning. Even with precautionary labeling and packaging of medication and household cleaning supplies, children display amazing ingenuity in opening

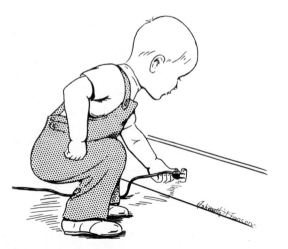

FIG. 8–3.   Electrical wall outlets should be covered with safety caps and electric cords should be kept out of reach of the toddler.

bottles and packages that catch their curiosity. A campaign began in 1972 to teach children to recognize substances unsafe for eating or drinking. This campaign features Mr. Yuk (Fig. 8–5), whose unhappy face appears on labels that can be placed on all containers of harmful substances. These labels are usually available from the nearest poison control center.

The following preventive measures should be observed by all parents with small children:

1. Medications should be kept in their original containers, well-labeled, in a locked cabinet. Even cupboards and cabinets that seem too high for a child to reach can appear as a challenge to be met.
2. Medications no longer in use should be discarded in an area to which children have no access, and where they will not damage other persons or animals.
3. Safety caps should not be regarded as child-proof. Although they have helped to reduce the incidence of childhood poisoning, they seem to be more easily mastered by children than by some adults.[2]
4. A bottle of syrup of ipecac (available without prescription) should be kept (in a locked cabinet) to induce vomiting if an ingestion of harmful substances does occur. There are instances where vomiting should not be induced, such as in the swallowing of corrosive substances or kerosene. Every household with small children should have a chart with emergency treatment for poisoning, and also the number of the nearest poison control center posted in a prominent place near a telephone or taped on the bottle of syrup of ipecac.
5. Household chemicals should be stored out of reach of small children, *not* under the kitchen sink or in a bathroom closet (Fig. 8–6).

The following medications are most frequently involved in cases of childhood poisoning:

- Salicylates—aspirin is still the leading cause of poisoning in small children
- Laxatives
- Sedatives
- Tranquilizers
- Analgesics
- Antihistamines
- Cold medicines
- Birth control pills

The importance of careful, continuous supervision of toddlers and other young children cannot be overemphasized.

TEACHING ORAL HYGIENE

Dental caries (cavities) constitute a major health problem among children and young adults. The average child has at least two cavities by age 2. Although sound teeth depend in part upon sound nutrition, the process of dental caries is linked to the effect of diet on the oral environment.

Tooth decay is caused by bacteria that act in the presence of sugar and form a film, or dental *plaque* on the teeth. Persons who frequently eat sweet foods accumulate

TABLE 8–3. FEEDING SKILLS OF THE TODDLER

Age	Skills
1 year	May need a toy to enhance attention while sitting for meals (enjoys holding cup); tilts head backward to drain last drop; enjoys finger feeding
15 months	Better gross motor control; able to sit through meals; finger feeding preferred method; increased desire to use spoon, however has difficulty "scooping up" foods (much spilling); grasps cup more with thumb and forefingers; now tilts cup with fingers rather than tilting head; child more insistent about feeding self
18 months	Appetite decreasing; refusals and preferences not clearly defined; better control of spoon; replaces spilled food back on spoon; holds cup with both hands; has good control with fingers and spills very little; often throws cup when finished if no one is there to take it
21 months	Easily distracted; enjoys pouring things from one container to another; rituals/patterns prevalent (*e.g.*, same spoon, cup)
2 years	Appetite fair to moderate; "finicky" or "fussy" (definite likes and dislikes); food jags; spoon grasped between thumb and index finger; able to place food on spoon without assistance of other hand; still considerable spilling; accepts no help ("Me do!")
30 months	Appetite fluctuates between very good and very poor; usually takes in *one* good meal (noon or evening); refusals and preferences still prevalent; rituals persist
3 years	Refusals and preferences less evident; spoon held between thumb and index finger (some hold it in adult fashion with palm turned inward); cup held by the handle in adult fashion; once again head tilts back to secure last drop

(Wieczorek RR, Natapoff JN: A Conceptual Approach to the Nursing of Children: Health Care From Birth Through Adolescence. Philadelphia, JB Lippincott, 1981)

plaque easily and are prone to dental caries. Sugars eaten at mealtime appear to be somewhat neutralized by the presence of other foods and are therefore not as damaging as between-meal sweets, and bedtime bottles.

At about age 2, the child should be taught to brush his teeth, or, if brushing is not possible, rinse his mouth after each meal or snack. Since this is an age at which he likes to imitate others, he is best taught by example. Plain water should be used until he has learned how to spit out toothpaste or toothpowder. In communities where the water is not fluoridated, the use of a fluoride toothpaste will strengthen tooth enamel and help prevent tooth decay. Fluoride can be applied during regular visits to the dentist.

The first visit to the dentist should occur at about this same time, just to get acquainted with the dentist, his staff, and his office. A second visit might be a good time for

TABLE 8–4.   A SAMPLE DAILY FOOD PLAN FOR CHILDREN 13 MONTHS TO 3 YEARS OF AGE

Foods	Daily Amount	Average Serving Size
Milk (whole, evaporated, skim, and so forth) (Cheddar cheese may be used occasionally in place of milk.)	2 to 3 cups	½ to 1 cup (4 to 8 ounces)
Meat, poultry, fish, eggs (As alternatives: cooked and mashed dried beans or dried peas, cottage cheese, smooth peanut butter may be used occasionally.)	1 to 2 servings	2 to 4 tablespoons (1 to 2 ounces)
Vegetables, fruits	4 or more servings	
A dark green or deep yellow vegetable for vitamin A	1 serving at least every other day	2 to 4 tablespoons
Fruit or vegetable high in vitamin C	1 serving	¼ cup juice
Other fruits and vegetables including potato	2 servings	2 to 4 tablespoons
Breads and cereals (whole grain or enriched) (Choose a cereal fortified with iron for the child 18 months of age or younger.)	4 or more servings	¼ cup cereal or ½ to 1 slice bread
Vitamin D (Present in vitamin-D-fortified milk or may be supplied as a concentrate if prescribed by a physician.)		
Other foods (Other foods such as margarine, butter, or other fats and simple desserts such as milk puddings and fruit desserts, may be used to satisfy the child's appetite and to provide energy.)		

(Wieczorek RR, Natapoff JN: A Conceptual Approach to the Nursing of Children: Health Care From Birth Through Adolescence. Philadelphia, JB Lippincott, 1981)

a preliminary examination, and subsequent visits twice a year for check-ups are recommended.

TOILET TRAINING

Learning control of bowels and bladder is an important part of the socialization process. In Western culture, a great sense of shame and disgust has been associated with body waste products. To function successfully in this culture, one must learn to dispose of body waste products in a place considered proper by society.

The toddler has no sense of shame about emptying his bowel and bladder; it simply gives him physical relief. For a year or more, he has been operating on the pleasure principle, accepting immediate satisfaction as his right. Now, as he is beginning to learn that he has some control over his environment and can cause or prevent certain happenings, he is asked to forego some of his gratifications. One of these is the satisfaction of emptying his bowels and bladder when he feels the urge to do so, regardless of time and place.

He must now not only learn to conform to please his parents; but in order to preserve his integrity, he must convince himself that he has voluntarily accepted the dictates of society. He already knows that he has the ability not to cooperate with his mother's wishes, which after all, make no sense to him.

TIMING

In order for a child to be able to cooperate in toilet training, he must have developed to the stage where he can control his sphincter muscles. Control of the rectal sphincter comes first. He also must be able to postpone his urge to defecate until he reaches the toilet or potty, and he must be able to signal his need *before* the event. This maturational development seldom takes place before the age of 15 to 18 months, and maybe later.

At the start of training the child has no understanding of the uses of the potty chair, but if his mother wishes him to sit there he is willing to please her, for a short time. If his bowel movements occur at approximately the same time every day, he will one day have a bowel movement in the potty. He has no sense of special achievement as yet, but he does like the praise and approval he receives. Eventually he will learn to connect this approval with bowel movement in the potty and will be happy that he has done something to please his mother.

SUGGESTIONS FOR BOWEL TRAINING

1. A potty chair in which a child can comfortably put his feet on the floor is preferable. Most small children are afraid of a flush toilet.
2. The child should be left on the potty chair for only a short time. If he has a bowel movement, approval is in order; if not, no comment is necessary.
3. During the beginning stages of training, the child will likely have a movement soon after he leaves the potty. This is not willful defiance and need not be mentioned.
4. The potty should be emptied unobtrusively after the child has resumed playing. He has cooperated and produced the product his mother desired. If she immediately throws it away, he may be confused, and not so eager to please her the next time.
5. The ability to feel shame and self-doubt appear at this age. Therefore, the child should not be teased about his reluctance or inability to conform. This could shake his confidence and make him doubt his worth.
6. The parent should not expect perfection, even after control has been achieved. Lapses inevitably occur, perhaps because the child is completely absorbed in play (Fig. 8–7), or because of a temporary episode of loose stools. Occasionally a child feels aggression,

TABLE 8–5. GUIDELINES FOR HEALTH PROMOTION IN THE TODDLER

Developmental Characteristics of Toddler (1–3 Yr)	Possible Deviations from Health	Nursing Measures to Ensure Optimal Health Practices

Self-feeding (foods/objects more accessible for mouthing, handling, and eating)	Inadequate nutritional intake
	Accidental poisoning
	Gastrointestinal disturbances:
	   Instability of GI tract
	   Infection from parasites (pinworm)
		Diet teaching
		Child-proofing the home
		Careful hand-washing (before meals, after toileting)
		   Avoidance of rich foods
		   Observe for perianal itching (Scotch tape test, Povan)

Toilet-training	Constipation (if too rigid training procedures initiated) Urinary tract infection (especially prevalent in girls due to anatomic structure and poor toilet habits)	Teaching regarding toileting procedures Urinalysis when indicated (*e.g.,* burning) Teaching hygiene (at the onset of training instruct girls to wipe from front to back, hand-wash—to prevent cross-infection)
Increased socialization	Increased prevalence of upper respiratory infections (immune levels still at immature levels)	Hygienic practices (*e.g.,* use of tissue or handkerchief, not drinking from same glass) Immunizations for passive immunity against communicable disease
Primary dentition	Caries with resultant infection or loss of primary as well as beginning permanent teeth	Initiation of oral hygiene, regular teeth brushing, dental exam at 21½ months– 3 yr Proper nutrition to ensure dentition
Sleep disturbances	Lack of sleep may cause irritability, lethargy, decreased resistance to infection.	Teaching regarding recommended amounts of sleep (10– 12 hr); need for rituals to enhance the transition process to bedtime; possibility of need for nap; setting bedtime limits

Wieczorek RR, Natapoff JN: A Conceptual Approach to the Nursing of Children: Health Care From Birth Through Adolescence. Philadelphia, JB Lippincott, 1981

TABLE 8–6. MORTALITY FROM LEADING TYPES OF ACCIDENTS AMONG CHILDREN AGED 1–4: UNITED STATES, 1972–73

Type of Accident	Average Annual Death Rate Per 100,000 Boys at Ages					Girls at Ages				
	1–4	1	2	3	4	1–4	1	2	3	4
Accidents—all types	38.0	44.5	40.7	36.5	30.1	25.4	32.9	27.9	21.9	18.9
Motor vehicle	13.6	12.7	13.3	14.7	13.9	10.2	10.8	11.2	9.3	9.4
Pedestrian (in traffic accidents)	6.5	3.6	6.3	7.9	8.3	3.3	2.3	3.5	3.6	4.0
Drowning*	8.3	8.8	10.2	8.4	5.6	3.6	5.1	4.6	2.8	1.8
Fires and flames	5.6	5.8	7.1	5.5	4.1	4.6	4.9	5.1	4.2	3.9
Inhalation and ingestion of food or other objects	1.8	4.1	1.8	0.9	0.5	1.4	3.2	1.2	0.7	0.6
Poisoning	1.6	3.8	1.4	0.9	0.5	1.1	2.4	1.2	0.6	0.3
Falls	1.5	2.8	1.4	1.2	0.8	1.2	2.1	1.0	1.1	0.5
Firearm missile	0.7	0.4	0.8	0.7	1.1	0.4	0.2	0.4	0.7	0.4
Accidental deaths as a percent of all deaths	42%	34%	44%	49%	49%	36%	30%	38%	40%	41%

* Exclusive of deaths in water transportation.

(Wieczorek RR, Natapoff JN: A Conceptual Approach to the Nursing of Children: Health Care From Birth Through Adolescence. Philadelphia, JB Lippincott, 1981)

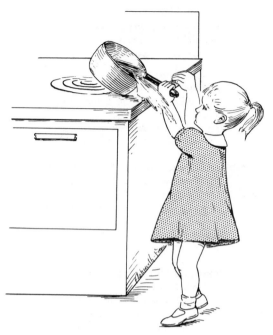

FIG. 8–4. The handles of pans on the stove should always be turned away from the reach of the toddler.

frustration, or anger and uses this method to "get even." As long as the lapses are occasional, they should be ignored. If frequent and persistent, the cause should be sought.

BLADDER TRAINING

Generally the first indication that a youngster is about ready for bladder training is when he begins to connect the puddle on the floor with something he did. Next, the child runs to his mother and indicates his need to urinate, but only after it has happened.

Not until the child has matured sufficiently to control his bladder sphincter and until he can reach the desired place is there much benefit to be gained from a serious program of training. One indication of this level of maturation is the child's staying dry for about 2 hours at a time.

Each child will follow his own individual pattern of development. No parent needs to be embarrassed or shamed because his or her child is still having accidents. Of course

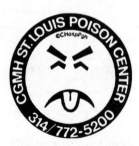

FIG. 8–5. Mr. Yuk labels. (Courtesy of Children's Hospital of Pittsburgh)

it is possible for a parent or caregiver to ignore the signs of readiness—no one should expect the child to train himself. Complete control, especially at night, may not be achieved until the fourth or fifth year.

psychosocial development

The toddler develops a growing awareness of himself as an entity, separate from other persons or objects. Intoxicated with his newly discovered powers, and lacking experience, the child tends to test his independence to the limit. This age has been called an age of *negativism.* Certainly the toddler's response to nearly everything is a firm "no," but this is more an assertion of individuality than of an intention to disobey. *Ritualism, dawdling,* and *temper tantrums* also characterize this age.

Ritualism is a compromising device employed by the young child to help him develop security. He must follow a certain routine, making rituals of simple tasks. At bedtime all toys must be in accustomed places, and his caregiver must follow an accustomed practice. This passion for a set routine is not found in every child to the same degree, but it does provide a comfortable base from which to step out into new and potentially dangerous paths.

Dawdling serves much the same purpose. The young child has to decide between following the wishes and routines of his parents, and asserting his independence by following his own desires. Being incapable of making such a choice, he compromises and tries both. If the matter is of any importance, the course for the parent to follow is to help the child along the way he should go, in a firm and friendly manner.

Temper tantrums spring from frustrations. The child's urge to do it himself naturally results in many frustrations. Add to this the fact that he is reluctant to leave the scene for necessary rest, and one can see that frequently the frustrations become too great. Even the very best of mothers may lose patience, showing a temporary lack of understanding. The child reacts with enthusiastic rebellion, but this too is a phase he must live through as he works toward becoming a person.

Reasoning with the child, scolding or punishing during the tantrum is useless. Someone he trusts needs to be nearby, calm, and patient until he gains control of himself. After the storm is over, it is best to help him relax by diverting his attention, but not yielding the point or giving in to the child's whim. That would tell him that he can get whatever he wants by throwing himself on the floor and screaming. He would have to learn, painfully, later in life that he cannot control others in this manner.

Admittedly it is not easy to handle a small child who throws himself down in a fit or screaming rage in the middle of the supermarket or the sidewalk; nor are comments from onlookers at all helpful. The best a mother can do is pick up the child as calmly as possible and carry him away to regain control of himself.

DISCIPLINE

Unfortunately the word *discipline* has come to mean *punishment* to many people. They are not the same. Discipline means to train or instruct in order to produce a particular behavior pattern, especially moral or mental improvement, and self-control. Though all small children need discipline, the need for punishment is much less frequent.

The toddler learns self-control very gradually. The development from an egotistic being, whose world exists only to give him satisfaction, into a person who understands and respects the rights of others is a long, involved process (Fig. 8–8). He cannot do this alone; he must be taught.

The first signs of responsibility for his own acts are even evident in the 2-year-old. He lacks inner controls and depends on adults to set limits. He still wants the forbidden thing, but realizes he is disobeying, even to the extent of repeating, "No, no, musn't," while he reaches for his father's valuable book. He understands very well what he must not do, but his desire is still too strong for him to resist. With proper guidance, he will soon incorporate the restraints into himself and develop control, or conscience.

In the meantime he needs much help. When he hits or bites another child, he is taken away from the situation. When he tries to "read" daddy's expensive book, it is taken away from him, gently but firmly.

The child needs to experience a sense of wrong-doing in order to develop self-control. However, adults need to make it clear that the action is "bad," not the child himself. He should not be criticized and shamed so much that his self-esteem is lowered to the point where he "can do nothing right," and, therefore, does nothing at all. Neither should his lapses of behavior be treated indulgently or overlooked, or else he will have great difficulty learning any self-control.

SHARING WITH A SIBLING

The toddler who is a first child has his parents' undivided attention until a new baby arrives. It is difficult to prepare a child just emerging from babyhood for this arrival. Although he can feel his mother's abdomen and understand that this is where the new baby lives, it does not prepare him for the real baby when it arrives. This real baby takes his place in his mother's attention.

As in many stressful situations, the toddler frequently will regress to more infantile behavior. If he has given up his bottle, he goes back to it. If he is on his way to being toilet-trained, he goes back to wetting and soiling.

The new infant doubtless creates considerable change in the home, whether he is the first child, or the fifth. In homes where the previous baby is being displaced by the newcomer, however, some preparation is necessary. Moving the older child to a larger bed some time before the new baby appears lets him take pride in being "a big boy" now. Preparation of the toddler for a new brother or sister is helpful but should not be intense until just before the expected birth.

Probably the greatest help in preparing the child of any age to accept the new baby is to make him feel that this is "our baby," not just "mommy's" baby (Fig. 8–9). If he can help care for the baby according to his ability, this contributes to his feeling that he is still important.

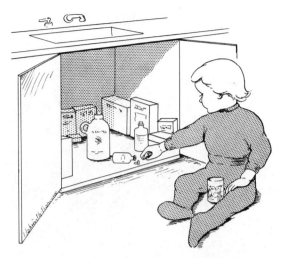

FIG. 8–6. The toddler playing with cleaning agents stored within his reach is in danger of accidentally poisoning himself.

The displaced toddler almost certainly will feel some jealousy. With careful planning, however, mother can reserve some time for cuddling and playing with the toddler just as before. Perhaps he may profit from a little extra parental attention for a time. He needs to realize that his parents love him just as much as ever, and there is plenty of room in their lives for both children.

The child should not be made to grow up too soon. He should not be shamed or reproved for reverting to babyish behavior, but understood and given a bit more love and attention. Perhaps the father could occasionally take over the care of the new baby while mother devotes herself to the toddler.

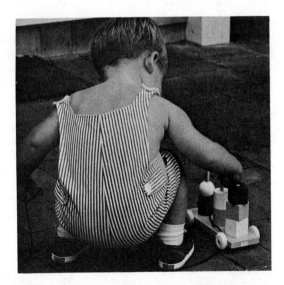

FIG. 8–7. The 2-year-old is capable of complete absorption in play and may forget or ignore the signals of a full bowel or bladder. (Photo by Carol Baldwin)

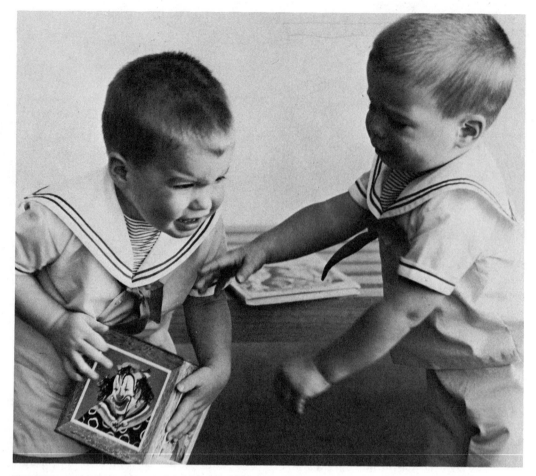

FIG. 8–8.   Learning to respect the rights of others, and to share, is a painful process for the toddler. (Photo by Carol Baldwin)

implications for hospital care

Much of the emotional effect of hospitalization is discussed in Physical Care of the Sick Child. The brief discussion here relates specifically to the hospitalized toddler.

The goal of a hospital pediatric staff is to get the child well and back with his parents as soon as possible. While the child is hospitalized, the staff must try to meet his needs under less than ideal circumstances. To meet those needs, one first must understand them.

The hospitalized toddler may have pain or be uncomfortable and ill at ease. He may have little incentive to carry on with his previous zest for living; his development continues, however. When his illness keeps him from obeying the demands of his nature, he becomes cross and irritable. If he must be confined to his crib, he becomes increasingly restless.

TOILET TRAINING

The toddler just learning sphincter control is still dependent on familiar surroundings and his mother's support. For this reason, some pediatric personnel automatically put toddlers back in diapers when they are admitted; this practice should be discouraged. Under the right circumstances, and especially with mother's help, many of these children can maintain control. They at least should be given a chance to try.

DISCIPLINE PROBLEMS

The nurse who feels a need to punish a child for nonconforming forgets one basic fact: the child is already being punished rather severely by his environment and by his discomfort. The nurse should think carefully before adding to this unpleasantness.

Certainly a sick child needs discipline. If pampered, indulged, and allowed to follow his own immature impulses, he is just as unhappy as the others he is making unhappy. He would be grateful to have limits set, if done with love and understanding.

The disciplinary problems of this age group are many and varied, and the solutions unclear. No two children come to the hospital from the same environment. Some have been ill for a long time and have been overindulged. Others have been severely disciplined or even rejected. Every child has a different capacity to withstand frustra-

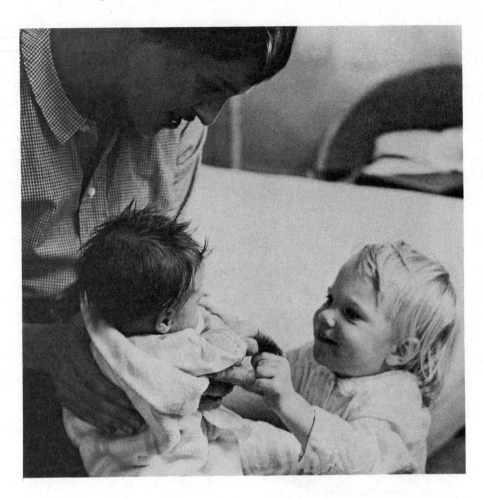

FIG. 8–9. The toddler meets the new baby. (Photo by Carol Baldwin)

tion, depending on his personality, his background, and his state of health.

EATING PROBLEMS

One problem that looms large in nurses' minds concerns the toddler's eating habits. In the hospital as at home, food can assume an importance out of all proportion to its value, and create an unnecessary problem.

EATING IS A SOCIAL ACTIVITY

In hospitals, the staff tends to forget that in our culture eating is a social activity. Many a toddler who sits in his crib playing with his food would eat with gusto if he were placed at the table with his peers. Few children have to stay in their cribs all the time, but even if a child must be confined to bed, he can be pulled over nearer to others for companionship.

Some pediatric wards serve meals family-style around a big table. A fortunate few allow the nurse to eat with the children. In hospitals where this is not the practice, children can eat with their friends, perhaps in another ward.

Some suggestions for avoiding eating problems are offered earlier in this chapter. Others are as follows:

1. A little calculated neglect at mealtime often works wonders. Hovering over the child, urging him to take just one more bite, makes it irresistible for the toddler to say "no." If it appears to the toddler that it makes no difference whether he eats or not, there is no need for him to resist. He can permit himself to be influenced by the attractiveness of the food and the behavior of his peers. An adult at the table eating in a businesslike manner also offers a helpful example.

2. Serve the dessert along with the rest of the meal. It doesn't matter whether he eats it first or last, because hospital desserts for children are usually as nourishing as other foods.

3. If the child is accustomed to other foods, such as Mexican tortillas or Italian spaghetti, find out if the hospital will allow his mother to bring in these foods. A small child finds it particularly difficult to eat strange foods, especially when illness takes away his appetite.

FLUIDS

"Push fluids" is an order that is frequently quite difficult to carry out in the toddler's department. A small child cannot take much fluid at any one time, so persistence seems to be the answer. Fluids should be offered in a small cup or glass.

A tea party with small cups and a pot to pour from provides entertainment as well as fluid. Taking turns pouring prolongs the party until everyone has had a turn. The

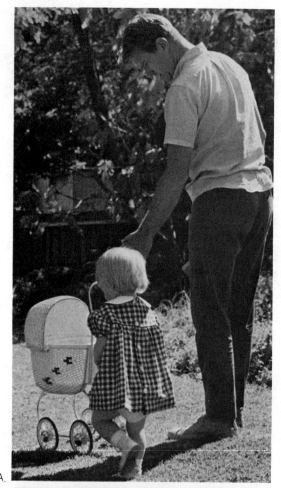

A.

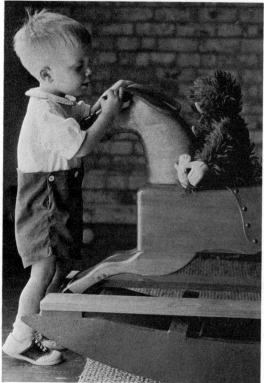

B

pot may need many fillings, but the fluid chart is going to look much better. Often a little imagination will help solve the problems of little people.

summary

No longer a baby, but not very "grown up" either, the toddler can be extremely difficult one moment, and totally lovable and loving the next. The ability to communicate, to imitate and imagine, makes this a fascinating stage for parents and caregivers to observe (Fig. 8–10A and B). The ability to walk, run, and climb makes this stage potentially dangerous for the toddler, demanding continuous supervision by a responsible person. If parents can summon sufficient patience and understanding to deal with the toddler's self-centered search for autonomy and the displays of temper that accompany that search, this time can be an especially close one for the family. Once the child begins to interact with persons outside the family, in a nursery school or daycare center, family influence is never again as strong.

review questions

1. What important points should the nurse teach parents of toddlers concerning safety measures and accident prevention in their home?
2. What suggestions should the nurse give to the parents concerning their toddler's developing feeding skills?
3. What medications are most frequently involved in childhood poisoning?
4. What causes dental caries?
5. What suggestions should the nurse give to parents concerning toilet training?
6. How should the parent handle temper tantrums?
7. During hospitalization how should the nurse deal with toilet training, discipline, and eating problems?

references

1. Wheatley G: Introduction: childhood accidents. Pediatr Ann 6, No. 11:12–25, 1977
2. Done AK, et al: Evaluation of safety packaging for the protection of children. Pediatr 48:631, 1971

bibliography

Brown JB: Infant temperament: a clue to childrearing for parents and nurses. Am J Mat Child Nurs 2:228–232, 1977

Chess S, Thomas A, Birch H: Your Child Is a Person. New York, Viking, 1965

Church J: Understanding Your Child From Birth to Three: A Guide to Your Child's Psychological Development. New York, Pocket Books, 1976

Garvey C: Play. Cambridge, Harvard University Press, 1977

FIG. 8–10. (*A*) The little girl imitates her mother. (*B*) The 2- to 3-year-old indulges in imaginative play. (Photo by Carol Baldwin)

Gesell A, Ilg F: Infant and Child in the Culture of Today. New York, Harper & Row, 1974

Maier HW: Three Theories of Child Development. New York, Harper & Row, 1978

Mayer GG: Choosing day care. Am J Nurs 81:346–348, 1981

Melichar MM: Using crisis theory to help parents cope with a child's temper tantrums. Am J Mat Child Nurs 5:181–185, 1980

Petrillo M, Sanger S: Emotional Care of Hospitalized Children, 2nd ed. Philadelphia, JB Lippincott, 1980

Piaget J: The Child's Conception of the World. Totowa, NJ, Littlefield Adams & Co., 1972

Pines M: Revolution in Learning: The Years From Birth to Six. New York, Harper & Row, 1966

Reinhard SC: Nursing responsibility in infant car safety. Am J Mat Child Nurs 5:26, 1980

Sigel IE, Coching RR: Cognitive Development From Childhood to Adolescence: A Constructual Perspective. New York, Holt, Reinhardt & Winston, 1977

Slattery J: Dental health in children. Am J Nurs 76:1159–1161, 1976

Snell B, McLellan C: Whetting hospitalized preschoolers' appetites. Am J Nurs 76:413–415, 1976

Wieczorek RR, Natapoff JN: A Conceptual Approach to the Nursing of Children: Health Care From Birth Through Adolescence. Philadelphia, JB Lippincott, 1981

Williams SR: Nutrition and Diet Therapy, 4th ed. St Louis, CV Mosby, 1981

health problems of the toddler

student objectives

The student successfully attaining the goals of this chapter will be able to

1 Define the following vocabulary terms:

  achylia   autism   autograft   celiac crisis   Curling's ulcer   diplopia
  ecchymosis   echolalia   orthoptics   pica   plumbism   strabismus

2 List five characteristics of infantile autism.

3 Describe the care of the child with cystic fibrosis, including dietary and pulmonary treatments, hospital and home care.

4 Describe the emergency treatment for the child who has ingested a toxic substance and list the four primary steps in the treatment in order of importance.

5 Describe the three different types of burns and discuss the appropriate treatment for each.

6 Identify five items the nurse should observe when monitoring vital signs.

The child from ages 1 to 3 years is likely to have a number of minor health problems, many of them caused by infection or environmental hazards. Most of these can be managed at home after a visit to the pediatrician's office or clinic. Some of the problems, however, are serious enough to require hospitalization, thus separating the toddler from his parents. This separation increases the seriousness of the health problem, and the need for loving and understanding attention to the child's emotional needs as well as his physical condition.

psychological problems

INFANTILE AUTISM

Although called infantile because it is thought to be present from birth, autism usually is not conclusively diagnosed until after 12 months of age. The word autism comes from the Greek word *auto* meaning "self" and was first used by Dr. Leo Kanner in 1943 to describe a group of behavioral symptoms in children. Autistic children are totally self-centered and unable to relate to others, and exhibit bizarre behaviors, often destructive to themselves and others.

Autism occurs in 1 out of every 2500 births, and twice as often in males as in females. Several theories exist about its cause as well as its treatment or management. Originally thought to result from an unsatisfactory early mother–child relationship (emotionally cold, detached mothers, sometimes described as "refrigerator mothers"), autism now appears to have organic, and perhaps genetic, causes, instead. Researchers suggest that autism may result from a disturbance in language comprehension, a biochemical problem involving neurotransmitters, or from abnormalities in the central nervous system, probably brain metabolism.

Since the cause of autism is not understood, treatment attempts have met with limited success. These children experience the normal health problems of childhood in addition to those that result from their behaviors. Therefore, it is important that nurses understand this tragic, unexplained disorder, and how it affects children and families.

CHARACTERISTICS

Kanner identifies characteristics of early infantile autism, among which, the following five are still generally accepted:

1. Inability to relate to and interact with other people
2. Inability to communicate with others through language
3. An obsession with preservation of sameness and a resistance to change
4. Preoccupation with objects instead of people
5. Occasional evidence of good potential for intelligence

These children do not develop a smiling response to others, or an interest in being touched or cuddled. In fact, they can react quite violently at attempts to hold them. Their blank expressions and lack of response to verbal stimulation can suggest deafness. They do not show the normal fear of separation from parents that most toddlers exhibit. Often they seem not to notice when parents are present.

During their second year, autistic children become completely absorbed in strange repetitive behaviors, such as spinning an object, flipping an electrical switch on and off, or walking around the room feeling the walls. Their bodily movements are bizarre: rocking, twirling, flapping arms and hands, walking on tip-toe, twisting and turning fingers. If these movements are interrupted, or if objects in the environment are moved, a violent temper tantrum may result. These tantrums may include such self-destructive acts as hand-biting and head-banging.

Though infants and toddlers normally are self-centered, ritualistic, and prone to displays of temper, autistic children show these characteristics to an extreme degree, coupled with an almost total lack of response to other persons. Standard intelligence tests indicate that many of these children are mentally deficient. Other tests, however, seem to contradict this indication because these children often show superior memory and advanced visual–motor coordination.

The autistic child is slow to develop speech, and any that does develop is primitive and ineffective in its ability to communicate. *Echolalia* (parrot speech) is typical of autistic children; they echo words they have heard but with no indication that they understand the words. Although autistic children are self-centered, their speech indicates that they seem to have no sense of self because they never use the pronouns "I" or "me."

DIAGNOSIS

The symptoms of autism can suggest other disorders such as lead poisoning, PKU, congenital rubella, and measles encephalitis. Therefore, a complete pediatric physical and neurologic examination is necessary, including vision and hearing testing, EEG, radiographic studies of the skull, urine screening, and other laboratory studies. In addition, the nurse usually will take a complete prenatal, natal, and postnatal history, including development, nutrition, and family dynamics. Other members of the health team may be involved in evaluation and treatment of the autistic child: audiologists, psychiatrists, psychologists, special education teachers, speech and language therapists, and social workers.

TREATMENT

Various approaches to treatment have been attempted, with limited success, even after intense involvement by parents and professionals in health care and education. Three principal approaches to treatment of autism are

1. Treating autism as if it were a halt in the developmental process, and attempting to activate the arrested developmental process.
2. Treating autism as an organic disorder, using electroconvulsive and insulin shock therapy, and drugs such as tranquilizers and other mood-altering drugs.
3. Behavior modification techniques that seek to eliminate inappropriate behaviors and replace them with other behaviors that are more acceptable.

NURSING CARE

Caring for the autistic child means recognizing that autism creates great stresses for the entire family of the sick child. The problems that cause parents to seek diagnosis are difficult to live with; diagnosis itself is usually a lengthy and expensive process, and the hope for successful treatment is slight. Most parents of autistic children feel guilty, despite the fact that current theories point to organic rather than psychological causes for this disorder. Frequently there are other children in the family who are normal, but who suffer from a lack of attention because the parents' energies are almost totally directed to solving the problems of the autistic youngster.

Nurses who care for these children in a hospital setting should consider the parents their most valuable source for information about the child's habits and communication skills. A private or semiprivate room is generally more satisfactory; visual and auditory stimulation should be minimized. Familiar toys or other valued objects from home reduce the child's anxiety about the strange environment. The nurse needs to learn what techniques have been used by the parents to communicate with the child and gain his cooperation.

central nervous system disorders

EYE CONDITIONS

CATARACTS

A cataract is an opacification of the crystalline lens. Congenital cataracts may be hereditary, or may be complications of maternal rubella during the first trimester of pregnancy. Cataracts may also develop later in infancy or childhood from eye injury or from metabolic disturbances such as galactosemia or diabetes.

The degree of opacity determines whether surgery should be performed. If the cataract is small and does not significantly impair vision, it is not usually removed. Following surgery, eyeglasses will be needed to provide light refraction. Surgical results are not as successful as in the adult patient; 20/20 vision is sometimes not attained.

GLAUCOMA

Glaucoma may be of the congenital infantile type, occurring in children under 3 years of age; juvenile glaucoma, showing clinical manifestations after the age of 3; or secondary glaucoma, resulting from injury or disease. Increased intraocular pressure due to over-production of aqueous fluid causes the eyeball to enlarge, the cornea to become large, thin, and sometimes cloudy. Untreated, the disease slowly progresses to blindness. Pain may, or may not, be present. Goniopuncture, which provides drainage of the aqueous humor, is effective in relieving intraocular pressure in a large number of cases. Goniotomy may improve the function of the filtration angle if it is defective.

STRABISMUS

Strabismus is the failure of the two eyes to direct their gaze at the same object simultaneously. Binocular (normal) vision is maintained through the muscular coordination of eye movements, so that a simple vision results. In strabismus, the visual axes are not parallel, and *diplopia* (double vision) results. In an effort to avoid seeing two images, the child suppresses vision in the deviant eye, causing a condition of *amblyopia ex anopsia* (dimness of vision from disuse of the eye), sometimes called "lazy eye."

A wide variation in the manifestation of strabismus exists; there are lateral, vertical, and mixed lateral and vertical types. There may be monocular strabismus, in which one eye deviates while the other eye is used, or alternating strabismus, in which deviation alternates from one eye to the other. The term *esotropia* is used when the eye deviates toward the other eye; *exotropia* denotes a turning away from the other eye (Fig. 9–1).

Treatment depends on the type of strabismus present. Occlusion of the better eye in monocular strabismus, to force the use of the deviating eye should be carried out early, and should be continued constantly for a period of weeks or months. The child should be stimulated to use the unpatched eye by such occupations as puzzles, drawing, sewing, and similar activities.

Glasses can correct a refractive error if amblyopia is not present. *Therapeutic exercises* (orthoptics) to improve the quality of vision may be prescribed to supplement the use of glasses or surgery.

Surgery on the eye muscle to correct the defect is necessary for those children who do not respond to glasses and exercises. Many children need surgery after amblyopia has been corrected. Early detection and treatment of strabismus is essential for a successful outcome.

EYE INJURY AND FOREIGN OBJECTS IN THE EYE

Eye injuries are fairly common, particularly in older children. *Ecchymosis* (black eye) is of no great importance unless the eyeball is involved. A penetrating wound of the eyeball is potentially serious—BB shots in particular are dangerous, and require the attention of an ophthalmologist. With any history of an injury, a thorough examination of the entire eye is necessary.

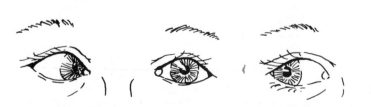

A   B

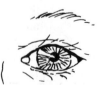

FIG. 9–1.   Strabismus. (*A*) esotropia, (*B*) exotropia.

Sympathetic ophthalmia may follow perforation wounds of the globe, even if the perforations are small. Sympathetic ophthalmia is an inflammatory reaction of the uninjured eye, showing phótophobia, lacrimation, pain and some dimness of vision. The retina may finally become detached, and atrophy of the eyeball may occur. Prompt and skillful treatment at the time of the injury is essential to avoid involvement of the other eye.

Small foreign objects such as specks of dust that have lodged inside the eyelid may be removed by rolling the lid back and exposing the object. Cotton-tipped applicators should not be used for this purpose because of the danger of sudden movement and of possible perforation of the eye. If the object cannot be easily removed with a small piece of moistened cotton or soft clean cloth, the child should be taken to the physician.

EYE INFECTIONS

A condition called properly *external hordeolum*, but known commonly as a *sty*, is a purulent infection of the follicle of an eyelash, generally caused by *Staphylococcus aureus*. Localized swelling, tenderness and pain are present, with a reddened lid edge. The maximum tenderness is over the infected site. The lesion goes on to suppuration, with eventual discharge of the purulent material. Warm saline compresses applied for about 15 minutes three or four times daily give some relief and hasten resolution, but recurrence is common. The sty should never be squeezed. Antibiotic ointment may help prevent accompanying conjunctivitis and recurrence.

HOSPITAL CARE FOR THE CHILD WITH EYE SURGERY

A person suffering any kind of sensory deprivation may find it difficult to stay in touch with reality. A child who must have his eyes covered is particularly vulnerable. The implications of not being able to see are not always appreciated by nurses who have not themselves experienced this. A young child who wakens from surgery to find himself in total darkness may well go into a state of real panic. If one observes such a child closely as he is returned to the unit, the panic may be quite evident; he trembles, and starts nervously if he is touched or spoken to. In hospitals that still limit visiting hours, eye surgery is seldom considered a condition serious enough to allow a mother to stay continuously. His mother may be at the bedside when he returns from surgery, but who is there beside him when he hears strange voices the next morning—but sees no one?

Preparation for the event, should, of course, be carried out as well as it is possible to do so, but the small child has no background experience to help him understand what actually is going to happen. The darkness, pain and total strangeness of the situation, can be overwhelming.

Restraints should not be used indiscriminately, but the majority of small children do need some reminder to keep their hands away from the sore eye, unless someone is beside them to prevent them from rubbing or from removing eye dressings. Elbow restraints are useful, although they do not prevent rubbing the eye with the arm. Flannel strips applied to the wrists in clovehitch fashion can be tied to the cribsides in such a manner as to allow freedom of arm movement, but to prevent the child from reaching his face.

The nurse should speak to the child before touching him, to make him aware of her presence. The child does need tactile stimulation though, so after speaking and identifying herself, the nurse would do well to stroke or to pat him, to pick him up, if this is allowed, or in some other way let him feel her presence.

Nurses caring for persons who are temporarily or permanently sightless should understand from first-hand experience what the loss of sight means. They should cover their eyes for a period and learn the difficulties involved in finding their way about, or in ordinary self-care.

Eye Dressings and Instillation.   An "eye tray" is usually kept in the treatment room on the pediatric department. The treatment room nurse is responsible for refilling all trays and checking expiration dates for medications or solutions, sterile trays, and dressings. The tray for eye care contains routine solutions for pupil dilatation, such as atropine and homatropine, vials or ampules of sterile saline solution, and other eye drops or ointments in common use.

The eye dressing tray should contain

1. Sterile eye pads
2. Sterile cotton balls
3. 4 × 4 gauze pads (flats)
4. A small sterile basin
5. Sterile scissors and small forceps
6. Adhesive tape
7. Container for water

The nurse may be expected to instill eye drops, particularly before eye surgery. When preoperative eye drops or drops prior to eye examination are ordered, timing must be exact. She will also have occasion to apply eye ointments and do eye dressings, as ordered by the physician.

Instillation of eye drops.   A small child cannot understand the necessity for having anything put in his eye, and cannot be expected to cooperate. It is usually necessary to apply a mummy restraint (Fig. 9–2) and have a second person hold the child's head still. The lower lid should be pulled down gently and the drops instilled into the inner canthus. Care must be used to prevent touching the eyeball with the dropper.

If a multiple dose bottle of solution is used, a clean dropper must be used for each patient. When the solution is in a sealed dropper vial, individual bottles for each patient will help prevent the spread of infection.

gastrointestinal system disorders

CELIAC SYNDROME *disorder*

Intestinal malabsorption with steatorrhea is a condition brought about by various causes, the most common being cystic fibrosis and gluten-induced enteropathy, the so-called idiopathic celiac disease. In 1889, the condition of malnutrition, abnormal stools, distended abdomen and retarded growth was described and named *celiac disease.*

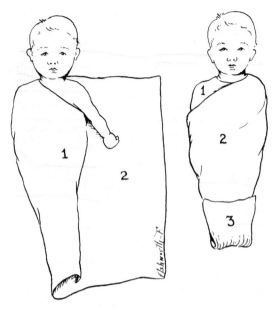

FIG. 9–2. Mummy restraint.

Not until the late 1930s was it recognized that several distinct entities were being described, with cystic fibrosis and celiac disease as two conditions of differing etiology. The term *celiac syndrome* is now used to designate the complex of malabsorptive disorders.

GLUTEN-INDUCED ENTEROPATHY

The "idiopathic celiac disease" is a basic defect of metabolism precipitated by the ingestion of wheat gluten or rye gluten, leading to impaired fat absorption. The exact etiology is not known; the most acceptable theory is that of an inborn error of metabolism with an allergic reaction as a contributing or possibly, the sole factor.

Severe manifestations of the disorder have become rare in the United States and in western Europe, but mild disturbances of intestinal absorption of rye, wheat, and sometimes oat gluten, are not uncommon.

Clinical Manifestations. Signs generally do not appear before the age of 6 months, and may be delayed until a year or later. Manifestations include chronic diarrhea with foul, bulky, greasy stools, and progressive malnutrition. Anorexia and a fretful, unhappy disposition are typical. The onset is generally insidious, with failure to thrive, bouts of diarrhea and frequent respiratory infections. If the condition becomes severe, the effects of malnutrition are prominent. Retarded growth and development, a distended abdomen and thin, wasted buttocks and legs are characteristic symptoms (Fig. 9–3).

CELIAC CRISIS

The chronic course of this disease may be interrupted by a *celiac crisis*. This is frequently triggered by an upper respiratory infection. The child commences to vomit copiously, has large, watery stools and becomes severely dehydrated. He becomes drowsy and prostrate, developing an acute medical emergency. Parenteral fluid therapy is essential to combat acidosis and to achieve normal fluid balance.

Diagnosis and Treatment. At present the only way to determine if a small child's failure to thrive is from this disorder is to place him on a trial gluten-free diet and to evaluate the results. Improvement in the nature of the stools and general well-being, with a gain in weight should follow, although several weeks may elapse before clear-cut manifestations can be confirmed.

Response to a diet from which rye, wheat and oats are excluded is generally good, although probably no cure can be expected; and dietary indiscretions or respiratory infections may bring relapses. The omission of wheat products in particular should continue through adolescence, because the ingestion of wheat appears to inhibit growth in sensitive persons.

Dietary Program. The young child is usually started on a starch-free, low-fat diet. If his condition is severe, this will consist of skim milk, glucose, and banana flakes. Bananas contain invert sugar and are usually well-tolerated. Additions to the diet of lean meats, pureed vegetables and fruits are made gradually. Eventually, fats may be added, and the child can be maintained on a regular diet with the exception of all wheat and rye products.

Commercially canned creamed soups, cold cuts, frankfurters, and pudding mixes, generally contain wheat products. The forbidden list also includes malted milk drinks, some candies, many baby foods and, of course, breads, cakes, pastries and biscuits, unless the latter are made from corn flour or corn meal. The list of ingredients on packaged foods should be read before purchasing. Vitamins A and D in water-miscible solutions will be needed in double amounts to supplement the deficient diet.

UMBILICAL HERNIA

Umbilical hernias are quite common among infants. Most of them disappear spontaneously during late infancy without treatment or manipulation. Incarceration is extremely rare, but does occur. The hernia is caused by an imperfect closure or weakness of the fibrous umbilical ring. It appears as a soft swelling covered by the skin at the site of the umbilicus. The hernia consists of omentum or portions of the small intestine, and can easily be reduced through gentle pressure.

The older method of applying adhesive to strap down the hernia is ineffective and may be injurious. The application of a coin or other rigid object over the site of the hernia serves to hold the fascial ring open.

Surgery is seldom indicated unless the hernia becomes strangulated or persists into early childhood.

respiratory system disorders

SPASMODIC LARYNGITIS (CROUP)

Spasmodic croup may occur in children between the ages of 2 and 4 years. The cause is undetermined; it may be of infectious or of allergic origin, but certain children seem to develop severe laryngospasm with little, if any, apparent cause. The attack may be preceded by coryza and hoarseness, or by no apparent signs of respiratory trouble during the evening. The child awakens after a few hours sleep with a barklike cough, increasing respiratory difficulty, and stridor. He becomes anxious and restless, and there is marked hoarseness. There may be a low grade fever and mild upper respiratory infection.

This condition is not serious, but is quite frightening, both to the child and his parents. The attack subsides after a few hours; little evidence remains the next day when an anxious mother takes him to the doctor. Attacks frequently occur two or three nights in succession.

TREATMENT

Humidified air is helpful in reducing the laryngospasm. Taking the child into the bathroom and opening the hot water taps, with the door closed, is a quick method for providing moist air—provided that the water runs hot enough. The pediatrician may prescribe syrup of ipecac in a dosage sufficient to produce vomiting, which usually gives relief. If repeated attacks occur, phenobarbital at bedtime may relax the child enough to prevent a recurrence.

ACUTE LARYNGOTRACHEOBRONCHITIS

Laryngeal infections are not uncommon in small children, and they frequently involve tracheobronchial areas as well. Acute laryngotracheobronchitis may progress very rapidly and become a serious problem within a matter of hours. The toddler is the most frequently affected member of the one to four age group. This condition is usually of viral origin, but bacterial invasion may follow the original infection. It generally occurs after an upper respiratory infection with fairly mild rhinitis and pharyngitis.

The child develops hoarseness and a barking cough, with a fever which may reach 104° F or 105° F. As the disease progresses, marked laryngeal edema occurs, and the child's breathing becomes difficult; the pulse is rapid, and cyanosis may appear. Congestive heart failure and acute respiratory embarrassment can result.

TREATMENT

The child is placed in a supersaturated atmosphere, such as that obtained in a croupette or some other kind of mist tent.

Close and careful observation of the child is important. Observation includes checking his pulse, his respiration, his color, listening for hoarseness and stridor, and noting any state of restlessness. Tepid sponge bath Tracheostomy.

TYPE OF RESPIRATION

Pull down the covers, and watch the child breathe. Observe the amount of chest movement, shallow breathing, and retractions. Listen with a stethoscope for breath sounds, particularly the amount of stridor, indicating difficult breathing.

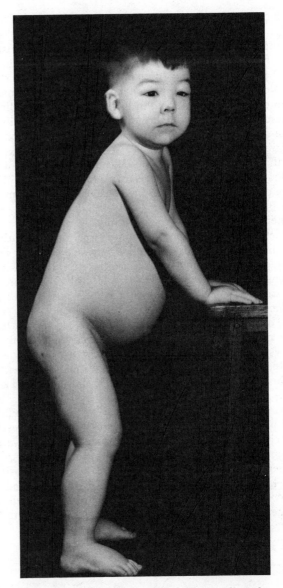

FIG. 9–3. Celiac disease showing protruding abdomen. (Wieczorek RR, Natapoff J: A Conceptual Approach to the Nursing of Children: Health Care From Birth Through Adolescence. Philadelphia, JB Lippincott, 1981)

HEARTBEAT

Listen for the rate, quality, strength, and regularity of the pulse. A rapid, weak pulse may indicate impending cardiac difficulty.

VOICE AND COLOR

Increasing hoarseness should be reported. Cyanosis of the nailbeds or lips, or increasing pallor signal impaired oxygenation of the blood, and should be reported promptly.

Difficult swallowing may limit the airway and prevent sufficient fluid intake.

Increasing restlessness and anxiety, are frequently signs of impending heart failure.

Intravenous fluids are usually needed, but they must be carefully monitored to prevent overloading the circulation and placing additional strain on the overworked heart.

Not all children with this type of infection become as acutely ill as their symptoms imply, but the possibility is present, and it should be understood. The majority of these infections are of viral origin, and do not respond to antibiotics.

If a tracheostomy becomes necessary because of respiratory difficulty, the surgeon will try to perform this in the operating room, under more ideal conditions than can be obtained at the bedside (Fig. 9–4). The decision as to when to perform a tracheostomy is a delicate one. Tracheostomy is a procedure not to be performed lightly or for insufficient reasons. The waiting period becomes a difficult one for the nurse, especially because her observations are used as partial basis for decision. The parents' anxiety, and her own feeling of helplessness add to her concern.

The nurse who is watching the child needs support from the other members of the nursing staff as well as from the physicians. She should not try to demonstrate her self-sufficiency or worry about the picture she may present to others. Her concern is for her patient, and she should seek help and advice without hesitation.

An emergency tracheostomy set is kept readily available for use if it is necessary, but because much better results can be obtained if the surgery is performed in the operating room—without the pressures of a last minute emergency procedure—the child will be taken there if possible. Postoperatively, humidified oxygen is administered by way of a tracheostomy mask rather than a croupette. When the child is in surgery, the nurse will prepare his room for his return. The bed can now be changed completely, the mist apparatus cleaned and checked for maximum efficiency, and the plastic tent checked for tears or holes.

Immediate postoperative care of the tracheostomy patient is generally done by a registered nurse. It includes continuous observation, frequent suctioning of the tube to keep the airway open, and maintenance of high humidity. Continuous observation is critically important because children with a tracheostomy are unable to speak, cry, cough, or gag and cannot signal their distress. Specific procedures for suctioning and care of the tracheostomy tube can be found in the procedure manuals of individual hospitals. Careful observation of the patient and strict aseptic techniques are the keystones of these procedures.

CYSTIC FIBROSIS

When first described, cystic fibrosis (CF) was called fibrocystic disease of the pancreas. Further research has revealed that this disorder represents a major dysfunction of all exocrine glands. The major organs affected are the lungs, pancreas, and liver. Because about one-half of all children with CF experience pulmonary complications, this disorder is discussed here with other respiratory conditions.

CF is hereditary, and transmitted as an autosomal recessive trait. Both parents must be carriers of the gene for CF to appear. With each pregnancy, the chance is one in four that the child will have the disease.

PATHOPHYSIOLOGY

Although the cause of CF is unknown, the basic defect is believed to be an inborn error of metabolism. Abnormal secretions of the mucus-producing glands throughout the body tend to accumulate; in some organs, particularly the pancreas and lungs, the mucus coagulates and forms obstructions in the pancreatic ducts and the bronchi (Fig. 9–5).

CLINICAL MANIFESTATIONS

In the newborn, meconium ileus is the presenting symptom of CF in 5% to 10% of the newborns who later develop additional manifestations. Depletion or absence of pancreatic enzymes before birth results in impaired digestive activity, and the meconium becomes viscid and mucilaginous. The inspissated (thickened) meconium fills the small intestine, causing complete obstruction. Clinical manifestations are bile-stained emesis, a distended abdomen, and an absence of stool. These babies taste salty when kissed, owing to high sodium concentrations in their sweat. Intestinal perforation with symptoms of shock may occur.

In older children, symptoms of CF may occur at varying ages during infancy or childhood. A hard, nonproductive chronic cough may be the first sign. Later, bronchial infections become frequent. Development of a barrel chest and clubbing of fingers indicate chronic lack of oxygen. Despite an excellent appetite, malnutrition is apparent and becomes increasingly severe. The abdomen becomes distended, and body muscles flabby (Fig. 9–6).

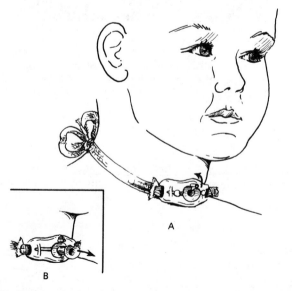

FIG. 9–4. A tracheostomy may become necessary if the child has respiratory difficulty. Note the tracheostomy tube in place (A) and the inner metal cannula unlocked and partially removed (B).

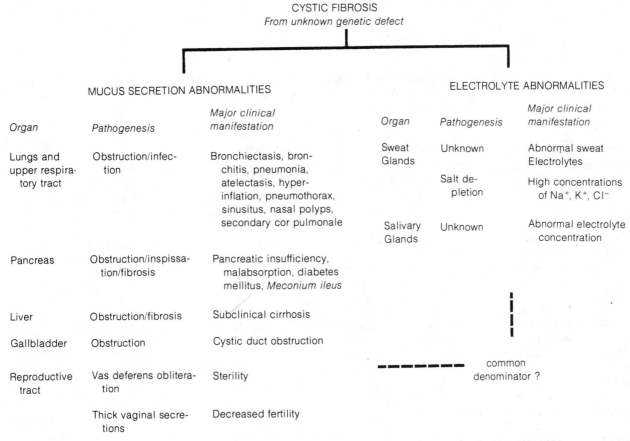

CYSTIC FIBROSIS
From unknown genetic defect

MUCUS SECRETION ABNORMALITIES

Organ	Pathogenesis	Major clinical manifestation
Lungs and upper respiratory tract	Obstruction/infection	Bronchiectasis, bronchitis, pneumonia, atelectasis, hyperinflation, pneumothorax, sinusitus, nasal polyps, secondary cor pulmonale
Pancreas	Obstruction/inspissation/fibrosis	Pancreatic insufficiency, malabsorption, diabetes mellitus, *Meconium ileus*
Liver	Obstruction/fibrosis	Subclinical cirrhosis
Gallbladder	Obstruction	Cystic duct obstruction
Reproductive tract	Vas deferens obliteration	Sterility
	Thick vaginal secretions	Decreased fertility

ELECTROLYTE ABNORMALITIES

Organ	Pathogenesis	Major clinical manifestation
Sweat Glands	Unknown	Abnormal sweat Electrolytes
	Salt depletion	High concentrations of Na^+, K^+, Cl^-
Salivary Glands	Unknown	Abnormal electrolyte concentration

——————— common denominator ?

FIG. 9–5. CF defects and manifestations. (Larter N: Cystic fibrosis. Am J Nurs 81:527–532, 1981

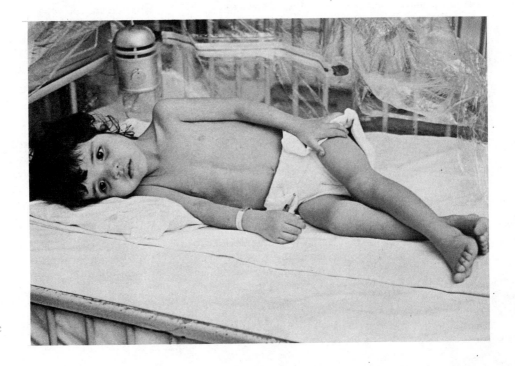

FIG. 9–6.   This child has cystic fibrosis.

Pancreatic Involvement. Thick, tenacious mucus obstructs the pancreatic ducts, causing the flow of pancreatic enzymes to be diminished (*hypochylia*) or absent (*achylia*). This achylia or hypochylia leads to intestinal malabsorption and severe malnutrition. Because of this malabsorption of fats, stools are frequent, bulky and greasy, with a distinctively foul odor. Anemia or rectal prolapse frequently occur if the pancreatic condition remains untreated. *Cotazym - pancreatic extract.*

Pulmonary Involvement. The degree of lung involvement determines the prognosis for survival. The severity of pulmonary involvement differs in individual children, a few showing only minor involvement. About one-half of the children with CF can be expected to live to age 18 or older.

Respiratory complications pose the greatest threat to children with CF. Abnormal amounts of thick viscid mucus clog the bronchioles and provide an ideal medium for bacterial growth. *Staphylococcus aureus coagulase* can be cultured from the nasopharynx and sputum of most patients. *Pseudomonas aeruginosa* and *Hemophilus influenzae* are also frequently found. The basic infection, however, appears most often to be caused by *S. aureus*.

Numerous complications arise from severe respiratory infection. Atelectasis and small lung abscesses are common early complications. Bronchiectasis and emphysema develop, with pulmonary fibrosis and pneumonitis, eventually leading to severe ventilatory insufficiency.

mucus 5-6y thicker

Other Affected Organs. The tears, saliva, and sweat of children with CF contain abnormally high concentrations of electrolytes, and the submaxillary salivary glands are enlarged in a majority of these children. In hot weather, the loss of sodium chloride and fluid through sweating produces frequent heat prostration. Additional fluid and salt in the diet, or salt tablets, should be given as a preventive measure.

DIAGNOSIS

Diagnosis is based on family history, evidence of elevated sodium chloride in the sweat, demonstration of hypochylia or achylia, a history of failure to thrive, pulmonary manifestations, and on radiologic findings.

Pilocarpine Iontophoresis. The principal diagnostic test to confirm CF is a sweat chloride test using the pilocarpine iontophoresis method. This method induces sweating by using a small electric current that carries topically applied pilocarpine into a localized area of the skin.

An area on the child's forearm (or on the infant's thigh) is washed with distilled water, dried, and covered with a 2×2 inch gauze square that has been saturated with a measured amount of .2% pilocarpine nitrate. A positive copper electrode is applied over the gauze and a negative electrode is placed elsewhere on the same arm, and both are attached with rubber straps of the type used for electrocardiography. Lead wires are connected and low current is applied for 5 minutes.

Following iontophoresis, the electrodes are removed, the gauze discarded, and the area again washed with distilled water. Dry gauze which has been weighed in a glass flask is removed from the flask with forceps, placed over the test area, and covered with a plastic square, firmly secured around the edges with tape. After 30 to 45 minutes, the gauze is removed with forceps, placed in the flask, weighed and analyzed in the laboratory for its sodium chloride content.

TREATMENT

In the newborn, meconium ileus is treated by surgical resection, employing one of several methods, but the mortality rate is high in spite of skillful surgery. The majority of infants who survive develop cystic fibrosis of varying degrees of severity.

In the older child, treatment is aimed at correcting pancreatic deficiency, and improving pulmonary function. If bowel obstruction does occur (meconium ileus equivalent), surgery may be necessary.

Dietary Treatment. Commercially prepared pancreatic enzymes given during meals, either in the form of granules sprinkled on the child's food, or as capsules, will aid digestion and absorption of fat and protein.

The child's diet should be high in carbohydrates and protein, with moderate restriction of fats. Unless acutely ill, these children have large appetites, but they can receive little nourishment without a pancreatic supplement. With proper diet and enzyme supplements, these children show evidence of improved nutrition, and their stools become relatively normal. Foods such as butter, ice cream, peanut butter, french fries, and mayonnaise should be restricted to occasional use, and then only when extra enzymes are given.

Because of the increased loss of sodium chloride, these children are allowed to use as much salt as they wish, even though onlookers may think it is too much. During hot weather, additional salt may be provided with pretzels, salt bread sticks, and saltines.

Vitamins, in water-miscible preparations, are needed in twice the normal daily amounts.

Pulmonary Treatment. The goal of treatment is to provide respiratory drainage by thinning the secretions, and by mechanical means such as postural drainage and clapping, to loosen and drain the secretions from the lungs. Antibacterial drugs for the treatment of infection are necessary as indicated. Immunization against childhood communicable diseases is extremely important for these chronically ill children. All immunization measures may be used, and should be maintained at appropriate intervals. Physical activity is beneficial, and should be restricted only to the extent of the child's endurance.

Inhalation therapy can be preventive or therapeutic for the child with CF. Intermittant inhalation of 10% propylene glycol in water or saline by nebulizer, in addition to a bronchodilator drug, is necessary three or four times daily. The addition of a mucolytic agent such as

Mucomyst may be prescribed during periods of acute infection.

Most of these children profit by continuous aerosol therapy during their naptime and through the night, using a 10% solution of propylene glycol.

A humidified atmosphere is achieved through use of a mist tent during sleep, a necessity for every child with CF. A heavy mist that raises humidity above 50% is essential. Various types of tents are available, which function through the use of a compressed air pump with an attach-

ment for a nebulizer provided in the event that oxygen becomes necessary. Children become quite accustomed to crawling inside their tents to sleep. During acute distress, the use of a mist tent becomes a necessary full-time treatment.

Postural drainage is performed routinely three or four times daily, even if little drainage is apparent (Fig. 9–7). Chest percussion, which is clapping and vibrating of the affected areas (Fig. 9–8), if done correctly, helps to loosen and move the secretions out of the lungs. The physical

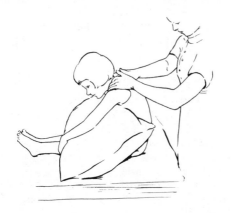
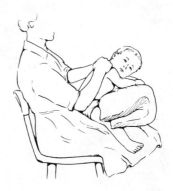

Upper lobes—posterior segments

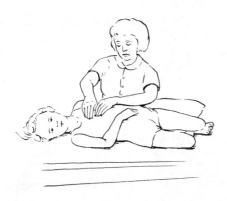
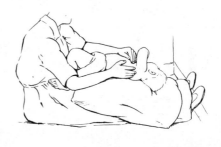

Left upper lobe—lingular segment

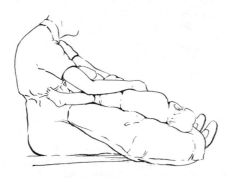
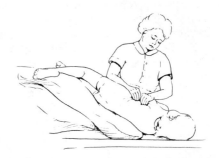

Left lower lobe—lateral segments

FIG. 9–7.   There are a number of positions for postural drainage in cystic fibrosis.

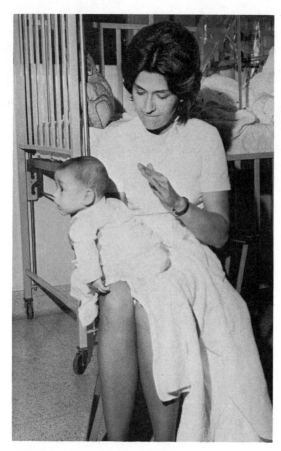

FIG. 9–8. "Clapping" of the affected areas in cystic fibrosis helps move the secretions.

therapist usually performs this procedure in the hospital and demonstrates it to parents, because they will have to perform it as an essential part of home care.

HOME CARE

The home care for these children places a tremendous burden upon the concerned families. This is not one-time hospital treatment, nor is there a prospect of cure to brighten the horizon. Each day, a large amount of time is spent in the performance of treatments. Parents must learn to manipulate the mist tent compressor and the nebulizer, perform postural drainage and clapping techniques. The child's diet must be planned, with the regulation of additional enzymes according to need. Great care is needed to prevent exposure to infections.

In addition, the parents must guard against overprotection and against undue limitation of their child's physical activity. Somehow, a good family relationship must be preserved, with time allowed for attention to other members of the family.

Physical activity is an important adjunct to the child's well-being, and is a necessary help in getting rid of secretions. The child soon learns his capacity for exercise, and can be trusted to become self-limiting as necessary, espe-

cially if he has had an opportunity to learn the nature of his condition. Small children may find postural drainage fun when daddy raises their feet in the air and walks them around "wheel-barrow" fashion.

Hot weather activity should be watched a little more closely, with additional attention directed toward increased salt and fluid intake during periods of exercise.

Caring for a child with CF places great stress on family financial resources. The expense of daily medications, frequent clinic or office visits, and sometimes lengthy hospitalizations can be devastating to an ordinary family budget, even with hospital–medical insurance coverage. Some financial assistance is available through such agencies as the Crippled Children's Service.[1]

As in many major health care problems, some of the most effective support comes from other parents and families facing the same situation. Parent groups are organized in most cities, and help in morale building, fund raising, and educational projects. The Cystic Fibrosis Foundation is active in research with established centers in a number of cities.

Camps for children with cystic fibrosis have proved quite successful. The camps are staffed with nurses and therapists who assist with necessary treatments and act as consultants. Children participate in the usual camping activities, such as nature walks, crafts, swimming, and sports, and return home enriched by the experience.

OUTCOME

The outlook for children with CF is improving but still bleak. Only one-half of them will live beyond age 18. The cause of the disease is still unknown, and no cure has been found. Early diagnosis and treatment can help prolong life and make it more normal, but until a cure is discovered that life may be painfully brief.

accidents

INGESTION OF TOXIC SUBSTANCES

When a child manifests symptoms that are difficult to assess, or which do not appear to relate specifically to any known cause, the possibility of poisoning should be suspected. Ingestion of a poisonous substance can produce symptoms that simulate an attack of an acute disease— vomiting, abdominal pain, diarrhea, shock, cyanosis, coma, or convulsions. If evidence of such a disease is lacking, acute poisoning should be suspected.

In cases of apparent poisoning, the child's parents will be asked to consider all medications in their home. Is it possible that any medication could have been available to the child, or did an older child or other person possibly give the child the container to play with? Or, could anyone have been negligent in supervising the child's actions? It is possible that a parent inadvertently gave a wrong dose or wrong medication to a child. All such possibilities need to be considered and perhaps investigated.

In the meantime, the most important priority is treatment for the child who shows symptoms of poisoning.

EMERGENCY TREATMENT

Except when corrosive or highly irritant poisons have been swallowed, the first measure is to induce vomiting. If the child is convulsing or unconscious, however, vomiting should not be induced because of the danger of aspiration.

The approved method for producing vomiting is to have the child swallow 15 ml of syrup of ipecac. A second 15 ml dose can be given if vomiting does not occur within 15 to 30 minutes. Vomiting may also be induced by stimulating the child's posterior pharynx with the adult's finger. The child's head should be allowed to droop forward or turned to the side to avoid aspiration of the vomitus.

All material vomited at home or on the way to the hospital or treatment center should be saved for analysis. If it is known that the child swallowed medication, the container should be taken along. If, in the panic and confusion, the container is left behind, someone will need to go to the home and retrieve the container.

Treatment Steps in Order of Importance

1. Remove the poison.
2. Prevent further absorption.
3. Administer antidote if known.
4. Administer general supportive and symptomatic care.

After vomiting has been induced, the child should be taken at once to the emergency department of the nearest hospital. Most cities have emergency numbers listed in the telephone book for assistance in a crisis, or the telephone operator can be asked to make the connection. If necessary, an emergency vehicle may be made available to take the child to the nearest emergency treatment center.

If the child cannot be moved immediately to a facility for treatment, a telephone call to the nearest poison control center will bring prompt information on how to treat the child. These centers are located in most cities, and many have toll-free numbers for the convenience of persons in remote areas.

If the substance the child has swallowed is known, the ingredients can be found on the label. The poison control center can suggest an antidote if the name of the drug or other substance is known. If the substance is a prescription drug, the pharmacist who filled the prescription or who is familiar with the drug can also be contacted for information. In some cases, it may be necessary to analyze the residual stomach contents.

The first procedure, however, is to try to remove as much of the ingested poison as possible. Gastric aspiration, performed by a skilled person, may be necessary.

There are specific antidotes for certain poisons, but not for all. Some antidotes react chemically with the poison to render it harmless; others prevent absorption of the poison. *Activated charcoal* given after vomiting absorbs many poisons. It is given in 6 to 8 ounces of water in a dose of 5 g to 10 g per gram of ingested poison.

Further specific treatment is given according to the kind and amount of the poison ingested. Examples of frequent types of poisoning and general treatment are listed here. Complete listings of poisonous substances with the specific treatment for each are available from poison control centers, clinics, and pharmacies.

ACETYLSALICYLIC ACID (ASPIRIN) POISONING

Although the incidence of aspirin poisoning in childhood has declined in recent years, it is still the most common cause of poisoning in young children. Other forms of salicylic poisoning do occur but less commonly.

Aspirin poisoning can result from ingestion of adult aspirin or from children's aspirin, even though the children's tablets are smaller dosage. Both are available without prescription and, therefore, are found in most medicine cabinets. *may cause ~~breath~~ bleeding.*

Symptoms of Overdose. Aspirin poisoning is signaled by *hyperpnea* (abnormal increase in depth and rate of breathing), followed by metabolic acidosis, hyperventilation, tinnitus, and vertigo. Dehydration, coma, convulsions, and death may follow in instances of heavy dosage.

Treatment. Vomiting should be induced even if some time has elapsed since ingestion. In severe cases, intravenous fluids may be needed to relieve the dehydration. Sodium bicarbonate may be given intravenously to combat the acidosis. Dialysis may be necessary if the child develops renal failure.

FERROUS SULFATE (IRON) POISONING

Ferrous sulfate is frequently used to treat iron deficiency in infants and children. It may be given in tablet or capsule form, as an elixir or syrup, or as drops. All preparations of iron marketed by reliable pharmaceutical firms bear the label "Keep out of reach of children." Unknowingly, parents may overdose their child, not realizing the potential dangers. Dosages prescribed by the physician should not be exceeded.

Symptoms of Overdose. Ingestion of an excessive amount has been fatal in many cases. Vomiting, lethargy, diarrhea, weak, rapid pulse, low blood pressure are common symptoms. Massive doses may produce shock, erosion of the small intestine, black, tarry stools, and bronchial pneumonia.

Treatment. Induced vomiting and gastric lavage containing sodium bicarbonate may be required. The child should be fed milk and eggs, if possible.

BARBITURATES

Ingestion of five or six times the average dose may be toxic, but any intake over the prescribed dosage should be reported.

Symptoms of Overdose. Respiratory, circulatory, and renal depression can occur and the patient may become comatose.

Treatment. Gastric lavage, establishment of an open airway if needed, oxygen, and artificial respiration may be required.

The patient should be watched closely even when consciousness returns after coma, as consciousness may be only temporary, and the child may again lapse into coma.

CORROSIVES (LYE, BLEACHES, DRAIN CLEANERS, TOILET BOWL CLEANERS)

A small child is likely to drink anything he finds in a bottle or other container. Ammonia, solutions containing silver nitrate, lye, or iodine cause severe symptoms when ingested, and can permanently damage the mouth and esophageal mucosa. Severe esophageal burns can cause nearly complete occlusion of the esophagus, and dilation of the esophageal tract may be required for a long period of time. Shock, followed by death, occurs in many patients.

The first mouthful of a corrosive substance causes intense burning and pain. Therefore, the child stops drinking, but damage has already occurred.

Emergency treatment for burns from alkali corrosives such as ammonia, lye, and household bleach, consists of oral administration of quantities of water, diluted acid fruit juices, or diluted vinegar.

Burns from acids (toilet bowl cleaners, iodine, silver nitrate) demand alkaline drinks such as milk, olive oil, mineral oil, or egg whites.

Lavage or emetics *should not be used* after ingestion of corrosive products as this will cause further damage.

Continuing treatment requires antidotes, usually gastrostomy or intravenous feedings, and specialized care. Severe burns may necessitate a tracheostomy. Esophageal dilations may be needed at regular intervals for long periods following corrosive burns.

HYDROCARBONS (KEROSENE, GASOLINE, FURNITURE POLISH)

These highly toxic substances are responsible for a number of childhood deaths when they are aspirated, inhaled, or swallowed. Although vomiting should not be induced because of the potential damage to the respiratory system, the child will usually vomit spontaneously.

Pneumonitis, bronchopneumonia, or lipoid pneumonia frequently follows ingestion or inhalation of these products. The child should be carefully observed for some time as symptoms of poisoning may be delayed.

LEAD POISONING (PLUMBISM)

Chronic lead poisoning has been a serious problem among children for many years. It is responsible for many childhood deaths, and leaves many other children with neurologic handicaps, including mental retardation, because of its effect on the central nervous system. Infants and toddlers are potential victims because of their propensity to mouth any object within their reach. In some children, this habit leads to *pica*, the ingestion of nonfood substances such as laundry starch, clay, tissue paper, and paint.

Causes of Chronic Lead Poisoning

Lead-containing paint used on the outside or inside of houses

Furniture and toys painted with lead-containing paint
Drinking water contaminated by lead pipes
Dust containing lead salts
Storage of fruit juices or other food in improperly glazed earthenware
Inhalation of motor fumes containing lead, or burning of storage batteries
Exposure to industrial areas with smelteries or chemical plants

There are other causes, but the most common cause has been the lead in paint. Children tend to nibble on fallen plaster, painted wooden furniture (including cribs), or painted toys because they have a sweet taste. They are also highly susceptible to harmful effects from inhalation of fumes from newly painted rooms or furniture. When the danger of lead poisoning became apparent, attempts were made to control the sale of lead-based paint. In 1973, Federal regulations banned the sale of paint containing more than 0.5% lead for interior residential use, or use on toys. This has not eliminated the problem, however, because many homes built prior to the 1960s were painted with lead-base paint, and they still exist, particularly in the inner-city areas.

Symptoms of Lead Poisoning. The onset of chronic lead poisoning is insidious. Some indications may be loss of weight, or failure to gain weight, weakness, and vomiting. The child's development may be slowed, or regression may occur. Because these symptoms also occur in other conditions, they are not conclusive indications of lead poisoning. Effects on the central nervous system can include hyper-irritability, clumsiness, and poor coordination.

The condition may progress to encephalopathy (degenerative disease of the brain) because of intra-cranial pressure. Acute manifestations include convulsions and coma. Acute episodes sometimes develop sporadically and early in the condition.

Diagnosis. The nonspecific nature of the presenting symptoms make it important that the environmental history of the child be examined closely.

Serum levels of lead are obtained, and a 24-hour urine specimen is examined for increased lead concentration. Blood levels are likely to be unstable as are single specimens of urine. Several laboratory tests are indicated for glycosuria, anemia, and a number of more sophisticated tests. Roentgenograms of the long bones that show broad bands of increased density at the metaphyses usually signify increased storage of lead but alone are not diagnostic.

Treatment. The use of a chelating agent, such as Calcium Disodium edetate, known as EDTA (ethylenediamine tetra-acetic acid), is the most important aspect of treatment. EDTA binds the iron ions with itself, preventing their entrance into the blood cells, and causes their excretion by the kidneys. This medication is preferably given intramuscularly to children.

BAL (2,3-dimercapto-1-propanol) may also be given, intramuscularly, to reduce the danger of increased intracranial pressure. Valium (diazepam) is useful in treatment of convulsions occurring in lead encephalopathy. None of these medications is innocuous, and should be prescribed, administered, and monitored very carefully.

Outcome. Prognosis is uncertain. Early detection of the condition and removal of the child from the lead-containing surroundings offers the best hope. Follow-up should include routine examinations to prevent recurrence and to assess any residual brain damage not immediately apparent.

Although the incidence of lead poisoning has decreased, it is still prevalent. Measures to educate the public on the importance of preventing this disorder are essential if the problem is to be eliminated.

BURNS

Among the many accidents that occur in the lives of children, burns are the most frequent and frightening. More than 80% of burn accidents happen to children under 5 years of age.[2] One tragic fact is that nearly all childhood burns are preventable, which causes considerable guilt for parents and the child.

Failure to explain dangers to the child, carelessness of an adult, the child's disobedience, all enter into the picture.

CAUSES

Scalds from Hot Liquids. This is a frequent type of burn in small children, resulting from a dangling electric percolator cord, pans of hot liquid on the stove with handles out, cups of hot tea or coffee, and bowls of soup, and small children left alone in bathtubs. Dangerous and sometimes fatal burns can occur from these conditions.

Burns from Fire. The second most frequent kind of burn results from children playing with matches, or being left alone in buildings that catch fire from any cause.

Electricity. Although not common in children, infants and toddlers do suffer severe facial or mouth burns requiring extensive plastic surgery from biting on electrical cords that are still plugged into a socket.

TYPES OF BURNS

Burns are divided into types according to the depth of tissue involvement; whether superficial, partial thickness, or total thickness (Table 9–1).

Superficial or First Degree Burns. The epidermis is injured, but there is no destruction of tissue or of nerve endings. Thus there is erythema, edema and pain, but prompt regeneration.

Partial Thickness or Second Degree Burns. The epidermis and underlying dermis are both injured and devitalized, or destroyed. There is generally blistering, with an escape of body plasma, but regeneration of the skin occurs from the remaining viable epithelial cells in the dermis.

Total Thickness or Third Degree Burns. Epidermis, dermis, and nerve endings are all destroyed. Pain is minimal, and there is no longer any barrier to infection, or any remaining viable epithelial cells.

EMERGENCY TREATMENT

Ice cold water or ice packs are excellent emergency treatments for burns. The immediate application of ice compresses or ice water to burn areas appears to inhibit capillary permeability and thus suppress edema, blister formation and tissue destruction. Immersion of a burned extremity in cold water alleviates pain and may prevent further thermal injury.

Superficial Burns. Superficial burns can usually be treated on an outpatient basis, as they heal readily unless infected. The area should be cleaned, an anesthetic ointment applied and covered with a sterile bandage or dressing. An analgesic may be needed to relieve pain.

Partial- and Full-Thickness Burns. It is not always possible to distinguish between partial- and full-thickness burns. In the presence of infection, a partial-thickness burn may be converted into full thickness; also, with extensive burns, there is often a greater amount of full-thickness burn than had been estimated.

Total-thickness burns require the attention, skill and conscientious care of a team of specialists. Children with mixed second- and third-degree burns, or with third degree burns involving 15% or more of body surface, require hospitalization.

TREATMENT OF SERIOUS BURNS

First Phase—48 Hours to 72 Hours. Shock is the major manifestation in the first phase of massive burns. As extracellular fluid pours into the burned area, it collects in enormous quantities, dehydrating the body. Edema becomes noticeable, and symptoms of severe shock appear. Intense pain seldom is a major factor.

Symptoms of shock are—

1. Low blood pressure
2. Rapid pulse
3. Pallor
4. Often, considerable apprehension

The physician's primary concern is to replace body fluids that have been lost or immobilized at the burn areas. Because there is a distinct relationship between the extent of the surface area burned and the amount of fluid lost, the physician needs to estimate the percent of the skin area affected (Fig. 9–9).

Intravenous fluids for the maintenance and the replacement of lost body fluids are estimated for the first 24 hours, with one-half of this calculated requirement to be given during the first 8 hours. The patient's needs may change rapidly, however, necessitating a change in the rate of flow, the amount, or the type of fluid. The physician must check frequently and carefully the urinary output, the vital signs, and the general appearance of the patient.

TABLE 9-1. CATEGORIES OF BURN DEPTH

Degree	Cause	Surface Appearance	Color	Pain Level	Histologic Depth	Healing Time
First all are considered minor unless under 18 months, over 65, or with severe loss of fluids	flash, flame, ultraviolet (sunburn)	dry, no blisters, edema	erythematous	painful	epidermal layers only	2 to 5 days with peeling, no scarring, may have discoloration
Second (partial thickness) Minor—less than 15% in adults, less than 10% in children. Moderate—15–30% in adults, or less than 15% with involvement of face, hands, feet, or perineum; minor chemical or electrical; in children, 10–30% Severe—more than 30%	contact with hot liquids or solids, flash flame to clothing, direct flame, chemical	moist blebs, blisters	mottled white to pink, cherry red	very painful	epidermis, papillary, and reticular layers of dermis; may include fat domes of subcutaneous layer	superficial—5 to 21 days with no grafting. deep with no infection—21 to 35 days. if infected convert to full thickness
Third (full thickness) Minor—less than 2% Moderate—2–10% any involvement of face, hands, feet, or perineum Severe—more than 10% and major chemical or electrical	contact with hot liquids or solids, flame, chemical, electricity	dry with leathery eschar until debridement, charred blood vessels visible under eschar	mixed white (waxy-pearly), dark (khaki-mahogany), charred	little or no pain, hair pulls out easily	down to and includes subcutaneous tissue; may include fascia, muscle, and bone	large areas require grafting that may take many months. small areas may heal from the edges after weeks

(Wagner MM: Emergency care of the burned patient. Am J Nurs 77:1788–1791, 1977)

Frequent hematocrit and hemoglobin readings indicate needs for blood transfusion or plasma.

Adequacy of the patient's airway must be assessed in terms of a possible need for a tracheostomy, and an aseptic environment must be rigidly maintained.

Oral fluids should either be omitted or kept to a minimum for the first day or two. Acute gastric dilatation is a common complication of burns, and can become a serious problem. The child's thirst, which is usually severe, should be somewhat relieved by the intravenous fluids, and sips of water may be allowed. The child needs considerable emotional support, however, to help him through this stage.

Antibiotics, if used, will probably be added to the intravenous fluids. Tetanus antitoxin or toxoid should be ordered according to the state of the child's previous immunization. If his inoculations are up to date, a booster dose of tetanus toxoid is all that will be required.

Nursing care. Burns units have been organized in hospitals in several areas of the country. Also, Shriner's Hospitals for Burned Children are functioning in several localities, providing total care for burned children. The burn units are usually self-contained, with treatment and operating areas, hydrotherapy units and patient care areas. Personnel wear gowns, caps and masks. If visitors are admitted to the unit, they also must scrub, gown and mask.

In hospitals where there is no specific burn unit, a private room with a door that can be closed should be set up as a burn unit. "Reverse isolation" exercising the strictest aseptic technique must be observed.

Immediate nursing care is demanding, with many things to be done at once, a fact which makes it important that, if possible, more than one nurse be available. The nurse in a sterile gown, a mask and a cap, can help to place the patient on the sterile sheet spread over the bed, and can adjust the cradle over his body.

The room temperature should be kept around 80° F, because evaporation of water through the denuded areas, and even through the leathery burn eschar, proceeds rapidly, with a consequent thermal evaporative loss.

First, in order of importance, is the assistance in starting intravenous fluids, and assisting in performing the cut-down procedure. Temporary fluid, such as 5% dextrose in water, may be started until the child's needs have been calculated; then the ordered intravenous fluid must be prepared and hung. Aqueous penicillin or other antibiotic may be ordered for addition to the intravenous fluid.

Monitoring fluids. Strict monitoring of all intake and output is essential, including the amount of fluid the child has received at any given time, the rate of flow, the time the present bottle was started and when it is due to be finished, and the contents of the present bottle. The bottle itself must be clearly labeled, with an indication of any additions to the original contents, such as antibiotics.

The physician carefully estimates the amount and kind of intravenous fluid necessary, relying on the nurse to keep an accurate record (Fig. 9–10).

After assisting with the insertion of a Foley catheter, the nurse should connect the catheter to a sterile drainage tube and allow drainage into a sterile, closed, calibrated container. Urinary drainage is recorded every hour, and specific gravity recorded. After the first hour, the volume of urine should be relatively constant. Any change in volume or specific gravity should be reported.

Monitoring vital signs. Vital signs should be checked and recorded at frequent intervals, ranging from every 15 minutes to every half to full hour, as the circumstances demand. Observation should include

1. Patency of the airway. Check for difficult breathing, stridor, and sternal retractions.
2. Pulse rate, rhythm, and character. State whether it is rapid, weak, or irregular.
3. Body temperature, to be taken rectally if possible.
4. Blood pressure.
5. Restlessness, anxiety, excessive thirst, or presence of pain.

Continuing care. After the initial fluid therapy has brought the burn shock under control, and after the extracellular fluid deficit has been made up, the patient faces another hazard with the onset of the diuretic phase. This occurs somewhere within the period of 24 to 96 hours after the accident. The plasma-like fluid is picked up and reabsorbed from the "third space" in the burn areas, and the patient may rapidly become hypervolemic (an abnormal increase in the blood volume in the circulatory system) even to the point of pulmonary edema. This is the principal reason for the extremely close check on all vital signs, and for the close monitoring of intravenous fluids, which must now be slowed or stopped entirely.

The nurse needs to be alert for any signs of the onset of this phase, in order to notify the physicians at once. Clues to the onset of the diuretic phase include:

1. Rapid rise in urinary output. May go up to 250 ml per hour, or higher.
2. Tachypnea, followed by dyspnea.
3. Increase in pulse pressure; mean blood pressure may also rise. Central venous pressure, if measured, will be found to be elevated.

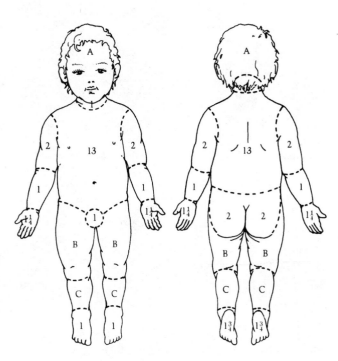

BURN SHEET

Name _____ Age _____ Number _____
Date of Observation _____

Relative Percentages of Areas Affected by Growth			
Area	Age 0	1	5
A = ½ of head	$9\frac{1}{2}$	$8\frac{1}{2}$	$6\frac{1}{2}$
B = ½ of one thigh	$2\frac{3}{4}$	$3\frac{1}{4}$	4
C = ½ of one leg	$2\frac{1}{2}$	$2\frac{1}{2}$	$2\frac{3}{4}$

% Burn by Areas		
Probable 3rd burn	Head _____ Neck _____ Body _____ Upper arm _____ Forearm _____ Hands _____ Genitals _____ Legs _____ Buttocks _____ Thighs _____ Feet _____	
Total burn	Head _____ Neck _____ Body _____ Upper arm _____ Forearm _____ Hands _____ Genitals _____ Legs _____ Buttocks _____ Thighs _____ Feet _____	
Sum of all areas _____	Probable 3rd _____	Total burn _____

Calculation of burn surface area.

FIG. 9–9. Calculation of burn surface area. (Wieczorek RR, Natapoff J: A Conceptual Approach to the Nursing of Children: Health Care From Birth Through Adolescence. Philadelphia, JB Lippincott, 1981)

FLUID BALANCE CHECK SHEET

Sol. #1	Gtt/ Min	cc/ hour	time started	time finished	flow checked
250 cc D/5/W (or ordered solution)					
500,000 units aqueous penicillin	12	48	9:00 AM		30 Min

		Intake			Output		
Time Checked	Gtt/Min	cc in Bottle	cc Given	Urine cc	Emesis		Checked by
9:00 AM	12	250	0				S N
9:30	12	226	24				S N
10:00	12	202	48	20			S N
10:30	12	178	72				
11:00	12	154	96	25			
11:30	12	130	120				
12:00	12	106	144	25			

FIG. 9–10.   Fluid balance check sheet.

If pulmonary edema becomes evident, vigorous action may be necessary, such as the use of rotating tourniquets, positive pressure respiration, and venisection. Morphine may be ordered.

Daily patient care through the first phases requires attention to positioning in order to help prevent contractures. This includes proper body alignment, the use of a footboard, keeping the head, the arms, and the legs in good position, as much as possible.

Frequent turning to prevent lung congestion and skin breakdown is extremely important, and extremely difficult. A Stryker frame, or a Circ-O-lectric bed on which a child may be turned quickly and painlessly, may be used. Children are, however, apt to become very frightened when being turned on the Stryker frame, requiring much reassurance and support.

Emotional support for child and parents.   Despite the physical and emotional shock of such a traumatic accident, most burn victims are not unconscious, but alert and able to talk. Thus, it is very important to explain to the child what is going to happen and what the various procedures are for. Often the urgency of performing physical care for the physiologic crises that burns create makes nurses and doctors overlook the frightened child's emotional needs. Meeting those needs throughout all phases of burn treatment usually results in better cooperation from the burned child.

The parents probably need greater support than their child during the first few hours, but they may get very little. No one has much time for them, unless nurses who are not directly involved with the burned child's treatment can show concern and be available to listen until the physicians can speak with the parents and counsel them.

These parents are dealing not only with the emotional shock of the accident but probably with guilt as well.

Emotional support for the attending staff.   Continuous nursing care of a burned child is an exceedingly traumatic emotional experience, as well as a most exhausting physical one. The child needs one individual to give him the support so important to his welfare, and the explanation and demonstration of complicated procedures take a disproportionate amount of time if these must be repeated to continually changing nurses. The nurse on each shift who has the care of the burned child needs a great deal of support from the personnel in the department.

Frequent checking to determine the nurse's needs, whether it is some article from outside the room, help with a procedure, or a few minutes relief, is most welcome. She needs prompt relief for meals, and coffee breaks are of great importance in order to get her away from the situation for a short time.

Second phase—48 Hours to 2 or More Weeks.   Many surgeons prefer to treat burns by the open, or exposure, method. The tough outer covering that forms over the burned area—called *eschar*—makes a satisfactory initial covering. When the burned crusts commence to separate from the underlying tissue, wet dressings and soaks will help loosen the eschar in preparation for skin grafts.

Infection is rarely a problem during the first 48 hours, if the proper aseptic environment is maintained. Normal skin bacteria invade the broken skin under the most careful management, however, so that every burn is potentially infected. Frequently *Staphylococcus aureus* and *Pseudomonas aeruginosa* infections are observed during the second phase in spite of stringent attempts at prevention of cross-contamination.

Infection poses the greatest threat to the burned child; therefore, cleanliness and aseptic technique are more significant than the topical medication prescribed. The physician is likely to choose from three commonly used agents: silver sulfadiazine (Silvadene), silver nitrate, and mafenide acetate (Sulfamylon). These agents are compared in Table 9–2.

Early debridement of the eschar to allow early skin grafting is considered important in controlling infection. After the initial shock phase, daily tub baths help remove the eschar. Gentle washing with a sterile washcloth or gauze during the bath hastens the process of debridement. Detailed instructions for this procedure can be found in any hospital's procedure manual.

Debridement and grafting. Eschar requires approximately 7 days to 2 weeks to slough off spontaneously, so debridement is frequently done mechanically in surgery under light anesthesia. If the area is clear of infection, grafts may be applied at the same time. Blood for transfusion should be ready because there may be considerable bleeding, especially if large areas are debrided.

Skin grafts. Grafts may be either homografts, allografts, or autografts. A *homograft* consists of skin taken from another person, and is eventually rejected by the recipient tissue, sloughing off after a period of three to six weeks. It provides a temporary dressing after debridement, and has proved a life-saving measure for children with extensive burns. Skin from cadavers is often used (*allograft*); it can be stored and used up to a period of several weeks, and permission for this use is seldom refused.

An *autograft,* consisting of skin taken from the child's own body, is the only kind of skin accepted permanently by recipient tissues, except for the skin from an identical twin. It is usually impossible to obtain enough healthy skin to cover a large area; therefore, homografts are of great value for immediate covering. If the donor site is kept free from infection, and grafts of sufficient thinness are taken, the site should be ready for use again in 10 to 12 days.

After grafting, donor as well as graft sites are kept covered with sterile dressings.

Complications. *Curling's ulcer.* Curling's ulcer (also called a "stress ulcer") is a gastric or duodenal ulcer that frequently occurs following serious skin burns. It can easily be overlooked when the attention of nurses and doctors is directed toward the treatment of the burn area and prevention of infection.

Symptoms are those of any gastric ulcer, but usually are rather vague, concerned with abdominal discomfort, with or without localization, or with relation to eating. Appearance of an ulcer, if it occurs, is during the first six weeks.

Blood may be present in the stools, an occurrence which, combined with abdominal discomfort, may be the basis for a diagnosis. If desired, roentgenograms can confirm the diagnosis.

TABLE 9–2. COMPARISON OF TOPICAL TREATMENTS FOR BURNS

Silver Sulfadiazine (1%) (Silvadene)	Silver Nitrate (0.5%)	Mafenide Acetate (Sulfamylon)
1. No acid–base complications; small systemic absorption	1. Causes hypochloremic *alkalosis*; depletes body of sodium and chloride through surface losses	1. Causes systemic *acidosis* due to carbonic anhydrase inhibitor; causes decreased bicarbonate reabsorption
2. Effective against gram-negative and gram-positive organisms; also against *Candida*	2. Most effective surface treatment in terms of antibacterial action	2. Effective against gram-negative and gram-positive organisms
3. Soothing when applied; keeps burn eschar soft, making debridement easier; easily removed before reapplication	3. Thick dressings necessary to minimize evaporative losses; dressings must be kept wet at all times, since drying strengthens the solution and will be toxic to new epithelium. Must keep child in high temperature, high humidity to prevent chilling through evaporative heat loss.	3. Painful on administration; discomfort may last 30 minutes to 1 hour. Adherence to burn wound makes daily removal of old preparation, before reapplication, painful.
4. Agent of choice for superficial to deep second-degree scald burns	4. Does not retard epithelialization	4. May delay eschar separation beneath the cream
5. No staining; no housekeeping problems	5. Black silver stains child, linen, floors, and clothing of those directly involved with care of child.	5. Easy to use; no housekeeping problems; no dressings required
	6. No sensitivity in 0.5% concentration	6. Some sensitivity reported

(Wieczorek RR, Natapoff J: A Conceptual Approach to the Nursing of Children: Health Care From Birth Through Adolescence. Philadelphia, JB Lippincott, 1981)

Treatment consists of a bland diet, the use of antacids and antispasmodics.

Nutritional needs.   The child who has received extensive deep burns must receive special attention regarding his nutritional needs. The nutritional problem is much more complex than simply getting a seriously ill child to eat. He is in negative caloric balance from a number of causes, including the following:

1. Poor intake, from anorexia, ileus, Curling's ulcer, or diarrhea.
2. External loss, due to exudative losses of protein through the burn wound.
3. Thermal losses from the burn itself; heat loss from the radiation of heat and from water loss, responsible for large caloric losses.
4. Hypermetabolism, from fever, infection, and from the state of "toxicity."

Hyperalimentation has been used for children with extensive burns to satisfy the 4,000 to 10,000 calorie daily requirement.[3]

A diet high in protein, for healing and for replacement, high in calories, and essentially bland in character, is an essential component of therapy. Great efforts must be made to interest the child in foods essential for tissue building and repair. Large servings are not acceptable because of anorexia as well as the physical condition of the child. Foods are going to be of no value if the child refuses to eat them. Colorful trays, foods with eye appeal, and any special touches to spur a child's appetite, should all be tried. A number of hints are suggested in the section on Care of the Child With Chronic Illness.

Some kinds of useful food are

Flavored milk shakes, ice cream shakes.
High protein drinks containing eggs and extra dried protein milk.
Ice cream, milk and egg desserts.
Pureed meats, and vegetables.

With the best efforts of nurses, dietitians, and of the child himself, the burn patient can seldom eat an amount of food sufficient to meet his increased needs. Tube feedings are frequently necessary as supplements to the daily intake. The dietary department can make up a supplementary formula that will meet the child's needs. Foods are liquified in a blender for tube feedings.

Great care must be used to avoid making tube feedings a threat. The child must understand what is to be done and why. If the nurse explains that the child needs extra food, more than he can eat by himself, to help his skin heal and make him strong, he is likely to be more cooperative. It is also helpful to demonstrate the tube feeding process with a doll.

Rehabilitation phase.   Occupational and physical therapy are frequently combined for the child in order to help maintain his normal functions, as well as to provide near normal situations for the child's continued growth and development.

One child's burns involved his chest, his axilla and his upper arm. It became essential for him to use his right arm in a variety of ways to prevent both contractures and permanent deformities, but Donny saw little sense in causing himself so much discomfort. Little by little, he was encouraged to use his arm for pushing along a wheeled toy, for coloring, for cutting pictures, and for similar activities. The real inspiration was the solitary fish in a small bowl. Bright yellow stones came in a bag for Donny to drop in, one by one, to provide a foundation, and every day he raised his arm to drop food into the bowl. Soon he became proud that he could feed his fish with his right hand, and willingly gave the fish loving care (Fig. 9–11).

INGESTION OF FOREIGN OBJECTS

Young children are very apt to put any objects small enough into their mouths. Unfortunately, these too often are swallowed. Normally, many of these will pass smoothly through the digestive tract and be expelled in the feces. Occasionally, however, somethings such as an open safety pin, nuts, or other objects may lodge in the esophagus and need to be extracted.

Unless symptoms of choking, gagging, or pain are present, it is usually safe to wait and watch the feces carefully for 3 or 4 days. Any object, however, may pass through the esophagus and stomach but become fixed in one of the

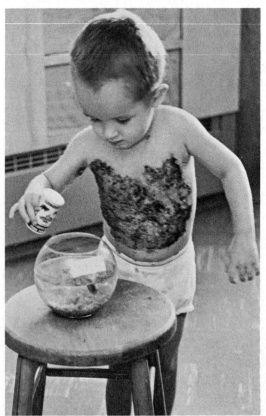

FIG. 9–11.   Feeding the fish is one way of motivating a child to move his right arm after chest and axillary burns.

curves of the intestine, causing an obstruction or fever due to infection. Also, sharp objects do present the danger of perforation somewhere within the digestive tract.

Diagnosis of a swallowed solid object may often, but not always, be made from the history. If a foreign object in the digestive tract is suspected, fluoroscopic and radiographic studies may be required.

TREATMENT

If a parent has seen the child swallow an object and begin choking, he should turn the child upside down and percuss his back. If this does not dislodge the object, the Heimlich maneuver can be attempted (Fig. 9–12). Lack of success with these measures means that the object will have to be removed by a physician. Objects in the esophagus are removed by direct vision through an esophagoscope. Attempts to push the object down into the stomach, or to extract it blindly can be dangerous. Some objects may need to be removed surgically.

Foreign objects aspirated into the larynx or bronchial tree may become lodged in the trachea or larynx. If it is not known that an object has been aspirated, the child may have choking or coughing spells without any realization that an object is causing the trouble, as edema at the site may prevent visualization of the object.

Adults should be made aware of the power of example. A child who sees an adult hold pins or nails in his mouth may quite well follow this example, with disastrous and often fatal results.

INSERTION OF FOREIGN BODIES INTO THE EAR OR NOSE

A child may insert small objects, such as peas or beans, crumpled paper, beads, or small toys, into his ear or nose. Irrigation of the ear may remove small objects, except paper, which will become impacted as it absorbs moisture. The physician generally uses small forceps to remove objects not dislodged by irrigation.

A foreign body in the nose may have been placed just inside the nares by the child, but manipulation may push it in further. If the object remains in the nose for any length of time, infection may occur. Inspection with a speculum and removal of the object by a physician should be done promptly when discovered.

child abuse

Maltreatment of children by their parents or caregivers has occurred for thousands of years. Growing concern for the rights of children in the United States has focused increased attention on this problem, resulting in laws passed for children's protection. Every state has laws that require health professionals to report child abuse and neglect. In 1974, The Child Abuse Prevention Act (PL 93-247) was signed into law, after which the National Center on Child Abuse and Neglect was established. This center has helped to promote research and education about child abuse, as well as offering crisis "hotlines" to assist high-risk children and families.

Despite all the efforts that have been made, child abuse

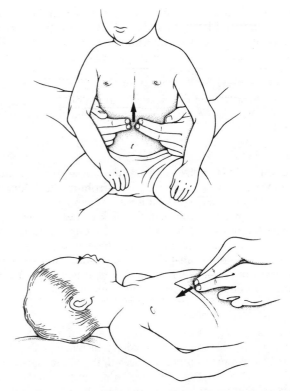

FIG. 9–12. Heimlich maneuver for infants and toddlers can be done either of two ways. (A) Place child in your lap, reach around and, with index and middle fingers of both hands place against abdomen, above naval and below rib cage, give quick upward thrust. (B) Position child face upward on a firm surface, face him, and deliver upward thrust with same fingers. (Adapted from Pinney M: Foreign body aspiration. Am J Nurs 81:521, 1981)

is increasing. More than 300,000 cases of abuse were reported in 1975, and approximately 2,000 deaths of suspicious origin occur annually. Various reasons are suggested for the increase in these tragic statistics: more cases are being reported; disappearance of the extended family leaves young parents feeling isolated; growing economic pressures place additional stress on parents, limiting their ability to cope.

BATTERED-CHILD SYNDROME

The term *battered child* was first used by C. Henry Kempe in 1961 to describe the increasing numbers of children being hospitalized with nonaccidental injuries: brain injuries, subdural hematomas, skull fractures, bruises, lacerations, burns, and fractures of the ribs and long bones. Most of these children are under the age of 3 years, and too young or too terrified to tell what really happened. Parents are vague about the "accident" that caused the child's injury. X-ray films of these children often reveal multiple fractures in various stages of healing.

Since Kempe's pioneering efforts to deal with the problem of child battering, other more subtle forms of abuse and neglect have gained attention. Though some children may show no signs of being physically battered, they ap-

Parents Anonymous +/or
Family Guidance center.

pear poorly nourished, physically neglected, and deprived of affection and love. This kind of abuse is not as easy to detect as battering, and, therefore, the children may suffer more because no one intervenes to change the situation.

TYPES OF ABUSE

Child abuse can be physical, sexual, emotional, or nutritional. Often more than one type is inflicted on a single child.

PHYSICAL ABUSE

When a child is brought to a physician or hospital because of physical injuries, parents may attribute the injury to some action of the child that is not in keeping with his age or ability. Bruises from being struck or beaten, head injuries, fractures and hematomas, cigarette burns on the body, burned hands that have been held on a hot stove, or even body burns from being immersed in a hot bath are common findings. When death occurs, it is usually due to subdural hematoma or intra-abdominal injuries.

SEXUAL ABUSE

In all ages and cultures, sexual abuse of children has existed but has seldom been admitted when it is perpetrated by parents or other relatives in the home. Estimates from the National Center on Child Abuse and Neglect indicate that incest (sexually arousing physical contact between family members not married to each other) occurs in 100,000 American families annually, and that number is growing each year. Like other forms of child abuse, sexual abuse is being recognized and reported more often.

This situation must be dealt with carefully for the child's sake to prevent further emotional trauma; yet, it can be difficult for the nurse caring for this child to deal with her own feelings of anger and disgust toward the abusing parent. Various community support groups have been established in California and other states to help families affected by child sexual abuse. One of the leading organizations in this effort is Parents United, with 46 chapters in 15 states. Information on local chapters can be obtained by writing Parents United, Box 952, San Jose, CA 95108. Counseling is available for victims and abusers, and some success has been achieved in helping both groups.

EMOTIONAL ABUSE

A child can be as seriously hurt by total emotional rejection as by physical battering. Indifference, deprivation of love, or total rejection can occur because the child does not fulfill the parents' expectations. A more drastic form of emotional trauma is that in which a child is locked in a cellar or closet when parents are away, isolated in one room for long periods of time, or abandoned in a strange place.

NUTRITIONAL ABUSE

Many children are underfed because of the mother's indifference or rejection, or because of her preoccupation with her own needs. Other parents deprive children of food or even water as punishment for some real or imagined misbehavior. Nutritional abuse can be due to lack of the right foods, or insufficient quantity of food.

THE ABUSED CHILD

Who are the abused children? Most of them are young, under 3 years of age. Often they have a problem—a behavior problem, a health problem, or something else that makes them fail to meet their parents' expectations. P.I. Tagg has identified several factors that increase the risk of child abuse and neglect. They are[4]

1. Low birth weight and prematurity
2. Unplanned or unwanted pregnancy
3. Parents with drug or alcohol addiction
4. Multiple births
5. Resemblance to a disliked person
6. Major birth defects
7. Parents who were abused as children

THE ABUSING PARENTS

Many studies have been done to try to discover why parents abuse their children; the conclusions differ. No consistent pattern, either cultural or ethnic, can be found. Child abuse occurs in affluent suburbia, in inner city ghettos, and all kinds of settings in between. Discovery is more likely in families from lower economic groups, however, because of their use of public clinics and emergency rooms, rather than private physicians.

Usually one or both of the parents of the abused child have long-standing emotional problems. Insecure parents look to the child for the love and comfort they have failed to find in their own lives, and become enraged when the young child does not respond.

Parents may expect the child to perform in areas beyond his ability, and when he fails to do so, he is punished. For example, parents may expect instant results when they begin toilet training a child, and punish the child when he fails to do as they wish. "He could do it if he wanted to; he is just being stubborn—or contrary—or lazy," is a frequently heard comment.

The actual abuse generally involves only one parent, but the other parent seldom reports the abuse. The nonabusive parent often collaborates to conceal the true state of affairs from authorities, fearing retaliation or loss of affection from the partner.

Child abuse is a vicious cycle; often abusive parents were abused children. As mentioned earlier, children learn to be parents when they are young by observing their own parents. These parents need help, but often do not know how or where to seek it. Some of the most effective help comes from community support groups such as Parents Anonymous, chapters of which exist in many cities across the country. Many of these groups are made up of parents who have faced this problem and conquered it, putting them in a better position to help without being judgmental. Crisis hot lines are available in many cities to offer advice and help to parents.

NURSING CARE

INTERVIEWING THE PARENTS

Before a nurse can work effectively with an abused child and his family, she needs to understand that child abuse is a symptom of family dysfunction, a problem that can often be dealt with effectively. It is also important that she try to be nonjudgmental and accepting of the parents, realizing that a punitive or rejecting attitude will not achieve beneficial results.

Although the usual goal in care of a hospitalized child is to restore health and return the child to his family, this is not always possible with abused children. In some cases, the child must be removed from the family temporarily or even permanently.

Tactful questioning of the parents about the child's habits and lifestyle is necessary to gain sufficient information to care for him effectively. Parents may be very uncertain and uneasy about their reception in the hospital, particularly if they have already been questioned by police, social workers, or others. It is important to reduce their anxiety by a nonjudgmental attitude before trying to question them.

CARE OF THE CHILD

Consistent nursing care, involving the least possible change in caregivers, is critically important to the welfare of the abused child. He is likely to view all adults with suspicion as potential punishers. Abused children need to re-establish their sense of trust, and the nurse can be a key figure in making that happen (Fig. 9–13).

The abused child needs to learn that the hospital is a safe place and that the care and treatment procedures will make him feel better, even though some of them may be

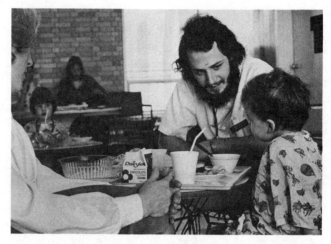

FIG. 9–13.   Honest discussions with the abused child help him rebuild his sense of trust and show him that the hospital is a safe place. (Reprinted with permission from the cover of J Nurs Educ, 17 No. 4, April, 1978)

painful. Honest explanations before performing examinations or painful procedures will help to establish trust. Providing support and reassurance during the stressful time, with loving care and cuddling before and after, can further strengthen the child's trust.

Treating the child's physical injuries, and meeting his emotional needs, are only symptomatic relief. The major treatment effort must be directed at the parents, and usually requires a team approach with social worker, mental health worker, community health nurse, and a self-help support group cooperating to help these troubled families break out of the vicious cycle of child abuse.

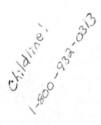

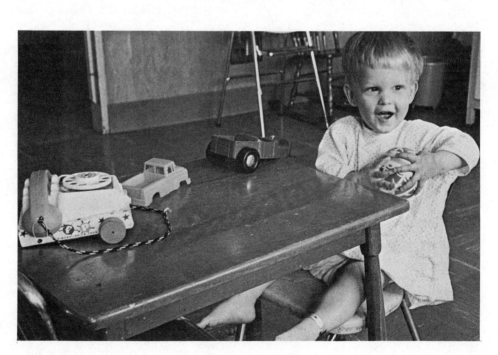

FIG. 9–14.   At 18 months of age even the hospital can be fun.

summary

The curious toddler ventures into a world full of hazards, protected only by the attention of caring adults. When accidents happen, or illness occurs, the toddler shows remarkable powers of recovery if proper care and treatment are given. Hospitalization can be a serious interruption in the toddler's growth and development, but competent, loving care can help make it a learning experience that is even fun at times (Fig. 9– 14).

review questions

1. What are the characteristics of autism?
2. What are cataracts?
3. What is an external hordeolum?
4. What metabolic defect occurs in idiopathic celiac disease?
5. What measures can the parents take in the home to relieve the laryngospasm that occurs with croup?
6. What should the nurse observe concerning respirations in children?
7. What organs are affected in cystic fibrosis?
8. Describe the appearance of a child with cystic fibrosis.
9. What diagnostic test confirms cystic fibrosis?
10. Describe the diet for cystic fibrosis.
11. Describe the pulmonary treatments for cystic fibrosis.
12. What response does syrup of ipecac produce?
13. Explain the emergency treatment for the ingestion of poisons and drugs?
14. How is lead poisoning treated?
15. Describe and differentiate between the different types of burns.
16. What is the emergency treatment for burns?
17. Define eschar.
18. Describe the nutritional needs following extensive burns.
19. Describe the different types of child abuse.
20. What factors increase the risk of child abuse and neglect?
21. How does the nurse approach the abused child? The abusing parent?

references

1. Larter N: Cystic fibrosis. Am J Nurs 81:527– 532, 1981
2. Herrin JT, Crawford JD: The seriously burned child. In Smith CA (ed): The Critically Ill Child: Diagnosis and Management. Philadelphia, WB Saunders, 1977
3. Pinney, M. Foreign body aspiration. AJN 81:522– 523, 1981
4. Borgen L: Total parenteral nutrition in adults. Am J Nurs 78:224– 228, 1978
5. Tagg PI: Nursing intervention for the abused child and his family. Pediatr Nurs 1, No. 5:36– 39, 1976

bibliography

Beckemeyer P, Bahr JE: Helping toddlers and preschoolers cope while suturing their minor lacerations. Am J Mat Child Nurs 5:326– 330, 1980

Campbell L: Special behavior problems of the burned child. Am J Nurs 76:220– 224, 1976

Croft H, Frenkel S: Children and lead poisoning. Am J Nurs 75:102– 104, 1975

Cystic Fibrosis Foundation, Rockville, Md

Czajka PA: Poisoning Emergencies: A Guide for Emergency Personnel. St Louis, CV Mosby, 1980

Dyer C: Burn care in the emergent period. J Emerg Nurs 6, No. 1:9– 16, 1980

Delacato CH: The Ultimate Stranger: The Autistic Child. Garden City, Doubleday, 1974

Evans M, Hansen B: Guide to Pediatric Nursing: A Clinical Reference. New York, Appleton-Century-Crofts, 1980

Harris M: Understanding the autistic child. Am J Nurs 78:1682– 1685, 1978

Johnson MP: Self-instruction for the family of a child with cystic fibrosis. Am J Mat Child Nurs 5:345– 348, 1980

Jones CA, Feller I: Burns: What to do during the first crucial hours. Nurs '77:23– 30, March, 1977

Killion SW, McCarthy SM: Hospitalization of the autistic child, parts I and II. Am J Mat Child Nurs 5:412– 423, 1980

Larter N: Cystic fibrosis. Am J Nurs 81:527– 532, 1981

Lybarger PM: Accidental poisoning in childhood: An ongoing problem. Issues Comp Pediatr Nurs 1, No. 6:30– 39, May 1977

Mennear JH: The poisoning emergency. Am J Nurs 77:842– 844, 1977

Neill K, Kauffman C: Care of the hospitalized abused child and his family: Nursing implications. Am J Mat Child Nurs 1:117– 123, 1976

Rush F: The Best-kept Secret: Sexual Abuse of Children. Englewood Cliffs, Prentice-Hall, 1980

Schmitt BD, Kempe CH: Child abuse and neglect. In Smith D (ed): Introduction to Clinical Pediatrics. Philadelphia, WB Saunders, 1977

Wagner MM: Emergency care of the burned patient. Am J Nurs 77:1788– 1791, 1977

Ward AJ: Childhood Autism and Structural Therapy. Chicago, Nelson Hall, 1976

growth and development of the preschool child: 3 years to 6 years

10

physical development
growth rate
facial growth and dentition
visual development
skeletal growth
nutrition
health maintenance
prevention of accidents
prevention of infection
psychosocial development
language development
development of imagination
sexual development
social development
implications for hospital care
summary
review questions
references
bibliography

student objectives

The student successfully attaining the goals of this chapter will be able to

1 Define the following vocabulary terms:

   associative play   castration   cooperative play   magical thinking
   masturbation   noncommunicative language   parallel play

2 Describe the growth and development of the preschool-age child in the following areas:
   personal–social development, fine motor skills, gross motor skills, language development,
   and cognition.

3 Discuss the dietary needs of the preschool-age child.

4 List eight precautions that the preschooler can be taught that can help prevent the spread of
   infection.

5 Describe six types of play common to the preschooler.

6 Describe three measures the nurse may take that can help to reduce the anxiety a preschooler
   may experience in the hospital.

Preschoolers are fascinating creatures. As their social circle enlarges to include peers and adults outside of the family, their language, play patterns, and appearance change markedly. Their curiosity about the world around them grows as does their ability to explore the world in greater detail and see new meanings in what they find (Fig. 10–1). "Why?" and "how?" are favorite words. This curiosity also means that accidents are still a serious concern.

Although he is a chubby, baby-faced toddler on his third birthday, by age 5 the child has developed into a leaner, taller, better coordinated social being (Fig. 10–2). He begins to enjoy being industrious, "making things," and telling everyone about it. Although he has some problem with separating fantasy from reality, he continues to explore and learn.

physical development

GROWTH RATE

The preschool period is one of slow growth. The child grows about 3 pounds to 5 pounds each year (1.8 kg) and grows about 2½ inches (6.3 cm) taller. Because the increase in height is proportionately greater than the increase in weight, the 5-year-old appears much thinner and less babyish than the 3-year-old. Boys tend to be leaner than girls during this time.

Gross motor and fine motor skills continue to develop rapidly. Balance improves and with that improvement the confidence to try new activities emerges. By age 5 the child is generally able to throw and catch a ball well, to climb effectively, and ride a bicycle. Important milestones for growth and development are summarized in Table 10–1.

FACIAL GROWTH AND DENTITION

By the time a child is 6 years of age, his skull is 90% of its adult size. Facial growth is downward and forward, so that the nose, chin, and jaw assume more adultlike proportions.

The deciduous teeth that emerged in late infancy and toddlerhood have begun to be replaced by permanent dentition. Pictures of smiling 5-year-olds and 6-year-olds typically show missing front teeth (Fig. 10–3).

The age at which teeth erupt varies with individual children, and with various ethnic and economic groups. Permanent teeth of American children of African ancestry erupt at least 6 months earlier than those of American children with European backgrounds. Teeth emerge sooner in children of higher economic backgrounds, and girls' dentition progresses faster than boys'.

VISUAL DEVELOPMENT

Although the preschooler's senses of taste and smell are acute, visual development is still immature at age 3. Eye–hand coordination is good, but judgment of distances generally is faulty, leading to many bumps and falls. Usually by age 6 the child has achieved 20/20 vision, but mature depth perception may not occur in some children until 8 to 10 years of age.

SKELETAL GROWTH

Between the third and sixth birthdays, the greatest amount of skeletal growth occurs in the feet and legs, another reason for the more slender appearance of the 6-year-old. In addition, the carpals and tarsals mature in the hands and feet, contributing to better hand and foot control.

nutrition

Because the preschool period is not a time of rapid growth, children do not need large quantities of food. Their appetites are erratic, however; one time they will devour everything on their plate, and the next time, be satisfied with just a few bites. Depending on their energy output, they may need to have meals supplemented with nutritious snacks, such as those listed in the boxed material on this page. Frequent, small meals with snacks in between are generally the best accepted by the preschooler.

Among the preschooler's favorites are sweets, soft foods, grain and dairy products, and raw vegetables. Television commercials for sugar-coated cereals, snacks, and fast-foods of questionable nutritional value exert a powerful influence on the preschooler, and can make supermarket shopping an emotional struggle between parent and child. Parents should read labels carefully before making a purchase.

Preschoolers need guidance in choosing foods, and are strongly influenced by the example of siblings, parents, and peers. Food should never be used as a reward or bribe; otherwise the child will continue to use food as a means to manipulate his environment and the behavior of others.

In order to meet the minimum daily requirements (Table 10–2), the preschooler should have 2 to 3 glasses of

---

Raw vegetables: such as carrots,* cucumbers, celery,* green beans, green pepper, mushrooms, turnips, broccoli, cauliflower, tomatoes
Fresh fruits: such as apples, oranges, pears, peaches, grapes,* cherries,* melons
Unsalted whole grain crackers
Whole grain bread: cut to finger-sized sticks; plain, toasted, or with peanut butter
Small sandwiches
Natural cheese: cut in cubes

Cooked meat: cut in small chunks or sliced thinly
*Nuts**
*Sunflower seeds**
Cookies: made with lightly sweetened whole grains
*Plain popped corn**
Yogurt: plain or with fresh fruit added

* Children under 2 years may choke on nuts, seeds, popcorn, celery strings, or carrot sticks. It is best to avoid offering these foods until the preschool years.

milk each day, and several small portions from each food group.

The preschooler shows growing independence and skill in eating. The 3-year-old tries to mimic adult behavior at the table but often reverts to eating with fingers, spilling liquids, and squirming. The 4-year-old is more skilled with the use of utensils, but sometimes misjudges his abilities and makes a mess. The 5-year-old uses utensils well, even cutting his own food, and can be taught to observe rather sophisticated table manners.

health maintenance

Preschoolers with up-to-date immunization schedules do not need boosters until age 6, but an annual health examination is recommended to monitor the child's growth and development and to screen for potential health problems. Children who attend nursery school or a daycare program are required to have an annual examination, but children who stay at home may not have this advantage. Particular attention should be paid to the child's vision and hearing, so that any problems can be treated before he enters school at age 6 (Table 10–3).

PREVENTION OF ACCIDENTS

Parents and caregivers of preschoolers need to be just as attentive as with toddlers, because a child's curiosity at this stage exceeds his judgment. Burns, poisoning, and falls are common accidents. Preschoolers are often victims of motor vehicle accidents, either because of darting into the street or driveway, or as passengers without proper restraints. Children should ride in the back seat of a car. If they weigh less than 50 pounds, a seat or harness for children should be used. Children who weigh 50 pounds or more should be restrained with adult seat belts, but *not* with the shoulder strap, because of the danger of strangulation.

PREVENTION OF INFECTION

Preschoolers who enjoy sound nutrition, adequate rest, exercise, and shelter, are not seriously affected by simple childhood infections. Less fortunate children, however, can be severely threatened even by a simple illness such as diarrhea or measles. Immunizations are available for many childhood communicable diseases; yet, some parents do not see that their children are immunized until it is required for entrance to school. As a result, some children suffer unnecessary illnesses.

Preschoolers are just learning to share, and that can mean sharing infections with the entire family. Teaching them the following basic precautions can help prevent spreading infections:[1]

- Cover the mouth when coughing or sneezing.
- Discard tissues used for blowing nose.
- Wipe well after bowel movements (girls should be taught to wipe from front to back to avoid urinary tract infections).
- Wash hands after toileting or blowing nose.
- Do not share partially eaten food.

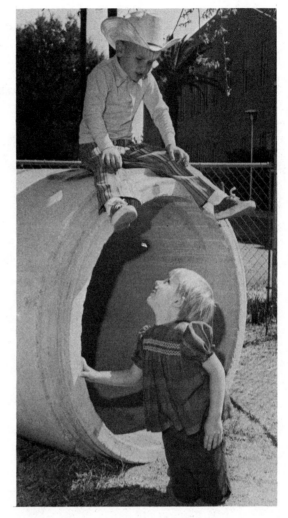

FIG. 10–1.   The preschool child has developed a sense of daring. (Photo by Carol Baldwin)

- Wash hands before eating.
- Wash dropped food or utensils.
- Do not drink from another person's cup.
- Do not share toothbrushes with others.

psychosocial development

LANGUAGE DEVELOPMENT

Between the ages of 3 and 5, language development is generally rapid. Most 3-year-olds can construct simple sentences, but they have many hesitations and repetitions as they search for the right word or try to make the right sound. Stuttering can develop during this period, but usually disappears within 3 to 6 months. By the end of the fifth year, preschoolers use long, rather complex sentences; their vocabulary has increased by more than 1500 words since age 2.

Preschoolers' use of language changes during this period. Three-year-olds often talk to themselves, to their toys or

TABLE 10–1.   GROWTH AND DEVELOPMENT CHART: THE PRESCHOOLER

Age (years)	Personal/Social	Fine Motor	Gross Motor	Language	Cognition
3	Begins Erikson's stage of "initiative vs guilt." It is at this time that conscience develops. Shy with strangers and inept with peers Sufficiently independent to be interested in group experiences with age mates (*i.e.,* nursery school)	Able to button clothes Copies ○ and + Uses pencils, crayons, paints Shows preference for right or left hand	Tends to watch motor activities before attempting them A jump from several feet is possible. Uses hands in broad movements Rides tricycle Negotiates stairs well	Vocabulary up to 1000 words Articulates all vowels accurately Talks a lot Sings and recites Asks many questions	Continues in pre-operational stage (2–7) characterized by: 1. *Centration* or the inability to attend to more than one aspect of a situation 2. *Egocentricity* or the inability to consider the perceptions of others 3. The static and irreversible quality of thought that makes the child unable to perceive the processes of change
4	Boisterous and inflammatory Aggressive physically and verbally but developing behaviors to become socially acceptable Becomes socially acceptable Accepts punishment for wrongdoings because it relieves guilt	Can use scissors; copies a square Adds three parts to stick figures	Has some hesitations but tends to try feats beyond ability Greater powers of balance and accuracy Hops on one foot; can control movements of hands	Vocabulary of about 1500 words Constant questions Sentences of 4–5 words Uses profanity Reports fantasies as truth	Reality and fantasy are not always clear to the preschooler Believes that words make things real—"magical" thinking
5	Initiates contacts with strangers and relates interesting vignettes Interested in telling and comparing stories about self Peer relations are important ("best friends" abound) Responds to social values by assuming sex roles with rigidity	Ties shoelaces Copies a diamond and a triangle Prints a few letters or numbers May print first name Cuts food	Will not attempt feats beyond ability Throws and catches ball well Jumps rope Walks backward with heel to toe Skips and hops Adept on bicycle and climbing equipment	Vocabulary of 3000 words 90% of speech is intelligible Asks meanings of words Enjoys telling stories	Thinks feelings and thoughts can happen Intrusions into the body cause fear and anxiety (fear of mutilation and castration)

pets, without any apparent purpose other than the pleasure of using words. Piaget called this egocentric or *noncommunicative* language. By age 4, children increase their use of communicative language, using words to transmit information other than their own needs and feelings. Development of preschoolers' verbal abilities is summarized in Table 10–4.

Delays or other difficulties in language development may be caused by one or more of the following:

- Hearing impairment or other physical problem
- Lack of stimulation
- Overprotection
- Lack of parental interest or rejection by parents

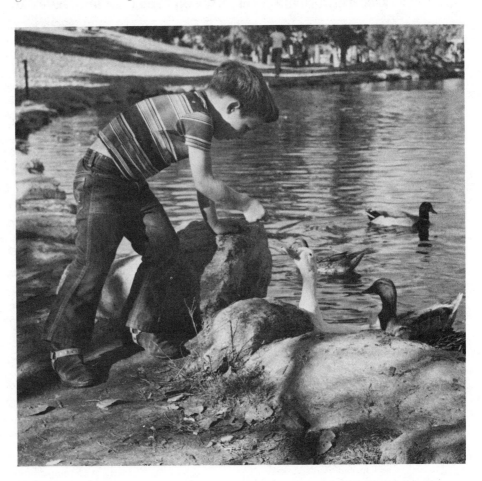

FIG. 10–2. A five-year-old enjoys feeding the ducks, but should not be left alone near the water. (Photo by Sylvia Mae Reeves)

TABLE 10–2.   RDA FOR PRESCHOOLERS

	1–3 Years (13 kg)	4–6 Years
Energy (kcal)	1300	1700
Protein (g)	23	30
Vitamin A (RE)	400	500
Vitamin D (mcg)	10	10
Vitamin E (mg α-TE)	5	6
Ascorbic acid (mg)	45	45
Folacin (mcg)	100	200
Niacin (mg)	9	11
Riboflavin (mg)	0.8	1.0
Thiamin (mg)	0.7	0.9
Vitamin B_6 (mg)	0.9	1.3
Vitamin B_{12} (mcg)	2.0	2.5
Calcium (mg)	800	800
Phosphorus (mg)	800	800
Iodine (mcg)	70	90
Iron (mg)	15	10
Magnesium (mg)	150	200
Zinc (mg)	10	10

(Food and Nutrition Board Recommended Dietary Allowances. Washington, DC, National Academy of Sciences/National Research Council, 1980)

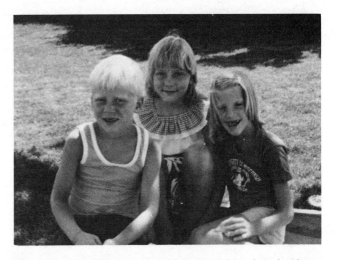

FIG. 10–3.   Five- and six-year-olds begin to lose their deciduous teeth. (Compliments of E Lundeen; Wieczorek RR, Natapoff J: A Conceptual Approach to the Nursing of Children: Health Care From Birth Through Adolescence. Philadelphia, JB Lippincott, 1981

TABLE 10-3. RECOMMENDED HEALTH MAINTENANCE FOR PRESCHOOLERS BY AGE

	36 Months (3 Years)	48 Months (4 Years)	60 Months (5 Years)	72 Months (6 Years)
Examinations *Immunizations*	Full physical examination First dental examination Bring up to date Tine	Full physical examination Dental examination Tine	Full physical examination Dental examination Tine	Full physical examination Dental examination Tine DPT booster OPV booster

Screening Procedures	Urinalysis
	Hematocrit
	Lead level (if indicated)
	Blood pressure
	Attempt vision
	  assessment
	Attempt hearing
	  assessment
	Denver Developmental
	  Screening Test
		Same as for 36 months	Same as for 36 months	Same as for 36 months
				(Omit lead unless
				indicated.)

TABLE 10-4. VERBAL ABILITIES OF PRESCHOOLERS

Age	Characteristics of Language Usage	Expected Language Comprehension	Expected Correct Speech Articulation	Language Rhythm
3-4 years	Enjoys talking and talks a lot. Makes up words or may sing or recite own version of a song or rhyme. Enjoys new and special words. Asks many questions and demands an answer. Sentences and concepts are not always logical. Comforts others with words. Vocabulary of 900-1000 words. Uses 4- to 5-word phrases. Aggression is displayed with words rather than physical force.	3 years—up to 3600 words 4 years—up to 5600 words	3½ years—all vowels and p, m, and b sounds 4 years—speech is 100% intelligible, even though misarticulations may occur.	3-5 year-olds may have many hesitations, repetitions, and revisions in an effort to produce adult speech. Stuttering may begin during this time. It disappears within 3-6 months but may continue as long as 2 years without permanent stuttering occurring.
4-5 years	Understands words outside of their usual context. Has difficulty finding the right word. Speech has high emotional content. Tells functions of things rather than names. Changes the subject rapidly. Boasts, brags, and quarrels. Fascinated with naughty words. Reports fantasies as truth. 90% of speech is intelligible. Uses complex phrase units. Vocabulary consists of 3000 words.	5 years—up to 9600 words	5½ years—f, v, y, th, l, and wh sounds	
5-6 years	Consistent use of pronouns and other parts of speech. Enjoys telling stories. Uses expressions such as "I forgot . . ." "I think . . . ."	6 years—up to 15,000 words	6½ years—r, s, z, ch, j, sh, and zh sounds	

(Data from Weiss CE, Lillywhite HS: Communicative Disorders: A Handbook for Prevention and Early Intervention. St Louis, CV Mosby, 1976; and McElroy CW: Speech and Language Development of the Preschool Child, pp 179-185. Springfield, Ill, Charles C Thomas, 1976)

The child who is not spoken to is unlikely to have adequate language skills. He must hear and understand words to learn to use them correctly. His attempts need to be praised, approved, and encouraged.

Family and cultural patterns also influence language development. Some children come from bilingual families and are trying to learn the rules of both languages. Others may come from geographic or social communities that have dialects quite different from the general population.

DEVELOPMENT OF IMAGINATION

Preschoolers have learned to think about something without actually seeing it—to visualize or imagine. This normal development, sometimes called *magical thinking*, makes it difficult for them to separate fantasy from reality. They believe that words or thoughts can make things real, and this can have positive and negative results. If, in a moment of anger, a child wishes that a parent or a sibling would die, and that person later is hurt, the child feels guilty as though he had made it happen. He needs reassurance that this is not so.

Imagination makes preschoolers good audiences for storytelling, simple plays, and television, as long as the characters and events are not too frightening or sad. When preschoolers see a television character die, they believe it is real and often cry.

During this stage, children often have imaginary playmates, who are very real to them. This occurs particularly with only children, probably because they desperately wish they had someone to play with. Parents need assurance that this is normal.

Dreams and nightmares are common during the preschool period. Parents need to explain that "it was only a dream" and offer love and understanding until the fear has subsided. Fear of the dark is another common problem during these years.

SEXUAL DEVELOPMENT

This is the stage that Freud termed the Oedipal or phallic (genital) period. During these years, children become acutely aware of their sexuality, including sexual roles and organs. They generally develop a strong emotional attachment to the parent of the opposite sex. Curiosity about their own genitals and those of peers and adults may make parents uncomfortable, and evoke responses that indicate that sex is dirty and something to be ashamed and guilty about.

This new sexual awareness creates fears of bodily mutilation. Boys fear *castration*, which is why circumcision delayed until this time can cause a severe emotional reaction. Girls discover that they do not have a penis and think perhaps something is "unfinished;" this has been called *penis envy.*

Despite today's abundance of sexually oriented literature, many parents find it difficult to deal with the questions and actions of the young child. Nurses can help parents understand that the child's sexual curiosity is a normal, natural part of his total curiosity about himself and the world around him. The informed, understanding parent can help children develop positive attitudes toward sexuality and toward themselves as sexual human beings.

MASTURBATION

It is as natural for the preschooler to explore his genitals and experience the resulting sensations, just as it is normal for an infant to suck his thumb. This is one way the child learns to perceive his body as a possible source of pleasure, and the beginning of acceptance of sex as natural and pleasurable.

Parents do have an obligation to teach their children that masturbation is private and not appropriate in public. Every child needs to learn that certain behaviors are not socially acceptable.

SOCIAL DEVELOPMENT

PLAY

Play activities are one way that children learn. Normally by age 3, children begin imitative play, pretending to be the mommy, the daddy, a policeman, a cowboy, an astronaut, or some well-known person (Fig. 10–4). Parents can gain good insight into the way their child interprets parental behavior by watching the child play. Listening to a preschooler scold a doll or stuffed animal for "bothering me while I'm busy talking on the telephone" lets parents hear how they sound to the child.

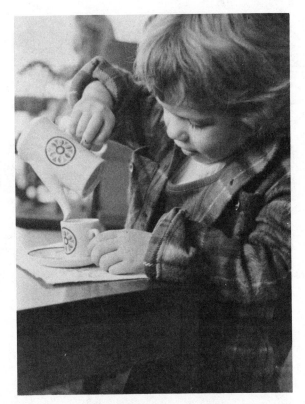

FIG. 10–4. A preschooler playing tea-party. (Compliments of E Lundeen; Wieczorek RR: Natapoff J: A Conceptual Approach to the Nursing of Children: Health Care From Birth Through Adolescence. Philadelphia, JB Lippincott, 1981

Dramatic play allows a child to act out troubling situations and to control the final solution to the problem. This is important in teaching children who are going to be hospitalized, perhaps for surgery. Use of dolls and puppets to explain procedures makes the experience less threatening.

Drawing is another form of play through which children learn to express themselves. During the preschool years, as fine motor skills improve, children's drawings become much more complex and controlled, and can be very revealing about the child's self-concept and perception of his environment (Fig. 10–5).

Preschoolers engage in various types of play: cooperative, associative, parallel, solitary independent, onlooker play, and unoccupied behavior.[2]

In *cooperative* play, children play *with* each other, as in team sports. *Associative* play means being engaged in a common activity, but without any sense of belonging. In *parallel* play, children play alongside each other, but independently. Although common among toddlers, parallel play exists in all age groups, for example, in a Scout troop where each member is working on an individual project or craft. *Solitary independent* play means playing apart from others without making an effort to be part of the group or their activity. Watching television is one form of *onlooker* play, in which there is an interest in observation without participation. In *unoccupied behavior*, the child may be daydreaming, fingering his clothes or a toy, without apparent purpose.

Children need all types of play to aid in their total development. Too much of one kind may signal a problem;

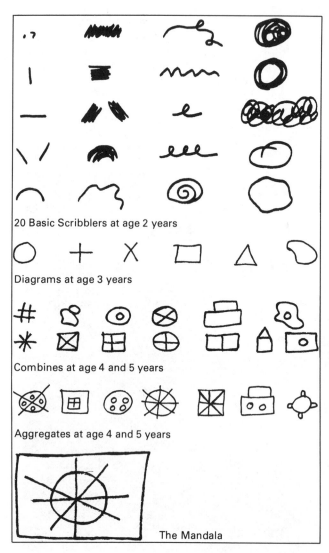

20 Basic Scribblers at age 2 years

Diagrams at age 3 years

Combines at age 4 and 5 years

Aggregates at age 4 and 5 years

The Mandala

FIG. 10–5. Components of children's drawings. (Kellogg R: Stages of development of preschool art. In Lewis HP (ed): Child Art—The Beginning of Self-affirmation. Berkeley, Diablo Press, 1966. Permission granted by Diablo Press, Inc., P.O. Box 7042, Berkeley, CA 94707. Copyright 1973 Diablo Press, Inc.)

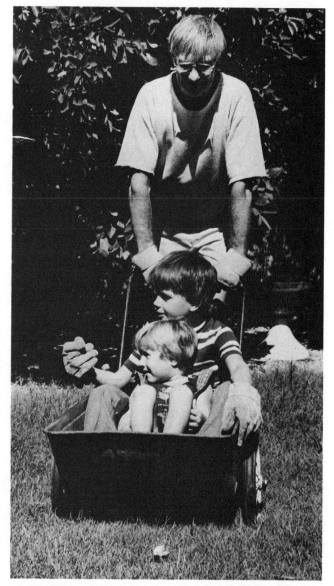

FIG. 10–6. This preschooler enjoys having his grandfather take him and his brother for a wheelbarrow ride. (Photo by Elizabeth McKinney Chmiel)

for example, a youngster who spends a great deal of time in unoccupied behavior may be troubled, depressed, or unstimulated. Cooperative play helps to develop social interaction skills, and often physical health as well.

Too much onlooker play, particularly television viewing, means that children are missing the benefits of other kinds of play, and may be forming strong, highly inaccurate impressions of people and their behaviors. Preschoolers watch an average of 54 hours of television per week, and are greatly influenced by television's portrayal of occupational, ethnic, behavioral, and sexual role stereotypes.[3]

AGGRESSION

Temper tantrums are an early form of aggression. The preschooler with his newly developed language skills uses words aggressively in name-calling and threats. Four-year-olds use physical aggression as well, pushing, hitting, and kicking, in an effort to manipulate the environment. The parents' task during these years is to help the child understand that the anger and frustration that result in aggressive behavior are normal, but need to be handled differently because aggressive behavior is not socially acceptable.

Children who come from unhappy home situations are likely to be more aggressive than those from a comfortable family situation. Their parents have served as role models and their aggressive behavior toward each other has said to the child, "this is acceptable."

DISCIPLINE

It is important for parents to remember that preschoolers are developing initiative, and a sense of guilt. They want
*and
inner control*

TABLE 10–5. METHODS OF DEVELOPING REPRESSION OF SOCIALLY UNACCEPTABLE BEHAVIORS

Method	Effect on Child	Effect upon Adult
Attending only to desired behaviors Calm reasoning with expression of dislike of behavior Physical restraint with adult present Isolation of child for a period of time Withholding of desired treats, excursions, presents Shaming in a calm manner	Development of inner control	Feelings of adequacy as parents
Yelling, screaming, and implying guilt and punishment Telling child he is bad Physical punishment	Development of fears and compulsive behaviors	Feelings of guilt and inadequacy
Giving treats, presents, or food for desired behavior Giving treats, presents, or food for lack of undesired behavior Physical punishment Threatening punishment from God	Development of control based upon external forces	Feelings of being manipulated by child

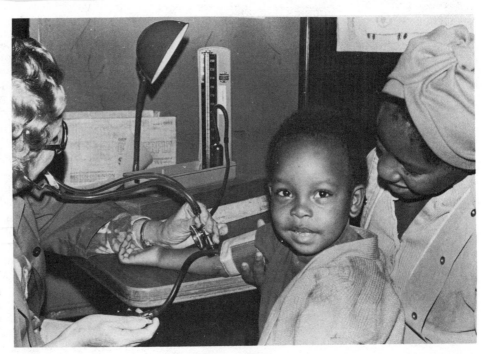

FIG. 10–7. If parents talk with preschoolers about hospitalization as an interesting adventure, it's less likely to seem frightening. (J Nurs Care, January, 1979)

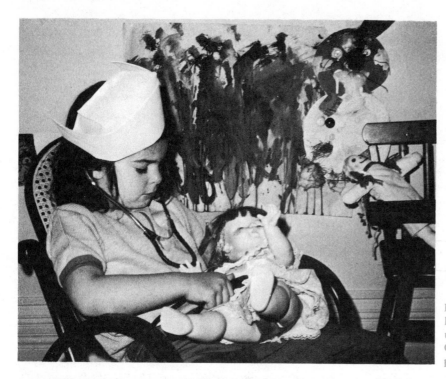

FIG. 10–8.   Using the stethoscope to listen to her doll's heart helps this preschooler to be unafraid. (Petrillo M: Sanger S: Emotional Care of Hospitalized Children, 2nd ed. Lippincott, 1980)

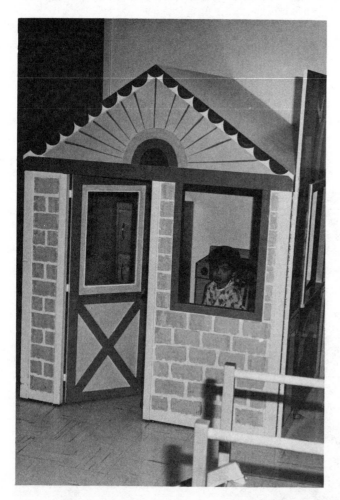

FIG. 10–9.   Five-year-old in the playhouse.

to be good and follow instructions, and they feel bad when they do not, even though they are not physically punished. Discipline during this time should strive to teach the child a sense of responsibility and inner control. Spanking and other forms of physical punishment remove the responsibility from the child. Taking away a privilege from a child who has misbehaved until he can demonstrate that his behavior has improved is much more effective. Since the child's concept of time is not clear, the time period should be comparatively brief (Table 10–5).

NURSERY SCHOOL OR OTHER DAYCARE FACILITY

Group experiences with peers and adults outside the immediate family are important to a child's development (Fig. 10–6). The transition to new experiences, new people, and new surroundings can be threatening to some preschoolers. Children vary in their willingness or ability to handle new situations, but being introduced gradually, according to individual readiness produces the most satisfactory adjustment. Some children spend only a few hours each week in a nursery school or other daycare program; others, because both parents work outside the home, must spend a great deal more time away from home and family. Parents should understand that this probably means the child will demand more of their attention during the hours when they are together. As the child grows older and the attachment to his own friends becomes stronger, parents will sense a decrease in the need for parental attention and a greater sense of independence in the child.

IMPLICATIONS FOR HOSPITAL CARE

The preschooler may look on hospitalization as an exciting new adventure or a frightening, dangerous experience, depending on how he has been prepared by parents and

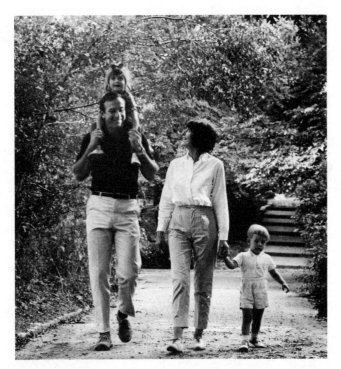

health professions (Fig. 10–7). As mentioned earlier, play is an effective way to let children act out their anxiety, and to learn what to expect from the hospital situation. Preschoolers are frightened about intrusive procedures; therefore, it is usually preferable to take the temperature orally. Children are less anxious about procedures if they are allowed to handle equipment beforehand, and perhaps "use" it on a doll or another toy (Fig. 10–8).

The hospitalized preschooler may revert to bedwetting and should not be scolded for it. The nurse should assure parents that this is normal. Explanations of where the bathrooms are and how to use the call light or bell to get help can help avoid problems with bedwetting. If a child is afraid of the dark, a night light can be provided.

Hospital routines should follow home routines as closely as possible. The child should be allowed to participate in his own care, even though this may take longer. All procedures should be carefully explained to the child in words that he understands, repeating if necessary.

If the child is ambulatory, he can be taken to the playroom (Fig. 10–9). If not, play materials can be provided for use in bed.

summary

Preschoolers can be delightful, yet frustrating to their parents and caregivers. Endless questions, boundless energy, and an ongoing struggle to separate fantasy from reality, make this small person stimulating to be with (Fig. 10–10). Parents and caregivers need to set limits within which the child can be free to explore and learn, and assert autonomy and initiative. They also need to serve as models for the kind of person they want the child to become, helping to build confidence and self-esteem that will make easier the child's entrance into school and participation in a continually enlarging world.

review questions

1. Describe the fine motor skills of the preschooler.
2. Describe the verbal ability of the preschooler.
3. Which immunizations are recommended for the preschooler?
4. What are the guidelines for helping children learn about food?
5. How do you help prevent accidents with preschoolers?
6. How should the parent deal with the child who masturbates?
7. What are the various types of play?
8. Why is regression normal for a hospitalized preschooler?

references

1. Wieczorek RR, Natapoff J: A Conceptual Approach to the Nursing of Children: Health Care From Birth Through Adolescence. Philadelphia, JB Lippincott, 1981
2. Whaley L, Wong D: Nursing Care of Infants and Children. St Louis, CV Mosby, 1979
3. Larrick N: A Parent's Guide to Children's Reading. Garden City, Doubleday, 1975

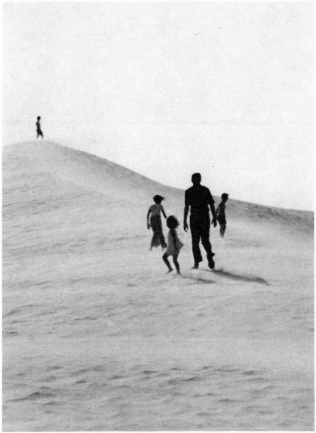

FIG. 10–10. Preschoolers and their parents can have good times together just walking, talking, and looking. (Compliments of F Duval; Wieczorek RR, Natapoff J: A Conceptual Approach to the Nursing of Children: Health Care From Birth Through Adolescence. Philadelphia, JB Lippincott, 1981)

bibliography

Carmichael C: Non-sexist Childraising. Boston, Beacon Press, 1977

Craig GJ: Human Development. Englewood Cliffs, Prentice-Hall, 1976

DeLeo JH: Child Development: Analysis and Synthesis. New York, Brunner Mazel, 1977

Heagerty M, Grass G, King H: Sex and the preschool child. Am J Nurs 74, 1479–1482, 1974

Hoekelman RA: The pediatric physical examination, In Bates B: A Guide to Physical Examination, 2nd ed. Philadelphia, JB Lippincott, 1979

Johnson JE, Kirchhoff KT, Endress MP: Easing children's fright during health care procedures. Am J Mat Child Nurs 1:206–211, 1976

Marion M: Guidance of Young Children. St. Louis, CV Mosby, 1981

McClinton BS, Meier BG: Beginnings: The Psychology of Early Childhood. St Louis, CV Mosby, 1978

Petrillo M, Sanger S: Emotional Care of Hospitalized Children, 2nd ed. Philadelphia, JB Lippincott, 1980

Pipes P: Nutrition in Infancy and Childhood, 2nd ed. St Louis, CV Mosby, 1981

Pomeroy W: Your Child and Sex: A Guide for Parents. New York, Delacorte, 1974

Stewart AC: Child Care in the Family. New York, Academic Press, 1977

Suitor CW, Hunter MF: Nutrition: Principles and Application in Health Promotion. Philadelphia, JB Lippincott, 1980

Taylor DC: The assessment of visual function in young children: An overview. Clin pediatr 17:226–232, 1978

Thomas A, Chess S: Temperament and development. New York, Brunner Mazel, 1977

Valett RE: Developing Cognitive Abilities: Teaching Children to Think. St Louis, CV Mosby, 1978

Weiss CE, Lillywhite HS: Communicative Disorders: A Handbook for Prevention and Early Intervention, 2nd ed. St Louis, CV Mosby, 1981

health problems
of the preschool child

student objectives

The student successfully attaining the goals of this chapter will be able to

1 Define the following vocabulary terms:

astigmatism   ataxia   athetosis   galactosemia   hemophilia   hyperopia
hypothermia   oliguria   sensorineural hearing loss   Snellen chart

2 Describe the four types of hearing loss and identify the possible causes of each.

3 Describe the three classifications of visual impairment.

4 Define the term cerebral palsy and list the prenatal, perinatal, and postnatal causes for this disorder.

5 Describe the four levels of mental retardation and discuss the nurse's role in the care of the mentally retarded child.

6 Describe the procedure for measuring the blood pressure of the preschool-age child.

Today's preschooler has a better opportunity for good health than ever before. Immunizations have dramatically reduced the threat of communicable childhood diseases. Antibiotics can minimize the dangers of infection. Early detection and proper nutrition can prevent certain kinds of mental retardation. Simpler, more effective screening techniques help identify vision and hearing problems that need early treatment. Surgical advances make possible the early repair of life-threatening heart problems. Yet serious health problems occur during the preschool period, some due to parental ignorance and negligence, others due to lack of understanding and knowledge about a disease or disorder. It is important that these problems be recognized and treated as soon as possible so that the child can be in optimum physical and emotional health when it is time to enter school, a landmark in the child's total development.

communicable diseases

Half a century ago, growing up meant being able to survive measles, mumps, whooping cough, diphtheria, and often poliomyelitis. They were expected almost as routinely as loss of the deciduous teeth. Immunization has changed that picture so drastically that some parents have become careless about having their children immunized until the immunization is required for entrance to school. Nevertheless, during 1980 the U.S. Center for Disease Control, in Atlanta, Georgia, reported that the five major childhood diseases—measles, mumps, rubella, tetanus, and diphtheria were at a record low in the United States.

Understanding the various communicable diseases, their prevention, symptoms, and treatment (Table 11–1), requires knowledge of the definitions of the following terms:

Some communicable diseases require isolation of the child in order to prevent spreading the infection. Specific isolation procedures can be found in the procedure manuals of individual hospitals. Guidelines for the kind of isolation required are summarized in Table 11–2.

It is important to explain to the child and the parents why isolation procedures are necessary, either to protect the child from the threat of infection or to protect others from the infection that the child has. Otherwise, the child may feel that the isolation is a form of punishment. Families are more likely to follow the correct procedures if they understand the need for them. Isolation increases the normal loneliness of being hospitalized, so that the child needs extra attention and stimulation during this time.

PREVENTION

The recommended schedule of infant immunization is found in Chapter 6. Immunizations for children who are not immunized according to this schedule should follow the schedule in Figure 11–1.

central nervous system disorders

HEARING IMPAIRMENT

Hearing loss is the most common handicap in the United States, affecting an estimated 3 million children and 13 million adults.[1] Depending on the degree of hearing loss and the age at which it is detected, a child's development can be moderately to severely impaired. Development of speech, human relationships, and understanding of the environment all depend on the ability to hear.

Hearing loss ranges from mild (hard of hearing) to profound (deaf) loss (Table 11–3). A child who is *hard of hear-*

Antibody. A protective substance in the body produced in response to the introduction of an antigen.

Antigen. A foreign protein that stimulates the formation of antibodies.

Antitoxin. An antibody that unites with and neutralizes a specific toxin.

Carrier. A person in apparent good health, who harbors in his body the specific organisms of a disease.

Carrier state is also a feature of the incubation period, the convalescence, and the postconvalescence of some infectious diseases.

Enanthem. An eruption upon a mucous surface.

Endemic. Habitual presence of a disease within a given area.

Epidemic. An outbreak in a community of a group of illnesses of similar nature, in excess of the normal expectancy.

Erythema. Redness of the skin produced by congestion of the capillaries.

Exanthem. An eruption appearing upon the skin during an eruptive disease.

Host. A man, an animal, or a plant that harbors or nourishes another organism.

Immunity. Passive—immunity acquired by administration of an antibody. Active—immunity acquired by an individual as the result of his own reactions to pathogens. Natural—resistance of the normal animal to infection.

Inapparent infection. Infection in a host without recognizable clinical signs.

Incubation period. The time interval between the infection and the appearance of the first symptoms of the disease.

Macule. A discolored skin spot not elevated above the surface.

Pandemic. A world-wide epidemic.

Papule. A small, circumscribed, solid elevation of the skin.

Pustule. A small elevation of the epidermis filled with pus.

Toxin. A poisonous substance elaborated by certain organisms such as bacteria.

Toxoid. A toxin that has been treated to destroy its toxicity but that retains its antigenic properties.

Vaccine. A suspension of attenuated or killed microorganisms administered for the prevention of a specific infection.

National Reye's Syndrome Foundation
441 Barker Drive
West Chester, PA 19380

PRIMARY IMMUNIZATION FOR CHILDREN NOT IMMUNIZED IN INFANCY

Schedule*	Immunization
Under 6 years of age	
First visit	DTP, TOPV, tuberculin test
1 month later	Measles† rubella, mumps
2 months later	DTP, TOPV
4 months later	DTP, TOPV‡
10–16 months later or preschool	DTP, TOPV
(6 years of age and over)	
First visit	TD, TOPV, tuberculin test
1 month later	Measles, rubella, mumps
2 months later	TD, TOPV
8–14 months later	TD, TOPV
(14–16 years of age)	TD (continue every 10 years)

* Physicians may choose to alter the sequence of these schedules if specific infections are prevalent at the time. For example, measles vaccine might be given on the first visit if an epidemic is underway in the community.
† Measles vaccine is routinely given before 15 months of age
‡ Optional

FIG. 11–1. Schedule for children not immunized as infants. (Courtesy American Academy of Pediatrics.)

ing has a loss of hearing acuity, but has been able to learn speech and language by imitation of sounds. A *deaf* child has no hearing ability. Children who are profoundly deaf are more likely to be diagnosed before 1 year of age than are children with mild to moderate hearing losses.

Deafness, mental retardation, and autism are sometimes incorrectly diagnosed because symptoms can be similar. Deaf children may fail to respond to sound or fail to develop speech because they cannot hear. Mentally retarded or autistic children may show the same lack of response and development even though they do not have a hearing loss.

TYPES OF HEARING IMPAIRMENT

There are four types of hearing loss: conductive, sensorineural, mixed, and central.

Conductive Hearing Loss. In this type of impairment, middle ear structures fail to carry sound waves to the inner ear. Most often conductive hearing loss is the result of chronic serous otitis media or other infection, and often makes hearing levels fluctuate. Chronic middle ear infection can destroy part of the ear drum or the ossicles, thus leading to conductive deafness. This type of deafness is seldom complete and responds well to treatment.

Sensorineural (Perceptive) Hearing Loss. This type of hearing loss may be caused by damage to the nerve endings in the cochlea, or to the nerve pathways leading to the brain. It is generally severe and unresponsive to medical treatment. Diseases such as meningitis or encephalitis, hereditary or congenital factors, or toxic reactions to certain drugs (such as streptomycin) may cause sensorineural hearing loss. Maternal rubella is believed to be the largest single cause of sensorineural deafness in children.

Mixed Hearing Loss. Some children suffer both conductive and sensorineural hearing impairment. In these cases, the conduction level determines how well the child is able to hear.

Central Auditory Dysfunction. Although this child may have normal hearing, damage or faulty development of the proper brain centers makes the child unable to use the auditory information he receives.

DETECTION AND EVALUATION OF HEARING LOSS

Mild to moderate hearing loss often remains undetected until the child moves outside the family circle into preschool, nursery school, or kindergarten. He may have had a gradual hearing loss, but may have become such a skilled lip reader that neither he nor his family is aware of the partial deafness. Parents and teachers should be aware of the possibility of hearing loss in children who appear to be inattentive, noisy, and creators of disturbances in class.

Certain reactions and mannerisms characterize a child with hearing loss. He may not be able to locate a sound, and may turn his head to one side when listening. He fails to comprehend when spoken to, giving inappropriate answers.

Audiological Assessment. The child who is suspected of having a hearing loss should be referred for a complete audiological assessment, including pure-tone audiometric testing, speech-reception loss, and speech-discrimination tests. Children with sensorineural impairment generally have a greater loss of hearing acuity in the high-pitched tones. The loss may vary from slight to complete. Those with a conductive loss are more likely to have equal losses over a wide range of frequencies.

A child's hearing should be tested at all frequencies in a

TABLE 11–1. CHILDHOOD DISEASES, IMMUNIZATION, AND NURSING CARE

Disease	Causative Agent	Incubation Period	Main Symptoms	Complications
diphtheria	*Corynebacterium diphtheriae*	• 2–7 days	pseudomembrane on pharynx, tonsils, and larynx nasal discharge swallowing and respiratory difficulty	bronchopneumonia respiratory and circulatory failure myocarditis nephritis
pertussis (whooping cough)	*Bordetella pertussis* *Hemophilus pertussis*	5–21 days	begins with nighttime cough three stages: catarrhal, spasmodic, convalescent paroxysmal cough with inspiratory whoop sticky phlegm	mental retardation convulsions hemorrhage pneumonia otitis media
tetanus (lockjaw)	*Clostridium tetani*	5–21 days	trismus muscular rigidity clonic convulsions difficulty swallowing irritability intramuscular hemorrhage cyanosis asphyxia	hemorrhage asphyxia malnutrition fluid & electrolyte imbalance
measles (rubeola)	rubeola virus (droplet infection)	7–21 days	Koplik spots photophobia conjunctivitis cough temperature elevation pruritic maculopapular rash that spreads down the body	encephalitis otitis media pneumonia cardiac damage neurological damage
rubella (*German* measles)	rubella virus	14–21 days	enlarged lymph glands of the head and neck rash—maculopapular begins on face and spreads downward rash disappears usually in three days	none in children birth deformities in the developing fetus
mumps (parotitis)	*Myxovirus mumps*	14–24 days	enlarged parotid glands sensitive to sour foods prodromal—fever, headache, pain on chewing, malaise	orchitis epididymitis deafness encephalitis myocarditis arthritis hepatitis
chicken pox (varicella)	varicella zoster	7–21 days	clear, oval vesicles in crops → crusts on trunk—all stages at same time pruritis lymphadenopathy irritability elevated temperature	viral pneumonia in adults shingles in adults encephalitis 2° infection from scratching
poliomyelitis (infantile paralysis)	poliovirus (3 types) (droplets from nose or throat, and in feces)	5–14 days	flaccid paralysis stiff neck and back nerve involvement	paralysis respiratory difficulty

(Selekman J: Immunization: What's it all about. Am J Nurs 80:140– 1445, 1980)

Roseola — cause by virus, high fever for 2–3 days, fever goes down break out in rash all over body (stomach + back), No vaccine.

Period of Contagion	Peak Incidence	Treatment and Nursing Measures	Immunization Available	Route	Possible Reactions
infectious for weeks if untreated 1–2 days in patients who have received treatment at least 4 weeks	2–5 years of age (passive protection 3–6 months)	antitoxin ice collars analgesics bed rest soft liquid diet high humidity possible tracheostomy	diphtheria toxoid diphtheria antitoxin	IM	no major ones
	0–3 months of age most severe in young infants (no passive protection)	maintain patent airway humidified oxygen quiet environment antibiotic therapy (ampicillin and erythromycin)	pertussis vaccine human pertussis immune serum globulin (minimal value)	IM	CNS involvement sterile abscess fever irritability anorexia
not transmitted man to man spores usually enter body during injury —puncture wound or burns	all ages having the disease does not provide immunity	decrease external stimulation seizure precautions sedation possible tracheostomy antibiotic therapy	tetanus toxoid absorbed (aluminum phosphate absorbed) tetanus immune globulin (Hypertet)	IM	sterile abscess— (if both types are given at same time, use different syringes and different sites) erythema stiffness tenderness fever (rare) slight rash
from 5th day of incubation to 1 week following symptoms	highest in school-age increase in adolescents (passive protection 15 months)	antipyretics dimly lit room tepid baths keep skin dry cool mist vaporizer	live measles attenuated measles immune globulin	SC	
1–7 days before rash and until rash has faded	older school-age children adolescents (passive protection first six months)	keep pregnant woman away from child symptomatic relief	live rubella attenuated	SC	rash peripheral neuritis arthralgia/ arthritis teratogenic effect
1–6 days before swelling and up to 9 days after swelling	school age	bed rest until swelling subsides analgesics for pain encourage fluids and soft foods hot or cold compresses antipyretics	live mumps attenuated	SC	none
1–5 days before eruption until vesicles are crusts (crusts are not contagious)	2–8 years of age (no passive protection)	antihistamines to prevent itching daily bath and linen change fingernails kept cut short mittens on hands if child scratches vesicles	none available for general use		
1 week before onset and as long as fever persists	all ages	complete bed rest general nursing care moist hot packs range-of-motion exercises	trivalent live oral polio vaccine (TOPV)	PO	rare

TABLE 11–2.　CLASSIFICATION OF CHILDHOOD COMMUNICABLE DISEASES REQUIRING ISOLATION OR PRECAUTIONS

Strict isolation (diseases–diphtheria, congenital rubella syndrome, smallpox)
Private room—necessary; door must be kept closed
Gowns—must be worn by all persons entering room
Masks—must be worn by all persons entering room
Hands—must be washed on entering and leaving room
Gloves—must be worn by all persons entering room
Articles—must be discarded or wrapped before being sent to central supply department for disinfection or sterilization

Respiratory isolation (diseases — chickenpox, measles [rubeola], mumps, pertussis [whooping cough], rubella [German measles])
Private room—necessary; door must be kept closed
Gowns—not necessary
Masks—must be worn by all persons entering room if susceptible to disease
Hands—must be washed on entering and leaving room
Gloves—not necessary
Articles—those contaminated with secretions must be disinfected
Caution—all persons susceptible to the specific disease should be excluded from patient area; if contact is necessary, susceptible persons must wear masks

Oral secretion precautions (disease–scarlet fever)
Private room—not necessary
Gowns—not necessary
Masks—not necessary
Hands—must be washed before and after patient contact
Gloves—not necessary
Articles—disposable handkerchiefs must be discarded in impervious bags, which should be sealed before being discarded in trash

Excretion precautions (disease—poliomyelitis)
Private room—not necessary
Gowns—not necessary
Masks—not necessary
Hands—careful hand washing after any patient contact and contact with secretions
Articles—no special precautions

(US Public Health Service: Isolation techniques for use in hospitals [Public Health Service Pamphlet No. 2054], Washington, DC, US Government Printing Office)

soundproof room by a pure-tone audiometer. Speech reception and speech discrimination tests measure the amount of hearing impairment for both speech and communication. Accurate measurements can usually be made on children of 5 years of age or older.

Infants and very young children must be tested differ-ently. An infant with normal hearing should be able to locate a sound at 28 weeks, be able to imitate sounds at 36 weeks, and associate sounds with people or objects at 1 year. A commonly used screening test employs noisemak-ers of varying intensity and pitch. The examiner stands beside or behind the child who has been given a toy. As the

TABLE 11–3.　EFFECTS OF HEARING LOSS

Threshold	Degree of Loss	Effects
0– 40 db	Mild (hard of hearing)	Difficulty hearing faint or distant speech; may require hearing aid; needs preferential seating in classroom
1– 55 db	Moderate (hard of hearing)	Difficulty hearing distant speech; requires amplification, preferential seating, auditory training, and probably speech therapy
6– 70 db	Moderate to severe	Difficulty with conversation unless loud; great difficulty in group/classroom discussion; requires hearing aid; may require special class for hard of hearing
1– 90 db	Severe (deaf)	May hear loud voice close to ear; may hear some vowels, recognize some sounds in environment; needs special education for the deaf, with specific training in speech and language
Over 90 db	Profound (deaf)	May hear some loud sounds; does not rely on hearing for communication; requires special education for the deaf

(Towne C: Disorders of hearing, speech and language. In Vaughan V, McKay R, Behrman R (eds): Nelson's Textbook of Pediatrics, p 155. Philadelphia, WB Saunders, 1979)

examiner produces sounds with a rattle, buzzer, bell, or other noisemaker, a hearing child is distracted and turns to the source of the new sound, whereas, the deaf child pays no heed.

TREATMENT AND EDUCATION

When the type and degree of hearing loss have been established, the child may be fitted with a hearing aid, even as young as 1 month of age.[2] Hearing aids are only helpful in conductive deafness, not in sensorineural or central auditory dysfunction. These devices only amplify sound; they do not localize or clarify it.

It is believed that deaf children can best be taught to communicate by a combination of lip reading, sign language, and oral speech (Fig. 11–2). His parents are his first teachers, and must be aware of all phases of development—physical, emotional, social, intellectual, and communicative—and then seek to aid this development.

A deaf child depends on sight to interpret his environment and to communicate. Thus, it is critically important to be sure that the child's vision is normal, and, if not, to correct that problem. The probability is twice as great that the child with a hearing loss will also have some vision impairment.

Training in the use of all his senses—sight, smell, taste, and touch—make the deaf child better able to use whatever hearing he may have, and it is believed that most deaf children do have some hearing ability.

Preschool classes for deaf children exist in many com-

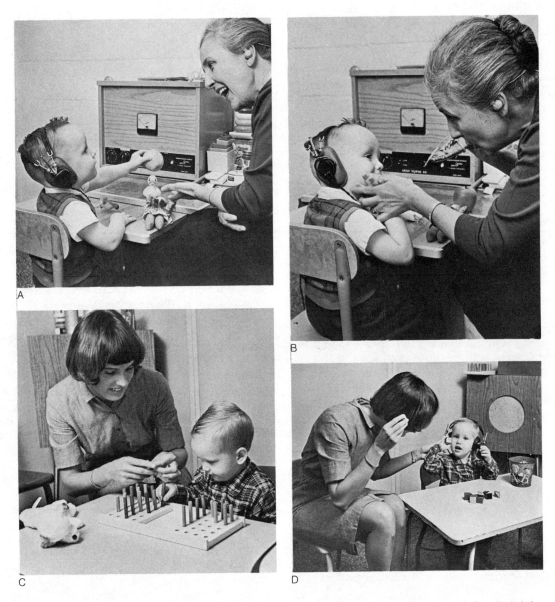

FIG. 11–2. The deaf child is taught to talk with the use of visual aids. (A) He learns the sound of apple, (B) the sound of shoe, (C) color and form, and (D) is helped to make use of his residual hearing.

munities. These seek to create an environment in which a deaf child can have the same experiences and activities that normal preschoolers have. Children are generally enrolled at age 2½.

The John Tracy Clinic in Los Angeles is concerned with the young child who has been born with a severe hearing loss or who has lost his hearing through illness before he has acquired speech and language.* The clinic's purpose is "to find, encourage, guide, and train the parents of deaf and hard of hearing children—first in order to reach and help the children, and second—to help the parents themselves."

All services to parents and children are given without charge. The clinic exists to help all deaf children. Consulting service, a nursery school and weekly clinic hours are offered. Of particular interest is the correspondence course available to parents of children 5 years old and under anywhere in the world. This is a 12-month course which includes first lessons in sense training, lip reading, language, auditory training and speech preparation. The clinic also suggests ways in which parents can help a younger child until he reaches the age of 20 months. Parent education films are also available for group viewing. Information concerning the many services offered by this clinic is available on request to the John Tracy Clinic.

Effective September 1977, Public Law 94-142 made free and appropriate education mandatory for all handicapped children. Children with a hearing loss who cannot successfully function in regular classrooms are provided with education in a residential school for deaf children. These schools provide speech therapy, lip reading, and auditory training.

NURSING CARE

When deaf children must be hospitalized, it is ideal for their parents to room-in with them, not as a convenience to the nursing staff, but for the child's benefit in being able to communicate his needs and feelings.

The deaf child's anxiety about unfamiliar situations and procedures probably is greater than that of the child with normal hearing. Therefore, it is even more important to demonstrate each procedure before it is performed, showing the child equipment or pictures of equipment to be used. Keeping a night light in the child's room is helpful, since sight is such a critical sense to the deaf child.

When speaking to the deaf child, the nurse should stand face to face with him, on his level. Explaining should be followed by showing, to be sure the child understands.

Nurses need to be familiar with the care and maintenance of hearing aids. They should also use parents as important resources about the child's habits and communication patterns.

VISION IMPAIRMENT

Like hearing, good vision is essential to a child's normal development. How well a child sees affects his learning process, social development, coordination, and safety. One

* John Tracy Clinic, 806 West Adams Blvd, Los Angeles, California, 90007

in every 1000 children of school age has a serious vision impairment. The sooner these impairments are corrected, if possible, the better a child's chances for normal or near-normal development.

Children with vision impairments are classified as sighted with eye problems, partially sighted, and legally blind.

TYPES OF VISION IMPAIRMENT

Eye Problems in Sighted Children. *Myopia (near-sightedness).* Among sighted children with eye problems, errors of refraction are the most common. Myopia means that the child can see objects clearly at close range but not at a distance. When proper lenses are fitted, vision is corrected to normal. If uncorrected, this defect may cause a child to be labeled inattentive or retarded.

Hyperopia (farsightedness). This is a common condition of young children, and frequently persists into the first grade or even longer. Whether corrective lenses are needed must be decided on an individual basis by the ocular specialist examining the child. Teachers and parents should be aware of the considerable eye fatigue that may result from efforts at accommodation for close work.

Astigmatism. This disorder may occur with or without myopia or hyperopia, and is caused by unequal curvatures in the cornea of the eye that bend the light rays in different directions, producing a blurred image. Slight astigmatism often does not require correction; moderate degrees usually require glasses for reading, television, and movies, and severe astigmatism requires that glasses be worn at all times.

Partial Sight. These are children with a visual acuity between 20/20 and 20/200 in the better eye after all necessary medical or surgical correction. These children also have a high incidence of refractive errors, particularly myopia. Eye injuries also cause loss of vision as do conditions such as cataracts that can be improved by treatment, but result in diminished sight.

Blindness. Blindness is legally defined as a corrected vision of 20/200 or less, or peripheral vision of less than 20 degrees in the better eye. Many of the causes of blindness have been reduced or eliminated, such as retrolental fibroplasia due to excessive oxygen concentrations in newborns and trachoma, a virus infection. Cataracts, amblyopia, and myopia are largely correctable. Maternal rubella is still a common cause of blindness, as are other maternal infections.

Somewhere between ages 5 and 7 years, children begin to form and retain visual images; they have memory with pictures. Children who become blind before age 5 are missing this crucial element in their development. Blindness seriously hampers the child's ability to form human attachments, to learn coordination, balance, and locomotion, to distinguish fantasy from reality, and to interpret the world around him. How well the blind child learns to cope with his problem depends on his parents' ability to communicate with him, teach him, and foster a sense of independence.

DETECTION AND EVALUATION OF VISION IMPAIRMENT

Squinting and frowning while trying to read a blackboard or other material at a distance, holding work too close to the eyes while reading or writing, and rubbing the eyes are all signs of possible vision impairment. While blindness is likely to be detected in early infancy, partial sightedness or correctable vision problems may go unrecognized until a child enters school, unless vision screening is part of routine health maintenance.

A simple test kit for preschoolers is now available for home use by parents or visiting nurses (Fig. 11–3). This kit is an adaptation of the Snellen E chart used for testing children who have not learned to read. The child covers one eye and then points his fingers in the same direction as the "fingers" on each E, beginning with the largest.

The Snellen Chart. This is the familiar test in which the letters on each line are smaller than those on the line above. If the child can read the lines standing 20 feet away from the chart, his visual acuity is stated as 20/20. If he can read only the line marked 100, acuity is stated as 20/100. The chart should be placed at eye level with good lighting and in a room free from distractions. One eye is tested at a time with the other eye covered.

Picture charts for identification are also used, but are not considered to be as accurate. A bright child can memorize the pictures and guess from the general shape without seeing distinctly.

TREATMENT AND EDUCATION

Significant medical and surgical advances have occurred in the treatment of cataracts, strabismus, and amblyopia. The earlier this treatment, the better the child's chances of adequate vision for normal development and function. Corrective lenses for minor vision impairments should be prescribed early and checked regularly to be sure that they are still providing adequate correction.

Children who are partially sighted or totally blind benefit from association with normally sighted children (Fig. 11–4). In some communities, education for these special children is provided within the regular school; in others, residential schools are available and may offer the child better equipment and instruction.

Special equipment for the use of children with sight impairment includes printed material with large print, pencils with large leads for darker lines, tape recordings, magnifying glasses, and typewriters. For children with a serious impairment whose participation in regular activities is sharply curtailed, talking books, raised maps, and braille equipment are needed as well. These devices prevent isolation of the handicapped child, and minimize his differences from the other children.

NURSING CARE

Blind and other handicapped children have the same needs as normal healthy children, and these should not be overlooked in dealing with the specific handicap. The blind child needs emotional comfort and sensory stimulation, much of which must be communicated by touch, sound, and smell. It is important for the nurse to explain sounds and other sensations that are new to the hospitalized child, and to let him touch equipment that will be used in any procedures. A tour of his room helps orient the child to the location of furniture and other facilities. Awareness of safety hazards is particularly important when caring for the blind or partially sighted child.

It is essential for the nurse and other personnel to identify themselves when they enter the child's room, and to tell the child when they leave. Explanations of what is going to happen reduce the child's fear and anxiety and the possibility of being startled by an unexpected touch.

The blind child should be involved with as many of his peers and their activities as possible. He should also be encouraged to do as much as possible for himself (Fig. 11–5).

CEREBRAL PALSY

Cerebral palsy is a term used to denote a group of disorders arising from a malfunction of motor centers and nerve pathways in the brain. It is one of the most complex of the common permanent handicapping conditions, and is often accompanied by seizures, mental retardation, various sensory defects, and behavior disorders.

Scientists predict that cerebral palsy can eventually be eliminated entirely from the group of diseases that threaten children, pointing to the significant reduction in the number of cases since the introduction of rubella vaccine in 1969. Research continues to find a means to protect against the infections that can cause cerebral palsy, and to prevent prematurity, another contributing factor.[3] Other research is directed at adapting biomedical technology to help persons with cerebral palsy cope with the activities of daily living, and gain maximum function and independence.

CAUSES

Cerebral palsy is caused by damage to the parts of the brain that control movement, and generally occurs during the fetal or perinatal period, particularly in premature infants. The brain damage is irreversible, making prevention the most important aspect of care. Improved prenatal care to prevent infection is one means; breastfeeding to give the infant the benefit of protective antibodies is another. Adequate nutrition can also help protect infants against infection. Poorly nourished children are more susceptible to infection and more likely to suffer central nervous system damage as a result. Causative factors are summarized as follows:[4]

Prenatal Causes

1. Any process that interferes with the oxygen supply to the brain such as separation of the placenta, compression of the cord, or bleeding
2. Maternal infection (*e.g.,* rubella)
3. Nutritional deficiencies that may affect brain growth

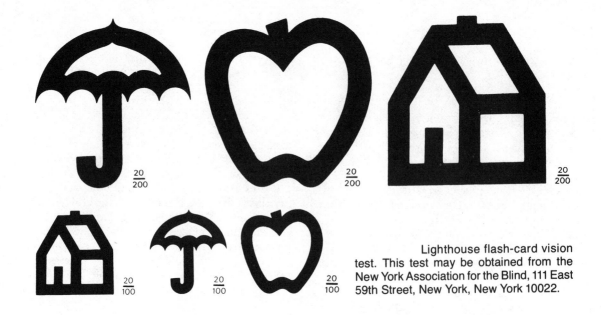

Lighthouse flash-card vision test. This test may be obtained from the New York Association for the Blind, 111 East 59th Street, New York, New York 10022.

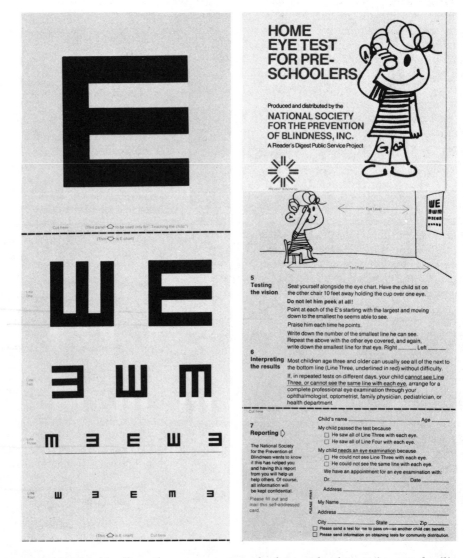

FIG. 11–3. Home testing kit. This kit allows the very young preschooler to take the test in more familiar surroundings. The best may be obtained from the National Society to Prevent Blindness, 79 Madison Avenue, New York, New York 10016.

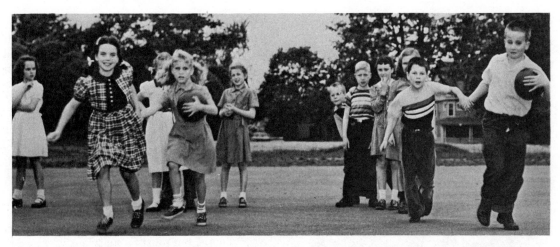

FIG. 11–4. Blind and sighted children play together. (Courtesy of American Foundation for the Blind)

4. Erythroblastosis fetalis or Rh incompatibility, which produces kernicterus resulting in anemia, liver damage, and a consequent interference with nutrition to the brain (Deaver, 1967)
5. Toxemia, because circulating toxins may cause brain damage and a predisposition to prematurity
6. Teratogenic factors such as radiation

Perinatal Causes

1. Anoxia immediately before, during, and after birth
2. Intracranial bleeding
3. Asphyxia or interference with respiratory function
4. Jaundice
5. Analgesia (*e.g.*, morphine) depressing the sensitive neonate's respiratory center
6. Birth trauma
7. Prematurity, since immature blood vessels predispose the neonate to cerebral hemorrhage

Postnatal Causes

1. Head trauma (*e.g.*, due to a fall)
2. Infection (*e.g.*, encephalitis or meningitis)
3. Neoplasms
4. Cerebral vascular accident

CLINICAL MANIFESTATIONS

Difficulty in controlling voluntary muscle movements is one manifestation of the central nervous system damage. Seizures, mental retardation, hearing and vision impairments, and behavior disorders frequently accompany the major problem. Delays in gross motor development, abnormal motor performance such as poor sucking and feeding behaviors, abnormal postures, and persistence of primitive reflexes are other signs of cerebral palsy. Diagnosis of cerebral palsy seldom occurs before 2 months of age and may be delayed until the second or third year.

There are several major types of cerebral palsy, each with distinctive clinical manifestations.

Spastic. This is the most frequent type, characterized by a hyperactive stretch reflex in associated muscle groups, an increased activity of the deep tendon reflexes, clonus, and contractures affecting the antigravity muscles, and scissoring. When scissoring is present, the child crosses his legs and points his toes when set on his feet.

Athetoid. Athetoid cerebral palsy is marked by involuntary incoordinate motion with varying degrees of muscle tension (Fig. 11–6). Children with this disorder are

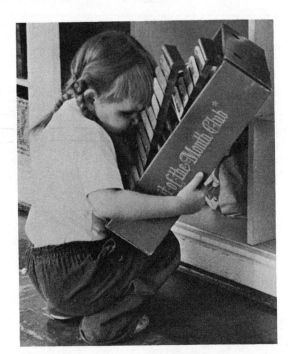

FIG. 11–5. The blind child learns by touch and should be encouraged to do things for herself. (Courtesy of American Foundation for the Blind; Charles Schuler, Dallas Services for Blind Children.

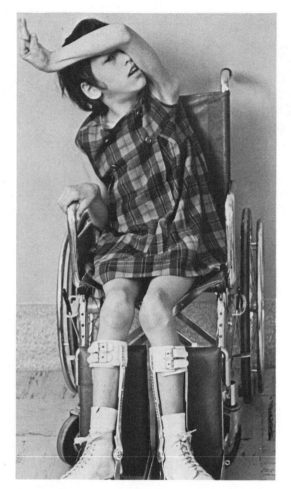

FIG. 11–6. This 11-year-old child with athetosis wears short leg braces and special shoes to keep her feet fairly flat. She shows the random movements characteristic of this type of cerebral palsy.

constantly in motion, the whole body in a state of slow, writhing, muscular contractions whenever voluntary movement is attempted. These children are most likely to have average or above average intelligence, despite their abnormal appearance. Hearing loss is most common in this group.

Ataxia. This is essentially a lack of coordination caused by disturbances of the kinesthetic and balance senses. The least common type of cerebral palsy, ataxia may not be diagnosed until children start to walk. Their gait is awkward and wide-based.

Rigidity. This type is characterized by rigid postures and lack of active movement.

Mixed. Children with signs of more than one type of cerebral palsy are usually severely disabled. The disorder may have been caused by postnatal injury.

TREATMENT AND SPECIAL AIDS

Treatment of cerebral palsy is directed toward helping the child make the most complete use of his residual abilities, and achieve maximum possible satisfaction and enrichment. It usually requires a team of professionals—physician, surgeon, physical therapist, occupational therapist, speech therapist, and perhaps a social worker—cooperating with the family. Dental care is important in the care of these children because enamel hypoplasia is common, and those children whose seizure disorders are controlled with Dilantin are likely to develop gingival hypertrophy.

Physical Therapy. Control of the body needed for purposeful physical activity is learned automatically by a normal child, but must be consciously learned by a physically handicapped child. Physical therapy attempts to teach a child to carry out an activity that he has been unable to accomplish. Methods must be suited to the needs of the individual child as well as to the general needs arising from his condition. These methods are based on principles of conditioning, relaxation, utilization of residual patterns, stimulation of contraction and relaxation of antagonistic muscles, and other pertinent principles. The major methods currently used are[5]

Bobath—A neurodevelopmental method directed toward the inhibition of abnormal reflex activity and the facilitation of normal movement.
Kabat, Knott, and Voss—A system of resistive exercises that facilitate voluntary control of movements through increased proprioceptive input to the brain.
Rood—Muscles area activated through application of an array of sensory stimuli such as heat, cold, and brushing.
Brunnstrom—Use of synergistic reflex movements to bring about active motion.
Doman–Delacato—An outgrowth of a theory proposed by Fay, this method training is carried out in basic patterns of movement according to an evolutionary sequence that progresses from fishlike swimming motions onward to the cross-pattern creeping of the anthropoid.

Orthopaedic Management. Braces are used as supportive and control measures to facilitate muscle training to reinforce weak or paralyzed muscles, or to counteract the pull of antagonistic muscles. Various types are available, each designed for a specific purpose. Orthopaedic surgery is sometimes used to improve function and correct deformities, such as the release of contractures and the lengthening of tight heel cords.

Technologic Aids for Daily Living. Biomedical engineering, particularly in the field of electronics, has perfected a number of devices to help make the handicapped person more functional and less dependent on others. They range from such simple things as wheelchairs and specially constructed toilet seats to completely electronic cottages, furnished with computer, tape recorder, typewriter, calculator, and other devices that facilitate independence and useful study or work. Many of these devices can be controlled by a mouth stick, an extremely useful feature for individuals with poor hand coordination.

A child who has had difficulty maintaining balance while he sits may need a high-backed chair with side pieces and a foot platform. Feeding aids include spoons with enlarged handles for easy grasping or with bent handles allowing the spoon to be brought easily to the mouth. Plates with high rims and suction devices to prevent slipping enable a child to feed himself. Covered cups, set in holders, with a hole in the lid to admit a straw, help a child who does not have hand control.

Manual skill can be aided by games such as pegboards, or cards that must be manipulated. Typing is an ego-boosting alternative for a child whose handicap is too severe to permit him to write legibly.

NURSING CARE

When a child with cerebral palsy is hospitalized, the nurse needs to learn as much as possible about the child's care and activities at home in order to minimize the changes in environment. Encouraging self-care activities, positioning to prevent contractures, providing modified feeding utensils, and opportunity for educationally sound play activities are important aspects of care. Both parents and child need emotional support and realistic explanations of what surgery or other treatment can be expected to accomplish.

OUTCOME

The basic defect of cerebral palsy is a fact that must be accepted by child and family. Like any chronic condition, it can become a devastating drain on the family's emotional and financial resources. The child's future depends on many variables—parental and sibling attitudes, economic and therapeutic resources, intelligence of the child, availability of competent, understanding professionals (Fig. 11–7). Some children, given the emotional and physical support they need are able to achieve a satisfactory degree of independence. Vocational training is available to an increasing number of these young people. Some will always need a significant amount of nursing care, with the possibility of institutionalized care when their family can no longer care for them. The picture is improving, but a great deal of work must be done to make it significantly brighter for these children and their families.

MENTAL RETARDATION

Mental retardation is doubtless as old as the human race, although it is difficult to find evidence of its existence prior to the 16th century when Paracelsus, a Swiss medical writer, wrote an entire treatise about mental deficiency. Later pioneers in the study of mental retardation included Jean Itard, Maria Montessori, and Samuel Howe.

During the 1960s the Kennedy family was responsible for greater acceptance of and increased research devoted to mental retardation. A change has gradually come about in the care of these children, recognizing that, given the proper care and attention, many of them can be helped to lead useful, productive lives. Institutions have become centers of learning and development rather than detention homes.

In 1968, a declaration of rights of the mentally retarded was proclaimed by the International League of Societies for the Mentally Handicapped (Fig. 11– 8).

CAUSES

Many factors can cause mental retardation. The most common are outlined as follows:

Prenatal Causes

Inborn errors of metabolism such as phenylketonuria (PKU)—damage can often be prevented by early detection and treatment.

Prenatal infection such as toxoplasmosis and cytomegalovirus infections—microcephaly, hydrocephalus, cerebral palsy, and other brain damage can result from intrauterine infections.

Teratogenic agents such as radiation or drugs—can have devastating effects on the central nervous system of a developing fetus.

Genetic factors—Inborn variations of chromosomal patterns result in a variety of aberrations, the most common of which is Down's syndrome (mongolism).

Perinatal Causes

Birth trauma, anoxia from various causes, prematurity, and difficult birth can all cause mental retardation. In some instances, prenatal factors may have influenced the perinatal complications.

Postnatal Causes

Poisoning such as lead poisoning—Children who develop encephalopathy from chronic lead poisoning usually suffer significant brain damage.

Infections and trauma such as meningitis, convulsive disorders, and hydrocephalus—often lead to mental retardation.

Impoverished early environment such as lack of sensory stimulation or adequate nutrition—can result in mental retardation. Emotional rejection in early life may do irreparable damage to a child's ability to respond to his environment.

THE MENTALLY RETARDED CHILD

About 3% of all children born in the United States are mentally retarded. Approximately one-fifth are so severely retarded that diagnosis is made at birth or during the first year. The majority of the other children are diagnosed as retarded when they begin school.

The mentally retarded child is one whose limited intelligence impairs his ability to learn and adapt to the demands of society. Intelligence is measured in terms of ability for abstract thinking. It includes causal reasoning, spatial comprehension, verbal expression, visual and auditory memory, and other adaptive adjustments. Adaptive ability is reflected in maturation, learning, and social adjustment. Therefore, the precise definition of mental retardation depends on the prevailing educational and cultural standards of society. A person who may function adequately in a

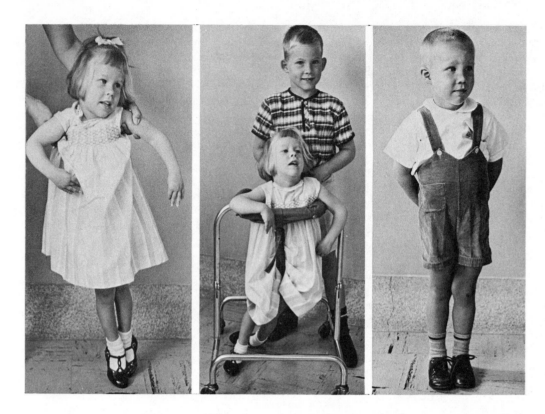

FIG. 11–7. (A) This 5-year-old girl with athetosis cannot stand alone and does not talk. (B) She uses a walker, and is shown here with one of her two healthy brothers who accept her naturally. (C) The other brother and the one shown in B show posture and general appearance indicating normal muscular control.

society that demands proficiency in certain skills may be totally unable to cope with the demands of a more complex culture.

The most common classification of mental retardation is based on intelligence quotients (IQ). Though controversy exists about the validity of tests that measure intelligence, this system is still the most useful for grouping these children.

Mildly Retarded (Educable).   IQ of 67 to 52. This child is a slow learner, but is capable of acquiring basic skills. He can learn to read, write, and do arithmetic to a 4th or 5th grade level. He is slower than average in learning to walk, talk, and feed himself, but retardation may not be obvious to casual acquaintances. With support and guidance, this child usually can develop social and vocational skills adequate for self-maintenance.

Moderately Retarded (Trainable).   IQ of 51 to 36. The moderately retarded child has little, if any, ability to attain independence and academic skills. Motor development and speech are noticeably delayed, but training in self-help activities is possible. This child may be able to learn repetitive skills in sheltered workshops. Some may learn to travel alone, but few become capable of assuming complete self-maintenance.

Severely Retarded (Totally Dependent).   IQ of 35 to 20. This child's development is markedly delayed during the first year of life. He is not capable of learning academic skills, but can perhaps learn some self-care activities if sensorimotor stimulation is begun early. Eventually this child will probably learn to walk and develop some speech; however, he needs a sheltered environment and careful supervision all his life.

Profoundly Retarded (Totally Dependent).   IQ below 20. This child has minimal capacity for functioning and needs continuing care. Eventually he may learn to walk and develop a primtive speech, but will never be able to perform self-care activities.

TREATMENT AND EDUCATION

Knowledge about mental retardation has increased dramatically during the past two decades, and exciting new teaching methods have begun to yield encouraging results. Mildly and moderately retarded persons are being taught in increasing numbers to perform tasks that will enable them to achieve·some degree of independence and usefulness. More and better services are being provided for all retarded children and adults.

Before effective treatment can begin, however, parents must accept the reality of their child's problem and want to cope with the difficult task of helping the child develop

DECLARATION OF GENERAL AND SPECIAL RIGHTS OF THE MENTALLY RETARDED

Whereas the universal declaration of human rights, adopted by the United Nations, proclaims that all of the human family, without distinction of any kind, have equal and inalienable rights of human dignity and freedom;

Whereas the declaration of the right of the child, adopted by the United Nations, proclaims the rights of the physically, mentally or socially handicapped child to special treatment, education and care required by his particular condition.

Now Therefore

The International League of Societies for the Mentally Handicapped expresses the general and special rights of the mentally retarded as follows:

ARTICLE I

The mentally retarded person has the same basic rights as other citizens of the same country and same age.

ARTICLE II

The mentally retarded person has a right to proper medical care and physical restoration and to such education, training, habilitation and guidance as will enable him to develop his ability and potential to the fullest possible extent, no matter how severe his degree of disability. No mentally handicapped person should be deprived of such services by reason of the costs involved.

ARTICLE III

The mentally retarded person has a right to economic security and to a decent standard of living. He has a right to productive work or to other meaningful occupation.

ARTICLE IV

The mentally retarded person has a right to live with his own family or with fosterparents; to participate in all aspects of community life, and to be provided with appropriate leisure time activities. If care in an institution becomes necessary it should be in surroundings and under circumstances as close to normal living as possible.

ARTICLE V

The mentally retarded person has a right to a qualified guardian when this is required to protect his personal wellbeing and interest. No person rendering direct services to the mentally retarded should also serve as his guardian.

ARTICLE VI

The mentally retarded person has a right to protection from exploitation, abuse and degrading treatment. If accused, he has a right to a fair trial with full recognition being given to his degree of responsibility.

ARTICLE VII

Some mentally retarded persons may be unable due to the severity of their handicap, to exercise for themselves all of their rights in a meaningful way. For others, modification of some or all of these rights is appropriate. The procedure used for modification or denial of rights must contain proper legal safeguards against every form of abuse, must be based on an evaluation of the social capability of the mentally retarded person by qualified experts and must be subject to periodic reviews and to the right of appeal to higher authorities.

ABOVE ALL—THE MENTALLY RETARDED PERSON HAS THE RIGHT TO RESPECT.

October 24, 1968.

FIG. 11–8. Declaration of general and special rights of the mentally retarded. (Mental Retardation 7:2, 1969).

to his full potential. Diagnosis made at birth or during the first year affords the greatest hope of early acceptance and beginning education and training.

Parents' first reaction to the tragedy of mental retardation is grief: this is not the perfect child they had wanted. Many feel shame at their inability to produce a perfect child. Some rejection of the child is almost inevitable, at least in the initial stages, but this needs to be worked through, for the family to cope.

Some parents compensate for their early hostile feelings by over-protection or over-concern, making the child unnecessarily helpless, and perhaps taking out their anger and frustration on the normal siblings. Only when the family accepts the child as another member of the family, to be helped, loved, and disciplined as the others, can they begin to function effectively.

Parents need to know that their feelings are normal. Talking with other parents of retarded children can offer some of the best support and guidance as they seek information to help them deal with the problem. One group that includes both parents and professionals is the National Association of Retarded Citizens, a volunteer organization with local chapters in many communities.

NURSE'S ROLE

Not all nurses are sufficiently educated or experienced to act as professional counselors for families with a retarded child. Every nurse, however, can listen, observe, and demonstrate caring acceptance of the child and the family. Knowing about community resources and other health professionals who can help parents is another important nursing function.

All but the most profoundly retarded children go through the sequence of normal development, with delays at each stage and leveling off of ability as they reach the limits of their capacity. A retarded child, however, proceeds according to his mental age rather than his chronological age. Thus, a 6-year-old retardate may be functioning on a mental level of 2 years, and the expected behavior must be essentially that of a 2-year-old. Adequate knowledge of the important landmarks of normal growth and development is essential to understanding the progressive nature of maturation.

Teaching Self-Help Skills. Teaching the mentally retarded child requires the same principles as teaching any child at a level appropriate to his stage of maturation, not his chronological age. If the child has physical handicaps in addition to retardation, the rate of development is also affected.

One factor that makes the retarded child different from the average child is the lack of ability to reason abstractly. This prevents transfer of learning or application of abstract principles to varied situations. Learning takes place by habit formation, emphasizing the three R's—routine, repetition, and relaxation. Most mentally retarded children increase in mental age, although slowly, and to a limited level. Therefore, each needs to be watched for evidence of readiness for a new skill.

Providing an Enriched Environment. Environmental stimulation is essential for everyone's development. Thinking that the retarded child does not need this stimulation, because he cannot learn, discourages further development. The retarded child needs much more environmental enrichment than the average child who can help provide his own stimulation. Suggested activities for providing this enrichment are summarized in Table 11–4.

Discipline. Whether the retarded child is at home or in the hospital, he needs to know which behavior is acceptable and which is unacceptable. Discipline is as important to this child as to any other.

The limited ability of these children to adapt to varying circumstances makes it essential that discipline be consistent, with instructions given in simple, direct, concise language. A positive approach that relies heavily on example and demonstration produces better results than a constant "don't touch" or "stop that." Obedience is an important part of discipline, especially for the child with faulty reasoning ability, but the objectives of discipline should be much broader. The child needs to know what to expect, and finds security and support in routines and consistency. Kindness, love, understanding, and physical comforting are also part of discipline.

If punishment is needed, it must follow the misdeed immediately, so that cause and effect is made clear. Taking the child away from the group for a short time can help restore his self-control. Retaliation can confuse and anger the retarded child. If he is using misbehavior to get attention, praise and approval for good behavior may eliminate the need for wrongdoing.

HOME CARE VERSUS INSTITUTIONAL CARE

The trend today is to keep retarded children at home with their families rather than place them in institutions. As more and better opportunities for help, education, and guidance emerge in the community, families gain confidence in their ability to cope.

The individual attention, security, and sense of belonging to a family are important factors in every child's programs and development. No institution, however progressive and well staffed, can entirely supply the experience a child gains from his own family.

Each family must decide individually whether they are able to manage the child at home. Depending on their physical, emotional, and financial resources, it may be better for the family to place the child in an institution. The profoundly retarded child can take so much time and strength from one or both parents that other children are neglected. A retarded child who is undisciplined, or improperly supervised, may become a nuisance in the home and the neighborhood. Caring for a retarded child may demand such sacrifice from other family members that the family eventually disintegrates. It is important for health professionals to be realistic in providing information on which the family can base their decision.

TYPES OF MENTAL RETARDATION

Only the most common conditions that include mental retardation are discussed here. For a complete list of mental deficiency disorders, a text specializing in such disorders should be consulted.

Down's Syndrome. Down's syndrome (mongolism) is the most common of the chromosomal anomalies. The condition was first described by Langdon Down in 1866, but its cause was a mystery for many years. In 1932 it was suggested that a chromosomal anomaly might be the cause, but the anomaly was not demonstrated until 1959.

Down's syndrome has been observed in nearly all countries and races. The term mongolism is not an appropriate name for the condition, and is going out of use. The majority of individuals with Down's syndrome have trisomy 21; a few have partial dislocation of chromosomes 15 and 21. All forms of the condition show a variety of abnormal

TABLE 11–4. EXAMPLES OF DEVELOPMENTAL STIMULATION AND SENSORIMOTOR TEACHING FOR RETARDED INFANTS AND YOUNG CHILDREN

Developmental Sequence	Possible Activities to Encourage Development
Sitting	
1. Sit with support in caretaker's lap	Hold child in sitting position on lap, supporting him under armpits. Do several times a day gradually lessening the support.
2. Sit independently when propped	Place child in sitting position against firm surface with pillow behind his back and on either side. Leave him alone several times a day.
3. Sitting with increasingly less support	Allow child to sit on equipment that provides increasingly less support such as baby swing, feeder, walker, high chair.
4. Sit in chair without assistance	Place child in a chair with arms. Provide balance support at first, then gradually withdraw. Leave for 10 minutes at a time.
5. Sit without support	Place child on floor. Gradually withdraw assistance.
Self-feeding	
1. Sucking	Encourage child to suck by putting food on pacifier, putting a drop on tongue, and so forth.
2. Drink from a cup	Put small amount of fluid in a baby cup. Raise cup to his mouth by placing hands under child's.
3. Grasp piece of food and place in mouth	Place bit of favorite food in child's hand. Guide hand and food to mouth. Gradually reduce support.
4. Transfer food from spoon to mouth	Move spoon to child's mouth with hand supporting baby's. Gradually withdraw support.
5. Scoop up food and transfer to mouth	Have child hold spoon by handle, scoop up food, and transfer to mouth. Do not allow child to use fingers. Progress from bowl to flat plate.
Stimulation of touch	
1. Body sensation	Hold, cuddle, rock child.
2. Explore environment through touch	Brush skin with objects of various textures (feathers, silk, sandpaper). Place objects of different textures near child. Move hand to object.
3. Explore environment through mouth	Give child objects which can be chewed. Guide hand to mouth at first.
4. Explore tactile sensations	Expose child to hard, soft, warm, and cold objects.
5. Explore with water	Place hands and/or feet in water.

(Johnson V, Werner R: A Step-by-Step Learning Guide for Retarded Infants and Children. Syracuse, Syracuse University Press, 1975; Eddington C, Lee T: Sensory-motor stimulation for slow to develop children. Am J Nurs 75(1):59– 62, 1975)

characteristics. Mental status is usually within the moderate to severe range of retardation with the majority moderately retarded.

The most common anomalies include: brachycephaly (shortness of head); retarded body growth; upward and outward slanted eyes (almond-shaped) with epicanthic fold at inner angle; short, flattened bridge of nose (Fig. 11–9). The child with Down's syndrome has a thick and fissured tongue; hair may be dry and coarse; hands are short, with an incurved fifth finger and a single palmar crease; wide space between first and second toes; very lax muscle tone (these children can assume relaxed positions difficult for normal persons). Frequently there are heart and eye anomalies. Susceptibility to leukemia is greater than in the general population.

Not all of these physical signs are present in all individuals with Down's syndrome. Some may have only one or two characteristics; others may show nearly all.

Cretinism (hypothyroidism) is associated with either a congenital absence of a thyroid gland or with the inability of the infant's thyroid gland to secrete the thyroid hormone. This disorder rarely appears in more than one member of the family.

The infant appears normal at birth, clinical signs and symptoms not being fully developed before 3 to 6 months. The symptoms are very similar to those of Down's syndrome and may cause some confusion. However, Down's syndrome is nearly always recognizable at birth. There are other dissimilarities: the eyes are not slanted but appear puffy. The voice is hoarse; the skin is dry; there is slow bone development. Two common features of cretinism are obstinate constipation and umbilical hernia. Radioactive iodine given by mouth fails to reach a normal concentration in the thyroid gland, and examination of the blood shows a low level of protein-bound iodine (PBI).

Some nurseries routinely perform T_3 and T_4 thyroid function tests on all newborns before discharge to diagnose cretinism early.

Outcome. Without treatment those cretins who live become mentally deficient dwarfs. Treatment consists of oral administration of desiccated thyroid tablets. This must be continued throughout the individual's lifetime,

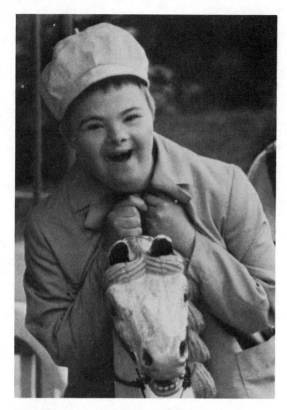

FIG. 11–9.   The typical facies of Down's syndrome is easily distinguished. (Courtesy of WHO; Photo by E Madelmann)

signs of mental arrest within a few weeks. It is therefore imperative that these infants be discovered as early in life as possible and placed immediately on a low phenylalanine formula.

Diagnosis.   A blood test devised in recent years gives good results as early as the third or fourth day after birth but is of no value until the infant has received dietary protein, which is present in his milk feedings. This screening procedure, called the Guthrie inhibition assay test, utilizes blood from a simple heel prick. It is standard procedure in most newborn nurseries, being performed just before the infant is discharged. A positive Guthrie test should always be followed by a blood test for tyrosine level. As many babies go home from the newborn nursery before they have ingested much milk, a urine test done a few weeks later is a good precaution.

Manifestations of the condition are neurologic. Many of these children develop aggressive and disagreeable traits. Convulsions may occur and eczema is common. There is a characteristic musty smell to the urine.

Treatment is dietary. A formula low in phenylalanine should be started as soon as the condition is detected. (Lofenlac is a low-phenylalanine formula produced by Mead Johnson.) Best results are obtained if the special formula is started before 3 weeks of age. A low phenylalanine diet is a very restricted one. Foods to be omitted are breads, meat, fish, dairy products, nuts and legumes. The diet should be carefully supervised by a nutritionist.

Galactosemia is a recessive hereditary metabolic disorder in which the enzyme necessary for converting galactose into glucose is missing. The infants generally appear normal at birth, but experience difficulties after the ingestion of milk—whether breast milk, cow's or goat's milk—because one of the component monosaccharides of milk lactose is galactose.

Early feeding difficulties, with vomiting and diarrhea severe enough to produce dehydration and weight loss, and jaundice, are primary manifestations. Unless milk is withheld early, other difficulties include cataracts, liver and spleen damage, and mental retardation, with a high mortality rate early in life.

The earliest diagnostic finding is the presence of galactose in the urine, but if vomiting or refusal to eat have been present, the test may be negative. Galactose tolerance tests have been used, but may present definite hazards to the infant. Recently, a blood test using the Guthrie inhibition assay method, has proved a reliable diagnostic test. It can be performed in conjunction with a test for phenylketonuria.

Treatment consists of omitting galactose from the diet, which, in the young infant, means a substitution for milk. Nutramigen and soybean preparations such as ProSobee or Mulsoy, are satisfactory substitutes.

with adjustments made in the dosage as needed. If treatment is begun as early as possible and in adequate dosage, physical growth will proceed normally, and mental development should be relatively normal.

Phenylketonuria (PKU) is a recessive hereditary defect of metabolism that if untreated causes severe mental retardation in most but not all affected children. It is an uncommon trait appearing in about one out of 10,000 births. In this condition, there is a lack of the enzyme that normally changes the essential amino acid, phenylalanine, into tyrosine.

As soon as the newborn baby with this defect begins to take milk, either breast or cow's milk, he begins to absorb phenylalanine in the normal manner. However, because of his inability to metabolize this amino acid, phenylalanine builds up in his blood serum to as much as 20 times the normal level. This takes place at such a rapid pace that increased levels of phenylalanine appear in the blood after a day or two of ingestion of milk. Phenylpyruvic acid appears in the urine of affected babies somewhere between the second and sixth week of life.

The majority of untreated children with this condition develop severe and progressive mental deficiency, apparently because of the high serum phenylalanine level. The infant appears normal at birth but commences to show

respiratory system disorders

TONSILLITIS AND ADENOIDITIS

PATHOPHYSIOLOGY

A brief description of the placement and the functions of tonsils and adenoids may be helpful before the difficulties of infection and the indications for removal are discussed.

A ring of lymphoid tissue encircles the pharynx, forming a protective barrier against upper respiratory infection. This ring consists of groups of lymphoid tonsils.

The faucial tonsils, the commonly known *tonsils*, are two oval masses attached to the side walls of the back of the mouth between the anterior and posterior pillars.

The pharyngeal tonsil, known as *adenoids*, is a mass of lymphoid tissue in the nasal pharynx, extending from the roof of the nasal pharynx to the free edge of the soft palate.

The lingual tonsils are two masses of lymphoid tissue at the base of the tongue.

There is a normal progression of enlargement of lymphoid tissue in childhood between the ages of two and eight or ten years, regressing during the pubertal period. If the tissue itself becomes a site of acute or chronic infection, it may become hypertrophied to the extent of interfering with breathing, causing partial deafness, or it may become in itself a source of infection.

TREATMENT

Tonsillectomies and adenoidectomies are not done as frequently today as in the past. No conclusive evidence has been found that a tonsillectomy, in itself, improves a child's health by reducing the number of respiratory infections, increasing the appetite, or improving his general well-being. Studies tend to show that incidence of colds may increase following removal of the tonsils.

It is generally agreed that absolute indications for removal of tonsils are: frequent attacks of acute tonsillitis; recurrent peritonsillar abscess (which has become rare); chronically infected tonsils with enlarged cervical nodes, which fail to yield to antibiotic therapy; and hypertrophy of tonsils to the extent of interfering with swallowing and breathing. Systemic disturbances, such as rheumatic fever or glomerulonephritis, are not considered as indications for tonsillectomy, unless the tonsils can be proved to be the source of an infection that fails to yield to antibiotic treatment.

Adenoids are more susceptible to chronic infection. Indication for adenoidectomy is hypertrophy of the tissue to the extent of impairing hearing or interfering with breathing. An increasingly common practice is to perform only an adenoidectomy if tonsil tissue appears to be healthy.

Tonsillectomy is postponed until after the age of four or five years, except in the rare instance when it appears urgently needed. Often, when a child has reached the acceptable age, the apparent need for the tonsillectomy has disappeared.

When the decision has been made to remove the tonsils, a period of two or three weeks following an acute infection should pass, although this is not always possible. On occasion, a surgeon, after several cancellations of surgery because of new infections, may decide that it is safer to operate while the child is relatively free from infection, rather than risk any more acute episodes.

Preoperative Care. In many hospitals, the child has had blood and urine tests performed before admission; if this has not been done, the nurse should make certain that the ordered tests are performed and the results entered on the chart. Written permission for surgery is then obtained, and the parents are notified of the time surgery is scheduled.

One unfortunate occurrence in busy hospitals is the failure to notify the parents of an advance in surgery time, so that the parent arrives to find her child has already left the ward. A concerned parent is justifiably angered, visualizing the child's fright and insecurity.

Emotional preparation for surgery has been discussed throughout this book. Acting out the forthcoming experience, particularly in a group, with the use of puppets, dolls, and play doctor or play nurse material helps the child to develop security. The amount and the timing of preparation before admission depends somewhat upon the child's age.

On the morning of surgery, the child is given no food or fluids, a fact that may well traumatize the child emotionally if he has to watch the others getting their breakfast trays. If surgery is to be late, there is no reason for keeping the child in his bed. He will be happier and better adjusted if he can spend this time in the playroom, with someone responsible for helping him resist the temptation to drink, if he should forget. As this is the age during which primary teeth become loose and fall out, the child should be checked carefully for loose teeth before surgery.

Postoperative Care. Immediately following a tonsillectomy, the child is placed in a partially prone position, with his head turned to one side, until he is completely awake. This position can be accomplished by turning the child partially over and by flexing his knee on which he is not resting to hold him in position. Pillows placed under the chest and abdomen may embarrass respiration, and so are usually forbidden.

Vital signs are checked every 10 to 15 minutes until the child is fully reacted, then every half-hour or every hour. The child is encouraged to expectorate any blood rather than swallow it and produce nausea and vomiting. The nurse should be aware of the normal rate of pulse and respiration for the child's age, in order to interpret the vital signs correctly (Table 11–5). Any unusual restlessness, frequent swallowing, or rapid pulse may indicate bleeding and should be reported. Vomiting of dark, old blood may be expected, but bright, red-flecked emesis or oozing indicates fresh bleeding. A tracheal suction machine, ready for use, should be available. Suctioning by the nurse must be performed with great care, and not extended beyond the front of the mouth. The nurse observes the pharynx with a flashlight each time vital signs are checked. Pale, cool, clammy skin.

TABLE 11–5.   NORMAL VITAL SIGNS FOR PRESCHOOLERS

Vital Sign	Age	Normal Value
Pulse rate	2–6 yr	68–138/min
Temperature	3 yr	37.5°C (99.4° F)
	4–6 yr	37°C (98.6° F)
Respirations	2–6 yr	20–40/min

(Bates BA: A guide to physical examination, 2nd ed. Philadelphia, JB Lippincott, 1980)

Fluids are encouraged as soon as the child's nausea has subsided. The thirsty child may be eager to drink, but painful swallowing probably will quell his enthusiasm, and encouragement will be needed. Jello water, fruit-flavored, uncarbonated drinks are allowed, with the oft-promised dish of ice cream in the afternoon.

Complications. *Epistaxis* (nosebleed) is a common occurrence after adenoidectomy. Hemorrhage is a frequent complication following tonsillectomy, and topical adrenalin may be prescribed for its vasoconstrictive action.

The child is discharged on the day after surgery if no complications are present. Parents are advised to keep him in bed for two days, and fairly quiet for about a week. Soft foods and nonirritating liquids should be given during the first few days. The parents are advised that a transient earache may be expected about the third day. If bleeding should occur, the pediatrician or clinic should be notified at once.

circulatory system disorders

BLOOD DYSCRASIAS

There are several abnormalities of the blood that may manifest themselves in the child of preschool age. Although leukemia, purpura, and hemophilia may be diagnosed at either an earlier or a later age they are commonly associated with the preschool years. Children with these disorders are often chronically ill and will require long-term care.

ACUTE LEUKEMIA

Leukemia has been considered a disease that is always fatal. In untreated children with this disease, death occurs rather quickly. Newer treatments and medications, however, have brought about remissions for many children that last for long periods, and there is now hope that some of these remissions may prove permanent. There are some patients, however, who do not respond to treatment. The disease has its highest peak of onset between the ages of 3 and 5 years.

Etiology. The cause of leukemia is still not known, although there are interesting clues. Recently, certain animal leukemias have been proved to be of viral origin. However, a simple infectious viral cause in childhood leukemia does not seem likely at this time. Leukemia also is frequently associated with Down's syndrome and other chromosomal disorders.

Pathophysiology. Immature white cells, called blast cells, are formed in large numbers in the blood-forming tissues throughout the body, while normal white cells are progressively reduced. Leukemia in childhood is nearly always the acute type in contrast to the chronic type sometimes found in adults. About 80% of childhood leukemias are of the acute lymphoblastic type. The overall leukocyte count is normal in half the cases, but the differential count shows a predominance of immature blast cells.

Clinical Manifestations. Clinical manifestations of the disease appear with surprising abruptness in many affected children, with few, if any, warning signs. Presenting manifestations are frequently lassitude, pallor and loss of appetite. Other early or presenting symptoms are fever, bone and joint pain, sore throat, widespread petechiae, and hemorrhages into the skin or the mucous membranes.

Nausea and vomiting, headache, diarrhea and abdominal pain, although seldom presenting signs, frequently occur during the course of the disease. Anemia and easy bruising are present, and enlargement of liver and spleen occurs. Ulceration of the gums and throat develops due to bacterial invasion. Intracranial hemorrhages are not uncommon. Anemia becomes increasingly severe.

Diagnosis. The diagnosis of acute leukemia is made by demonstration of leukemic blast cells in the bone marrow, blood and other tissues (Table 11–6).

Treatment. In addition to symptomatic, palliative measure, certain drugs have been successful in bringing about remissions during which period the child feels and acts quite well (Fig. 11–10). Remissions may last for a period of several weeks, and some children have had 2 or 3 remissions, under sustained medical therapy. These drugs include prednisone, 6-mercaptopurine, methotrexate, Cytoxan, and vincristine, all of which may cause *alopecia* (loss of hair), a common problem with chemotherapy or radiotherapy. It may boost the child's self-image if he wears a wig.

Home Care. Hospitalization for leukemic children is limited to diagnostic procedures and to the institution of therapeutic measures whenever possible. The child at home is allowed to live a normal life as much as he is able. The family needs to unite to make the home pleasant and cheerful, and should make a particular effort to keep anxiety and discouragement away from the child. Parents may need special encouragement about this, and may appreciate an understanding, sympathetic friend for support.

Overindulgence and undue permissiveness tend to make the child anxious and confused, however, and are not in his best interest. Short periods of hospitalization for exacerba-

TABLE 11–6.   FINDINGS FROM HISTORY, PHYSICAL ASSESSMENT, AND LABORATORY ANALYSIS AT DIAGNOSIS OF LEUKEMIA

History	Physical Assessment	Laboratory Findings

Fatigue
Fever
Purpura
Bone pain
Weight loss
Infection
	Enlarged spleen
	Enlarged liver
	Lymphadenopathy
	Bone tenderness
	Skin or mucous membrane bleeding
		WBC is elevated, low, or normal.
		Neutrophils (also called polys, segs, PMNs, or granulocytes) are <1000/m³.
		Platelets are <50,000/mm³.
		Bone marrow
		  Markedly hypercellular
		  Lacking fat globules and bone particles
		  Blast cells over 5% (25% needed for diagnosis, but usually 60–100% blasts)

(Wieczorek RR, Natapoff J: A Conceptual Approach to the Nursing of Infants and Children: Health Care From Birth to Adolescence. Philadelphia, JB Lippincott, 1981)

tions quite possibly are going to be necessary, as well as admission for terminal care.

Nursing Care.   Physical care for a child in the terminal stages of a wasting disease (such as leukemia) is aimed at providing all possible comfort for the patient. Frequent turning is necessary, but painful, and is dreaded by the child. Unhurried movement, a soft, gentle touch, and careful handling, help minimize the pain. Abrupt movements should be avoided, and necessary analgesics should be used as indicated. Cleansing of bleeding, ulcerated areas in the mouth must be very gentle in order to prevent further trauma.

Emotional care of the child and his parents is equally important and is discussed in the chapters on chronic and terminal illness.

IDIOPATHIC THROMBOCYTOPENIC PURPURA

Purpura is a blood disorder associated with a deficit of platelets in the circulatory system. The most common type of purpura is the idiopathic thrombocytopenic purpura.

This condition is preceded by a viral infection in about half of the diagnosed cases.

Clinical Mainifestations.   The onset is frequently acute. Bruising and a generalized rash occur. In severe cases, hemorrhage may occur in the mucus membranes, epistaxis, which is difficult to control, or hematuria may be present. Rarely, a serious complication of intracranial hemorrhage occurs. In the majority of cases, spontaneous disappearance of symptoms occurs in a few weeks without serious hemorrhage. A few may continue in a chronic form of the disease.

Diagnosis.   The platelet count is reduced to below 40,000 per cu mm. Bleeding time is prolonged and clot retraction time is abnormal. White cell count remains normal, and anemia is not present unless excessive bleeding has occurred.

Treatment and Nursing Care.   Corticosteroids are useful in reducing the severity and shortening the duration of the disease in some, not all, cases. Nursing care consists in protecting the affected child from falls and trauma, regular diet and general care.

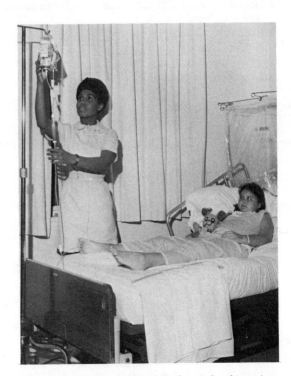

FIG. 11–10.   This child with leukemia has been given steroids, causing edema and moonface features.

HEMOPHILIA

Hemophilia is one of the oldest hereditary diseases known to mankind. Dispensation of the rites of circumcision to the sons born subsequent to the birth of an older son who bled uncontrollably was mentioned in the Talmud.[6]

Recent research has demonstrated hemophilia as a syndrome of several distinct inborn errors of metabolism, all resulting in the delayed coagulation of blood. Defects in the synthesis of protein give rise to deficiencies in any of the factors in the blood plasma needed for thromboplastic activity. The principal factors involved are factor viii (AHG), factor ix (PTC), and factor xi (PTA).

Mechanism of Clot Formation.   The mechanism of clot formation is complex. In a simplified form, it can best be described as occurring in three stages.

1. Prothrombin is formed through plasma–platelet interaction.
2. Prothrombin is converted to thrombin.
3. Fibrinogen is converted into fibrin by thrombin.

Fibrin forms a mesh that traps red and white cells and platelets into a clot, closing the defect in an injured vessel. A deficiency of one of the thromboplastin precursors may give rise to hemophilia. This progression of events is diagrammed in Figure 11–11.

Reference to one of the specialized texts on the circulatory system is necessary for a detailed discussion and for better understanding of the clot-forming mechanism.

Clinical Manifestations.   Hemophilia is characterized by prolonged bleeding, with frequent hemorrhages into the skin, the joint spaces, the intramuscular tissues and externally. Bleeding from tooth extractions, brain hemorrhages, and crippling deformities are serious complications. Circumcision is contraindicated when hemophilia is present. Death during infancy or in early childhood is not unusual in severe hemophilia, and results from a great loss of blood, intracranial bleeding, or from respiratory obstruction caused by bleeding into the neck tissues.

A young infant beginning to creep or walk bruises easily, and may often cause serious hemorrhages from minor lacerations. Bleeding frequently occurs from lip biting, or from sharp objects put in the mouth. Tooth eruption seldom causes bleeding, but extractions require specialized handling, and should be avoided by preventive care, if at all possible.

Clinical manifestations in any type of hemophilia are similar, and are treated by transfusions to supply the deficient factor, and by measures to prevent or treat complications. In severe bleeding, the quantities of fresh blood needed may easily overload the circulatory system. It therefore becomes important to know the type of deficiency, in order that concentrated plasma containing the necessary factor may be administered when a transfusion is considered necessary.

Diagnosis of hemophilia is made by a careful examination of family history and of the type of bleeding the patient presents. Abnormal bleeding dating from infancy, in combination with a family history, suggests hemophilia. A markedly prolonged clotting time is characteristic of severe AHG or PTC deficiency, but mild conditions may have only a slightly prolonged clotting time. It must be kept in mind that in a number of instances, no family history may be obtained.

Recognized Types of Hemophilia.   *Factor VIII deficiency* (*hemophilia A; AHG deficiency; classic hemophilia*).   Classic hemophilia is inherited as a sex-linked recessive mendelian trait with transmission to affected males by carrier females.

Hemophilia A (classic hemophilia) is the most commonly found type, and is also the most severe. It is caused by a deficiency of antihemophilic globulin (AHG)—the factor viii necessary for blood clotting.

Factor IX deficiency (*hemophilia B; PTC deficiency; Christmas disease*).   Christmas disease was named after a 5-year-old boy who was one of the first patients diagnosed as having a deficiency of factor *ix*.

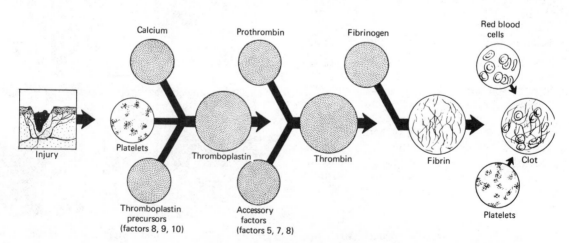

FIG. 11–11.   The mechanism of the formation of a blood clot is complex.

This deficiency constitutes about 15% of the hemophilias. It is a sex-linked recessive trait appearing in male offspring of carrier females, caused by a deficiency of one of the necessary thromboplastin precursors, factor ix, the plasma thromboplastin component (PTC). In either hemophilia A or hemophilia B, as many as 25% or more of the affected persons can trace no family history of the disease. It is assumed that spontaneous mutations have occurred in some of these cases. Hemophilia B (Christmas disease) is indistinguishable from classic hemophilia in its clinical manifestations, particularly in its severe form. It may also exist in a mild form, probably more frequently than in hemophilia A.

Factor XI deficiency (hemophilia C; PTA deficiency). This exists as an autosomal dominant trait, appearing in both males and females. Sporadic cases may also be observed, as in the other hemophilias. The deficient factor is plasma thromboplastin antecedent (PTA), factor xi. Bleeding is generally milder than in the AHG and the PTC deficiencies, hemorrhage usually being by trauma, and rarely spontaneous.

Von Willebrand's syndrome (vascular hemophilia; pseudohemophilia). Von Willebrand's syndrome is classified with the hemophilias. It is a mendelian dominant trait present in both sexes, and is characterized by prolonged bleeding time.

Treatment. For many years the only treatment for bleeding in hemophilia was the use of fresh blood or plasma. When fresh frozen plasma came into use it became the mainstay in the management of hemophilia. Great improvements have been made possible in the treatment of hemophilia through the use of fresh frozen plasma. It has been particularly helpful in emergency situations.

It does however have shortcomings. One major problem has been the large volumes needed to control bleeding. Another is the danger that injections of large amounts of plasma may lead to congestive heart failure.

In 1952, a method was found for separating hemophilia A and B, and a suitable procedure developed for identifying the antihemolytic factor for hemophilia A.; Factor viii. This basic laboratory procedure known as the *partial thromboplastin time* (PTT) is now commonly used for assay and diagnosis of both hemophilia A and hemophilia B.

Several factor viii concentrates for the treatment of hemophilia are now available. One of these, called cryoprecipitate, resulted from the discovery that the precipitate remaining undissolved when frozen plasma thawed slowly could be used to stop bleeding. A procedure was developed by which blood banks can collect this material and use it in the treatment of hemophilia A.

A newer preparation is now available which is said to supply higher potency AHG than previous preparations.*

This means that only a small volume of fluid is needed for treatment, and it can be administered intravenously by syringe.

A concentrate for hemophilia B is also now available.†

These concentrates are supplied in dried form together with diluent for reconstitution. Directions for mixing and administration are included with the package. They can be given either by slow intravenous drip or injected into the vein by syringe.

Continued research has produced some progress in the treatment of hemophilia. Table 11–7 summarizes therapeutic and nontherapeutic drug interventions for the child with hemophilia.

Bleeding into the joint cavities frequently occurs following some slight injury, and seems nearly unavoidable if the child is to be allowed to lead a normal life. Pain, caused by the pressure of the confined fluid in the narrow joint spaces, is extreme, requiring the use of sedatives or of narcotics. Prompt immobilization of the involved extremity is essential to prevent contractures of soft tissues and the destruction of the bone and joint tissues (Fig. 11–12). Emergency splints are available, and should be kept in every hemophiliac's home. Ice packs should also be available for instant use. Before leaving for the hospital, a splint and cold packs should be applied, and if any great length of time is required for transportation, a transfusion of plasma should be given.

A bivalve plaster cast may be applied in the hospital for the immobilization of the affected part. Orthopaedic surgeons disagree as to whether collected blood in the affected joint should be aspirated.

After bleeding has been stopped, the cast may be removed, and gentle traction may be applied to restore motion and alignment. Passive physiotherapy is used to help prevent the development of joint contractures. A fairly large number of patients who have had repeated hemarthroses, however, have developed functional impairment of their joints despite careful treatment.

Most children with hemophilia have their lives interrupted by frequent hospitalization. Nurses and auxillary personnel should be well informed concerning general care of a hemophilia patient, as well as the care needed by a particular child.

Nursing Care. Particular attention must be paid to treatments and procedures in order to avoid pain or additional bleeding. Medication should be given orally, if possible, but if injections are ordered, sites must be carefully chosen and rotated, avoiding bruised areas or hematomas. Medication should be injected slowly, after which manual pressure should be applied for 5 or more minutes. A pressure dressing and an ice pack may be used instead. Venipunctures should be done by experienced persons.

During daily hygiene, the nails should be trimmed to prevent scratching, and adequate skin care given to prevent irritation. Oral hygiene is important, and if a tooth brush is used, it should have very soft bristles.

---

* Antihemophilic Factor (Human) Method Four, Dried, Hemofil. Hyland Division Travenol Laboratories.

† Hyland Proplex Factor Complex (Human). Factors ii, vii, ix and x. Hyland Division Travenol Laboratories.

TABLE 11-7.   THERAPEUTIC AND NONTHERAPEUTIC DRUG INTERVENTIONS FOR THE HEMOPHILIAC

Recommended	Not Recommended	
Non-narcotic agents	Analgesics	
Tylenol ⎫ (acetaminophen)	Aspirin	
Tempra ⎭	Aspirin-containing compounds	
Darvon (plain) (propoxyphene)	Bufferin	Empirin
Talwin (pentazocine)	Anacin	Percodan
Narcotic agents	Alka-Seltzer	APC tablets
Codeine	Darvon Compound	Excedrin
Demerol (meperidine)	Antihistamines	
Morphine (morphine sulfate)	Periactin (cyproheptadine)	
Methadone (methadone	Chlor-trimeton (chlorpheniramine)	
hydrochloride)	Cough syrup	
	Robitussin (glycerol guaiacolate)	
	Anti-inflammatory agents	
	Butazolidine (phenylbutazone)	
	Indocin (indomethacin)	
	Motrin (ibuprofen)	

(Hilgartner MW: Hemophilia in Children: Progress in Pediatric Hematology/Oncology, p 165. Littleton, Massachusetts, Publishing Sciences Group, 1976)

If internal bleeding is present, vital signs must be watched carefully for signs of shock, and excretions should be examined for the presence of blood. If the bleeding is into the joints, the nurse should take care to avoid additional pain or injury. A bed cradle can keep the weight of the blanket off painful areas. The knee is the most commonly affected joint, and only a slight degree of motion may lead to more bleeding. Careful turning and handling are essential.

Emotional Support.   A small child may be placed in a crib with padded sides to protect him from bruises. This isolates him from the rest of the world, however. Coming at the same time as separation from his mother, this isolation is especially hard to bear. His choice of toys is going to be quite limited, because anything that could possibly cause injury must be avoided. Even if he is feeling well, he will likely be kept in his crib, because no one will have enough time to watch him carefully. His prospects are rather dismal, and they present a strong point in favor of allowing his mother to stay with him.

If a mother has been understandably apprehensive about her child's condition, he will quite possibly enter the hospital determined to get his own way. He does not expect any one to cross him too much, because he can always have a temper tantrum.

The nurse may frequently avoid such occasions if she uses a little forethought. If the dispute is not particularly important, as is often the case, flexibility is in order. Failure to make necessary restrictions because a child might react is not in his best interest, nor will it contribute to his emotional welfare.

For an older child, frequent hospitalizations, treatments and school absences are difficult to accept, and he needs considerable help. He can learn to understand his condition, and can learn the need for caution in his life. Occupational activities suitable for his age, and placement in the ward with others of his age and with his interests, are important adjuncts to his emotional well-being.

Home Care.   A child with hemophilia is perfectly well between bleeding episodes, but the fact that bleeding may occur as the result of very slight trauma, or often without any known injury, causes considerable anxiety. For an un-

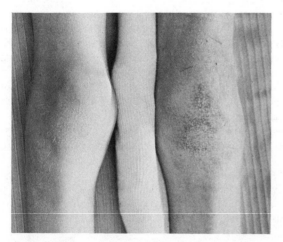

FIG. 11-12.   The hemophiliac can suffer from bleeding into the joints and painful swollen knees.

known reason, bleeding episodes are more common in the spring and fall. There also appears to be some evidence that emotional stress can initiate bleeding episodes.

Topical fluoride applications to the teeth are of particular importance to these children. Particular attention should be paid to proper oral hygiene, well-balanced diet and to proper dental treatment. Although parents may be aware of the benefits to the teeth from a well-balanced diet and from the avoidance of in-between snacks without toothbrushing, damage frequently occurs before the patient's first visit to the dentist. Parents should be encouraged to bring their affected children to the dentist very early, in order that they may secure assistance in establishing good dietary habits. In this manner, the child also becomes familiar with the dental office before any care is actually needed. Parents may also appreciate help in the selection and use of proper equipment such as a toothbrush, toothpaste and dental floss. The parents need to carefully select a dentist who understands the problems presented, and who will set up an appropriate program of preventive dentistry.

Nosebleeds in affected children are frequent, but can usually be controlled with a Gelfoam pack soaked in topical thrombin solutions and maintained by gentle pressure. Bleeding from any source in a hemophiliac, however, indicates the titer of AHG or other deficient factor is below a critical level; therefore, transfusion of whole blood, fresh frozen plasma, or plasma concentrate is necessary.

Parents experience continual anxiety over how much activity to allow their child, how to keep from overprotecting, how to help him achieve a healthy mental attitude, and yet prevent mishaps that may cause serious bleeding episodes. In some way, they must help him toward autonomy and independence within the framework of his limitations. There certainly will be times when the emotional effect of social deprivation and restrained activity must be weighed against possible physical harm.

The financial strain on the family is considerable, as is so frequently the case when a child has a long-term chronic condition. Children who have had several episodes of hemarthrosis may be crippled to the extent of needing crutches and braces, or wheelchairs. Measures toward rehabilitation require hospitalization, with possible surgery, casts, and other orthopedic appliances. Rehabilitative measures have been remarkably successful when in the hands of competent orthopedists, but they take long periods of time and cannot be hurried.

A hemophilic child usually suffers much loss of school time. The child who must frequently interrupt his schooling, for whatever reason, suffers a considerable handicap. Each child should be considered individually, with as normal an environment as possible planned for him.

Both a child and his family must accept his limitations, and yet realize the importance of normal social experiences. School, health, and community agencies must be prepared to assist the family with counseling and encouragement, and enable them to bring up their affected child in a healthy manner, both emotionally and physically.

Rehabilitation. Extensive crippling resulting from hemophilic arthropathies presents a difficult task for rehabilitation. Prompt and thorough care of any injuries as they arise helps minimize crippling. Many children, however, develop deformities severe enough to limit successful daily living.

Rehabilitation for the correction of flexion deformities requires hospitalization for periods of weeks for treatment with corrective casts. When the best possible correction has been obtained, braces usually are fitted for maintenance of the correction.

Braces are frequently needed for a period of years, during which, they must be kept in perfect repair, adjusted to the patient's growth, and replaced as necessary. Rehabilitation of the severely crippled patient requires a long period under specialized orthopedic care, but the results have been eminently worthwhile.

The nurse should be aware of the resources in her community, both for family counseling and for financial assistance. State chapters of the National Hemophilia Foundation provide information, form parent groups, support the establishment of special clinics, and provide a diversity of other services.

genitourinary system disorders

NEPHROTIC SYNDROME

A number of different types of nephrosis in the nephrotic syndrome have been identified. The most common in children is *lipoid nephrosis.* All forms of nephrosis have early characteristics of edema and proteinuria, so that definite clinical differentiation cannot be made early in the disease.

The chief clinical manifestation of lipoid nephrosis is a generalized edema that becomes so great the child may double his normal weight. It has a course of remissions and exacerbations, usually lasting for months. Although the mortality rate remains high, present-day management has allowed many more children to survive until the disease disappears spontaneously than had previously been the case. Previously, before the availability of effective antibacterial agents and corticosteroid therapy, recovery rates were estimated as low as 30%. Presentday estimates place the recovery rate as high as 75% with the use of intensive steroid therapy and protection against infection.

The cause of lipoid nephrosis is not known. It is in rare cases associated with other specific diseases. The nephrotic syndrome is present in about 7 children per 100,000 population under 9 years of age. The lipoid form has its onset, on the average, at 2½ years.

CLINICAL MANIFESTATIONS

Edema is usually the presenting symptom, appearing first around the eyes and ankles. As the swelling advances, the edema becomes generalized, with a pendulous abdomen full of fluid. Respiratory embarrassment may be severe, and edema of the scrotum is characteristic. The edema shifts with change of position of the child when lying quietly or walking about. Anorexia, irritability, and loss of appetite develop. Malnutrition may become severe. The generalized edema masks the loss of body tissue, causing the child to present a chubby appearance, but after diuresis, the malnutrition becomes apparent. These children are usually susceptible to infection, and repeated acute respiratory conditions are the usual pattern.

DIAGNOSIS

Laboratory findings include marked proteinuria, with large numbers of hyaline and granular casts in the urine. Hematuria is not usually present. Blood serum protein is reduced, and the total serum globulin level is normal or increased, with a reversed serum-globulin ratio.

TREATMENT

Management of nephrosis is a long process, with reversals and reappearance of symptoms. Use of corticosteroids has induced remissions in most cases and reduced recurrences. Corticosteroid therapy usually produces diuresis in about 7 to 14 days, but the drug is continued until a remission occurs. Prednisone is the most commonly used. Intermittent therapy is continued every other day, or for three days a week. Daily urine testing for protein is continued whether the child is at home or in the hospital.

Antibiotic therapy using a broad spectrum antibiotic such as ampicillin is used to protect the child against infection. The use of diuretics may not be necessary when diuresis can be induced with steroids.

A general diet, appealing to the child's poor appetite, is recommended. Salt should be kept to a minimum. Parents will need encouragement and support for the long months ahead. The course of the disease is seldom less than about 18 months.

CONTINUING CARE

Children with nephrosis are usually hospitalized for diagnosis, thorough evaluation of their general health and specific condition, and for the institution of therapy. A course of antibiotic therapy is given to clear up any concurrent infection, and unless unforeseen complications develop, the child is discharged with complete instructions for management.

A written plan is most useful to help parents follow the program successfully. They must keep a careful record of home treatment, and bring it to the clinic or to the physician's office at regular intervals.

Parents must be aware of reactions that may occur with the use of steroids, and the adverse effects of abrupt discontinuance of these drugs. If these things are well understood, the incidence of forgetting to give the medication, or of neglecting to refill the prescription, should be reduced or eliminated entirely. Parents also need to feel free to report promptly any symptoms that they consider caused by the medication.

Special care to keep the child in optimum health is important, and intercurrent infections must be reported promptly. Exacerbations are common, and parents need to understand that these will probably occur, and to report rapidly increasing weight, increased proteinuria or signs of

infections for a possible alteration of the therapeutic regimen and the specific antibiotic agents as indicated.

Caring for the child at home follows the same pattern as that for any chronically ill child. Bed rest is not indicated except in the event of an intercurrent illness. Activity is restricted only by the edema, which may slow the child down considerably, but otherwise normal activity is beneficial. Sufficient food intake may be a problem, as it is in other types of chronic illness. Fortunately, there are usually no food restrictions, and the appetite can be tempted by attractive, appealing foods.

Complications from kidney damage necessarily alter the course of treatment. Failure to achieve satisfactory diuresis, or the need to discontinue the use of steroids because of adverse reactions, will call for a re-evaluation of treatment. The presence of gross hematuria suggests renal damage. Persistence of abnormal urinary findings following diuresis presents a less hopeful outlook. Reagent strips are available for determining presence of various substances in the urine such as glucose, albumin, protein, and several others.

PROGNOSIS

The course of nephrosis is generally characterized by recurrent episodes of edema of varying length. With present-day methods of treatment, recovery rates have been estimated at 75%.

ACUTE GLOMERULONEPHRITIS

Acute glomerulonephritis is a condition that appears to be an allergic reaction to a specific infection, most often a group A beta hemolytic streptococcal infection, as in rheumatic fever.

Acute glomerulonephritis occurs most frequently in children between the ages of three and seven years. As a rule, the child is not very ill, and it is often difficult to impress on parents the seriousness of this condition.

Pathophysiology. The kidneys are slightly enlarged and pale, with changes in the glomerular capillaries, which permit the passage of blood cells and protein into the glomerular filtrate. In a majority of cases, these changes are reversible, but there is no way to predict which cases will show complete recovery or will instead develop into chronic nephritis.

CLINICAL MANIFESTATIONS

Presenting symptoms appear 1 to 3 weeks after the onset of a streptococcal infection. Most frequently, the presenting symptom is grossly bloody urine; periorbital edema may accompany or precede the hematuria. Fever may be as high as 103° F or 104° F at the onset but falls in a few days to about 100° F. Slight headache and malaise are usual, and there may be vomiting. A transient hypertension appears in 60% to 70% of patients during the first 4 or 5 days, returning to normal in about 1 week.

Oliguria (production of a subnormal volume of urine) is usually present, and the urine has a high specific gravity and contains albumin, red and white blood cells and casts.

The blood urea nitrogen level is elevated, and the serum albumin is usually low.

COMPLICATIONS

Cerebral symptoms occur in connection with hypertension in a small percentage of cases, consisting mainly of headache, drowsiness, convulsions and vomiting. When the blood pressure is reduced, these symptoms disappear. Cardiovascular disturbance is present in many patients, but has few clinical manifestations in the majority and is apparent only in electrocardiographic tracings. In most children, this condition is transient, but in some, it goes on into cardiac failure.

TREATMENT

Although the child usually feels well in a few days, it is important that he be kept in bed until clinical manifestations subside. This generally occurs 2 to 4 weeks after the onset. Penicillin during the acute stage is given to eradicate any existing infection. A fluid diet may be offered for the first few days, followed by a soft to full diet as acute symptoms subside. Low-salt, low-protein diets, or limited fluid intake is not prescribed, except in the presence of edema or renal failure. The treatment for complications is symptomatic.

NURSING CARE

Bed rest must be enforced until acute symptoms and gross hematuria have disappeared. The child should be protected from chill and from contact with persons with infections. When he is allowed out of bed, he should be prevented from becoming fatigued.

Urinary output must be carefully checked and recorded every 8 hours. The amount of fluid allowed the child will be based on his output, as well as on evidence of continued hypertension and oliguria. Careful recording of the child's fluid intake is essential and careful attention paid to keep it within prescribed limits.

Blood Pressure Readings. Accurate blood pressure readings are difficult to obtain from infants and from young children. Readings are taken usually only on specific order of the physician.

Blood pressure readings in infancy and in early childhood are essentially the same as those of a 4-year-old.

If hypertension becomes a problem, a diuretic such as reserpine may help reduce the pressure to normal levels. Apresoline may be added if needed. A diastolic level of 100 or over is an indication for the administration of hypertensive drugs. Specific gravity of the voided urine, as well as tests for any urinary protein are also part of nursing procedure. Tests such as the Addis count or urine concentration require preparation.

Specific Gravity Determination.   Fill the cylinder with urine to within 1 inch of the top (25 ml). Grasp the float at the tip and insert slowly until it is immersed in the urine to near the top of the graduation marks. Give the float a slight twirl, and note the reading as it comes to rest. While reading, keep the float away from the sides of the container. Avoid wetting the stem above the water line be-

MEASUREMENT OF BLOOD PRESSURE

Average Blood Pressures

Age	Systolic	Diastolic
4 years	85	60
6 years	90	60
8 years	95	62
10 years	100	65
12 years	108	67
14 years	112	70
16 years	118	75

Principles

1. A child should be at rest for accurate reading. Excitement or exercise may significantly raise the systolic rate.
2. Fright, discomfort, or distrust of the examiner, causes resistance and excitement.
3. The proper size cuff is essential for an accurate reading. Too wide or too narrow a cuff gives an erroneously high or low reading. The cuff should cover two-thirds of the upper arm.
4. If strict accuracy is important, use of the same cuff for each reading will be necessary.

Technique

1. Ascertain the latest reading for comparison.
2. Choose the proper size cuff. If possible, use the same cuff each time.
3. Approach the child with a gentle manner and with slow, deliberate movements. Establish good rapport. Avoid tightening the cuff beyond a necessary point. For an older child, prepare him with an explanation, and with an opportunity to explore the equipment. Give the reasons for the procedure.
4. Apply the cuff to arm. Raise the manometer gradually to a point above the obliteration of the radial pulse.
5. Deflate the cuff slowly. The *systolic* pressure reading is made when the first sound is heard with each heart beat. The *diastolic* pressure reading is made when the sound suddenly diminishes in volume. A sudden muffling of the sound denotes a pressure equal to the diastole.
6. Compare this reading with previous readings. If there is a significant discrepancy, have the pressure checked by second person.
7. Remove the cuff. Reassure and console the child as it seems necessary.
8. Report any significant variation from the previous reading.
9. Record the time and the reading on the patient's chart.

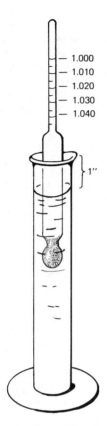

— 1.000
— 1.010
— 1.020
— 1.030
— 1.040

1″

FIG. 11–13. A urinometer is used for determining the specific gravity of urine.

cause this gives an inaccurate reading. A normal specific gravity is 1.015–1.025 (Fig. 11–13).

CONTINUING CARE

Traces of protein in the urine may persist for months after the acute symptoms disappear, and an elevated Addis count, indicating urinary red cells, persists as well. Parents are taught to test for urinary protein routinely, and to collect the urine for an Addis count about every 3 months, until all evidence of kidney damage disappears. If the urinary signs persist for more than a year, the disease has probably assumed a chronic form.

OUTCOME

In spite of such grave implications, a recovery rate of 82% or higher is reported. In an additional small number of children, the condition progresses into chronic nephritis. Mortality rate for the acute condition is about 2%.

summary

Most preschoolers encounter minor health problems during this period, but with proper care and nutrition, recover rather quickly. Some children in this age group are less fortunate, however, and must undergo lengthy, sometimes painful treatment for major health problems. This is a period when congenital conditions such as mild hearing or vision impairment and central nervous system disorders become quite apparent.

Many preschoolers are quite independent in feeding, dressing, toileting, and other activities of daily living. This independence should be encouraged during illness and hospitalization, so that interruption of normal development is minimized.

TABLE 11–8. PRESCHOOLERS' REACTIONS TO DEVIATIONS FROM HEALTH

Theorist	Psychodynamic Process	Emotional Response
Erikson Autonomy vs shame and doubt	Loss of independence alters self-esteem.	Denial of the problem too painful to face
Erikson Initiative vs guilt	Interference with ability to control situations alters self-esteem.	Anger at inability to continue life as usual
Erikson Industry vs inferiority	Altered ability to "produce" alters self-esteem.	Feelings of inadequacy
Piaget Preoperational thought	Egocentric view of events; lack of ability to comprehend "cause and effect" or "chance" occurrence	Guilt due to belief they caused problem
Freud Oedipal stage	Desire for attention from parent of opposite sex creates fear of retribution from parent of same sex.	Fear of illness or body mutilation as punishment

The preschooler's magical thinking can lead to many anxieties and fears about illness and treatment. He may feel that adults are capable of "fixing" any health problem if they want to; therefore, he needs to be good. The preschooler's reactions to health problems are summarized in Table 11-8.

review questions

1. What are the five major childhood diseases?
2. What are the symptoms, treatment, and prevention of these major childhood diseases?
3. Describe the four types of hearing impairment.
4. What nursing measures are important when caring for blind or other handicapped children?
5. What are the causes of cerebral palsy?
6. Why is dental care especially important when a child is taking Dilantin?
7. What are the causes of mental retardation?
8. How many chromosomes are present in Down's syndrome?
9. Describe the child with Down's syndrome.
10. What clinical manifestations indicate fresh bleeding following a tonsillectomy?
11. What type of leukemia is most common in children?
12. What nursing measures are important in caring for a child with hemophilia?
13. What classification of drugs is used to treat lipoid nephrosis?
14. What appears to be the cause of acute glomerulonephritis?

references

1. Hearing alert, Washington, DC. Alexander Graham Bell Association for the Deaf.
2. Schmitt BD: Ear, nose and throat. In Kempe CH, Silver HC, O'Brien D (eds): Current Pediatric Diagnosis and Treatment, 4th ed. Los Altos, Lange Publications, 1976
3. Preventing cerebral palsy and mitigating its disabling effects: A research imperative for the 80s. In Research Report, Vol 4. New York, United Cerebral Palsy Research and Educational Foundation, 1980
4. Wieczorek RR, Natapoff J: A Conceptual Approach to the Nursing of Children: Health Care From Birth Through Adolescence, p 534. Philadelphia, JB Lippincott, 1981
5. Whaley L, Wong D: Nursing Care of Infants and Children, pp 1509–1510. St Louis, CV Mosby 1979
6. Bearn AG: Hemoglobin, hemophilia and agammaglobulinemia, p 231. In Fishbein M: Birth Defects. Philadelphia, JB Lippincott, 1963

bibliography

American Academy of Pediatrics. Report of the committee on infectious diseases. Evanston, Ill, 1977

Azarnoff M, Hardgrove C: The Family in Child Health Care. New York, John Wiley & Sons, 1981

Bleek E: Integrating the physically handicapped child. J School Health 49:3, 141–146, 1979

Bouchard-Kurtz R, Speese-Owens N: Nursing Care of the Cancer Patient, 4th ed. St Louis, CV Mosby, 1981

Conway BL: Pediatric Neurological and Neurosurgical Nursing. St Louis, CV Mosby, 1977

Curry JB, Peppe KK (eds): Mental Retardation: Nursing Approaches to Care. St Louis, CV Mosby, 1978

Desotill S: A brighter future for leukemia patients. Nurs 77 7, No. 1:19–23, 1977

Giaquinta B: Helping families face the crisis of cancer. Am J Nurs 77:1585–1588, 1977

Hussey CG: Surviving a handicap in everyday life: How to help. Am J Mat Child Nurs 4:46–50, 1979

Killilea M: Karen. New York, Dell, 1960

Killilea M: With Love From Karen. New York, Dell 1964

Krugman S, Katz S: Infectious Diseases of Children, 7th ed. St Louis, CV Mosby, 1980

Kruse LC, Reese JL, Hart LK (eds): Cancer Pathophysiology, Etiology and Management. St Louis, CV Mosby, 1979

Leahy IM, St Germain JM, Varricchio CG: The Nurse and Radiotherapy: A Manual for Daily Care. St Louis, CV Mosby, 1979

Meehan RM: Isolation—To be or not to be afraid. Am J Mat Child Nurs 5:257–261, 1980

O'Neil SM, McLaughlin BN: Behavioral Approaches to Children with Developmental Delays. St Louis, CV Mosby, 1977

Selekman J: Immunization: What's it all about? Am J Nurs 80:1440–1445, 1980

Sutow WW, Vietti TJ, Fernbach DJ (eds): Clinical Pediatric Oncology. St Louis, CV Mosby, 1977

Towne CC: Disorders of hearing, speech and language. In Vaughan V, McKay R, Behrman R (eds): Nelson's Textbook of Pediatrics, 11th ed. Philadelphia, WB Saunders, 1979

Walker P: Bone marrow transplant: A second chance for life. Nurs 77 7, No 1: 24–25, 1977

Wolman IJ: The "T and A" status in 1976. In Wolman IJ (ed): Clinical Pediatrics. Philadelphia, JB Lippincott, 1976

Younger J: Detecting visual problems in children. Pediatr Nurs 5, No. 6:45E–45F, 1979

Zelle R: The developmentally disabled child and the family. In Hymovich D, Bain M: Family Health Care, Vol 2. New York, McGraw-Hill, 1979

growth and development of the school-age child: 6 to 10 years

12

student objectives

The student successfully attaining the goals of this chapter will be able to

1 Define the following vocabulary terms:

   conservation   classification   decentration   epiphysis   molars   reversibility

2 Describe the growth and development of the school-age child in the following areas: personal–social development, fine motor skills, gross motor skills, language development, and cognition.

3 Describe the elements of proper dental hygiene and explain why it is particularly important for the school-age child to acquire good hygiene habits.

4 List five actions that can be taught to school-age children and their parents that will help them become more responsible health-care consumers.

5 Discuss the points that should be considered when offering sex education to school-age children.

6 Describe four measures that may help to make hospitalization a more tolerable experience for the school-age child.

The first day of school marks a major milestone in a child's development, opening a whole new world of learning and growing. Between the ages of 6 and 10, dramatic changes occur in the child's thinking process, social skills, activities, attitudes, and use of language. The squirmy, boisterous 6-year-old with a limited attention span bears little resemblance to the more reserved 10-year-old who can become absorbed in a solitary craft activity for several hours.

Moving from the small circle of family into school and community, children begin to see differences in their own lives and the lives of others. They constantly compare their parents and siblings with other children's parents and siblings, and observe the way other children are disciplined, the foods they eat, the way they dress, and the houses they live in. Every aspect of lifestyle is subject to comparison with that of other children.

Most children reach school age with the necessary skills, abilities, and independence to function successfully in this new environment. They are able to feed and dress themselves, use the primary language of their culture to communicate their needs and feelings, and separate from their parents for extended periods of time. They show increasing interest in group activities and in making things. Erikson called this the period of industry versus inferiority.

The health of the school-age child is no longer the exclusive concern of the family, but of the community. Prior to entrance, most schools require that children have a physical examination, and that immunization records be supplied. Generally this is a healthy period in the child's life, although minor respiratory disorders and other communicable diseases can spread quickly within a classroom. Few major diseases have their onset during this period. Accidents still pose a serious hazard; therefore, safety measures are an important part of learning.

physical development

GROWTH

Between the ages of 6 and 10, growth is slow and steady. Average annual weight gain is about 7 pounds (3 kg to 3.5 kg). By age 7, the child generally weighs 7 times as much as he did at birth. Annual height increase is about 2½ inches (6 cm) per year. This period ends in the preadolescent growth spurt—in girls at about age 10 and in boys at about age 12 (Figs. 12–1 and 12–2).

DENTITION

At about age 6, the child starts to lose the deciduous (baby) teeth, usually beginning with the incisors. At about the same time, the first permanent teeth, the 6-year molars appear directly behind the deciduous molars (Fig. 12–3).

These 6-year molars are of the utmost importance; they are the key or pivot teeth that help to shape the jaw, and affect the alignment of the permanent teeth. If they are allowed to decay so severely that they must be removed, the child will encounter dental problems later on.

Education for the care of the teeth, with particular at-tention to the 6-year molars, is important (Fig. 12–4). Proper dental hygiene includes a routine inspection with cleaning and application of a fluoride, at least twice a year, and conscientious brushing after meals. A well-balanced diet with plenty of calcium and phosphorus and minimum sugar is important to healthy teeth. Foods containing sugar should be limited to mealtimes, and should be followed immediately by proper brushing.

SKELETAL GROWTH

The 6-year-old silhouette is characterized by a protruding abdomen and lordosis (swayback). By the time the child has reached age 10, the spine is straighter, the abdomen flatter, and the body generally more slender and long-legged (Fig. 12–5).

Bone growth is gradual during the school years. Cartilage is being replaced by bone at the *epiphyses* (growth centers at the end of long bones, and at the wrists). Skeletal maturation is more rapid in girls than in boys, and in blacks than in whites. Growth and development of the school-age child is summarized in Table 12–1.

nutrition

As the child's coordination improves, he becomes increasingly active, and requires more food to supply the necessary energy. Increased appetite and a tendency to go on food "jags" are typical of the 6-year-old. This stage soon passes and is unimportant if the child generally gets the necessary nutrients. It does not matter greatly if a child dislikes or refuses a certain food; he is apt to learn to like it later if his dislike is not emphasized too much. Children are more likely to learn to eat most foods if everyone else accepts them in a matter-of-fact way.

Children learn by the examples parents and others set for them. They will accept more readily the importance of manners, soft voices, and the customs associated with gracious living if they see them carried out consistently at home. Mealtime should never be used for nagging, finding fault, or correcting a child's manners. It is important to teach hygiene in a cheerful but firm manner, even if the child must leave the table more than once to be sure that his hands are clean.

Most children prefer simple, plain foods, and are good judges of their own needs if they are not coaxed, nagged, bribed, rewarded, or influenced by television commercials. Even in sickness, an average child knows enough not to eat more than is good for him. Disease or strong emotions may cause loss of appetite, but force helps little and can have harmful effects.

Parents need to carefully supervise children's snacking habits to be sure that snacks are nutritious and not too frequent, avoiding junk food and continual nibbling that can cause lack of interest at mealtime. Children need a clearly planned schedule that allows time for a good breakfast and brushing of teeth before leaving for school.

Health teaching at school should reinforce the importance of a proper diet (Table 12–2). Family and cultural food patterns are strong, however, and tend to persist despite nutritional education. Most school lunches are

Text continues on page 223.

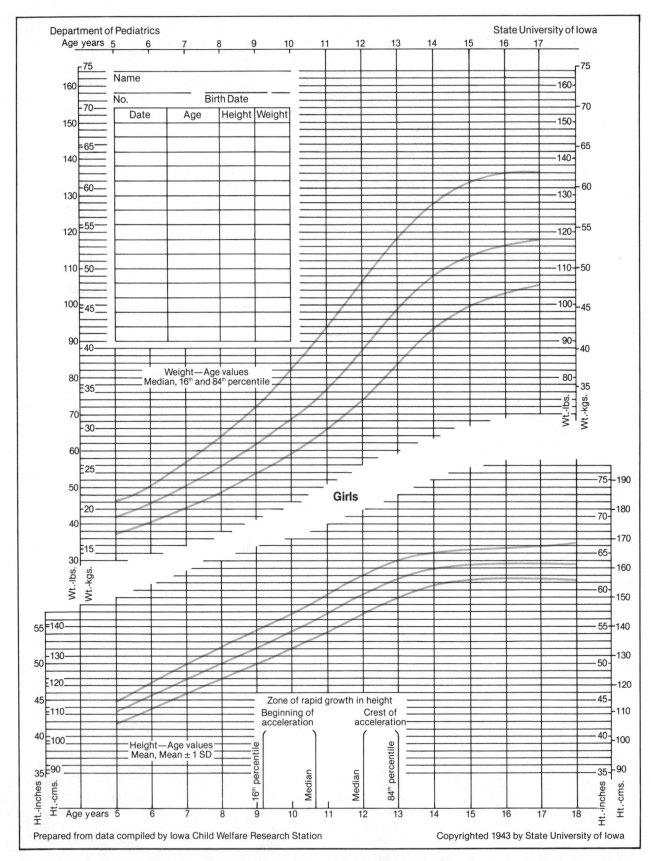

FIG. 12–1. Iowa growth chart for girls. (University of Iowa)

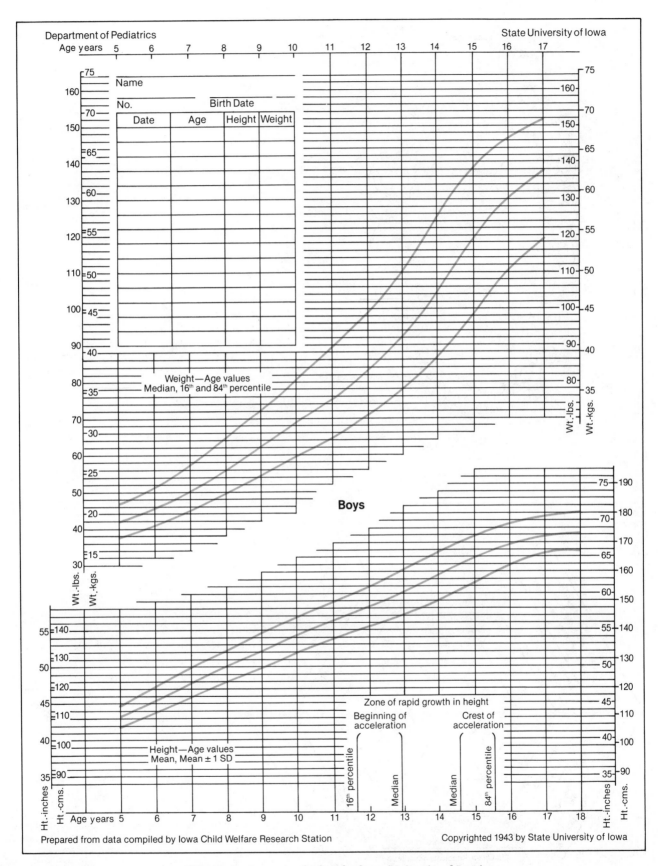

FIG. 12–2. Iowa growth chart for boys. (University of Iowa)

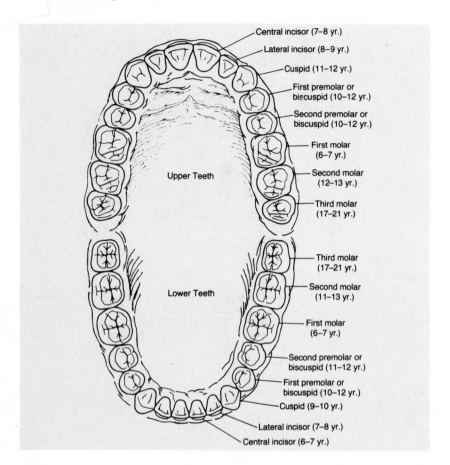

FIG. 12–3. Chart showing sequence of eruption of permanent teeth.

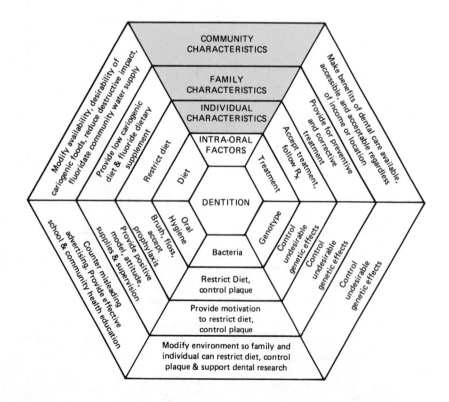

FIG. 12–4. An ecological model for preventing dental disease: intra-oral factors and individual, family, and community characteristics affecting children's dentition. (Jenny J: Preventing dental disease in children: An ecological approach. Am J Public Health 64:1152, 1974)

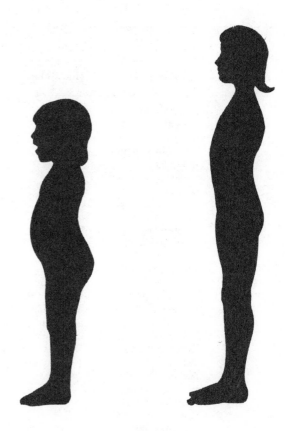

FIG. 12–5. (*Left*) Profile of a 6-year-old showing protuberant abdomen. (*Right*) Profile of a 10-year-old showing flat abdomen and four curves of adultlike spine. (Courtesy of S. Robbins)

TABLE 12–1.   GROWTH AND DEVELOPMENT CHART: THE SCHOOL-AGE CHILD

Age (years)	Personal/Social	Fine Motor	Gross Motor	Language	Cognitive
6–7	Beginning Erikson's stage of "industry vs inferiority" Adheres to predetermined rules Becoming ready to enter the larger society; to venture out into the world of peer groups, school, clubs Interacts with a small number of neighborhood youngsters in loosely organized groups Able to handle basic impulses, separate from parents, adapt to new situations	Painting, cutting, pasting Not able to control small muscles precisely Copies diamond and square Prints words, starting with name Draws a man with 12–16 parts	Improved capabilities Larger, stronger muscles Unable to sit for prolonged periods Knows right from left Can walk a chalk mark	Major speech patterns and syntax are established Able to speak the culture's dominant language Large increases in new grammatical constructions take place Can tell stories about monsters and other threats but nothing is done about them	Egocentric—believe everyone thinks as they do Continues preoperational thinking until age 7 Wants to learn all about the body: interested in functions of activities like growing, running, sneezing Sees health in concrete terms
7–8	Groups become firmly established, often sex and race segregated	Eye–hand coordination not fully developed Seems a little "clumsy"	Cautious when attempting new gross motor activities May be able to swim and ride bicycle Balance improving	Vocabulary continues to increase	Thinking becomes operational Cause and effect are now understood

(*continued*)

TABLE 12–1. *(Continued)*

Age (years)	Personal/Social	Fine Motor	Gross Motor	Language	Cognitive
7–8 *(cont.)*	Sets own elaborate rules and moral codes Looks for structure and order Spends many hours with peers Hierarchy emerges with leaders and followers rigidly determined and relatively stable over time			Story characters begin to respond to threat or trouble but do not really do much for themselves The trouble just goes away	Will learn to understand that others have thoughts and intentions; that if you hurt someone you may be hurt in return Begins to see the relationship between part and whole
8–10	Organized sports become popular Adheres rigidly to rules Fantasy and aimlessness decrease Becomes increasingly concerned with techniques and formal activities like model building	Increasing capabilities with fine motor control Uses both hands independently Draws a man with 18–20 parts	Very energetic Jumps, chases, skips, runs Tends to be more graceful and coordinated Engages in organized sports	Vocabulary continues to increase Story characters begin to react to the danger with specific and successful actions	The child's ability to get along with peers coincides with cognitive growth and the ability to understand the other's point of view Can understand weight changes Reversibility—cognitive processes can take place in opposite directions Can go through a chain of events backward to the beginning and understand how it is possible to undo something Ability to classify objects into a hierarchical arrangement growing Can recognize subclasses of a larger group (dog → animal) Concepts of birth and death become clearer but are still thought of in concrete terms Interest grows in the intricasies of bodily functions, in internal organs, and how things work Health: able to consider internal factors such as feeling states

(Wieczorek RR, Natapoff J: A Conceptual Approach to the Nursing of Children: Health Care From Birth Through Adolescence. Philadelphia, JB Lippincott, 1981)

TABLE 12–2.   RECOMMENDED FOOD INTAKE FOR THE SCHOOL-AGE CHILD

Food Group	Servings Per Day	Average Size of Servings
Milk and cheese	4	¾ = 1 cup
(1.5 oz cheese = 1 cup milk)		
(1 cup = 8 oz or 240 g)		
Meat group (protein foods)	3 or more	
Egg		1
Lean meat, fish, poultry		2–3 oz
(liver once a week)		(4–6 Tbsp)
Peanut butter		2–3 Tbsp
Fruits and Vegetables	At least 4	
Vitamin C source		1 medium orange
(twice as much tomato as citrus)		
(citrus fruits, berries, tomato, cabbage, cantaloupe)		
Vitamin A source	1 or more	¼ cup
(green or yellow fruits and vegetables)		
Other vegetables (potato and legumes, *etc*)	2	⅓ cup
or		
Other fruits (apple, banana, *etc*)		1 medium
Cereals (whole-grain or enriched)	At least 4	
Bread		1–2 slices
Ready-to-eat cereals		1 oz
Cooked cereal		½ cup
(including macaroni, spaghetti, rice, *etc*)		
Fats and carbohydrates	To meet caloric needs	
Butter, margarine, mayonnaise, oils:		2 tbsp
1 Tbsp = 100 calories (kcal)		
Desserts and sweets: 100-calorie portions as follows:		3 portions
⅓ cup pudding or ice cream		
2–3 cookies, 1 oz cake, 1⅓ oz pie,		
2 Tbsp jelly, jam, honey, sugar		

(Vaughan V, McKay J, Nelson W (eds): Nelson's Textbook of Pediatrics, p 159. Philadelphia, WB Saunders, 1976)

well-balanced meals, but often children eat only part of what they are offered.

health maintenance

DISEASE PREVENTION

Despite immunization efforts, communicable diseases still make the rounds of the schoolroom among children not immunized earlier, either by inoculation or by the disease itself. Minor respiratory diseases spread quickly and easily; therefore, children with head colds, coughs, or sore throats should be kept home from school, kept indoors during cold weather, and encouraged to rest as much as possible.

Although they dislike taking time for it, children need 10 or 11 hours of sleep during school years. Six-year-olds may need rest periods during the day as well.

Skin diseases, such as ringworm or scabies, as well as pinworm infestations, are also easily spread, although present-day school health supervision and teaching have reduced their incidence.

During the school years, children should have regular physical examinations, with hearing and vision assessments (Table 12–3). Immunizations should be brought up to date (Table 12–4).

School health programs have traditionally been concerned with disease prevention, safety, nutrition, and hygiene. Today, some innovative programs are teaching children how to take an active role in their own health care. One of these programs is Project Health PACT (Participatory and Assertive Consumer Training), developed by the faculty of the School Nurse Practitioner Program at the University of Colorado.[1] This program teaches school-age children to be responsible health-care consumers during their visits to the school nurse, physician, clinic, or hospital, by taking the following actions:

- Asking questions.
- Telling the health professional about themselves.
- Asking the health professional for health instructions.
- Participating in decisions about health; telling the health professional whether the advice is acceptable so the plan developed meets the individual's needs.
- Clarifying responsibilities for day-to-day health care before leaving the facility.

TABLE 12–3.   RECOMMENDED HEALTH-MAINTENANCE PROCEDURES FOR CHILDREN FROM AGES 6 TO 10

| Procedure | Age of Child | |
	6–8 Years	8–10 Years
Health history	Update health history with particular attention to school readiness.	Continue to update history with particular attention to school progress and indications of beginning puberty.
Physical examination	Complete physical exam with attention to neurologic development indicating school readiness or dysfunction	Complete physical examination
	Include the following:	
	Height	Same
	Weight	Hearing test may be omitted if child has had one and hearing presents no problems.
	Review of systems	
	Dental examination	
	Vision testing	
	Hearing testing	
Immunizations	None if immunizations completed prior to age 6	TB testing
Teaching and counseling	Safety	Same, with addition of anticipatory guidance about changes of puberty
	Nutrition	
	Anticipatory guidance about changes that will occur with school	
	Encourage participation in school activities by family.	
	Stress importance of peer relationships.	
	Limit-setting and regulation of after school activities	
	Assignment of chores (simple) to child to assist in establishing a sense of independence	
	Provide increasing independence and decision-making.	
	Provide activities which child can complete satisfactorily.	
	Allow regular schedule of physical activities.	

(Wieczorek RR, Natapoff J: A Conceptual Approach to the Nursing of Children: Health Care From Birth Through Adolescence. Philadelphia, JB Lippincott, 1981)

TABLE 12–4.   RECOMMENDED IMMUNIZATION SCHEDULE FOR CHILDREN 6 YEARS OF AGE AND OLDER

Schedule of Immunizations	Immunization
First visit	Tetanus-diphtheria (Td), polio
1 month after first visit	Measles, rubella, mumps
2 months after first visit	Tetanus–diphtheria (Td), polio
8–14 months after first visit	Tetanus–diphtheria (Td), polio
14–16 years	Tetanus–diphtheria (Td)—repeat every 10 years

(Public Health Service: Parents' Guide to Childhood Immunization. Washington, DC, Department of Health, Education and Welfare, 1977)

Project Health PACT has three objectives: (1) To enable students to communicate and negotiate more effectively with health professionals; (2) to develop reciprocal relationships between health consumers and providers so that health-care plans may be mutually formulated and approved; (3) to tailor the delivery of health services to the consumers' needs. Persons involved with this project believe that it contributes to better health attitudes and behaviors throughout life, thereby reducing the cost of health care and helping to control major health problems such as heart disease, cancer, stroke, alcoholism, and obesity.

SAFETY

Accidents are a leading cause of childhood death during this period. Even though school-age children do not require constant supervision, they must be taught certain safety rules, and practice them until they are routine (Fig. 12–6). They should understand the function of traffic

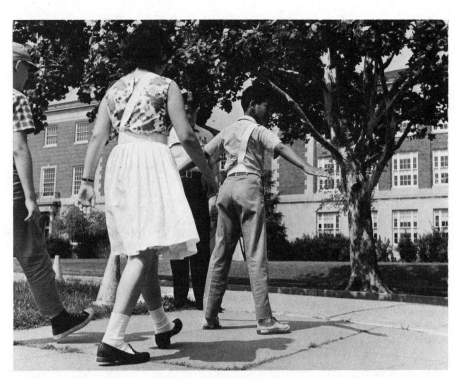

FIG. 12–6. School safety patrols in action, supervised by a police officer. (Provided by the American Automobile Association)

lights and should have watched family members obeying them as a matter of course. Children should know their full name, their parents' names, their home address and telephone number. It is helpful for them to have met and become acquainted with police officers to understand that police officers have a duty to help small children, not to punish them.

SEX EDUCATION

Children learn about femininity and masculinity from the time they are born. The mother's gentle touch, soft voice, and the smell of her body help the child associate these qualities with being a female. The father's actions toward the child, and the parents' respect and love for each other are also a part of the child's sex education and preparation for adult sexuality. Sex education means more than information about reproduction. It means helping children develop desirable attitudes toward their own bodies, their own sex and sexual role, in order to achieve optimum satisfaction in being a boy or a girl.

As children move from the *phallic* (genital) *stage* into the period described as *latency*, their range of interest broadens, but their sexual interest is still present. This interest doubtless is stimulated by the frank and frequent emphasis on sex in movies, television, and magazines. Children's questions about sex need to be answered honestly and simply; if parents do not provide answers, children seek information elsewhere, often from their peers, certainly not an authoritative source.

Parents who feel uncomfortable discussing sex with their children may find it helpful to use books or pamphlets available for various age groups. Generally, daughters and mothers find it easier to discuss sex with

each other, as do sons and fathers. This can pose special problems for the single parent with a child of the opposite sex. Here again, printed materials may be helpful.

Controversy surrounds the question of where sex education should take place, and when. Many authorities believe that it can be taught most effectively by parents who are relaxed and natural, fitting the teaching into the context of daily living. Because not all parents can meet this standard, it is important that sex education be part of the school curriculum, beginning in the early grades, rather than waiting until just before puberty.

Teachers, often aided by school nurses, can offer sex education based on what the children want to know, their developmental level, and their present knowledge of and feelings about sex. It is also important to consider each child's culture and family environment. Children who grow up on a farm are more likely to understand the process of reproduction than a child from an urban setting.

psychosocial development

The sense of duty and accomplishment occupies the years from 6 to 12. This is the period Erikson calls *industry* versus *inferiority*, during which the child is interested in engaging in real tasks and seeing them through to completion. These children direct all their energies toward mastering problems as they arise, aware that they are still children and not capable of taking an equal part in the adult world. This tends to give children a feeling of inferiority, and spurs them on to learning and experimenting more diligently. Effective completion of several personality developmental tasks should take place during these

TABLE 12–5.   PERSONALITY DEVELOPMENTAL TASKS—SCHOOL-AGE CHILD

Task	Environmental Support
Development of coping mechanisms	Stable home environment
	Examples of positive coping by caretakers and peers
Development of a sense of right and wrong by	Consistent limits with gradual lessening of restrictions
Gaining a sense of the future	Future-oriented home environment
Recognition of authority	Exposure to authority outside the home
Feeling guilty about acts not sanctioned by authority	Delineation of "rules of the game" by authority figures
Validation of feelings and actions with others	Opportunity to question the rules
in environment	Opportunity to validate own feelings and actions with others
Strengthening of a feeling of self-esteem by	Exposure to different ways of living
Gaining a sense of fit with the outside world	Opportunity to discuss these ways with peers and family
Learning when to accommodate with these forces	Positive reinforcement for opinions and actions
Gaining a feeling of satisfaction through the completion	Opportunity to adjust ways of living to fit with others despite differences
of projects	Exposure to new experiences and activities
	Development of competence in some of these activities
	Opportunity to complete projects of own choosing
Assuming body independence through	Demonstration of faith in ability to care for self
Unconscious control of bladder	Opportunity for self-care
Ability to care for own body	Pleasant eating experiences
Independence in eating and satisfaction with food itself	Role modeling

(Wieczorek RR, Natapoff J: A Conceptual Approach to the Nursing of Children: Health Care From Birth Through Adolescence. Philadelphia, JB Lippincott, 1981)

years, providing that the environmental support is adequate (Table 12–5).

No child is innately good or evil, but becomes good or bad because of the impact of his heredity, his environment, his ability to understand, and his physical health. Every child needs love and acceptance, with understanding support and concern when he makes mistakes. Children thrive on praise and will work to earn more praise and recognition.

THE CHILD FROM AGE 6 TO 7

Children in this age group are still characterized by magical thinking—the tooth fairy, Santa Claus, the Easter Bunny, and others. Keen imaginations contribute to fears, especially at night, about remote, fanciful, or imaginary events. Trouble distinguishing fantasy from reality can contribute to lying in order to escape punishment or boost self-confidence.

Children who have attended nursery school, kindergarten, or a Head Start program usually make the transition into first grade with pleasure, excitement, and little anxiety. Those who have not may find it helpful to visit school, and to experience separation from home and parents and getting along with other children on a trial basis. Most 6-year-olds are able to sit still for short periods of time and understand about taking turns. Those who have not matured sufficiently for this experience will find school unpleasant and may not do well.

Group activities are important to most 6-year-olds, even if the groups are comprised of only two or three children. They delight in learning, and show an intense interest in

every experience. Judgment about good and bad behavior is not precise, resulting in name calling and the use of vulgar words.

Between the ages of 6 and 8, children begin to enjoy participating in real-life activities, helping with gardening, housework, and other chores (Fig. 12–7). They love making things—drawings, paintings, craft projects.

THE CHILD FROM AGE 7 TO 10

Between the seventh and eighth birthdays, children begin to shake off their acceptance of parental standards as the ultimate authority, and become more impressed by the behavior of their peers. Interest in group play increases, and acceptance by the group or gang is tremendously important. These groups quickly become all boy or all girl groups, and are often project-oriented, such as Scouts or athletic teams. Secret codes and languages are popular. Individual friendships also are formed, and "best friends" are intensely loyal. Table games, and arts and crafts requiring skill and dexterity are popular, as well as more active pursuits (Fig. 12–8).

Even though parents are no longer considered the ultimate authority, their standards have become part of the child's personality and conscience. Although the child may cheat, lie, or steal on occasion, he suffers considerable guilt if he has learned that these are unacceptable behaviors.

Important changes occur in a child's thinking processes at about age 7, when there is movement from preoperational, egocentric thinking to concrete, operational, decentered thought. For the first time, children are able to see the world from someone else's point of view. *Decentration* means being able to see several aspects of a problem at the same time, and understand the relationship of various parts to the whole situation. Cause-and-effect relationships become clear; consequently, magical thinking begins to disappear.

During the seventh or eighth year, children begin to understand *conservation* of continuous quantity; for example, the volume of liquid does not change when it is poured from a tall beaker or glass to a shorter, wider container. Using concrete thinking, children can remember the previous state and compare it with the changed state of the liquid.

Understanding conservation depends upon *reversibility*, the ability to think in either direction. Children of 7 can add and subtract, count forward and backward, and see how it is possible to put something back the way it was. A child of 7 or 8 can understand that illness is probably only temporary; whereas, a 6-year-old may think it is permanent.

Another important change in thinking during this period is *classification*, the ability to group objects into a hierarchical arrangement. Children in this age group love to collect—baseball cards, insects, rocks, stamps, and coins. These collections may be only a short-term interest, but some can develop into lifetime hobbies.

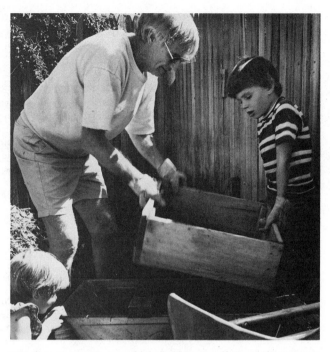

FIG. 12–7. An 8-year-old helps his grandfather sift compost while 4-year-old sister looks on. (Photo by Elizabeth McKinney Chmiel)

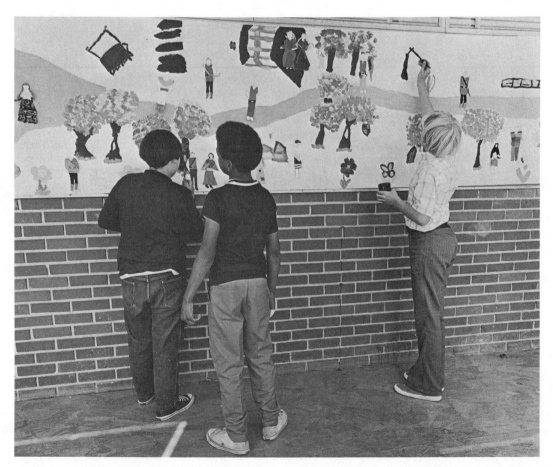

FIG. 12–8. Cooperation and creativity are achieved. (Photo by Carol Baldwin)

TABLE 12–6.   CHILDREN'S CONCEPT OF BIOLOGY

Concept	6 to 8 Years	8 to 10 Years	Implications for Nursing
Birth	Gradually see babies as the result of three factors—social, sexual intercourse, and biogenetic fusion Tend to see baby as emerging from female only; many still see baby as manufactured by outside force—created whole Boys are less knowledgeable about baby formation than girls	Begin to put three components together; recognize that sperm and egg come together but may not be sure why Less discrepancies in knowledge based on sex differences	Cultural and educational factors play a part in development of where babies come from Nurse should assess children's ideas about birth and whether they can understand where babies come from and how before teaching Explanations about role of both parents can begin but the ideal of sperm and egg union may not be understood until 8 or 9 years of age
Death	May be viewed as reversible Animism (attribution of life) may be seen in some children—death viewed as result of outside force Experiences with death facilitate concept development	Considered irreversible Ideas about what happens after death unclear—related to concreteness of thinking and socioreligious upbringing	Change from vague view of death as reversible and caused by external forces to awareness of irreversibility and bodily causes Fears about death more common at 8—adults should be alert to this Explanations about death, the fact that their thoughts will not cause a death, and they will not die (if illness is not fatal) are needed
The human body	Know body holds everything inside Use outside world to explain inside Aware of major organs Interested in visible functions of body	Can understand physiology; utilize general principles to explain body functions; interested in invisible functions of body	Cultural factors may play a part in ability and willingness to discuss bodily function. Educational programs can be very effective because of natural interest Assess knowledge of body by using diagrams before teaching.
Health	See health as doing desired activities List concrete practices as components of health Many do not see sickness as related to health; may not consider cause and effect	See health as doing desired activities Understand cause and effect Believe it is possible to be part healthy and part not at the same time; can reverse from health to sickness and back to health	Need assistance in seeing cause and effect Capitalize on positiveness of concept—health lets you do what you really want to do Young children who are sick may feel they will never get well again
Illness	Sick children may see illness as punishment; evidence suggests that healthy children do not see illness as punishment Highly anxious children more likely to view illness as disruptive Sickness is a diffuse state; rely on others to tell them when they are ill	Same as 6–8 years of age; can identify illness states; report bodily discomfort; recognize illness is caused by specific factors	Social factors play a part in illness concept Recognize that some see illness as punishment. Encourage self-care and self-help behavior, especially in older children

(Wieczorek RR, Natapoff J: A Conceptual Approach to the Nursing of Children: Health Care From Birth Through Adolescence. Philadelphia, JB Lippincott, 1981)

THE DEPRIVED CHILD

Discussions of normal growth and development assume that children come from a secure, well-adjusted home in which there is ample opportunity for social, cultural, and intellectual enrichment. This assumption unfortunately ignores a sizable population that, for many reasons, is deprived of such a background. This population is the one most likely to have health problems and needs for health services.

Children who have not been able to achieve a sense of security and trust, because of inadequate parents, broken homes, or placement in foster homes, need special understanding, warm acceptance, and intelligent guidance in order to grow into self-accepting individuals. Society seems to be gradually awakening to the needs of these children and trying to provide enriched nursery school and kindergarten experiences for those whose home life cannot do this for them.

HEAD START PROGRAMS

Recognition that environmental enrichment is frequently not available in families of limited social, cultural, and economic resources, has led to the establishment of Head Start programs. Children in such programs have an opportunity to broaden their horizons through varied experiences. Their understanding of the world they live in is increased, and they are better prepared for a successful entry into the schoolroom. Parent participation is encouraged, although this is frequently difficult for working parents.

implications for hospital care

Increased understanding of their bodies, continuing curiosity about how things work, and development of concrete thinking all contribute to helping school-age children tolerate hospitalization better than younger children. They can communicate better with caregivers, understand cause and effect, and tolerate longer separations from parents and family.

Nurses who care for school-age children should understand how concepts about birth, death, the body, health, and illness change between the ages of 6 and 10 (Table 12–6). It is important to explain all procedures to children and parents, show the equipment and materials to be used (or pictures of these), and outline realistic expectations of procedures and treatment. Children's questions should be answered truthfully, including those about pain. School-age children need privacy more than younger children, and may not want to have physical contact with adults, a wish that should be respected. They too may regress, but this regression should not be encouraged. Opportunity for interaction with peers, learning experiences, crafts, and projects can help make hospitalization more tolerable for these children (Fig. 12–9 A and B).

summary

The years between 6 and 10 are an exciting time for children and parents. Growth and development are steady at

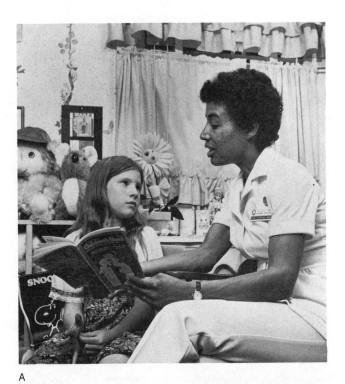

A

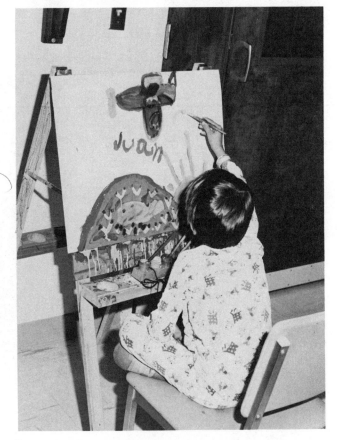

B

FIG. 12–9. (A) Eight-year-olds still like to listen to stories. (B) Young artist in the hospital playroom. (A, courtesy of J Nurs Care, Westport, Ct)

all levels—emotional, social, intellectual, and physical. Normally this is a less turbulent time than either the preschool period, or the adolescent period that is soon to follow. The school-age child gains a real sense of self, with individualized moral standards and conscience. Although much time is spent with peers in activities outside the home, the family is still the major sustaining force. Whether a child succeeds or fails in his efforts during this period can have life-long impact on attitudes and performance.

review questions

1. What are the recommended immunizations for the school-age child?
2. Proper dental hygiene includes what measures?
3. What is the leading cause of death for school-age children?
4. What points should be included in sex education?
5. What are the nursing implications concerning hospitalization of the school-age child?

references

1. Igoe JB: Project health PACT in action. Am J Nurs 80:2016–2021, 1980

bibliography

Campbell JD: Illness is a point of view: The development of children's concept of illness. Child Development 46:92–100, 1975b

Chinn PL: Child Health Maintenance: Concepts in Family Centered Care, 2nd ed. St Louis, CV Mosby Company, 1979

Chow M, Durand B, Feldman M, Mills M: Handbook of Pediatric Primary Care. New York, John Wiley & Sons, 1979

Doress B: Society's impact on families. In The Boston Women's Health Book Collective: Ourselves and Our Children. New York, Random House, 1978

Friedman S, Hoekelman R: Behavioral Pediatrics. New York, McGraw-Hill, 1980

Fong B, Resnick M: The Child: Development Through Adolescence. Menlo Park, Addison-Wesley, 1980

Hymovich D, Barnard MU: Family Health Care. New York, McGraw-Hill, 1979

Igoe JB: Project health PACT in action. Am J Nurs 80:2016–2021, 1980

Kaluger G, Kaluger MF: Human Development: The Span of Life, 2nd ed. St Louis, CV Mosby, 1979

McFarlane J, Whitson BJ, Hartley LM: Contemporary Pediatric Nursing: A Conceptual Approach. New York, John Wiley & Sons, 1980

Miller JR, Janosik EH: Family-focused Care. New York, McGraw-Hill, 1980

Natapoff J: Children's ideas about health: A developmental study. Am J Public Health 68:995–1002, 1978

Pearson G: Nutrition in the middle years of childhood. Am J Mat Child Nurs 2:378–384, 1977

Pipes P: Nutrition in Infancy and Childhood, 2nd ed. St Louis, CV Mosby, 1981

Rogaff ML: Sexual attitudes and behaviors. In Hoekelman RA (ed): Principles of Pediatrics: Health Care of the Young. New York, McGraw-Hill, 1978

Southall C: Family life and sex education. Am J Nurs 77:1473–1476, 1977

Suitor CW, Hunter MF: Nutrition: Principles and Application in Health Promotion. Philadelphia, JB Lippincott, 1980

Swarman K: Brain development in the middle childhood years. J School Health 48:289–292, 1978

Tackett JJM, Hunsburger M: Family Centered Care of Children and Adolescents. New York, McGraw-Hill, 1981

Talbot NB: Raising Children in Modern America. Boston, Little-Brown & Co, 1976

Wold SJ: School Nursing: A Framework for Practice. St Louis, CV Mosby, 1981

health problems of the school-age child

13

Devdope: industry, sense of accomplishment + duty.
Physical + motor devdopement: rate of weight gain increased + rate of height is decreased.

student objectives

The student successfully attaining the goals of this chapter will be able to

1 Define the following vocabulary terms:

acidosis agoraphobia allergen aura encopresis enuresis glycosuria
hyposensitization ketones orchiopexy polydipsia polyphagia polyuria

2 Describe the problem of school phobia and explain why early recognition and treatment is important.

3 Identify the two forms of scoliosis and explain the differences between them.

4 Identify the five types of generalized seizures and the four types of partial (focal) seizures that may be characteristic of epilepsy.

5 Describe three major clinical manifestations of rheumatic fever and discuss the treatment and nursing care of the child with this disorder.

6 Identify four complaints of a diabetic child that may lead the nurse to suspect impending insulin shock.

Entering school is a stressful time for every child, but especially for the child with a chronic health problem. Imitation of one's peers is important during this time, but sometimes impossible for the child with a learning disorder, severe allergies, or a problem that limits physical mobility. These children must cope with all the normal developmental stresses and the additional stress of being different.

School-age children can learn to manage their health problems. Given enough information and guidance, children can understand and cope with such problems as diabetes and asthma. Nurses and parents who care for these children should foster maximum independence and a life as normal as possible.

behavioral problems

SCHOOL PHOBIA

Absenteeism from school is a major national problem. For example, in New York City, 200,000 children are absent from school each day.[1] Some of these absences are due to illness, some to truancy, and others to school phobia, a reluctance to go to school, due either to fear of the school situation, fear of leaving home and parents, or both. No statistics are available on how many absences are due to truancy, but one authority estimated that 3 children per 1000 experienced severe school phobia, and another 7 per 1000 were affected by mild school phobia.[2] This problem affects more girls than boys, but no particular age group predominates.

Children who develop school phobia are usually good students, unlike truant children whose academic performances are generally below average. School phobic children have a strong attachment to one parent, usually the mother, and fear separation from that parent. Parents unconsciously can reinforce the school phobia by permitting the child to stay home. These children learn quickly that illness is the most valid reason for staying home from school, and show very genuine symptoms such as vomiting, diarrhea, abdominal or other pain, and even a low-grade fever. The symptoms disappear as soon as the parent has given permission to stay home.

School phobia needs to be recognized and treated early; otherwise, serious problems can develop in later life, such as agoraphobia (fear of going out in open places), frequent absenteeism in the work setting, and frequent job changes.[3]

Treatment includes complete medical examination to rule out any organic cause for the symptoms, followed by return of the child to school, after conferences with child and parents. The school nurse, the teacher, and other health professionals such as a social worker, psychologist, or psychiatrist may all contribute to the resolution of this problem. If a specific factor in the school setting is feared, such as an overcritical teacher, the child may need to be moved to another class or another school.

CHILDHOOD SCHIZOPHRENIA (LATE-ONSET PSYCHOSIS)

Psychosis that develops in children between the ages of 6 and 10 has some of the same characteristics as infant autism: poorly developed speech or no speech, ritualistic, self-stimulating behaviors, intolerance for change in the environment, temper tantrums, and the absence of a sense of self. Like autism, childhood schizophrenia limits the child's personality and cognitive development, and threatens the integrity of the family.

Many theories exist about the causes of childhood schizophrenia, ranging from biochemical or other organic cause, to inadequate parent–child relationships. It is known that children of parents with schizophrenia are much more likely to develop the disorder than children of mentally healthy parents. Controversy exists about whether childhood schizophrenia is a single disorder or a group of disorders that includes both organic and environmental factors.

Since the cause or causes are unknown, treatment of this disorder is based on modifying the child's behavior to help him organize his thinking and cope with reality.[4] The bizarre behavior of these children is tremendously difficult for parents and professionals to deal with, and requires long, intensive, and expensive therapy with no guarantee that the children will become functional adults. Characteristics of these children and their families are summarized in Table 13–1.

Three principal types or models of treatment for childhood psychosis have been identified by Hageman as follows:[5] the *medical model* (diagnosis and short-term treatment in hospitals); the *educational model* (structured educational program in residential or day-school setting); and the *social service model* (supportive home environment for children without family support). Home care is preferable whenever possible, unless it proves too disruptive for other family members. Interim-care centers in the community afford temporary relief for families who want to care for their child at home most of the time.

Drug therapy may be part of the total treatment; tranquilizers and antidepressants are most commonly used. These drugs do not cure the disorder, but can enable the therapist to break through to the child, making possible other forms of treatment.

allergic reactions in children

Millions of Americans suffer from allergic diseases, most of which begin in childhood. An allergic ailment is caused by sensitivity to a specific substance, such as pollen, mold, certain foods, and drugs. That substance is called an *allergen*. Many areas of the body are sensitive to allergens, the most common being the nose, throat, eyes, bronchial tissues in the lungs, the skin, and the digestive tract. When an allergen comes into contact with one of these sensitive areas, it causes a release of certain substances, such as histamine, which produces the symptoms known as allergy. Common allergic reactions in children are summarized in Table 13–2.

One national survey suggests that one third of all chronic childhood conditions are due to allergy.[6] Millions of children with allergies are hampered by poor appetite, poor sleep, restricted physical activity in play and at school, often resulting in altered physical and personality development.

TABLE 13–1. HYPOTHESIZED CHARACTERISTICS OF CHILDREN WITH CHILDHOOD PSYCHOSIS (SCHIZOPHRENIA) AND THEIR FAMILIES

Children*	Families†
Ritualistic behavior	One parent schizophrenic in 10–16% of cases
Whirling, dancing, robotlike walking	Two parents schizophrenic in 35–45% of cases
Self-mutilation	High incidence of emotional disorders in siblings
Self-stimulating behaviors	Parental perplexity, paralysis
Intolerance of change	Failure to define clear boundaries
Faulty use of self	Rigid relationships
Faulty perceptual processing	Failure to maintain appropriate roles
Absent sense of self-boundaries	Use child to satisfy need not met by other parent
Rigid stereotyped speech	History of trauma during early life of child
Echolalia	Marital discord
Mutism	Cold, distant, "frozen"
Faulty time orientation	Failure to impart cultural techniques
Strange memory feats	Confused communications with double messages
Compulsive behaviors	Some evidence of increased catecholamines in identical twins
Hallucinations	
Assumes nonhuman identity	
Temper tantrums	
Impaired human relationships	
Evidence of increased dopamine and	
Serotonin levels (catecholamines)	

* Represents consensus of literature

† Frequently cited but not proven

(Wieczorek RR, Natapoff J: A Conceptual Approach to the Nursing of Children: Health Care From Birth Through Adolescence. Philadelphia, JB Lippincott 1981)

Children whose parents or grandparents have allergies are more likely to become allergic than other children. There are hundreds of allergens; some of the most common are pollen, mold, dust, animal danders, nuts, chocolate, milk, fish, and shellfish. Drugs can be allergens too, particularly aspirin and penicillin. Some plants and chemicals cause allergic reactions on the skin.

Diagnosis of the allergic ailment requires a careful history and physical examination, and possibly skin tests and blood tests. Skin testing is generally done when removal of obvious inhalants is not possible or has not brought relief. If a food allergy is suspected, an "elimination" diet may help to identify the allergen. When specific allergens have been identified, patients can either avoid them, or if this is not possible, undergo immunization therapy by injection, called *hyposensitization* or immunotherapy.

Hyposensitization is performed for those allergens that produced a positive reaction on skin testing. The allergist sets up a schedule for injections in gradually increasing doses until a maintenance dose is reached. The patient should remain in the doctor's office for 20 to 30 minutes following injection, in case any reaction occurs. Reactions are treated with adrenalin. Severe reactions in children are uncommon, and hyposensitization is considered a safe procedure with considerable benefit for some children.

Symptomatic relief in allergic reactions can be gained through antihistamine or steroid therapy; however, the best treatment is prevention.

ALLERGIC RHINITIS (HAY FEVER, ROSE FEVER)

Allergic rhinitis in children is most often due to sensitization to animal danders, house dust, pollens, and molds. Pollen allergy seldom appears before 4 or 5 years of age.

Symptoms. A watery nasal discharge, postnasal drip, sneezing, and allergic conjunctivitis are the usual symptoms of allergic rhinitis. Continued sniffing, itching of the nose and palate, and the "allergic salute" (Fig. 13–1) are common complaints. Discoloration under the eyes is typical (Fig. 13–2).

Treatment. When possible, offending allergens are avoided or removed from the environment. Antihistamine–decongestant preparations such as Dimetapp or Actifed can be very helpful for some patients. Hyposensitization can be implemented, particularly if antihistamines are not helpful or are needed chronically.

ASTHMA

Asthma is a spasm of the bronchial tubes due to hypersensitivity of the airways in the bronchial system. This reversible obstructive airway disease affects at least 9 million people in the United States, of which more than 1 million are children under age 15.

TABLE 13-2. COMMON ALLERGIC REACTIONS IN CHILDREN

Allergic Manifestation	Description
Allergic rhinitis	Usually called *hayfever* by lay public. Seasonal rhinitis is a symptom complex of sneezing, rhinorrhea, nasal obstruction, itching of nose, palate, pharynx, and ears in response to pollens.
	Perennial rhinitis is present all year round with same symptoms as seasonal variety. House dust and molds, foods, and pets are common offenders. The allergy begins during pre-school years in many children.
Asthma	Leading cause of school absence from a chronic respiratory problem, characterized by bronchospasm, expiratory wheezing, dyspnea, cyanosis, tachypnea, and excessive mucus production. Pollens, irritant fumes, changes in air temperature, exercise, house dust and molds, and similar inhalants are common causes. It begins in early childhood (2 to 3 years of age), peaks during school years, and may decrease slightly after puberty.
Eczema	Atopic dermatitis is characterized by erythema, pruritis, exudation, crusting and scaling of face, neck, wrists, and hands. May cover extensor surfaces of extremities and trunk in severe cases. Begins in first months of life and continues for several years. Food is the most common allergen.
Food	Called the "great masquerader" because any system of the body can become involved.
Urticaria (Hives)	Skin reaction characterized by erythematous, raised, pruritic skin lesions. Inhalants, drugs, and some foods are common allergens.
Insect bites	Respiratory, local cutaneous, or anaphylactic reaction to an insect bite (most commonly a bee in the United States)
Anaphylaxis	Immediate reaction to a foreign substance, frequently a drug. Characterized by facial tingling, feeling of warmth, tightness in chest, respiratory stridor, sneezing, wheezing, abdominal cramps, contractions of smooth muscles, cardiopulmonary arrest, and possible death. It is rare in childhood.
Drug sensitivity	Adverse reaction to a drug involving all or any one of the body systems. Common during neonatal period, then rare during childhood. Rashes, nausea, vomiting, and diarrhea are the most common effects. Anaphylaxis is rare, but can occur. Drug reactions may be divided into toxic reactions, side-effects, and allergies.
Tension–fatigue syndrome	Most important reaction in central nervous system, triggered by inhalant and food allergy. Characterized by motor fatigue, listlessness, irritability, motor and sensory tension, inability to please, and sometimes abdominal pain and headache. It is rare in infancy, but increases in frequency with age.

(Wieczorek RR, Natapoff J: A Conceptual Approach to the Nursing of Children: Health Care From Birth Through Adolescence. Philadelphia, JB Lippincott, 1981)

Etiology.   Asthma attacks are often triggered by an allergic response to allergens; in young children, asthma may be the response to certain foods. Asthma can frequently be triggered by exercise, exposure to cold weather, or such irritants as cigarette smoke. Infections, such as bronchitis or a urinary tract infection, can frequently cause asthma attacks. In children who have asthmatic tendencies, emotional stress or anxiety can trigger an attack.

Pathophysiology.   Spasms of the smooth muscles cause the lumina of the bronchi and bronchioles to narrow. Edema of the mucous membrane lining these bronchial branches, and increased production of thick mucus within them, combine with the spasm to cause respiratory obstruction.

Clinical Manifestations.   The onset of an attack may be very abrupt, or it may progress over several days, evidenced by a hacking cough, wheezing, and difficult breathing. Asthmatic attacks frequently occur at night, waking the child from his sleep. The child has to sit up and is totally preoccupied with his efforts to breathe. Attacks may last for only a short time or may continue for several days. Thick, tenacious mucus may be coughed up. In some asthmatic patients, coughing is the major symptom, and wheezing occurs rarely, if at all. tight chest

Diagnosis.   Pulmonary function tests are the most valuable diagnostic tools. These tests indicate the amount of obstruction in the bronchial airways, especially in the smallest airways of the lungs. A definitive diagnosis of asthma is made when the obstruction in the airways is reversed with bronchodilators.

Treatment. *Bronchodilators* are the drugs of choice for treatment of asthma. These drugs are divided into two groups: theophylline preparations and adrenergic, or sympathomimetic, drugs.

Theophylline preparations are available in short-acting and long-acting forms. The short-acting forms such as Theon and Elixicon liquids and aminophylline rectal suppositories are given approximately every 6 hours. These are most effective when used by the patient, as needed, for intermittent episodes of asthma, because they enter the bloodstream quickly.

Long-acting preparations of theophylline, such as Theo-Dur tablets and Theophyl SR capsules are given every 8 to 12 hours. They are helpful in patients who continually need medication because these drugs sustain more consistent theophylline levels in the blood than the short-acting forms. Patients hospitalized for status asthmaticus receive theophylline intravenously.

The adrenergic, or sympathomimetic, drugs used with theophylline preparations include metaproterenol sulfate (Alupent or Metaprel) and terbutaline sulfate (Brethine). They are short-acting and available in liquid or pill form. These drugs are administered every 6 to 8 hours if breathing difficulty continues despite theophylline. In severe attacks, adrenalin by subcutaneous injection often affords quick relief of symptoms. Also, some bronchodilators can be given in inhalant form, such as Metaprel or Bronchosol.

Side effects of these medications are usually dose-related. Theophylline can cause nausea, vomiting, loss of appetite, and headaches if the dose is too high for the patient to tolerate or if the patient is particularly sensitive. Diuresis is sometimes a side effect, and can result in enuresis during drug use. In very high doses, these medications can cause seizures. In some patients, restlessness or agitation may occur. In most patients these side effects disappear if the dosage is decreased.

Terbutaline can cause tremors in skeletal muscles and increased awareness of one's heartbeat. These are normal side effects, and not a cause for alarm. Often these effects will diminish with continued use of the medication or a decrease in dosage.

Steroids are used in severe or very chronic cases of asthma, but must be used with great care, and are prescribed only after other medications have failed to produce the desired effects.

Combination medications, such as Tedral and Marax, are of little value in the modern treatment of asthma.

Breathing Exercises. Because asthma has multiple causes, treatment and continuing management of the disease require more than medication. Studies have shown that breathing exercises to improve respiratory function and help control asthma attacks can be an important adjunct to treatment. Although not taught routinely, these exercises teach children how to help control their own symptoms, and thereby build self-confidence, sometimes lacking in asthmatic children. If the exercises can be taught as part of play activities, children are more likely to

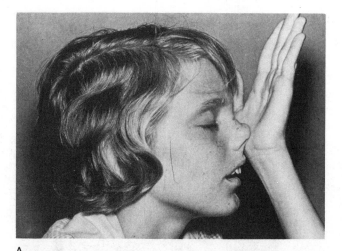

A

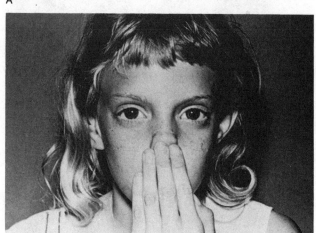

B

FIG. 13–1.   Allergic salute—(A) The allergic child often pushes his nose upward and backward to relieve itching and to free edematous turbinates from contact with the septum. This allows for free passage of air. (B) The allergic salute induces transverse nasal crease. (The Upjohn Company, Kalamazoo, Michigan, and M.B. Marks, M.D., Miami, Florida)

find them fun and to practice them more often.[8] Figure 13–3 shows three examples.

Families who must cope with asthma or other allergies need to be aware of national and community resources. Some of these are summarized in the boxed material.

Skin disorders thought to be allergic in origin are discussed later in this chapter; infantile eczema is discussed in Health Problems of the Infant, Chapter 7.

gastrointestinal system

APPENDICITIS

Appendicitis is rare in infancy. Most cases in childhood occur after the fourth year. In young children the symptoms may be difficult to evaluate.

Obstruction of the lumen of the appendix is the primary

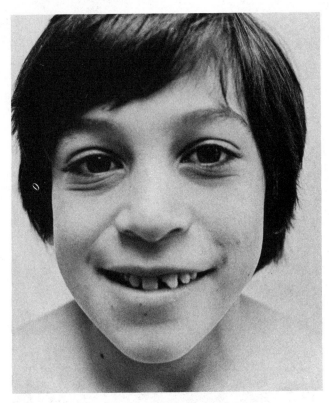

FIG. 13–2. Typical facies of allergic rhinitis. (Photo by Marcia Lieberman)

cause. The obstruction may follow a generalized infection or occasionally an infestation of pinworms.

Clinical Manifestations. Symptoms in the older child may be the same as in an adult: pain and tenderness in the right lower quadrant of the abdomen, nausea and vomiting, fever, and constipation. These symptoms are infrequent in young children, many of whom have a ruptured appendix when first seen by the physician. The young child has difficulty localizing pain, may act restless and irritable, have a slight fever, flushed face, and rapid pulse. Usually the white cell count is slightly elevated. It may take several hours to rule out other conditions and make a positive diagnosis. Laxatives and enemas are contraindicated because they increase peristalsis, and thereby enhance the possibility of rupturing the appendix.

Treatment. Surgical removal of the appendix is the necessary procedure and should be performed as soon as possible after diagnosis.

If the appendix has not ruptured previous to surgery, the operative risk is nearly negligible. Even after perforation has occurred, mortality rate is less than 1%.

Food and fluids by mouth are withheld prior to surgery. If the child is dehydrated, intravenous fluids will be ordered. If fever is present, temperature should be reduced to below 102° F.

Recovery is rapid and usually uneventful. The child is ambulated early and is able to leave the hospital a few days after surgery. In the unusual case where peritonitis or a localized abscess is a complication, gastric suction, parenteral fluids, and antibiotics may be ordered.

complication is peritinitis

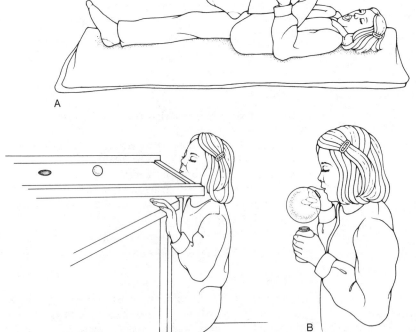

FIG. 13–3. Breathing exercises for asthmatic children, being taught as part of play activities. *A* demonstrates one exercise that introduces a child to the technique of breathing exercises. During this exercise the child raises her knee slowly to her chest, at the same time breathing out and tightening her abdominal muscles. *B* illustrates that bubble blowing can be incorporated into exercising. *C* shows a game as an exercise which is scored by the number of breaths it takes to get the ball through the hole. The lowest number wins. All these activities help to increase lung capacity and respiratory control. (McCaully HE: Breathing exercises as play for asthmatic children. Am J Maternal Child Nurs 5:340–344, 1980)

RESOURCES FOR PERSONS WHO LIVE WITH ALLERGIES

Allergy Identification Items

American Medical Association
535 N. Dearborn Street
Chicago, Illinois 60610

EMI, Inc
P.O. Box 5114
Englewood, Florida 33533

Medic Alert Foundation
P.O. Box 1009
Turlock, California 95380

National Identification Company
3955 Oneida Street
Denver, Colorado 80207

Insect Sting Kits

Center Laboratories
35 Channel Drive
Port Washington, New York 11050
  (immunity kit available by prescription)

Hollister-Stier Laboratories
P.O. Box 19957
Atlanta, Georgia 30325
  (emergency treatment kit available
  by prescription)

Non-Allergic Products

Allergen-Proof Encasings
1450 E. 363rd Street
Eastlake, Ohio 44094

General Allergy Information

Asthma and Allergy Foundation of America
19 W. 44th Street
New York, New York 10036

National Institutes of Allergy and Infectious Disease
National Institutes of Health
Bethesda, Maryland 20014

American Lung Association
1740 Broadway
New York, New York 10019
  (contact local association)

Cooking Aids

Chicago Dietetic Supply, Inc.
405 E. Shawmut Avenue
LaGrange, Illinois 60525

Wuest Laboratories and Diet Bakeries, Inc.
176 Sherman Avenue
Jersey City, New Jersey 07307

U.S. Department of Agriculture
Consumer and Food Economics Research Division
Agricultural Research Services
Bureau of Home Economics
Beltsville, Maryland 20705

INTESTINAL PARASITES

ENTEROBIASIS (OXYURIASIS, PINWORM INFECTION)

Etiology. The pinworm, *Enterobius vermicularis*, is a white, threadlike worm which invades the cecum and may enter the appendix.

Epidemiology. Pinworms are spread from person to person by articles contaminated with pinworm eggs. The infestation is common among children.

Infestation occurs when the pinworm eggs are swallowed. The eggs hatch in the intestinal tract and grow to maturity in the cecum. The female worm, when ready to lay her eggs, crawls out of the anus and lays the eggs on the child's perineum.

Itching around the anus causes the child to scratch and trap new eggs under his fingernails, where frequently he reinfects himself when he puts his fingers in his mouth. Clothing, bedding, food and other articles become infected, and the infestation spreads to other members of the family.

The life cycle of these worms is from 6 to 8 weeks, after which reinfestation commonly occurs unless treated. The condition appears most frequently in school-age children and next highest in the preschool age. Other members of the family are also susceptible.

Identification. Capturing the eggs from around the anus by the use of scotch tape, and examining under a microscope is the usual method. As they emerge from the anus, adult worms may also be seen when the child is lying quietly or sleeping.

The Scotch-tape test for identifying worms is carried out as follows:

1. Wind Scotch tape around the end of a tongue blade, sticky side outward.
2. Spread the child's buttocks and press the tape against the anus, rolling from side to side.
3. Transfer the tape to a microscope slide and cover with a clean slide to send to the laboratory.
4. Tape is examined microscopically in the laboratory for eggs.

The most favorable time for finding pinworms or their eggs is in the early morning before the child wakens.

weight loss, anorexia, grinds teeth hs, scratching.

Prevention and Treatment. The child should be taught to wash his hands after bowel movements and before eating, and to observe other hygienic measures such as regular bathing and frequent change of underclothing. Fingernails should be kept short and clean. Bedding should also be changed frequently to avoid reinfestation.

Treatment consists in the use of vermifuge medications. Povan and Antepar are most commonly used.

antihelmetic.

ROUNDWORMS

Ascaris lumbricoides is a large intestinal worm found only in humans. Infestation is from the feces of infested persons. It is usually found in areas where sanitary facilities are lacking and human excreta is deposited on the ground.

The adult worm is pink and from 9 to 12 inches in length. The eggs hatch in the intestinal tract and the larvae migrate to the liver and lungs. The larvae reaching the lungs ascend up through the bronchi, are swallowed and reach the intestines where they grow to maturity and mate. Eggs are then discharged into the feces. Full development requires about 2 months. In tropical countries where infestation may be heavy, bowel obstructions may present serious problems. Generally, however, no symptoms are present in ordinary infestations.

Identification. Microscopic examination of feces for eggs.

Treatment. Antepar is the specific medication. Improved hygienic conditions are necessary to prevent infestation.

HOOKWORMS

Etiology. The hookworm lives in the human intestinal tract where it attaches itself to the wall of the small intestine. Eggs are discharged in the feces of the host.

These parasites are prevalent in areas where infected human excreta is deposited on the ground and the soil, moisture and temperature are favorable for the development of infective larvae of the worm. In the southeastern United States and tropical West Africa the prevailing species is *Necator americanus.* In other parts of the world both this species and *Ancylostoma duodenale* are present.

Epidemiology. After feces containing eggs are deposited on the ground, larvae hatch. Usually they penetrate the skin of barefoot persons. They produce an itching dermatitis (ground itch). The larvae pass through the bloodstream to the lungs and into the pharynx where they are swallowed and reach the small intestine where they attach themselves to the intestinal wall. Heavy infestation may cause anemia through loss of blood to the worms. Chronic infestation produces listlessness, fatigue and malnutrition.

Identification is made by examination of the stool under the microscope.

Treatment. Specific medications to control the infection will be ordered by the physician.

The infected child will need a well-balanced diet with additional protein and iron. Transfusions are rarely necessary.

musculoskeletal system

SCOLIOSIS

Scoliosis is a lateral curvature of the spine that appears most frequently in young girls during the rapid growth period before puberty. It occurs in two forms, *structural* and *nonstructural* (functional), the latter being the more common. Structural scoliosis is caused by rotated and malformed vertebrae. Nonstructural scoliosis can have several causes: poor posture, muscle spasm due to trauma, an unequal length of legs. When the primary problem is corrected, elimination of the functional scoliosis has begun.

Most cases of structural scoliosis are idiopathic; a few are due to congenital deformities or infection. Treatment is by application of braces, casts, traction, and spinal fusion, which may include internal fixation with rods. The brace most commonly used is the Milwaukee brace, which exerts pressure on certain areas to maintain correct posture or immobilization. Other devices include the turnbuckle cast and the Risser jacket, discussed more fully in Chapter 19, The Child with Mobility Problems.

SYNOVITIS

A condition of unknown causes, synovitis of the hip occurs more frequently in boys than girls of early school age. Symptoms are pain in the hip or knee, and a limp. The joint later fills with fluid, causing additional pain that is relieved by lying down with the hip in a position of flexion, abduction, and external rotation. Bedrest and avoidance of weight-bearing will usually clear up the condition within 2 weeks, after which, activity may be gradually increased. If pain and spasm persist, Buck's traction may be applied. This condition is likely to recur, and about 5% of these children will develop Legg-Calvé-Perthes disease.

LEGG-CALVÉ-PERTHES DISEASE (OSTEOCHRONDROSIS OF THE HIP)

Legg-Calvé-Perthes disease is an aseptic necrosis of the head of the femur, occurring four to five times more often in boys than in girls and ten times more often in whites than in blacks. It can be caused by trauma to the hip but generally the cause is unknown. Symptoms that mimic synovitis make immediate diagnosis difficult. Radiographic examination is necessary for definitive diagnosis.

There are three stages of the disease. In the first, radiographic studies show opacity of the epiphysis. In the second, the epiphysis becomes mottled and fragmented, and during the third stage, reossification occurs. Each stage lasts from 9 months to 1 year.

Blood supply to hip joint is temporarily disturbed.

Immobilization of the hip is essential for recovery without deformity; therefore, the most important aspect of treatment is avoidance of weight-bearing. Several methods can be employed to achieve this, including the use of braces and crutches, bedrest with traction, or casting. Recent advances have made surgical correction possible and enable the child to return to normal activities within 3 to 4 months, as compared with 2 to 3 years for conservative treatment. Complete recovery without difficulty later in life depends on the age of the child at the time of onset, the amount of involvement, and the cooperation of the child and parents.

OSTEOMYELITIS

Osteomyelitis is an infection of the bone usually caused by the *Staphylococcus aureus*. Acute osteomyelitis is twice as common in boys and results from a primary infection such as a staphyloccocal skin infection. The bacteria enter the bloodstream and are carried to the metaphysis of a bone, where an abscess forms, ruptures, and spreads the infection along the bone under the periosteum.

Symptoms usually begin abruptly with fever, malaise, pain and localized tenderness over the metaphysis of the affected bone. There is limitation of joint motion.

Diagnosis is based on laboratory findings of leukocytosis of 15,000 to 25,000 cells or more, and on positive blood cultures. Radiographic examination does not reveal the process until 5 to 10 days after the onset.

Treatment for acute osteomyelitis must be immediate. Antibiotic therapy is started at once, and surgical drainage of the involved metaphysis is performed. If the abscess has ruptured into the subperiosteal space, chronic osteomyelitis follows.

Prognosis can be favorable if prompt specific antibiotic treatment, vigorously employed, brings acute osteomyelitis under rapid control and prevents the extensive bone destruction of chronic osteomyelitis. Relief of pain and immobilization of the affected joint are other aspects of treatment. If extensive destruction of bone has occurred before treatment, surgical removal of necrotic bone becomes necessary.

There are many orthopaedic conditions that occur infrequently among children and young people. These are discussed more fully in orthopaedic texts, some of which are listed in the bibliography at the end of this chapter.

MUSCULAR DYSTROPHY (MD)

The most common form of muscular dystrophy is Duchenne (pseudohypertrophic) muscular dystrophy. An X-linked recessive hereditary disease, it occurs almost exclusively in males and is carried by females. When muscular dystrophy has been diagnosed in a child, the mother and the siblings should be tested to see if they have the disease, or are carriers.

Can be detected by amnioscentesis.
Progressive wasting away of muscles

First signs are noted in childhood or infancy when the child finds it difficult to stand or walk; later, trunk muscle weakness develops. Mild mental retardation often accompanies this disease. The child is unable to rise easily to an upright position from a sitting position on the floor. He rises by "climbing up" his lower extremities with his

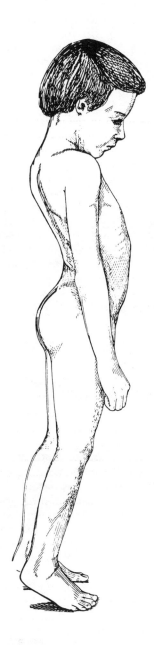

FIG. 13–4. Characteristic posture of a child with Duchenne muscular dystrophy. Along with the typical toe gait, the child develops a lordotic posture as Duchenne dystrophy causes further deterioration. (Brady MH: Lifelong care of the child with Duchenne muscular dystrophy. Am J Mat Child Health 4, No. 4: 227–230, 1979)

TABLE 13–3.   NATURAL COURSE OF DUCHENNE MUSCULAR DYSTROPHY

Approximate Age (Yr)	Progression of Muscular Involvement	Result	Adaptation
2–5	Weakness of gluteus maximus	Lumbar lordosis Gower's sign	Increasing use of hamstring muscles
	Weakness of tensor fascia lata and iliotibial tract	Shortening of iliotibial tract	Widening of gait and standing posture
	Weakness of quadriceps	Knee stabilization compromised	Rising on toes to stand and walk with knees flexed so that weight line is in front of knee and behind hips.
	Imbalance of muscles of feet	Falling	Inversion of the feet
	Flexion of knees	Extension of trunk	Increased lumbar lordosis and flexion of head to maintain weight line
	Ankle flexion	Head resting on chest	This is the final adaptation to maintain a standing posture. A wheelchair is necessary when this no longer works.
8–12	*In Wheelchair* Lateral flexion of trunk toward the nondominant extremity as shoulder muscles become weak	Elevation and abduction of shoulders and dominant extremity	Scoliosis with convexity toward dominant extremity

(Wieczorek RR, Natapoff J: A Conceptual Approach to the Nursing of Children: Health Care From Birth Through Adolescence. Philadelphia, JB Lippincott, 1981)

hands. Weakness of leg, arm, and shoulder muscles progresses gradually (Table 13–3). The victim becomes progressively weaker and usually succumbs to cardiac failure or pneumonia in early adult life (Fig. 13–4).

The patient is encouraged to be as active as possible to delay muscle atrophy and contractures. Physiotherapy, diet to avoid obesity, and parental encouragement help keep the child active.

Once a child becomes bound to a wheelchair, respiratory function decreases and infections increase. Breathing exercises are a daily necessity for these children.

Parents are advised to make the child's life as normal as possible, which is certainly not an easy task. This disease can drain the emotional and financial reserves of the entire family. Some assistance can be found through The Muscular Dystrophy Association of America, 810 Seventh Avenue, New York, New York 10019, through local chapters of this organization, and through talking with other parents who face the same problem. No effective treatment for the disease has been found.

genitourinary system

CRYPTORCHIDISM

Shortly before or soon after birth, the male gonads (testes) descend from the abdominal cavity into their normal position in the scrotum. Occasionally one or both of the testes do not descend, a condition called *cryptorchidism* (Fig. 13–5). The testes are usually normal in size; the cause for nondescent is not clearly understood.

The testes may descend any time before puberty. A testis that has not descended before puberty will begin to degenerate and become nonfunctioning. If both testes remain undescended the male will be sterile.

A surgical procedure called *orchiopexy* is used before puberty to bring the testis down into the scrotum and anchor it there. Some physicians prefer to try medical treatment before doing surgery. This consists of administration of a gonadotropic hormone, usually given during the preschool period. If this is not successful in bringing the testis down, orchidopexy will be done. Surgeons differ in their opinion as to when this operation should be performed, some preferring to wait until the child is 10 or 11 years old. *between 2–3 yrs.*

The testis will be held in position in the scrotum by a suture placed there during surgery. This suture will be attached to a rubber band which has been secured to the child's thigh with adhesive tape. This attachment will be removed 5 to 7 days after surgery. However, the child is encouraged to resume normal activity on recovery from anesthesia. Prognosis for a normal functioning testicle is good if no degenerative action has taken place before treatment.

Hope they descend by 1 yr.

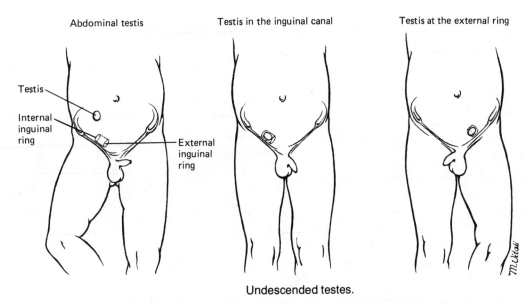

Abdominal testis   Testis in the inguinal canal   Testis at the external ring

Testis

Internal inguinal ring

External inguinal ring

Undescended testes.

FIG. 13–5. Undescended testes. (Wieczorek RR, Natapoff J: A Conceptual Approach to the Nursing of Children: Health Care From Birth Through Adolescence. Philadelphia, JB Lippincott, 1981)

ENURESIS

Enuresis is a term used for involuntary urination beyond the age when control of urination should have been acquired. Many children do not acquire complete nighttime control before 5 to 7 years of age, and an occasional bed wetting may be seen in children as late as 9 or 10 years of age. Boys have more difficulty than girls, and in some cases enuresis may persist into the adult years.

Persistent bed wetting in a child of 5 or 6 is often due to too vigorous toilet training before the child is physiologically ready. Neurotic enuresis in the older child may express resentment toward parents or a desire to regress to an earlier level in order to receive more care and attention. Occasionally persistent bed wetting may have a physiologic cause. It is also believed that the child is a very sound sleeper and not aware of the signal to empty the bladder. The child should have an examination to rule out any abnormality.

Nagging and punishment will only increase the child's anxiety. Efforts should be made to discover the cause of emotional stress. If the child is interested in achieving control, as for instance in order to go to camp or visit friends overnight, waking him during the night to go to the toilet, or limiting fluids before retiring may be helpful. These measures should not be used as a replacement for searching for the cause, however. In deeply disturbed persons, help from a psychiatrist may be needed.

ENCOPRESIS

Encopresis is the chronic involuntary fecal soiling beyond the age when control is expected (about age 3). Speech and learning disabilities may accompany this problem. If there is no organic cause, encopresis indicates a serious emotional problem and the need for counseling the child and the parents. It is believed that parental overcontrol or un-

dercontrol can cause encopresis. Recommendations for treatment differ; the most important aspect, however, is recognition of the problem and referral for treatment and counseling.

central nervous system

MINIMAL BRAIN DYSFUNCTION

Minimal brain dysfunction (MBD) has been used interchangeably with the terms *learning disability* or *learning disorder* (LD), and there is little agreement on a precise definition among professionals in education and health care. The cause or causes of minimal brain dysfunction are also surrounded by controversy. Some theories suggest biochemical disturbance or actual brain injury, others state that MBD results from impaired parent–child interaction or an adverse reaction to food additives. Although the cause is still in question, MBD is a common problem that surfaces during the school years and affects from 5% to 20% of school-age children, and more than five times as many boys as girls. These are children with normal or above normal intelligence.

Wieczorek and Natapoff describe MBD as a syndrome characterized by certain behavioral and perceptual disturbances and psychomotor difficulties in varying degrees and combinations.[9] These include hyperactivity, perceptual–motor impairment, coordination difficulties, language and symbolic impairments, and "soft" neurologic signs (manifestations normal for a younger child, but indicative of dysfunction when seen at an older age, such as clumsiness and involuntary minor movements).

Treatment is complex, multi-disciplinary, and highly individualized, and includes family education and counseling, educational management, psychotherapy, and drug and diet therapy. Children who remain untreated continue to perform poorly in school, resulting in feelings of isolation, frustration, and lowered self-esteem. These feelings can have serious consequences throughout the individual's life.

CONVULSIVE DISORDERS

Convulsive disorders are not uncommon in children, and may result from a variety of causes. A common form of seizure is the febrile convulsion that occurs with fevers and acute infections.

EPILEPSY (RECURRENT CONVULSIVE DISORDERS)

Approximately 700,000 people in America have been diagnosed as epileptic.[10] Epilepsy can be classified as *primary* (idiopathic) with no known cause, or *secondary*, resulting from infection, head trauma, hemorrhage, tumor, or other organic or degenerative factor. Primary epilepsy is the most common, its onset generally between ages 4 and 8 years.

Seizures are the characteristic clinical manifestation of both types of epilepsy, and may be either *generalized* or *partial* (focal).

Generalized Seizures. Types of generalized seizures include *grand mal* (major motor), *petit mal* (absences), *akinetic, myoclonic,* and *infantile spasms.*

Grand mal (major motor) *seizures* consist of a sudden loss of consciousness, with generalized tonic and clonic movements. The seizure may be preceded by an *aura* (a sensation that signals impending attack), although young children may have difficulty describing it. The initial tonic rigidity changes rapidly to generalized jerking movements of the muscles (clonic phase). The child may bite his tongue or lose control of bladder and bowel functions. The jerking movements gradually diminish, then disappear, and the child relaxes. The seizure can be brief, lasting less than a minute, or can last 30 minutes or more. Following the attack, some children return rapidly to an alert state, while others go into a prolonged period of stupor.

Petit mal (absence) seizures last for only a few seconds, rarely longer than 20 seconds. The child loses consciousness and stares straight ahead but does not fall. He becomes immediately alert following the seizure and continues conversation, but does not know what was said or done during the attack. Absences recur frequently, sometimes as often as 50 to 100 in a single day. They often decrease significantly or stop entirely at adolescence.

Akinetic seizures cause a momentary loss of consciousness, muscle tone, and postural control, and can result in serious facial, head, or shoulder injuries. They recur frequently, particularly in the morning.

Myoclonic seizures are characterized by a sudden jerking of a muscle or group of muscles without loss of consciousness. Myoclonus occurs in persons who are nonepileptic during the early stages of falling asleep.

Infantile spasms occur between 3 and 12 months of age and almost always indicate a cerebral defect, and poor prognosis despite treatment. These seizures occur twice as often in boys as in girls, and are preceded or followed by a cry. Muscle contractions are sudden, brief, and symmetrical, accompanied by rolling eyes. Loss of consciousness does not always occur.

Partial (Focal) Seizures. Types of partial (focal) seizures include *psychomotor seizures, focal motor seizures,* and *focal sensory seizures.*

Psychomotor seizures are difficult to recognize. They consist of purposeful but inappropriate, repetitive motor acts. The child gradually loses postural tone and falls to the floor. After a few minutes of unconsciousness he may fall asleep or resume his former activity.

Focal motor seizures are characterized by involuntary, unilateral convulsive movements that begin in the extremities, such as the fingers, and progress up the limb to the body. These are of short duration, sometimes with undisturbed consciousness. However, a typical grand mal seizure may follow at times if the spread has been rapid and extensive. These are common in hemiplegic children.

Focal sensory seizures produce such sensations as tingling, numbness, prickling, pain, or paresthesia, which originates in one area and spreads to other parts of the body.

Diagnosis. Differentiation between types of seizures may be made through the use of electroencephalograms, skull radiography, CT scan, brain scan, and physical and neurologic assessment.

Treatment. Complete control of seizures is the main goal, and can be achieved for the majority of persons through the use of anticonvulsant drug therapy. A number of anticonvulsant drugs are available and are used according to their effectiveness in controlling seizures and to their degree of toxicity (Table 13–4). The most popular of these is Dilantin, which can cause hypertrophy of the gums after prolonged use.

Education and counseling of the child and the parents are important parts of treatment. They need complete, accurate information about the disorder, and the results that can be realistically expected from treatment. It is important to emphasize that epilepsy does not lead inevitably to mental retardation, but that continued and uncontrolled seizures increase the possibility of mental retardation. This points up the importance of early diagnosis and control of seizures.

Although the outlook for a normal, well-adjusted life is favorable, the child and family need to be aware of the restrictions that may be encountered. In many states a person with epilepsy is legally forbidden to drive a motor vehicle. This could limit choice of vocation and lifestyle. Despite attempts at educating the general public about epilepsy, many persons remain prejudiced about this disorder, which can limit social and vocational acceptance.

cardiovascular system

RHEUMATIC FEVER

Acute rheumatic fever is a chronic disease of childhood, affecting the connective tissue of the heart, joints, lungs,

TABLE 13–4. ANTIEPILEPTIC DRUGS

	Indications	Side-Effects and Adverse Reactions
Drugs of Choice		
Phenytoin (new generic name for diphenylhydantoin) (Dilantin)	Generalized convulsive seizures; all forms of partial seizures; often used in combination with primidone or phenobarbital	Drowsiness; gastric distress; gingival hyperplasia; rash; megaloblastic anemia; ataxia; diplopia, fever; hirsutism
Phenobarbital (Luminal)	Generalized convulsive seizures; all forms of partial seizures; often used in combination with phenytoin	Drowsiness; rash; ataxia
Primidone (Mysoline)	Generalized convulsive seizures; all forms of partial seizures; often used in combination with phenytoin or phenobarbital	Drowsiness; dizziness; rash; megaloblastic anemia; ataxia; diplopia; nystagmus
Ethosuximide (Zarontin)	Generalized nonconvulsive seizures, especially petit mal; used in mixed seizure states with phenytoin	Gastric distress; nausea; vomiting; anorexia; dermatitis; drowsiness; dizziness; blood dyscrasia
Alternative Drugs		
Carbamazepine (Tegretol)	Generalized convulsive seizures; partial seizures, especially psychomotor; also used for treatment of trigeminal neuralgia	Headache; drowsiness; dizziness; feelings of inhibition; gait disturbance; blood dyscrasia
Mephenytoin (Mesantoin)	Generalized convulsive seizures; all forms of partial seizures	Drowsiness; rash; blood dyscrasia
Mephobarbital (Mebaral)	Same as phenobarbital	Drowsiness; irritability; rash
Trimethadione (Tridione)	Generalized nonconvulsive seizures—petit mal, myoclonic, and akinetic; often used with phenytoin and phenobarbital	Drowsiness; gastric distress; rash; hemeralopia; blood dyscrasia; nephrosis
Paramethadione (Paradione)	Generalized nonconvulsive seizures, especially petit mal; sometimes useful for psychomotor seizures	Gastric distress; rash; photophobia; blood dyscrasia
Methsuximide (Celantin)	Generalized nonconvulsive seizures, especially petit mal; sometimes useful for psychomotor seizures	Drowsiness; headache; anorexia; blood dyscrasia; ataxia
Phensuximide (Milontin)	Generalized nonconvulsive seizures; sometimes useful for psychomotor seizures	Dizziness; hematuria; nausea; rash
Phenacemide (Phenurone)	Only used in resistant cases because of toxicity; all types of seizures, especially psychomotor	Liver damage; psychotic behavior; nausea; rash
Acetazolamide (Diamox)	Sometimes useful for petit mal seizures; in all seizure disorders as an adjuvant to control seizures related to menstrual cycle	Anorexia; dizziness; drowsiness
Dextroamphetamine	Used with some antiepileptics to counteract sedative effects; some therapeutic effect in petit mal	Anorexia; irritability; insomnia

(Bruya M, Bolin R: Epilepsy: a controllable disease, copyright © 1976, American Journal of Nursing Company. Adopted with permission from the American Journal of Nursing, March, Vol 76, No 3)

and brain. One of the sequelae of Group A beta-hemolytic streptococcal infections, rheumatic fever occurs throughout the world, particularly in the temperate zones. During the past 30 years, its incidence has declined markedly in the United States, but it is still the leading cause of acquired heart disease in children. Rheumatic fever rarely occurs before the age of 5, but is a leading cause of heart failure and death in children between the ages of 5 and 15 years.

Etiology. Rheumatic fever appears to be a sensitivity reaction precipitated by streptococci. The initial streptococcal infection may be inapparent or unrecognized, and the resultant rheumatic fever manifestation may be the first indication of trouble. An elevation of antistreptococcal antibodies, indicative of recent streptococcal infection, however, can be demonstrated in about 95% of the rheumatic fever patients tested within the first 2 months of onset. An hereditary influence is also recognized.

Clinical Manifestations. Following the initial infection, a latent period of 1 to 5 weeks ensues; in certain cases, such as chorea, the period may be longer. The onset is frequently insidious. The child may be listless, anorexic, pale, and may lose weight, complaining of vague muscle, joint, or abdominal pains. Frequently a low grade, late afternoon fever occurs. None of these is diagnostic by itself but if such signs persist, the child merits medical examination.

Major manifestations of rheumatic fever are *polyarthritis, chorea,* and *carditis.* The onset may be acute rather than insidious, with severe carditis or arthritis as the presenting symptom. Chorea, generally, has an insidious onset.

Polyarthritis. This is a migratory arthritis that moves from one major joint to another, the ankles, knees, hips, wrists, elbows, and shoulders. The joint becomes hot, swollen, and painful to either touch or movement. Body temperature is moderately elevated; the sedimentation rate is increased. Although extremely painful, this type of arthritis does not lead to the crippling deformities that occur in rheumatoid arthritis.

Chorea (Sydenham's chorea). This manifestation affects the central nervous system. Emotional instability, purposeless movements, and muscular weakness are characteristic. The onset is gradual, with increasing incoordination, facial grimaces, and repetitive involuntary

---

TABLE 13–5.   REVISED JONES CRITERIA FOR DIAGNOSIS OF RHEUMATIC FEVER

Major Manifestations	Minor Manifestations
Carditis	Previous rheumatic fever
Polyarthritis	Arthralgia
Chorea	Fever
Erythema marginatum	Elevated sedimentation rate
Subcutaneous nodules	Elevated C-reactive protein
	Prolonged P-R interval
	Evidence of preceding streptococcal infection
	Increased ASO or other streptococcal antibody titer

(Wieczorek RR, Natapoff J: A Conceptual Approach to the Nursing of Children: Health Care From Birth Through Adolescence. Philadelphia, JB Lippincott, 1981)

---

movements. Movements may be mild and remain so, or they may become increasingly violent. Active arthritis is rarely present when chorea is the major manifestation. Carditis occurs, although less frequently than when polyarthritis is the major condition. Attacks tend to be recurrent and prolonged, but rare after puberty. It is seldom possible to demonstrate a rise in antistreptococcal antibodies, because of the generally prolonged latency period.

Corticosteroids and salicylates are of little value in the treatment of uncomplicated chorea. Sedation with phenobarbital for relaxation, or the use of a tranquilizer such as chlorpromazine (Thorazine) helps to relax the child. Bedrest is necessary, and with protection such as padding the bed sides if the movements are severe. When the chorea is complicated by a heart condition, the treatment should include therapy for that condition too.

Carditis is a serious manifestation because it is the major cause of death or of permanent disability among children with rheumatic fever. Carditis may occur singly, or it may occur as a complication of either arthritis or chorea. Presenting symptoms may be vague enough to be missed. A child may have a poor appetite or pallor, perhaps a low-grade fever, listlessness, and a moderate degree of anemia. Careful observation may reveal slight dyspnea on exertion. Physical examination shows a soft systolic murmur over the apex of the heart. Unfortunately, such a child may have been in poor physical health for some time before the murmur is discovered.

Acute carditis may be the presenting symptom, particularly in young children. An abrupt onset of high fever, perhaps as high as 104° F, tachycardia, pallor, poor pulse quality, and a rapid fall in hemoglobin are characteristic. Weakness, prostration, cyanosis, and intense precordial pain are frequently present. Cardiac dilatation usually occurs. The pericardium, the myocardium, or the endocardium may be affected.

Diagnosis. Rheumatic fever is difficult to diagnose, and sometimes impossible to differentiate from other diseases. The possible serious effect of the disease demands early and conscientious medical treatment. It is unfortunate, however, to cause apprehension and disrupt the patient's life if the condition proves to be something less serious. The nurse should naturally not attempt a diagnosis, but should understand the criteria on which a presumptive diagnosis is based.

The Jones criteria (modified), a guide based on criteria formulated in 1944, is generally accepted as a useful rule for guidance when making a decision as to whether to treat the patient for rheumatic fever. Criteria are divided into major and minor categories (Table 13–5).

The presence of two major, or one major and two minor, criteria is accepted as an indication of a high probability of rheumatic fever if supported by evidence of a preceding streptococcal infection. It is not infallible, because no one criterion is specific for the disease, and other additional manifestations are helpful aids toward a substantiation of the diagnosis.

Treatment. The chief concern in caring for a patient with rheumatic fever is prevention of residual heart disease. As long as the rheumatic process is active, progressive heart damage is possible. Bedrest, therefore, is essential in order to reduce the work load of the heart. How long the period of bedrest should last cannot be arbitrarily stated. It is generally agreed that a child should be kept in bed until both laboratory and clinical evidence of the acute stage of the disease have disappeared (Table 13–6).

Bedrest is essential during the acute stage. Strict bedrest, including feeding of the child by the nurse or mother, is essential for patients with cardiac enlargement or congestive failure. Gradual ambulation may be started when the clinical and laboratory signs of the acute stage have subsided. This may be as early as 7 to 10 days where there is no evidence of cardiac disease. Bedrest from 3 weeks to 3 months may be prescribed for patients with cardiac involvement. Residual heart disease is treated in accordance with its severity and its type with digitalis, restricted activities, diuretics and a low-sodium diet as indicated.

Laboratory appraisal tests, although they are non-specific, are useful for an evaluation of the activity of the disease. Two commonly used indicators are the *erythrocyte sedimentation rate,* and the presence of *C-reactive protein.* The erythrocyte sedimentation rate (ESR) is elevated in the presence of an inflammatory process, and is nearly always raised in the polyarthritis or in the carditis manifestations of rheumatic fever. It remains elevated until clinical manifestations have ceased, and any subclinical activity has subsided. It seldom rises in uncomplicated chorea. Therefore, ESR elevation in a choreic patient may point toward cardiac involvement.

C-reactive protein is not normally present in the blood of healthy persons, but it does appear in the serum of acutely ill persons, including those ill with rheumatic fever. As the patient improves, C-reactive protein disappears.

Leukocytosis is also an indication of an inflammatory process. Until the leukocyte count returns to a normal level, the disease probably is still active.

Drug therapy. Medications used in the treatment of rheumatic fever include salicylates and corticosteroids. Salicylates are given in the form of acetylsalicylic acid (aspirin) to children, with the daily dosage calculated according to the child's weight. Remarkable relief from polyarthritis is afforded by the use of this drug. It is used for its analgesic as well as its antipyretic effect. The continued administration of a relatively large dosage may cause toxic effects, because individual tolerance differs greatly. The nurse must note any signs of toxicity and report them promptly. Tinnitus, nausea, vomiting, and headache are all signs of toxicity. Aspirin administered after meals or with a glass of milk causes less gastrointestinal irritation. Enteric-coated aspirin is also available for patients who are sensitive to its effects. Large doses may alter the prothrombin time and thus interfere with the clotting mechanism.

In the presence of mild or severe carditis, corticosteroids appear to be the drug of choice because of their prompt, dramatic action. Neither drug is expected to alter the course of the disease, but the control of the toxic manifestations enhances the patient's comfort and sense of well-being, and helps reduce the burden on the heart. This is of particular importance in acute carditis with congestive failure. Because premature withdrawal of a steroid drug is likely to cause a relapse, its use is continued until any evidence of activity has subsided. It is then gradually discontinued. Toxic reactions are naturally to be watched for and reported as well.

Because the presence of group A streptococci prolongs the rheumatic activity, a course of penicillin should be given to eliminate these organisms from the child's body.

TABLE 13–6. SUGGESTED REGULATION OF PHYSICAL ACTIVITY IN RHEUMATIC FEVER

Cardiac Status	Management
No carditis	Bedrest for 3 weeks; then gradual ambulation (even if on aspirin)
Carditis but no cardiomegaly and no heart failure	Bedrest for a month after carditis is detected; then gradual ambulation (even if on aspirin)
Carditis with cardiomegaly but no failure	Strict bedrest first 2 weeks after detection of cardiomegaly; then modified bedrest for 4 weeks; then gradual ambulation (even if on treatment); modified bedrest again during the "rebound period" (first 2 weeks after cessation of treatment); then gradual ambulation
Carditis with cardiomegaly and heart failure	Strict bedrest as long as heart failure is present; if failure is severe, patient should be washed and fed by aides; after subsidence or control of failure, modified bedrest until a month after cessation of treatment if no rebound ensues; or until 2 weeks after spontaneous subsidence of rebound; then gradual ambulation

(Stollerman G: Rheumatic Fever and Streptococcal Infection, p 242. New York, Grune & Stratton, 1975)

Nursing Care. A child who has developed rheumatic fever may be hospitalized for diagnosis and beginning therapy, and then returned home for continuing care, depending on the particular circumstances.

The severity of the condition, the home circumstances, and the availability of care outside the home should all be considered. If the family is able to provide adequate physical care and emotional support, and if medical supervision is obtainable, home care would seem to best meet the child's needs.

A child may be willing to accept total dependency when he is in pain and is acutely ill, but any prohibition of all activity when he feels better may be extremely traumatic emotionally—with the trauma possibly outweighing the adverse physical effects. The nurse and the family need to understand the physical limitations imposed, and the child patient needs limitations clearly explained to him in terms suited to his understanding and his ability to accept.

Outcome. Outcome is related primarily to the presence or absence of heart disease. Most chronic disabilities and most deaths occur in the presence of repeated attacks. Supportive prophylactic therapy has greatly reduced the incidence of death and chronic disability.

Prevention. Because rheumatic fever is a condition that has its peak of onset in school-age children, health services for this age group assume an added importance. The overall approach is to promote continuous health supervision for all children, including the school-age child. Establishment of well child conferences or clinics, and encouragement of the general population to use them needs to increase among school-age children to provide continuity of care.

Clinic services in the area of prevention and treatment are available from crippled children's agencies, public health agencies, and the Heart Association, through its state associations.

Registration with a state heart association is a helpful way of keeping in touch with persons who have had one or more attacks of rheumatic fever. Through the association, prophylactic drugs may be purchased at wholesale prices, a service that also makes possible guidance and encouragement during the continuation of self-care.

endocrine system

DIABETES MELLITUS IN CHILDREN (INSULIN-DEPENDENT DIABETES)

At least 10 million Americans have been diagnosed as diabetic; a significant number of these are children. Although specific statistics are not available, it is estimated that diabetes mellitus affects 1 out of every 600 children between the ages of 5 and 15 years. Incidence of this condition continues to increase.

Diabetes mellitus should not be confused with *diabetes insipidus*, a relatively rare disorder of the pituitary or the hypothalamus, which has no relation to diabetes mellitus. Diabetes insipidus is designated by its entire name; diabetes mellitus usually is called simply diabetes. If onset occurs during childhood, it may be called *juvenile diabetes*, although use of this term is declining in favor of *youth-onset* or *growth-onset diabetes*.

Diabetes is often considered an adult disease, but at least 5% begins in childhood, with the greatest incidence at approximately 6 and 12 years of age.[11] Management of diabetes in children is quite different from adults, and demands a fresh approach on the part of health professionals and families (Table 13–7).

Classification of diabetes includes four types:

Type I   Insulin dependent diabetes mellitus (IDDM)
Type II   Non-insulin dependent diabetes mellitus (NIDDM)
Type III Impaired glucose tolerance (IGT)
Type IV Gestational (elevated blood sugar [glucose] only during pregnancy)

As noted in the classification, diabetes in children is Type I (IDDM).

Pathogenesis. The exact pathophysiology of diabetes is not completely understood; however, it is known to result from dysfunction of the beta (insulin-secreting) cells of the islets of Langerhans in the pancreas. It is believed that the

TABLE 13–7. DIFFERENCES BETWEEN JUVENILE AND ADULT-ONSET DIABETES

Characteristic	Juvenile	Adult
Onset	Rapid	Slow, insidious
Weight	Thin	Predisposing factor
	Evidence of weight loss	
Dietary treatment	Not adequate alone; insulin required	Possible in one-half of cases
Oral antidiabetic agents	Contraindicated	Probably not indicated
Hypoglycemia and ketoacidosis	Common	Uncommon

(Adapted from Weill W, Kohrman A: Diabetes mellitus. In Rudolph A (ed): Pediatrics, p 699. New York, Appleton-Century-Crofts, 1977)

presence of an acute infection during childhood may trigger a mechanism in genetically susceptible children, activating beta cell dysfunction, thus disrupting insulin secretion.

Normally the sugar derived from digestion and assimilation of foods is burned to provide energy for the body's activities. Excess sugar is converted into fat or glycogen and stored in the body tissues. Insulin, a hormone secreted by the pancreas, is responsible for the burning and storing of sugar. In diabetes, the supply of insulin is inadequate, allowing sugar to accumulate in the bloodstream and spill over into the urine. In children, diabetes causes an abrupt, pronounced decrease in insulin production, resulting in decreased ability to derive energy from the food eaten. This combination of failure to gain weight and lack of energy prompts parents to bring in the child to the physician or clinic for a check-up.

Diagnosis. *Symptoms.* Classic symptoms of diabetes mellitus are *polyuria* (dramatic increase in urinary output, probably with enuresis), *polydipsia* (abnormal thirst), and *polyphagia* (increased food consumption). These symptoms are usually accompanied by weight loss or failure to gain weight, plus lack of energy.

If the child's symptoms are not noted and referred for diagnosis, the disorder is likely to progress to diabetic acidosis, and eventually to diabetic coma.

Because of inadequate insulin production, carbohydrates are not converted into fuel for energy production. Fats are then mobilized for energy, but, in the absence of glucose, are incompletely oxidized. Ketone bodies (acetone, diacetic acid, and oxybutyric acid) accumulate. They are readily excreted in the urine, but in this excretion the acid–base balance of body fluids is upset, resulting in acidosis.

Diabetic acidosis is characterized by drowsiness, dry skin, flushed cheeks, and cherry-red lips, acetone breath with a fruity smell, and hyperpnea (abnormal increase in the depth and rate of the respiratory movements). Nausea and vomiting may occur. If untreated, the child lapses into coma and exhibits *Kussmaul breathing* (paroxysms of dyspnea or labored breathing), rapid pulse, and subnormal temperature and blood pressure.

Treatment for acidosis includes keeping the patient warm. Blood and urine are tested to evaluate the degree of acidosis. If the child is unable to urinate, a catheter will be inserted. Gastric lavage may be performed to relieve abdominal distention. Regular insulin is given subcutaneously or intramuscularly, followed by intravenous fluids.

Tests. Children in families with a history of diabetes can have their urine tested by their parents. Although the presence of sugar in the urine does not necessarily indicate a diabetic state, it should be reported to the physician. (See boxed material.) The physician will probably follow up with a *glucose tolerance test* (GTT). The presence of sugar in the urine or an elevated blood sugar is indicative of diabetes, but occasionally is due to other causes. A postprandial (after a meal) blood specimen is often ordered for the determination of glucose metabolism. Normal blood

glucose is 70–140 mg per 100 ml blood. Only a GTT will give a definite diagnosis of diabetes mellitus; however, it is not indicated when obvious symptoms are present and fasting blood sugar levels are extremely high.

Nurse's role. Children of families in which there is or has been diabetes should be tested routinely. This is particularly important during or after an infectious disease.

When the nurse is aware of diabetes in a family history, she should observe carefully for suggestive symptoms in every family member, regardless of age. She should also help educate parents to observe their children for frequent thirst, urination, and weight loss. All relatives of diabetics should be considered a high-risk group and should have periodic testing.

Early detection and control are of critical importance in postponing or minimizing later complications.

Treatment. Diabetic children have little or no residual ability to produce insulin; thus, it is probable, according to present knowledge, that they will always need to take insulin. Their treatment includes diabetic stabilization through regulation of diet and insulin, and education for both children and their parents.

After it has been determined that a child is diabetic, he is usually hospitalized for a period of time, to stabilize his condition under supervision. The nurse must remember that this is a trying time for the parents as well as for the child, especially if he is old enough to understand its significance. The parent sees his child as someone who "will always be different," and who will need to take special care of himself all his life. The idea of giving insulin injections is in itself appalling. The combination of giving insulin, checking urine daily, and regulating diets can seem overwhelming.

Insulin. Although oral medications can be useful in maintaining a satisfactory blood sugar level for an adult who has diabetes late in life, the child must have insulin supplied to him; and, to date, insulin is effective only when injected because it is a protein substance and will be broken down by the gastrointestinal enzymes. The type of insulin ordered is determined by the individual child's needs. Table 13–8 outlines the various types of insulin and their action.

Insulin reaction (insulin shock) is caused by insulin overload, resulting in too-rapid metabolism of the body's glucose. This may be due to a change in the body's requirement, carelessness in diet such as failure to eat proper amounts of food, an error in insulin measurement or excessive exercise. Because diabetes in children is very labile, the child is subject to insulin reactions.

Some of the symptoms of impending insulin shock in children are—any type of odd, unusual, or antisocial behavior, headache and malaise, blurred vision and faintness, and undue fatigue or hunger. One small child complained of hunger just before evening tray time, and before the nurse could bring the supper tray, the child went into a convulsion. After two such episodes, the nurse learned to

TABLE 13–8. ONSET, ACTION, AND DURATION OF INSULIN PREPARATIONS IN HOURS

Action	Preparation	Onset	Peak Action	Duration
Short	Regular	½–1	2–4	6–8
	Actroped Pork	½–1	2–7	8–9
	Semilente	½–1	2–4	8–10
Intermediate	NPH	1–2	6–8	12–14
	Lente	1–2	6–8	14–16
	Globin zinc	1–2	6–8	12–14
Long	Protamine zinc	4–6	14–24	36–72
	Ultralente	4–6	8–12	24–36

(Wieczorek RR, Natapoff J: A Conceptual Approach to the Nursing of Children: Health Care From Birth Through Adolescence. Philadelphia, JB Lippincott, 1981)

have orange juice readily available at the bedside for the child whenever she complained of hunger.

Frequently children go into shock during the early morning hours. The night nurse must observe the child at least every 2 hours, note the tossed bedding that would indicate restlessness, note any excessive perspiration, and if necessary, try to arouse the child. As the child becomes regulated and observes a careful diet at home, parents need not watch so closely but should have a thorough understanding of all aspects of this condition.

Treatment of insulin reaction should be immediate, allowing the child to take sugar, candy, orange juice, or one of the commercial products designed for this emergency. Repeated reactions, or impending reactions call for a checkup by the physician.

If the child is unable to take sugar orally, glucagon should be administered subcutaneously to bring about a prompt rise in blood sugar. Every adult responsible for a diabetic child should clearly understand the procedure for administering this drug and should have easy access to it.

Glucagon is a hormone produced by alpha cells of the pancreatic islets. Whereas an elevation of blood glucose results in an insulin release (in a normal person), a fall in blood sugar stimulates glucagon release. The released glucagon in the blood stream acts on the liver to promote glycogen breakdown and glucose release.

Glucagon is now available as a pharmaceutical product, packaged as a powder in individual dose units. A person preparing the dose need only add the diluent, which comes with the powdered drug, by using a sterile syringe and needle. The solution is then drawn up into the syringe and administered in the same manner as insulin.

Glucagon acts within minutes to restore a child to consciousness, after which he can take candy or sugar. This treatment prevents the long delay in waiting for a doctor to come and administer glucose intravenously, or waiting for an ambulance to reach the hospital emergency department. It is, however, one form of emergency treatment, and not a substitute for proper medical supervision.

Teaching the Child and the Family. The diabetic teaching program in a hospital is concerned primarily with a sound, basic concept of the condition itself. A child can assimilate facts and concepts at a very young age if he is psychologically ready to learn. As time goes on, his parents must be his principal teachers; therefore, they must have a satisfactory acceptance and understanding of the condition. The success of any subsequent teaching about diet, insulin, exercise, and control depends largely on the degree to which the child and parents have worked through their feelings. The child who is mature will gradually take responsibility for his own management.

Teaching programs for diabetics usually require the cooperative efforts of nurses and dieticians or nutritionists. The nurse is more than an educator; she is an important listener to whom the patient and family can express fears, concerns, and other feelings. The nurse must not only assess their level of understanding, but also their level of acceptance before beginning any teaching program.

Patient and family need to learn what diabetes does to the body, how to test for the presence of sugar in the urine, how to inject insulin, and how to regulate diet, exercise, and insulin to meet the child's needs as they change.

If the hospital does not have a regular instruction program outlined for patients and parents, the nurse can use a number of books and articles to assist her in teaching and to give or loan to the family.

Diet. Prior to diagnosis, the diabetic child's nutritional stores are depleted. In the initial phase of management, he needs additional calories and nutrients to rebuild body tissues and reserves. He will also need insulin to take care of the additional calories. This is one of the important reasons for hospitalization and involvement of the dietician.

Understanding the principles of a diabetic diet is an important aspect of the teaching program in the hospital. The dietician should be principally responsible for this, but the nurse is the person who ultimately is going to have the

DIABETES DIAGNOSTIC TESTS

When testing for the presence of sugar (glucose) or acetone (ketone bodies) in the urine, the most accurate results can be obtained when
1. A second-voided* specimen is used
2. Reagent tablets or strips are fresh and have been stored away from direct light, moisture, and heat
3. The specific testing material is used according to the manufacturer's instructions for that specific product and the results compared to the color chart provided for that product
4. All equipment, such as test tubes, is clean

Tests for Sugar in the Urine

Clinitest. *Two-drop method:* This method allows for an estimated concentration of sugar up to 5% and is more accurate at higher glucose concentrations.
1. Hold dropper vertically and place 2 drops (0.1 ml) of urine in test tube.
2. Rinse the dropper. Add 10 drops (0.5 ml) of water in test tube.
3. Add 1 Clinitest reagent tablet. Do not shake test tube.
4. Wait 15 seconds after boiling stops.
5. Compare color of urine with appropriate color chart. Use only the 2-drop method color scale, which has 7 colors, ranging in value from 0–5 percent.

Five-drop method:
1. Hold dropper vertically and place 5 drops of urine in the test tube.
2. Rinse dropper. Add 10 drops of water in test tube.
3. Add 1 Clinitest tablet in test tube.
   a. Watch while reaction takes place. Do not shake test tube during reaction or for 15 seconds after boiling inside test tube has stopped.
   b. Observe the solution in the test tube *while the reaction takes place and during the 15-second waiting period to detect pass-through color changes caused by glucosuria over 2%.*
      (1) If the solution passes through orange and dark shades of green brown, it indicates that more than 2% (4+) urine sugar is present.
      (2) Record as such without reference to color scale.
4. After 15-second waiting period, shake test tube gently and compare with the color scale. Record the results.

Diastix, Clinistix, Labstix, TesTape. These enzyme-impregnated tapes/strips are used to test for glucose in the urine. The strip is moistened with the urine, any excess is shaken off, and the resulting color compared to the closest matching color block on the chart of the product being used.

Tests for Ketone Bodies (Acetone)

Acetest tablets contain a chemical reagent that reacts with ketone in the urine to change its color, depending on the concentration of ketone bodies.
Ketostix (reagent strips) are dipped into the urine; after the time specified on the information sheet, a lavender color appears if the urine contains ketones.
Keto-Diastix (reagent strips) are a combination product, designed to detect ketones *and* glucose in the urine

After Brunner LS, Suddarth DS: Textbook of Medical–Surgical Nursing, 4th ed. Philadelphia, JB Lippincott, 1980

* The patient empties the bladder 30 minutes before the specimen is due, drinks fluids, and voids again at the specified time. It is the second-voided specimen that is used for testing.
CAUTION: Reagent tablets are caustic and should be kept away from small children.

task of reinforcing this information, as well as the possibility of having to interpret it.

The present tendency with respect to diet is to put the child on a diet best suited to his nutritional needs for his weight and for his age. The measured diet provides a nutritionally adequate diet with the emphasis on protein and vitamin-rich foods. Exchange foods lists are used with this diet, and the standard measuring cups and spoons can usually be used.

It is important that the diabetic child's diet be a nutritionally well-balanced combination of protein, carbohydrates, and fats. To accomplish this, it is necessary to find out how much the family understands about basic nutrition and to fill in the gaps.

Urine testing. The parents, as well as the child, need instruction in urine testing. A child of 5 or 6 years is not too young to learn, under supervision, the mechanics of urine testing. The parents must be reminded that the tablets, if they are used, are corrosive and harmful, if by chance they are swallowed. The color may be attractive to the child who might want to investigate further. Perhaps the parents should feel the test tube while the tablet is dissolving to discover how hot the solution actually becomes. Any reagent, of whatever type, should be stored away when it is not in use, in order to keep it out of the hands of small children.

A young child in the hospital can watch the nurse while she does the test, and help count the drops of urine as they are added. He will be proud of his ability to count, and fascinated over the change of color. Soon he should be able to do it himself under the watchful eye of his mother and should be able to keep his own chart by coloring-in the correct color change.

A child of 3 or 4 years very quickly learns that there is a relationship between voiding and urine testing, and accepts this as a way of life.

Youth-onset diabetes is extremely labile, making it important that urine be tested before each meal, at least until control is established. A second, or double-voided, specimen, voided 20 to 30 minutes after the first, will be more accurate and should be obtained, if at all possible. It does present a problem to little tots who have only recently been toilet-trained. When asked to "go potty" they are apt to protest, "But I did go potty," and to feel quite injured that they are not considered to have performed satisfactorily. Usually, it is best to test a toddler's urine every time he voids, because it is entirely unpredictable as to whether he will go at the designated times. After the child leaves the hospital, urine tests are usually continued 3 or 4 times daily. Tests for acetone, using acetest tablets, are made at the same time as a blood sugar monitoring device. Any appearance of acetone in the urine should be reported immediately.

A school-age child may have difficulty, or may experience embarrassment over noon-time urine tests. If he does not go home at noon, the physician may allow him to skip the noon test, or a child may go to the school nurse's office to do the test. One girl collected urine in a tightly corked test tube, carried it in her purse and tested it at home after school.

A child should be taught to keep a record of urine tests, making a color chart or using one of the prepared charts. Some supervision from the parents is necessary, particularly if the chart is repeatedly negative. Children frequently get bored or angry over the whole thing, and the testing of tap water in place of urine is not unheard of. Charts have even been made up neatly for a week in advance. Parents need to understand the child's emotions, however. Probably some scheme of a routine check—perhaps a weekly test—would be more acceptable than a check based on doubt or suspicion.

Insulin regimen. Most newly diagnosed diabetic children show a decreased need for insulin during the first weeks or months after control is established. This is a natural reaction, and it should be explained to avoid the false hope that the diabetic is "getting better." As the child grows, his need for insulin increases and continues to do so until he reaches full growth. Again, this needs to be explained; the child's condition is not "getting worse."

Another matter that merits discussion is the use of insulin during illness or an infection in a diabetic child. When an ill child is unable to eat his prescribed diet, his mother rather naturally assumes that his insulin dose should be reduced. This is not the case, however; his insulin may actually need to be increased during this period.

This all points up the importance of close supervision by the physician. Parents need to understand this, and should have no hesitancy about reporting any change in the child's health, any recurring insulin reactions, the persistence of more than a small amount of urine sugar, and, in particular, any positive urine acetone reaction.

Methods of giving insulin. The child will not be able to take over the management of his insulin dose as early as he learned to test his urine, but he can watch the preparation of the syringe, and learn the technique for drawing up the dosage. If he can watch until it becomes routine, it might be helpful. By the time he is 8 or 9, he should be thinking out his dose and getting the feel of the syringe. He should be drawing up his own dose and preparing for the time when he will be caring for himself. Just when that comes cannot be stated arbitrarily. No two children mature at the same rate; some may be able to do this quite early. For others, this may be an act of love on the mother's part, showing her concern and care for him. A child should be encouraged, however, to take over the management of his therapy as soon as he is ready. *He can learn the importance of the routine and accept the restrictions his disease imposes if he has helped to make the decisions.*

Manner of injection. The child and his parents should be taught the correct way to give insulin, and supervised until it is certain that they are injecting the insulin correctly. Disposable syringes are preferable for home use.

Rotating injection sites is also a matter of considerable importance. If insulin is given frequently in the same location, the area is apt to become indurated and is eventually fibrosed, hindering proper insulin absorption. The atrophic hollows in the skin, or the lumps of hypertrophied tissue, are unsightly as well. Some people, however, appear to have a greater skin sensitivity than others.

Definite instruction should be given concerning the importance of rotating sites (Fig. 13–6). Areas on both the upper arms and the upper thighs can be used, allowing several weeks between the use of the same site, if a plan is carefully mapped out. Starting from the inner, upper corner of the area, each injection is given one-half inch below the preceding one, going down in a vertical line, with the next series starting one-half inch outward at the upper level. The lower abdomen and the buttocks may also be used if necessary. If there is any sign of induration, the local site should be carefully avoided for a period of weeks after all signs of irritation have disappeared.

Continuing Care. A diabetic child should carry some form of sugar with him at all times. Candy is useful, although perhaps it presents more temptation to the child than does pure sugar. In cases of doubtful insulin reactions, it is undoubtedly better to give sugar than to withhold it, but frequent reactions indicate a need for a physician's attention.

It is extremely important that a child wear a Medic Alert identification medal or a bracelet, with information about his diabetic status. Identification cards, such as those carried by many adult diabetics, are seldom practical for a child diabetic.

Some of the difficulty encountered in regulating blood sugar stability stems from the variations in an average child's activity. His school day contains many hours of sitting still, interspersed with sports or gymnastics, whereas on weekends and vacation periods, he may be much more active. Theoretically, his greatest periods of activity should come at the time of day when his blood sugar is highest; in practice, this is not always possible for a school child. Many physicians advocate a diet increase for those days when the child is more active physically. This calls for good judgement and understanding on the part of the child's parents.

A diabetic child should participate in normal activities for his age, and should consider himself a normal child. He should, however, make his diabetic condition known to at least one friend, and should not go swimming or hiking without a responsible individual nearby, who knows what to look for and who knows what to do if the child should have a reaction.

Some older children are quite sensitive about their condition, and fear that they seem "different" from their friends. Even with the best of instruction and preparation they may feel this way, and wish to keep their condition secret. They must understand that a teacher or some other adult in their environment should be acquainted with their condition. Classroom teachers should know which of their students have such a condition, and should understand the signs of an impending reaction.

Diabetic children under good control need not be kept from such activities as campouts, overnight trips with the school band, or other, similar activities away from home. Exercise increases the metabolism of carbohydrates and thereby reduces the need for insulin. Of course, these children must be capable of measuring their insulin and giving their own injections. Some young people report that a desire to participate in such an activity was the factor that overcame their reluctance to measure and administer their own insulin.

The relatively inexpensive disposable insulin syringes and needles simplify traveling for the diabetic. A diabetic must keep in mind, however, that in a number of states insulin syringes and needles are sold only on prescription—a fact that a young person might not realize if syringes have been bought in only one drug store.

When traveling, the diabetic should take a prescription with him for presentation, if, for any reason, he needs to buy equipment. He must also make sure that a responsible person on the trip knows about his diabetes, the symptoms of insulin reaction and diabetic acidosis, and what to do in these emergencies. If the diabetic visits another family for a weekend, they must also have this information.

Home blood glucose monitoring. Advances in technology have made it possible for diabetics to monitor blood glucose levels at home and thus achieve greater con-

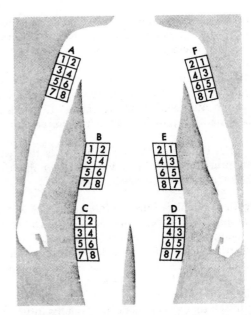

FIG. 13–6.   Possible sites for administration of insulin. (Brunner LS, Suddarth DS (eds): The Lippincott Manual of Nursing Practice, 2nd ed. Philadelphia, JB Lippincott, 1978)

trol over their disorder and prevent complications. This is particularly important to the following diabetics:[12]

1. Patients whose renal threshold is abnormal or unstable
2. Patients in renal failure
3. The unstable diabetic child
4. Patients with impaired color vision
5. Patients who have difficulty recognizing true hypoglycemia
6. The pregnant diabetic

These diabetics can use one of several glucose meters, or test strips (Dextrostix, Chemstrip bG). The meters are large, and expensive, but generally more accurate than the strips. The Dextrometer (Ames Corporation, division of Miles Laboratories) is the most lightweight and least expensive of the systems available. Chemstrip bG appears to be more accurate than Dextrostix but takes slightly longer to use.

Traditionally urine tests have been used as a basis for regulation of insulin. By the time sugar appears in the urine, it has had at least 4 hours to affect the body. Home blood glucose monitoring gives a blood sugar measurement that is accurate to the moment so diabetics can adjust more precisely their insulin–exercise–diet combination.

Laboratory monitoring of blood glucose. The standard GTT measures blood-glucose levels at the moment of testing. It is traumatic, expensive, and can be inaccurate. Its principal use is diagnosing early diabetes, primarily in adults who do not present the acute symptoms. Recently a test has been devised that will measure blood-glucose levels throughout a period of 120 days. This test is called Hemoglobin A_1C, and can be administered at any time of day, no matter what the patient has just eaten. It requires only a few milliliters (one tube) of blood and offers more accurate measurement of glucose than ever before possible.

Although this new test is quite useful, it cannot replace the standard GTT for diagnosis of diabetes because Hemoglobin A_1C is not sensitive enough to detect minor GT abnormalities, possible risk factors for cardiovascular disease.

The chief benefit of Hemoglobin A_1C is that patients who monitor glucose at home will be better able to compare long-range control of glucose levels.

Long-Term Implications. *Adolescence.* Adolescence is an extremely trying period for many diabetics, as it is for other young people. Just as a normal child has to work through from dependence to independence, so does the diabetic child. Even when a child has accepted much of his own care, he may rebel against the control that this condition places on him, become impatient, and seem to convince himself that he does not care about his future health. He may skip meals, drop diet controls, or neglect urine testing. Going barefoot and neglecting proper foot care can also cause problems for the diabetic adolescent. It can be a difficult time for both the parents and their child. The parents naturally become concerned, and are apt to give the child more controls to rebel against. Special care should be taken by the family, teachers, nurses, and doctors to see that these young people find enough maturing satisfaction in other areas, and do not need to rebel in this vital area.

If a child completely understands all aspects of his condition (especially if he has been allowed to assume control of his treatment previously) he should be allowed to continue. Should he run into difficulty, this is a time when an adolescent clinic can be of great value. Here he can discuss his own problems with understanding people who treat him with dignity and listen to him.

Future health. According to present knowledge, a person who develops diabetes during childhood will always have the disorder. About one-half of these persons will die from kidney disease within 25 years after the onset of clinical symptoms.[13] No way has been found to stimulate the nonfunctioning islets of Langerhans in the pancreas to produce insulin.

Research continues into the cause and treatment of diabetes, making possible such improvements as the systems for home blood glucose monitoring, the Hemoglobin A_1C test, and the insulin pump, an automated, lightweight device that acts as an artificial pancreas, feeding a steady flow of insulin through an attached needle into the abdomen. The insulin pump is still in the experimental stage, but may eventually offer many diabetics better control and more effective prevention of complications such as eye and kidney damage.

Pregnancy. Prospects for the health of the diabetic mother and her infant have improved markedly during the past few years; stillbirth or perinatal death is still a serious threat, however. (See Chapter 3.) Early adequate prenatal care and conscientious adherence to the diabetic regimen affords mother and infant the best chance for a healthy life.

skin disorders

FUNGUS INFECTIONS OF THE SKIN

TINEA OR RINGWORM OF THE SCALP

This infection is called *tinea capitis* or *tinea tonsurans.* The most common cause is *Microsporum audouini*, transmitted from person to person. A less common type, *Microsporum canis*, is transmitted from animal to child.

Tinea capitis begins as a small papule on the scalp and spreads, leaving scaly patches of baldness. The hairs become brittle and break off easily. Examination under ultraviolet light (Wood's light) is helpful for diagnosis. Griseofulvin, an antifungal antibiotic, is the medication of choice. As treatment may be prolonged, it is not recommended that children who are being properly treated be kept out of school.

RINGWORM OF THE BODY

The lesions of tinea corporis occur on any part of the body and resemble the lesions of scalp ringworm. Ointment applied to the area relieves the itching. Griseofulvin is also used in this condition.

RINGWORM OF THE FEET (TINEA PEDIS)

Tinea pedis is the scaling or cracking of the skin between the toes commonly known as athlete's foot. Examination under a microscope of scrapings from the lesions is necessary for diagnosis. Transmission is by direct or indirect contact with skin lesions from infected persons. Contaminated sidewalks, floors, and shower stalls spread the condition to those who walk with bare feet.

Treatment includes washing the feet with soap and water, removing scabs and crusts, and applying a topical agent. Tinactin is useful after the acute inflammatory stage begins to subside. Griseofulvin by mouth is also useful. During the chronic phase, use of ointment, scrupulous foot hygiene, and frequent changing of socks are helpful. Desenex foot powder may also be useful.

PEDICULOSIS

Lice are a common infestation of the scalp, or of the hairy parts of the body. The most common condition seen in children is infestation with head lice. The infesting agent is *Pediculus capitis.* Animal lice are not transferred to man.

Head lice are passed around from child to child by direct contact or indirectly by contact with combs and other headgear. Lice lay their eggs, called *nits*, on the head, attaching them to strands of hair. The nits hatch in about 1 week, and the lice become sexually mature in approximately 2 weeks.

Clinical Manifestations. Severe itching of the scalp is the most obvious symptom. Combing the hair with a fine-toothed comb will remove lice, but nits are difficult to remove.

Treatment. Use of Kwell shampoo, which is prescribed by a physician, gives the most satisfactory results. After wetting the hair with warm water, the Kwell is applied like any ordinary shampoo: about 1 ounce is used. The head should be lathered for 4 minutes, rinsed thoroughly and dried. Shampooing may be repeated if necessary in 24 hours, but Kwell should not be used more than twice a week. Care must be taken to avoid getting Kwell into the eyes or on mucous membranes.

SKIN ALLERGIES

One of the most common allergic skin reactions is *eczema* (atopic dermatitis), which is discussed in Chapter 7. Other skin disorders of allergic origin include hives (urticaria) and giant swellings (angioedema), rashes caused by poison ivy, poison oak, and other plants, or by drug reactions.

HIVES (URTICARIA) AND GIANT SWELLINGS (ANGIOEDEMA)

Hives appear in different sizes, on many different parts of the body, and are usually caused by foods or drugs. They are bright red and itchy, and can occur on the eyelids, tongue, mouth, hands or feet, or in the brain or stomach. When affecting the mouth or tongue, hives can cause difficulty in breathing; in the stomach, the swelling can produce pain, nausea, and vomiting. Swelling in brain tissue causes headache and other symptoms.

Foods such as chocolate, nuts, shellfish, berries or other raw fruit, fish, and highly seasoned foods are likely to cause hives. Possible drug allergens include aspirin and related drugs, laxatives, anti-inflammatory drugs, tranquilizers, and antibiotics (penicillin is the most common allergen of this group). Sometimes it is impossible to identify the cause.

Skin rashes are common in school-age children. Some are caused by infectious diseases and others by allergy. Whatever the cause, rashes are usually treated with topical preparations such as lotions, ointments, or greases, plus cool soaks. It is important to relieve the itching as much as possible because scratching can introduce additional pathogens to the affected area. Table 13–9 summarizes some of the skin rashes likely to affect the school-age child.

Treatment is aimed at reducing the swelling and relieving the itching. If the allergen can be identified, it can be removed from the child's environment, and hyposensitization performed. Antihistamines are used to relieve itching and reduce swelling. Cool soaks also help relieve itching. Fingernails should be kept short and clean. In severe cases, corticosteroids may be necessary. If the allergen is a certain food, diet will need to be planned to eliminate this food.

PLANT ALLERGIES

Poison ivy is the worst offender among the plant allergens in North America, particularly during the summer months. Its effects vary from slight inflammation and itching to severe, extensive swelling that virtually immobilizes the child. This disorder causes intense itching (pruritus) and forms tiny blisters that weep and continue to spread the inflammation. Antihistamines or oral steroids help the child not to scratch; cool soaks and Calamine lotion or topical steroids help minimize the discomfort.

BITES

Because school-age children are active, inquisitive, and not completely inhibited in their actions, they commonly suffer bites, both animal and human, as well as insect stings and bites. Many of these are minor, particularly if the skin is not broken. Some, however, can have life-threatening implications if proper care is not given.

Children enjoy pets, especially dogs; yet, they are not always taught how to care for them and to avoid unfamiliar dogs. Thus, dog bites are a common occurrence. Any dog or other pet who bites should be held until it can be determined whether the animal has been vaccinated against rabies. If not, it will be necessary for the child to undergo a painful series of injections to prevent this usually fatal disease.

All animal and human bites should be thoroughly washed with soap and water. An antiseptic should be applied after the wound has been thoroughly rinsed; Zephiran is a compound active against rabies virus and an agent of choice in the treatment of animal bites. Animal bites should be reported to the proper authorities.

Spider and tick bites can cause serious illness if untreated. Bites of black widow and brown recluse spiders, and scorpions demand medical attention. Absorption of their poison can be slowed by applying ice to the affected area.

Tick bites can cause Rocky Mountain spotted fever; persons living in areas where ticks are common can be immunized against this disease. Ticks should be carefully removed by placing a drop of nail polish remover, alcohol, gasoline, or other volatile substance onto the tick.

Snake bite demands immediate medical intervention. The wound should be washed, and ice applied, and the body part involved should be immobilized.

Insect stings or bites can prove fatal to children who are sensitized. Swelling may be localized or include an entire extremity. Circulatory collapse, airway obstruction, and anaphylactic shock can cause death within 30 minutes if the child is untreated. Immediate treatment is necessary, and may include injection of epinephrine, antihistamines, or steroids. These children should wear a MedicAlert bracelet and carry an anaphylaxis kit that includes a plastic syringe of epinephrine and an antihistamine.

TABLE 13–9.　COMMON SKIN RASHES IN THE SCHOOL-AGE CHILD

Rash	Description	Signs and Symptoms	Care
Infections			
Measles (Rubeola)	Maculopapular rash, reddish brown, first on face and neck, then spreads to trunk and extremities; lasts 5–6 days; some desquamation; may coalesce on head and neck	Incubation period of 10–21 days; prodromal period with fever, conjunctivitis, and cough; Koplik's spots in mouth; pruritus	Bed rest until fever subsides on 5th or 6th day; dim lights for photophobia; rinse eyes with warm saline or water; use calamine location for itching. Watch for complications such as encephalitis; keep child home from school.
Rubella	Maculopapular rash, pinkish red with discrete lesions; appears first on face and neck then spreading to trunk and extremities. Rash lasts 2–3 days; the face clears first.	Prodromal period of 1–4 days with some malaise and fever; lymphadenopathy in children	Mild or no symptoms; keep home from school until rash disappears; do not expose pregnant women to child.
Erythema infectiosum (Fifth disease)	Red, flushed cheeks and circumoral pallor; slapped face appearance; maculopapular rash on extremities follows; rash may reappear and disappear several times.	Viral origin; prodromal period may include fever and malaise, but is frequently absent; mild pruritus	Child comfortable, only mildly infectious; may be kept home from school
Scarlet fever	Punctiform rash, erythematous, yellowish red, first on flexural surfaces; most intense on neck, axillary, and popliteal skin folds, becomes diffuse and may then cover whole body; desquamates	Prodromal of 12–48 hours, fever, sore throat, vomiting caused by group A beta-hemolytic streptococcus; red strawberry tongue on 4th or 5th day, exudative tonsillitis, elevated antistreptolysin titer O	Penicillin should be given to prevent complications such as nephritis and rheumatic fever—encourage parents to give drug and fluids; keep quiet activities during febrile phase; keep child home from school.
Rocky Mountain spotted fever	Maculopapular and petechial rash; centrifugal distribution, first on wrists and ankles, palms and soles	Presence of tick bite; prodromal period of 3–4 days with spiking fever, chills, malaise, anorexia, headache, mental confusion, restlessness	Measures to relieve high fever; fluids, rest, and sedative may be needed to relieve anxiety and restlessness; keep home from school until child feels well (not contagious).
Chickenpox	Maculopapular rash with vesicles forming later; vesicles rupture leaving crusts; rash appears first on chest and spread to face, trunk and scalp; lesions found in all stages	Prodromal period of 24–48 hr with headache and anorexia in older children; caused by variola-zoster virus; infectious until lesions heal; pruritus	Relieve itching with calamine lotion, ointments, cool soaks and sedatives; may need mits at night; keep child home from school until lesions have crusted and scabs are well formed.
Contact Dermatitis			
Poison Ivy (Rhus dermatitis)	Red vesicular and sometimes bulbous rash; occurs first on exposed skin areas; may eventually cover large areas	Intense pruritus, weeping	Cool soaks to relieve itching; calamine lotion, topical steroids; oral steroids if severe. Replace fluid loss if lesions are weeping and cover large areas; may need mitts at night and some sedation; keep child home from school until bulbous lesions clear.
Shoe allergy	Scaling, red; some vesicles seen on feet, first in toe region; macerations	Pruritus; painful if irritated	Change shoes, expose to air, topical steroids if severe

Handwritten annotations:

Scarlet fever: Strep throat c̄ fine red rash on body. Cause: strain of strep. Infectious till symptoms subside.

Rocky Mountain spotted fever: Treatment: Bedrest, antibiotics, encourage fluids.

TABLE 13–9. (*Continued*)

Rash	Description	Signs and Symptoms	Care
Food Allergies and Drug Reactions Urticaria	Maculopapular rash, bright red, found anywhere on body; may see wheals	Pruritus	Eliminate cause: stop all but life-threatening drugs; get accurate diet history; if severe and repetitious, try elimination diet; use cool soaks to relieve itching; if severe and prolonged, use antihistamines and steroids.
Erythema multiforme	Erythematous and erosive lesions on skin and mucous membranes; lesions have red periphery and cyanotic looking center.	Slight fever; secondary infection possible; may be triggered by hypersensitivity reaction	Remove offending antigen if known; prevent scratching of lesions; cut nails; use mitts at bedtime; oral steroids may be given early in process.
Stevens-Johnson syndrome (severe variant of erythema multiforme)	Circular, erythematous lesions become confluent and form vesicles or bullae. Lesions appear on extensor surfaces of extremities and dorsum of hands and feet; in severe cases, they will be found on trunk, neck, head, palms, and soles.	Stomatitis, pharyngitis, conjunctivitis, painful swallowing, cough, and possible pneumonia; myocarditis, pericarditis, arthritis, or encephalitis may occur.	Ensure fluid and protein intake; pulmonary care; mouth care for stomatitis; eye care, including frequent eye washes with saline; administer medications including corticosteroids and analgesics if needed.

(Wieczorek RR, Natapoff J: A Conceptual Approach to the Nursing of Children: Health Care From Birth Through Adolescence. Philadelphia, JB Lippincott, 1981)

summary

The school years are a time of intense learning for every child. Children with health problems must learn even more; for instance, how their problem affects their bodies and how to care for themselves. For some, the years from 6 to 10 can be a period of growth and improvement in general health, minimizing the specific problem. For others, it can be a time of deterioration, frequent hospitalization, and painful procedures. Nurses can be valuable resources for these children and families during the school years, offering supportive, understanding care, acceptance, and education. School nurses can be particularly helpful to children and families who must cope with health problems.

review questions

1. What is an allergen?
2. What is the pathophysiology of asthma?
3. What are the classifications of drugs used to treat asthma?
4. Why are breathing exercises necessary in the management of asthma?
5. What are the two forms of scoliosis?
6. What is an essential factor for recovering from Legg-Calvé-Perthes disease?
7. What is cryptorchidism?
8. Differentiate between the types of general and the types of partial (focal) seizures, including the diagnosis and treatment.
9. What are the major manifestations of rheumatic fever?
10. What is the chief concern in the treatment of rheumatic fever?
11. What drugs are used to treat rheumatic fever?
12. What are the symptoms of diabetes mellitus?
13. What are the clinical manifestations of diabetic acidosis and how are they treated?
14. What are the causes of insulin reaction?
15. What are the symptoms of impending insulin shock, or reaction, and how are they treated?
16. What is the role of the nurse in teaching the diabetic child and his family?
17. Why is it essential to rotate insulin injection sites?
18. Why is adolescence a particularly trying period for the diabetic?
19. What foods and drugs are likely to cause urticaria?

references

1. Fromer MJ: Community Health Care and the Nursing Process. St Louis, CV Mosby, 1979

2. Leton DA: Assessment of school phobia. Mental Hygiene 46:256–264, 1962
3. Kahn JH, Nursten JP: Unwillingly to School. Elmsford, Pergamon Press, 1964
4. Wieczorek RR, Natapoff J: A Conceptual Approach to the Nursing of Children: Health Care From Birth Through Adolescence. Philadelphia, JB Lippincott, 1981
5. Hageman MB: Childhood psychosis: Residential treatment and its alternatives. In Wolman B (ed): Handbook of Treatment of Mental Disorders in Childhood and Adolescence. Englewood Cliffs, Prentice-Hall, 1978
6. National Health Survey. U.S. Public Health Service, Washington, DC, U.S. Government Printing Office, 1970
7. Asthma and Allergy Foundation. Handbook for the Asthmatic. New York, The Foundation, 1980
8. McCaully HE: Breathing exercises as play for asthmatic children. Am J Mat Child Nurs 5:340–344, 1980
9. Wieczorek RR, Natapoff J: A Conceptual Approach to the Nursing of Children: Health Care From Birth Through Adolescence. Philadelphia, JB Lippincott, 1981
10. Heilbrunn G: Disorders of mental function. In Leitch C, Tinker R: Primary Care. Philadelphia, FA Davis, 1978
11. Weil WB, Korman A: Diabetes mellitus. In Rudolph A (ed): Pediatrics. New York, Appleton-Century-Crofts, 1977
12. Christiansen C, Sachse M: Home blood glucose monitoring: Benefits for the patient and educator. Diabetes Educ, 13–21, Fall 1980
13. Malone J: Newer aspects of diabetes. Advances Pediatr 1–42, 1977

bibliography

Asthma and Allergy Foundation of America. Allergy in Children. New York, The Foundation, 1980

Asthma and Allergy Foundation. Skin Allergy. New York, The Foundation, 1979

Bowers JE: Can you recognize childhood learning disorders? Nurs 77 7, No. 11:26–29, 1977

Bridgewater SC, Voignier RR, Smith CS: Allergies in children: Recognition, testing, treating and teaching. Am J Nurs 78:613–621, 1978

Bruya MA, Bolin RH: Epilepsy: A controllable disease. Am J Nurs 76:388–397, 1976

Cohen S, Glass G: Skin rashes in infants and children. Am J Nurs 78:1–32, 1978

Evans M, Hansen B: Guide to Pediatric Nursing: A Clinical Reference. New York, Appleton-Century-Crofts, 1980

Feingold BF: Hyperkinesis and learning disabilities linked to artificial food flavors and colors. Am J Nurs 75:797–803, 1975

Friedland G: Learning behaviors of a preadolescent with diabetes. Am J Nurs 76:59–61, 1976

Goldfarb W, Mahres H: The causes and treatment of childhood schizophrenia. In Segal S (ed): The Mental Health of the Child. Public Health Service pamphlet No. 1268. Washington, DC, U.S. Government Printing Office, 1971

Guthrie DW, Guthrie RA (eds): Nursing Management of Diabetes Mellitus. St Louis, CV Mosby, 1977

Hall VA, Shaw PK, Smith EB: Could that itching be scabies? Nurs Update 7, No. 8:1, 13–16, 1976

Hilt, NE, Schmitt EW: Pediatric Orthopedic Nursing. St Louis, CV Mosby Company, 1975

Hilt NE, Cogburn SB: Manual of Orthopedics. St Louis, CV Mosby, 1979

Lawson BA: Chronic illness in the school-age child: Effects on the total family. Am J Mat Child Nurs 2:49–56, 1977

Muehl JN: Seizure disorders in children: Prevention and care. Am J Mat Child Nurs 4:154–160, 1979

Nadar PR, Bullock D, Caldwell B: School phobia. Pediatr Clin N Am 22:605–617, 1975

Nysather JO, et al: The immune system: Its development and functions. Am J Nurs 76:1616, 1976

Rogers M: Early identification and intervention of children with learning problems. Pediatr Nurs 2:21–26, 1976

Rosser PL: The learning-disabled child. J Nurs Care 11, No. 1:14–15, 1978

Simonds JF: Enuresis. Clin Pediatr 16:79–82, 1977

Stewart WD, Danto JL, Maddin S: Dermatology: Diagnosis and Treatment of Cutaneous Disorders, 4th ed. St Louis, CV Mosby, 1977

Tamborlane WV Jr, Sherwin RS: Man-made. Diabetes Forecast 18–21, January–February 1981

Welch N: Recent insights into the childhood "social diseases:" Gonorrhea, scabies, pediculosis, ringworm. Clin Pediatr 17:318–322, 1978

Whaley L, Wong D: Nursing Care of Infants and Children. St Louis, CV Mosby, 1979

growth and development of the adolescent: 11 to 18 years

14

physical development
height and weight
secondary sexual characteristics
vital signs
nutrition
food choices
health maintenance
physical examinations, screening, and immunization
health education and counseling
psychosocial development
personality development
body image
implications for hospital care
summary
review questions
references
bibliography

student objectives

The student successfully attaining the goals of this chapter will be able to

1 Define the following vocabulary terms:

   anorexia nervosa   ejaculation   intimacy   lacto-ovo-vegetarian diet   menarche
   nocturnal emissions   puberty

2 Describe the growth and development of the adolescent in the following areas: personal–
   social development, fine motor skills, gross motor skills, language development, and
   cognition.

3 List six nutrients that are commonly deficient in the adolescent's diet and identify good food
   sources for each.

4 Describe the recommended immunizations for adolescents.

5 Describe the guidelines for contraceptive teaching and discuss five contraceptive methods
   that are currently available.

6 List twelve guidelines that are designed to help adolescents adjust to hospitalization.

Knowing

by Karen Haynes

There are times
when I have to know
who I am,
what I am,
where I am
but really,
who I am.
I have to know
for
a cat just knows she's a cat,
a dog just knows she's a dog;
I must know what I am
for a flower must know it belongs to a plant,
a grain of sand must know it belongs to
a beach.
I must know
where I am
for
a leaf must know it is among thousands
of others,
a tree in a forest must know it is
one in a thousand of others.
Since they all know,
Why can't I?

Adolescence comes from the Latin word meaning "to grow up," an apt description of this stage of life. The adolescent is maturing physically and emotionally, "growing up" from childhood toward adulthood and seeking to know and understand what it means to be grown-up.

Early adolescence (preadolescence, pubescence) begins at about age 10 with a dramatic growth spurt that signals the advent of puberty (reproductive maturity). During this stage, the child's body begins to take on adultlike contours, primary sex organs enlarge, secondary sexual characteristics appear, and hormonal activity increases (Table 14–1). By the end of adolescence, the bone growth that began during intrauterine life is completed.

Adolescents are fascinated, and sometimes fearful and confused, by the changes occurring in their bodies and in their thinking processes (Table 14–2). They begin to look grown-up, but do not have the judgment or independence to participate in society as a grown-up. These young people are strongly influenced by their peer group, and often resent parental authority. Roller-coaster levels of emotion characterize this age group, as does intense interest in the opposite sex (Fig. 14–1).

The adolescent years can be a time of conflict between parents and children. If these conflicts are successfully resolved, normal development can continue. Unresolved, the conflicts can foster delays in development and prevent the young person's maturing into a fully functioning adult.

Body image is critically important to adolescents. Health problems that threaten body image—acne, obesity, dental or vision problems, traumatic accidents—can seriously interfere with development.

Girls generally begin adolescence before boys and mature faster during this period; therefore, their development is discussed separately.

TABLE 14–1. GROWTH AND DEVELOPMENT CHART: THE PREADOLESCENT

Age (years)	Personal–Social	Fine Motor	Gross Motor	Language	Cognitive
10–12	Distinct need for close peer relationships Constant desire to be with "best friend" Shares innermost thoughts, secrets, opinions, and emotions with "best friend": provides a sense of acceptance, significance, and security Intolerance for violations of group norms; strong identification with peers, increased concern with body, self-understanding, urge for independence In group interaction: a. Is able to follow rules b. Is able to make independent judgments by utilizing stored knowledge c. Can adapt to another opinion or point of view	May have difficulty with some fine motor coordination due to growth of large muscles prior to that of small muscles Hands and feet are first structures to increase in size; therefore, actions may appear uncoordinated during early preadolescence.	Physical activity intensifies with apparently inordinate amounts of energy. Increasingly absorbed in athletic sports	Fluent in spoken language Utilizes slang words and terms, vulgarities, jeers, jokes, and sayings Paradigmatic associated responses (to language tests) are more logically related and more formal.	Continues in stage of concrete operations Evidences many transitional trends in cognitive processes including moral development (level II—conventional); understands the viewpoint of others Abilities to sympathize, love, and reason are all evolving. Right and wrong become logically clear.

(Wieczorek RR, Natapoff J: A Conceptual Approach to the Nursing of Infants and Children: Health Care From Birth Through Adolescence. Philadelphia, JB Lippincott, 1981)

physical development

HEIGHT AND WEIGHT

FEMALES

Early adolescence begins in the female some time between the ages of 9 and 11 years, and is marked by a growth spurt that lasts about 18 months. Girls grow about 3 inches each year until *menarche* (beginning of menstruation), after which growth slows considerably. Normally by age 16 girls have reached about 98% of their adult height.

Weight gain increases markedly about 6 months after height is accelerated, and continues for approximately 3 years.

MALES

Boys enter adolescence between 11 and 13 years, and their growth spurt lasts almost 3 years. Height increases about 4 inches annually until puberty, after which it continues to increase, but at a slower rate. Between 12 and 16 years of age, boys almost double in weight.

SECONDARY SEXUAL CHARACTERISTICS

FEMALES

Early in adolescence, girls begin to develop "a figure;" breast development starts, the pelvis widens, pubic hair appears; and a little later, axillary hair. The wide variance in individual rates of development (Fig. 14–2) means that

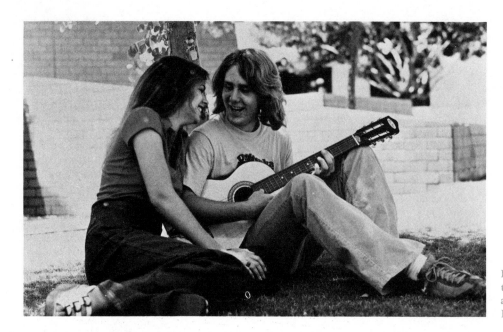

FIG. 14–1. Intense interest in the opposite sex characterizes adolescence. (Am J Mat Child Nurs, May–June 1980)

some girls may be embarrassed by their undeveloped breasts, while others may feel out of place with their womanly figures. Since acceptance by the peer group is so vital, adolescents do not appreciate being different in any way.

MALES

The earliest pubescent changes in boys occur between 11 and 13, and include enlargement of the penis, testes, and scrotum; appearance of pubic hair, and then axillary and facial hair. After age 13, muscle strength and coordination develop rapidly. The voice changes gradually, becoming deeper and more resonant.

Puberty for the male begins officially with the first ejaculation, even though sperm usually is not present until between age 13 and 16. Often these ejaculations occur spontaneously at night and are referred to as *nocturnal emissions* or "wet dreams." They normally begin about 1 year after the appearance of secondary sexual characteristics.

VITAL SIGNS

During adolescence, respiratory capacity increases in both boys and girls, and respiratory rate decreases. Pulse rates decrease slightly (Table 14–3) and blood pressures increase (Table 14–4).

nutrition

Even though adolescents understand something about nutrition, they may not relate this understanding to their dietary habits. Their accelerated growth rate, and, for some, increased physical activities mean that they need more food to supply their energy requirements. Because adolescents are seeking to establish their independence, their food choices are sometimes not wise ones, but tend to be influenced by peer preference rather than parental advice. The era of fast-food has given adolescents easy access to high-calorie but nutritionally unbalanced meals. Too many fast-food meals and nutritionally empty snacks can result in nutritional deficiencies (Table 14–5).

FOOD CHOICES

When good nutritional habits have been established in early childhood, adolescent nutrition is likely to be better

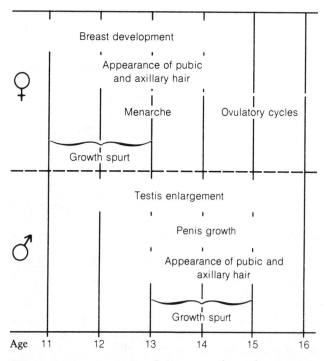

FIG. 14–2. Average timing of the events of sexual maturation.

TABLE 14–2. GROWTH AND DEVELOPMENT CHART: THE ADOLESCENT

Personal–Social	Fine Motor	Gross Motor	Language	Cognition
Positive peer relationships are sought out and valued. Early adolescents place emphasis on becoming sophisticated and feeling "grown-up." Adolescents want authority over themselves and their own environment, dignity, hetereosexual intimacy, and self-respect. Most adolescents want the reciprocal reinforcement of the peer group. Peer cliques are usually homogeneous in social class, race, age, and academic achievement. The adolescent enjoys recognition from his fellow classmates. Peer group is used for emotional support. The extent of the pressure exerted on adolescent males concerning their vocational choice is influenced by socioeconomic class, ethnic background, peer pressure, cultural factors, and community resources. In moral development, beliefs of ideas are evaluated for their logic. Sexual identity becomes fully matured.	The abilities to see, hear, touch, taste, and smell become more refined.	Growth is a continuous process until the end of adolescence. Boys catch up to girls in maturity. Adolescents become more efficient and more adaptable in getting work done. Adolescents walk, run, bend down, swing their bodies into various positions in sport activities.	Intensive use of slang terms Excessive use of "dirty" words, symbols, and gestures Affinity toward rock 'n' roll and hard rock, and use of colloquialisms Logic can function on either verbal or symbolic language Academic study of a second language may be started.	A central task of adolescence involves the young person moving away from dependency on family to establishing self an an independent person. Superego develops. The adolescent can rely less on parental directions and more on internal thoughts and ideas. Peer groups are established to assist in the establishment of personal identity. Adolescents reason on an abstract or symbolic level. They can develop and apply generalizations. Teenagers have the ability to move back and forth between the stages of concrete and abstract reasoning. They have the ability to find discrepancies or inconsistencies within complex materials. Adolescents are cognitively able to interpret and integrate their sensations and impressions into an internalized self-concept. Stage of formal operations occurs where youngsters are able to reason using hypothesis and proposition. Making generalities is common, as is stereotyping.

(Wieczorek RR, Natapoff J: A Conceptual Approach to the Nursing of Infants and Children: Health Care From Birth Through Adolescence. Philadelphia, JB Lippincott, 1981)

balanced than in cases where insufficient nutritional teaching has occurred. Being part of a family that practices sound nutrition assures that occasional lapses into sweets, fast-foods, and other peer-group food preferences will not create serious deficiencies.

In their quest for identity and independence, some adolescents experiment with food fads and diets, such as organically grown fruits and vegetables, health foods, and vegetarian diets. Others snack continually. If the snacks are nutritious, such as fresh fruits, milk, juices, and grain products, this can provide a better balanced diet than some other choices.

VEGETARIAN DIETS

Several types of vegetarian diets have become a way of life for middle and late adolescents. The *lacto-ovo-vegetarian*

TABLE 14–3. AVERAGE PULSE RATES AT REST DURING ADOLESCENCE

	Age	Lower Normal	Average	Upper Normal
Females	14	65	85	110
	16	60	80	105
	18	55	75	95
Males	14	60	80	100
	16	55	75	95
	18	50	70	90

(Adapted from Vaughan V, McKay R, Behrman R: Nelson's Textbook of Pediatrics, 11th ed, p 1252. Philadelphia, WB Saunders, 1979)

diet includes dairy products, eggs, fruits, vegetables, and grain products, and can meet all the daily requirements of an adolescent. A *fruitarian diet* includes principally fruits and nuts, and can contribute to vitamin deficiencies. Strict vegetarian diets include only fruits, vegetables, and grains, and can cause deficiencies of vitamin D, calcium, riboflavin, zinc, iron, and niacin.[1]

ORGANICALLY GROWN FOODS AND HEALTH FOODS

Recent attention focused on pollution and other environmental issues has prompted a "back-to-nature" movement, particularly among young people. Health food restaurants and retail stores now offer a variety of fresh foods grown without chemicals, and foods processed without

TABLE 14–4. BLOOD PRESSURE IN EARLY AND MID-ADOLESCENT MALES AND FEMALES BY AGE, SEX, AND WEIGHT PERCENTILE

Age	Sex	Weight Percentile	Systolic Rate (mmHg)	Diastolic Rate (mmHg)
13	M	50	118	75
13	F	50	116	75
14	M	50	120	77
14	F	50	119	76
15	M	50	122	78
15	F	50	120	77
16	M	50	124	78
16	F	50	120	78
17	M	50	126	79
17	F	50	122	78

(Adapted from Task Force on Blood Pressure Control in Children. National Heart, Lung and Blood Institute: Percentiles in blood pressure report from the Task Force. Pediatrics (Suppl) 59:803, 1977. Copyright American Academy of Pediatrics)

additives. These foods are more expensive than ordinary supermarket foods; however, many persons feel that the superior taste and nutritional benefit warrants the additional expense.

SNACKS

Adolescents' needs for refuelling their energy supply lead them to eat whatever is most handy. Thus, it behooves parents and school nutritionists to see that the most available snacks are also the most nutritious, such as fruits, milk, yogurt, grain products, and other foods high in iron, calcium, and vitamins A and C.

ETHNIC INFLUENCES

Culture also influences adolescent food choices and habits. For example, Mexican-Americans are accustomed to having their big meal at noon. When school lunches do not provide such a heavy meal, the Mexican-American adolescent may supplement with sweets or fast-foods. Within the Chinese community, milk is not a popular drink, and this can result in a calcium deficiency. Addition of ice cream, custard, and cheese to the diet of Chinese adolescents can help overcome this problem.

health maintenance

Adolescents have much the same need for regular health checkups, protection against infection, and prevention of accidents as do younger children. They also have very special needs that can best be met by health professionals with in-depth knowledge and understanding of adolescent needs and concerns (Fig. 14–3). During recent years, the number of adolescent clinics and health centers has increased, along with such innovative health services as crisis hotlines, homes for runaways, and rehabilitation centers for adolescents who have been involved with alcohol or other drugs, or with prostitution.

PHYSICAL EXAMINATIONS, SCREENING, AND IMMUNIZATION

Annual physical examinations are recommended for healthy adolescents, with more frequent visits for those in groups at risk. Recommended immunizations are summarized in Table 14–6. School and community health services conduct screening programs to detect the presence of such health problems as scoliosis, vision and hearing deficits, hypertension, anemia, venereal disease (VD), and kidney disease.

Adolescents need to be assured of privacy, individualized attention, confidentiality, and the right to participate in decisions about their health care. They feel out of place in a pediatrician's waiting room where most of the patients are 3 feet tall, or in a waiting room filled with adults.

Continuity of care helps to build the adolescent's confidence in the service and the caregivers. Professionals dealing with this group should recognize that the physical symptoms offered as the reason for seeking care are often not the most significant problem about which the adolescent is concerned. An attitude of unjudging acceptance on

TABLE 14–5. FOOD SOURCES OF NUTRIENTS COMMONLY DEFICIENT IN PREADOLESCENT AND ADOLESCENT DIETS

Common Nutrient Deficiencies	Foods High in These Nutrients
Vitamin A	Direct sources: liver, fish liver oils, butter, cheese, eggs, and milk Sources of carotene: yellow vegetables, green leafy vegetables, tomatoes, yellow fruits
Vitamin C	Citrus fruits, strawberries, broccoli, bell peppers, tomato juice, rose hips
Calcium	Milk, cheese, yogurt, ice cream, soybeans, mustard, and turnip greens
Iron	Red meats, especially liver, wheat germ, brewer's yeast, egg yolks, dark green leafy vegetables, apricots, whole grain cereals, fish
Riboflavin	Milk, liver, brewer's yeast, whole grains, green leafy vegetables, fish and eggs
Thiamine	Brewer's yeast, wheat germ, rice polish, pork, milk, nuts, whole grains, liver, peas, lentils

(The American Journal of Maternal Child Nursing, 2, No. 2: 120, 1977. Copyright March/April 1977, The American Journal of Nursing Company)

the part of the nurse or physician can frequently encourage the adolescent to share questions, feelings, and concerns about the matter that is troubling him.

HEALTH EDUCATION AND COUNSELING

Before adolescents can take an active role in their own health care, they need information and guidance on the need for health care and how to most effectively meet that need. Education and counseling about sexuality, venereal disease, contraception, substance abuse, and mental health are a vital part of adolescent health care. Some of this teaching should, and sometimes does, come from parents, but often the parents' lack of information, or their discomfort in discussing these topics, means that the job will have to be done by health professionals.

SEXUALITY

Ideally sex eduation begins at home and is continued as a part of the school curriculum, so that children understand the basics of sexuality and reproduction before puberty. Proper preparation can help the adolescent be proud to have reached sexual maturity. If this is not the case, puberty can be a frightening, shameful experience. Girls who have not been taught about menstruation until it occurs are understandably alarmed. Those who have been taught to regard it as "the curse" rather than as an entrance into womanhood will not have positive feelings about this part of their sexuality.

Boys who are unprepared for nocturnal emissions may feel guilty, believing that they have caused these "wet dreams" by sexual imaginings or masturbation. They need to understand that this is a normal occurrence and simply the body's method of getting rid of surplus semen.

Assuming that adolescents are adequately prepared for the events of puberty, sex education during adolescence can deal with the important issues of responsible sexuality, contraception, and venereal disease. Adolescents today are more sexually active than ever, resulting in an alarmingly rapid increase in teenage pregnancies and venereal disease.

Girls need to learn the importance of regular pelvic examinations and Pap smears, and should learn the technique for self-examination of the breast, a monthly self-care procedure (Fig. 14–4).

Masturbation. Growing awareness of their sexuality, sexually provocative material in the media, and lack of acceptable means to gratify sexual desires make masturbation a common practice during adolescence. Unlike young children's genital exploration, adolescent masturbation can produce orgasm in the female and ejaculation in the male. Generally it is a private, solitary activity, but occasionally occurs with one or more members of the peer group.

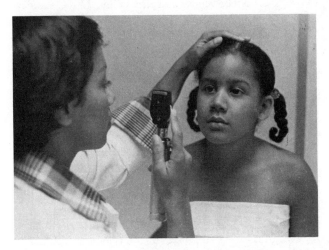

FIG. 14–3. Clinic nurse examining a preadolescent. (Brunner LS, Suddarth DS (eds): The Lippincott Manual of Nursing Practice, 2nd ed. Philadelphia, JB Lippincott, 1978)

TABLE 14–6.   RECOMMENDED IMMUNIZATIONS IN ADOLESCENCE IN THE UNITED STATES

Immunization Type	Characteristics
Td-Tetanus toxoid	Given at 14 to 16 years, then repeated every 10 years
Tuberculin testing	Repeated every 1 to 3 years depending on the youngster's living environment
Rubella vaccine	Given to sexually active adolescent females with low rubella titers whether or not they state they have received rubella vaccine before. These young women are instructed to avoid pregnancy for at least 2 months following the immunization to prevent congenital rubella syndrome in their offspring.
Typhoid	Given to adolescents during epidemics, those that are residents of rural endemic areas, or foreign travelers
Influenza (bivalent A and B)	Given to adolescents with chronic debilitating diseases like congenital heart diseases, chronic bronchopulmonary disease, or diabetes
Yellow fever	Given to adolescents who are going to travel to Southeast Asia. It should not be given simultaneously with smallpox. If both immunizations are required, a 3-week waiting period is advised.
Smallpox	Given to adolescents who are traveling to very underdeveloped areas of Africa or Asia
Malaria prophylaxis	Given to adolescents who are traveling to places where infestations are present such as Southeast Asia
Cholera	Given to adolescents who are traveling to foreign countries where exposure is a possibility

(Wieczorek RR, Natapoff J: A Conceptual Approach to the Nursing of Infants and Children: Health Care From Birth Through Adolescence. Philadelphia, JB Lippincott, 1981)

Attitudes toward masturbation have changed during recent years so that many persons, particularly health professionals, recognize it as a positive way to release sexual tension and increase one's knowledge of body sensations. Frequency may be reduced if sexual intercourse occurs with some regularity.

Contraception.   Not all adolescents are sexually active, but the increasing number who are need to be aware of the currently available methods of contraception (Table 14–7), their effectiveness and risk (Table 14–8). Adolescents who seek contraceptive services are entitled to con-fidentiality; consequently, the trend is to provide these services free or at a nominal fee so teenagers will not need to tell their parents.

Every contraceptive method carries some risk, but none so great as the risk associated with pregnancy. Adolescents must understand the risks in order to give informed consent. (See boxed material.) Girls in this age group tend to favor "the pill" over any other method because it requires little effort to use.

Adolescent boys should be taught about various contraceptive methods as well, and should be aware that the condom affords reliable contraception as well as limited protection against venereal disease.

GUIDELINES FOR CONTRACEPTIVE TEACHING

Informed consent is the voluntary, knowing assent from the individual on whom any procedure is to be performed after she or he has been given

1. a fair explanation of the procedures or method;
2. a description of attendant discomforts and risks, including all major (life-threatening) and all common minor risks;
3. a description of the benefits to be expected;
4. an explanation of alternative methods and effectiveness rates with indication that nothing is 100 percent, and that sterilization is permanent;
5. an offer to answer any questions about procedures or method;

6. an instruction that the individual is free to withdraw consent to the procedure or method at any time prior to the procedure, or to discontinue the method, without affecting future care or loss of benefits;
7. a written consent document detailing the basic elements of informed consent and the information provided. This should be signed by the patient, an auditor-witness of the patient's choice, and by the person obtaining the consent.

(Reeder SJ, Mastroianni L, Martin LL: Maternity Nursing, 14th ed. Philadelphia, JB Lippincott, 1980)

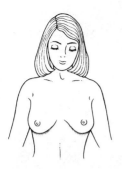

1. Careful examination of the breasts before a mirror for symmetry in size and shape, noting any puckering or dimpling of the skin or retraction of the nipple.

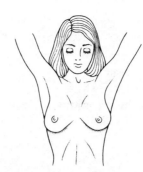

2. Arms raised over head, again studying the breasts in the mirror for the same signs.

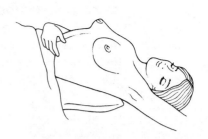

3. Reclining on bed with flat pillow or folded bath towel under the shoulder on the same side as breast to be examined.

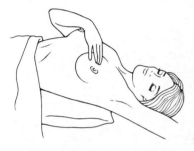

4. To examine the inner half of the breast the arm is raised over the head. Beginning at the breastbone and, in a series of steps, the inner half of the breast is palpated.

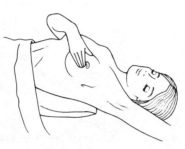

5. The area over the nipple is carefully palpated with the flat part of the fingers.

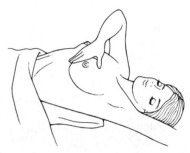

6. Examination of the lower inner half of the breast is completed.

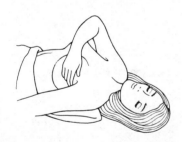

7. With arm down at side self-examination of breasts continues by carefully feeling the tissues which extend to the armpit.

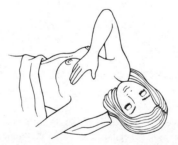

8. The upper outer quadrant of the breast is examined with the flat part of the fingers.

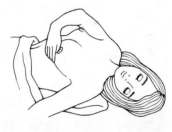

9. The lower outer quadrant of the breast is examined in successive stages with flat part of the fingers.

FIG. 14–4. Breast self-examination.

Venereal Disease (VD). Increased early sexual activity and use of oral contraceptives have made venereal disease so prevalent among teenagers that its incidence is second only to the common cold. Syphilis and gonorrhea are the most common of these diseases, but herpes simplex, type 2 is increasing rapidly in all age groups.

Prevention of venereal disease is the ideal method of care. When prevention has proved ineffective, the most important factor is referral for treatment. Many adolescents are reluctant to seek treatment, fearing that their parents will discover their activity. Crisis hotlines can be valuable resources to assure adolescents that treatment is vital for them and their partner, and that confidentiality is assured.

Health professionals who work with adolescents seeking treatment for VD should assume a nonjudgmental, understanding attitude, and provide sufficient information to help prevent recurrence of the infection.

SUBSTANCE ABUSE

In today's culture, the use of alcohol and some illicit drugs is considered adult recreation until use becomes abuse.

TABLE 14–7.   METHODS OF CONTRACEPTION CURRENTLY AVAILABLE

Male and Female	Male	Female
ABSTINENCE	WITHDRAWAL	SPERMICIDES*
Total	CONDOMS	Foam, Cream, Gels
Periodic	VASECTOMY	Diaphragm with Gel or Cream
Rhythm		OVULATION PREVENTION†
Basal Body		Oral
Temperature (BBT)		Injectable
Nonvaginal Variations		Implanted
Masturbation		UNKNOWN ACTION
Solitary		Minipill
Mutual		Morning-After Pill
Oralgenital		Intrauterine Device
Anal Intercourse		Mechanical
		Chemical
		Hormonal
		Heavy Metals (Copper)
		TUBAL STERILIZATION‡

* Douching is not a contraceptive method.

† Breast-feeding is not a contraceptive method.

‡ Abortion is not a contraceptive method.

(Pierson EC: Sex is Never an Emergency, 3rd ed, p 5. Philadelphia, JB Lippincott, 1973)

TABLE 14–8.   EFFECTIVENESS AND RISKS OF CONTRACEPTIVES, PREGNANCIES PER 100 WOMEN PER YEAR

Method	Theoretical Effectiveness	Use Effec- tiveness	Continuing Pregnancies	Deaths Due to Pregnancy	Deaths Due to Contra- ceptive	Major Morbidity (%)	Minor Morbidity (%)
No contraception	—	—	80	0.016	0	—	—
Oral contraceptives	0.1	3–4	0.5	0	0.003	1	40
IUD	2	5	3	0.001	0.001	1	40
Diaphragm	3	13–17	12	0.002	0	—	—
Rhythm	14	35–40	25	0.005	0	—	—
Early abortion*	0	0	0	0	0.003	1	8
Laparoscopic tubal ligation	0	0.04	0.15	0	0.03	0.6	1
Vasectomy	0	0.15	0.15	0	0	1	5
Condom†	3	15	—	—	—	—	—
Spermicides†	3	13–17	—	—	—	—	—
Coitus interruptus†	3	15–25	—	—	—	—	—

* Abortion is not a method of contraception, but is included here for comparison.

† Data on continuing pregnancies, deaths due to pregnancy are not available, but use effectiveness figures indicate these would be in the range found for the diaphragm.

(Adapted from Hatcher RA, et al: Contraceptive Technology 1976–1977, pp 25, 100. New York, Halstead Press, 1976; and Romney SL, et al: Gynecology and Obstetrics: The Health Care of Women, pp 551, 552. New York, McGraw-Hill, Blakiston, 1975)

Striving to be an adult, the adolescent often sees these practices as sophisticated, and indulges in them as rites of passage. Prescription drugs, particularly those that alter mood or awareness, are part of many family medicine cabinets, and accessible to adolescents. Abuse of these substances is common among teenagers, and sometimes, among parents as well.

Adolescents need counseling about the immediate and long-term effects of alcohol, marijuana, cocaine, heroin, and other "street drugs" as well as improper use of pre-scription medications. Health professionals can help dispel the myths that these drugs enhance sexual experiences because in reality most of them interfere with sexual per-formance. Moralizing will not help, but only makes the forbidden seem more attractive. Accurate presentation of facts about consequences can permit adolescents to make informed choices. Despite the age limit on purchase of alcoholic beverages, and the illegality of many narcotics, these substances are readily available to children of school age who have the money to purchase them.

TABLE 14–9.   DEATHS AND DEATH RATES FOR THE 10 LEADING CAUSES OF DEATH FOR MALES AND FEMALES 5 TO 14 YEARS OF AGE: 1976

Rank	Age, Sex, Cause of Death, and Category Numbers of the Eighth Revision International Classification of Diseases, Adapted, 1965		Number	Rate Per 100,000 Population in Specified Group
	5–14 Years, Both Sexes			
	All causes		12,901	34.7
1	Accidents	E800–E949	6,308	17.0
2	Malignant neoplasms, including neoplasms of lymphatic and hematopoietic tissues	140–209	1,849	5.0
3	Congenital anomalies	740–759	745	2.0
4	Homicide	E960–E978	392	1.1
5	Influenza and pneumonia	470–474, 480–486	362	1.0
6	Diseases of heart	390–398, 402, 404, 410–429	332	0.9
7	Cerebrovascular diseases	430–438	206	0.6
8	Suicide	E950–E959	163	0.4
9	Benign neoplasms and neoplasms of unspecified nature	210–239	112	0.3
10	Anemias	280–285	98	0.3
	5–14 Years, Male			
	All causes		8,068	42.6
1	Accidents	E800–E949	4.343	22.9
2	Malignant neoplasms, including neoplasms of lymphatic and hematopoietic tissues	140–209	1,105	5.8
3	Congenital anomalies	740–759	367	1.9
4	Homicide	E960–E978	240	1.3
5	Influenza and pneumonia	470–474, 480–486	177	0.9
6	Diseases of heart	390–398, 402, 404, 410–429	174	0.9
7	Suicide	E950–E959	126	0.7
8	Cerebrovascular diseases	430–438	118	0.6
9	Benign neoplasms and neoplasms of unspecified nature	210–239	72	0.4
10	Anemias	280–285	50	0.3
	5–14 Years, Female			
	All causes		4,833	26.5
1	Accidents	E800–E949	1,965	10.8
2	Malignant neoplasms, including neoplasms of lymphatic and hematopoietic tissues	140–209	744	4.1
3	Congenital anomalies	740–759	378	2.1
4	Influenza and pneumonia	470–474, 480, 486	185	1.0
5	Diseases of heart	390–398, 402, 404, 410–429	158	0.9
6	Homicide	E960–E978	152	0.8
7	Cerebrovascular diseases	430–438	88	0.5
8	Anemias	280–285	48	0.3
9	Meningitis	320	43	0.2
10	Benign neoplasms and neoplasms of unspecified nature	210–239	40	0.2

(Department of Health, Education, and Welfare, Public Health Service, National Center for Health Statistics. Facts of life and death [PHS 79-1222]. Washington, DC, U.S. Government Printing Office, November 1978)

MENTAL HEALTH

Adolescents often feel like strangers in a strange land, with countless questions, concerns, and anxieties, and no one with whom to share them except peers who are equally uninformed. A common complaint of this group is that no one really listens or takes them seriously. The attitude of adults seems to be, "This is just a phase you're going through, and you'll soon get over these unimportant worries." Evidence that their problems are very real and that some adolescents don't "get over" them can be found in the suicide statistics in Table 14–9 and 14–10.

Mental health counseling, sometimes available in free clinics, offers adolescents listeners who respect their worries and are concerned about their problems. These young people are anxious about many things: their changing bodies, particularly external appearance such as skin, figure, and hair; they also worry about grades, school ac-

TABLE 14–10. DEATHS AND DEATH RATES FOR THE 10 LEADING CAUSES OF DEATH FOR MALES AND FEMALES 15 TO 24 YEARS OF AGE: 1976

Rank	Age, Sex, Cause of Death, and Category Numbers of the Eighth Revision International Classification of Diseases, Adapted, 1965		Number	Rate Per 100,000 Population in Specified Group
	15–24 Years, Both Sexes			
	All causes		46,081	113.5
1	Accidents	E800–E949	24,316	59.9
2	Homicide	E960–E978	5,038	12.4
3	Suicide	E950–E959	4,747	11.7
4	Malignant neoplasms, including neoplasms of lymphatic and hematopoietic tissues	140–209	2,659	6.5
5	Diseases of heart	390–398, 402, 404, 410–429	1,072	2.6
6	Influenza and pneumonia	470–474, 480–486	611	1.5
7	Congenital anomalies	740–759	568	1.4
8	Cerebrovascular diseases	430–438	506	1.2
9	Diabetes mellitus	250	159	0.4
10	Anemias	280–285	138	0.3
	15–24 Years, Male			
	All causes		34,253	167.7
1	Accidents	E800–E949	19,214	94.1
2	Homicide	E960–E978	3,907	19.1
3	Suicide	E950–E959	3,786	18.5
4	Malignant neoplasms, including neoplasms of lymphatic and hematopoietic tissues	140–209	1,628	8.0
5	Diseases of heart	390–398, 402, 404, 410–429	690	3.4
6	Influenza and pneumonia	470–474, 480–486	336	1.6
7	Congenital anomalies	740–759	329	1.6
8	Cerebrovascular diseases	430–438	281	1.4
9	Anemias	280–285	86	0.4
10	Nephritis and nephrosis	580–584	76	0.4
	15–24 Years, Female			
	All causes		11,828	58.6
1	Accidents	E800–E949	5,102	25.3
2	Homicide	E960–E978	1,131	5.6
3	Malignant neoplasms, including neoplasms of lymphatic and hematopoietic tissues	140–209	1,031	5.1
4	Suicide	E950–E959	961	4.8
5	Diseases of heart	390–398, 402, 404, 410–429	382	1.9
6	Influenza and pneumonia	470–474, 480–486	275	1.4
7	Congenital anomalies	740–759	239	1.2
8	Cerebrovascular diseases	430–438	225	1.1
9	Complications of pregnancy, childbirth, and the puerperium	630–678	137	0.7
10	Diabetes mellitus	250	85	0.4

(Department of Health, Education and Welfare, Public Health Service, (PHS 79-1222). National Center for Health Statistics, Washington, DC, United States Government Printing Office, November, 1978)

tivities, dating, and vocational choices. If parents cannot or will not act as understanding counselors, or if the problems are so serious that professional help is needed to augment parents' efforts, mental health counseling can often help the adolescent work through troublesome situations and avoid chronic mental health problems.

psychosocial development

Adolescence is a time of transition from childhood to adulthood. During the years between 10 and 18, these young people move from latency to the genital stage, from industry versus inferiority to identity versus role confusion, and from concrete operational thinking to formal operational thought (Table 14–11). They develop a sense of moral judgment, and a system of values and beliefs that will influence their entire adult life. The foundation provided by their family, school, and community experiences is still a strong influence, but tremendous power is exerted by the peer group. Trends and fads among adolescents dictate clothing choices, hairstyles, music, and other recreational choices (Fig. 14–5). The adolescent whose parents make it difficult for him to conform are adding another stress to an already emotion-laden period. Peer pressure to experiment with potentially dangerous practices such as drugs, alcohol, and reckless driving, can also be strong, and adolescents may need careful guidance and understanding support to help them resist this peer influence.

PERSONALITY DEVELOPMENT

Erikson considered the central task of adolescence to be the establishment of identity. Adolescents spend a lot of time asking themselves, "Who am I as a person? What will I do with my life? Marry? Have children? Will I go to college? If so, where? If not, why not? What kind of career should I choose?"

Today's adolescents are confronted with a greater variety of choices than ever before. Sex-role stereotypes have been shattered in many careers and professions. More women are becoming lawyers, doctors, plumbers, and carpenters; more men are entering nursing or are choosing to become house-husbands while their wives earn the family income. Transportation has made greater geographic mobility possible, so that many youngsters can spend summers or a full school year in a foreign country; plan to attend college thousands of miles from home, and begin a career in an even more remote location. Making decisions and choices is never simple, and with such a tremendous variety of options, it is understandable that adolescents are often preoccupied with their own concerns.

When identity has been established, generally between ages 16 and 18, adolescents seek intimate relationships, usually with members of the opposite sex. Intimacy means mutual sharing of deepest feelings with another person, impossible unless both persons have established a sense of trust and a sense of identity. Intimate relationships are a preparation for marriage, and persons who fail to achieve intimacy may develop feelings of isolation and

TABLE 14–11. COMPARISON OF PIAGET'S STAGES OF CONCRETE AND FORMAL OPERATIONAL PATTERNS OF REASONING

Concrete Operations (5 or 7 to 11 Years)	Formal Operations (12 Years through Adulthood)
Can perform complex mental operations using personal experiences or objects actually seen	Can perform complex mental operations going from the actual to the possible.
Ability to organize and classify things that have been experienced or seen	Ability to imagine and organize unseen or unexperienced possibilities
	Ability to organize possibilities
Randomly and unsystematically uses problem-solving techniques	Systematically applies problem-solving techniques
Capable of coming to correct solutions only occasionally	Capable of coming to correct solutions consistently
Uses inductive logic (particular to general)	Uses deductive logic (general to particular)
Occasionally arrives at general principles	Arrives at general principles
Does not draw inferences from general principles	Draws inferences from general principles

(Wieczorek RR, Natapoff J: A Conceptual Approach to the Nursing of Infants and Children: Health Care From Birth Through Adolescence. Philadelphia, JB Lippincott, 1981)

experience chronic difficulty in communicating with others.

Most intimate relationships during adolescence are heterosexual. Sometimes, however, young people form intimate attachments with members of the same sex, or homosexual relationships. Because our culture is predominately heterosexual, these relationships can cause great anxiety for parents and children. Although some areas of American society are beginning to accept homosexual relationships as no more than another life-style, prejudice still exists. So great a stigma has been attached to homosexuality that many adolescents fear they are homosexuals if they are uncomfortable about heterosexual intimacy, which is a normal problem as adolescents move from same-sex peer group activities to dating peers of the opposite sex. Until 1973, homosexuality was officially listed as a psychiatric disorder; small wonder that adolescents who discovered a strong sexual attraction for persons of the same sex felt that they were "bad" or even "sick." These feelings still force many homosexuals to keep their relationships hidden ("in the closet").

BODY IMAGE

An individual's concept of body image is closely related to self-esteem. Seeing one's body as attractive and functional

Influenced By: (affects your identity)

Peers press body changes   religion, race, culture

Parents   environment

Money   what you want to do or be.

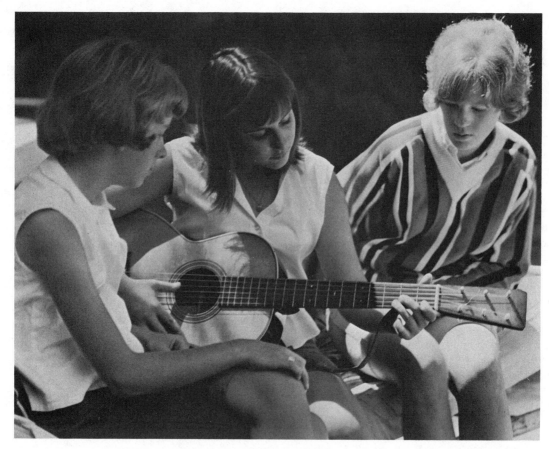

FIG. 14–5.   Adolescents are interested in music, and enjoy singing together. (Photograph by Carol Baldwin)

contributes to a positive sense of self-esteem. During adolescence, the desire not to be different can extend to feelings about one's body and cause young people to feel inadequate about their bodies even though they are really healthy and attractive.

American culture tends to equate a slender figure with female beauty and acceptability, and a lean, tall, muscular figure with virility and strength. Adolescents who feel that they are underdeveloped suffer great anxiety, particularly males. Adolescent girls have even undergone plastic surgery to augment their breasts to relieve this anxiety. Girls in this age group often feel that they are too fat, and try strange, nutritionally unsound diets in order to reduce. Some literally starve themselves, even after their bodies have become emaciated, truly believing that they are still fat and therefore unattractive. This condition is called *anorexia nervosa* and is discussed further in the next chapter.

It is important that adolescents establish a positive body image by the end of this developmental stage. Since bone growth is completed during adolescence, an individual's height will remain basically the same throughout adult life, even though weight can fluctuate greatly. Tall girls who long to be petite and short boys who would like to be 6 feet tall may need guidance to bring their expectations in

line with reality, and learn to have positive feelings about their bodies the way they are.

implications for hospital care

Adolescents are usually hospitalized because of a major health problem such as a traumatic injury from a motor vehicle accident, substance abuse, attempted suicide, an unsupported pregnancy, or a chronic health problem intensified by the physiological changes of adolescence. These young people must cope with the stress of hospitalization, possible dramatic alterations in body image, being partially or totally unable to conform with peer group norms, and an interruption in their search for identity.

Caregivers who work with hospitalized adolescents need to thoroughly assess the individual's developmental level, to listen carefully with empathy to the adolescent's concerns, to encourage maximum participation in self-care, and to provide sufficient information to make this participation possible. As with all patients, clear, honest explanations about treatments and procedures are essential. Adolescents need to know what limits are set, what the rules and regulations are for their behavior while hospitalized. They will often find it helpful to discuss their health problem with a peer who has had the same or a related problem, to share feelings and gain information.

Long offers twelve guidelines to help adolescents adjust to hospitalization:[2]

1. Know the patients' bill of rights.
2. Learn how to protect yourself from petty annoyances such as 5 a.m. blood pressures.
3. Guard against regression.
4. Demand respect.
5. Don't allow yourself to be treated as a child.
6. Avoid feeling dependent.
7. Don't be apologetic to hospital personnel for the performance of services for which they are assigned and paid.
8. Realize you have a right to know what health-care providers are doing and why.
9. Don't be treated as an object.
10. Constantly seek data about your treatment and progress.
11. Don't think "sick."
12. Ask for occasional periods of privacy, even if it means pretending to be asleep.

The adolescent's health problem may require a lengthy hospitalization and intense rehabilitation efforts. Adequate preparation and guidance can help make that difficult experience easier and less damaging to normal growth and development.

summary

No longer a child, not yet an adult, the adolescent wanders through a kind of never-never land, moving toward an unknown destination seeking directions that, if found, may be ignored or defied in the name of independence. Today's adolescents tread a path fraught with more numerous and serious hazards than ever before. Those strengthened by a warm, accepting family environment, positive school experiences, and good health have the best chance of reaching adulthood with a positive sense of self, the ability to form close relationships, and the capacity to make sound decisions about their lives. Nurses play an increasingly important role in adolescent health by providing education, guidance, and concerned caring, in clinics, schools, physicians' offices, adolescent health centers, and hospitals.

review questions

1. What are the common nutritional deficiencies in the preadolescent and adolescent?
2. Which snacks are the most nutritious?
3. What are the recommended immunizations for the adolescent?
4. What are the guidelines for contraceptive teaching?
5. What are the guidelines to help adolescents adjust to hospitalization?

references

1. Gutierrez Y: Nutrition and the adolescent. In Mercer RT (ed): Perspectives on Adolescent Health Care. Philadelphia, JB Lippincott, 1979
2. Long ES: How to survive hospitalization. Am J Nurs 74:486–488, 1974

bibliography

Bee H: The Developing Child. New York, Harper & Row, 1978

Caghan SB: The adolescent process and the problem of nutrition. Am J Nurs 75:1728–1731, 1975

Chinn PL: Child Health Maintenance: Concepts in Family-centered Care. St Louis, CV Mosby, 1979

Chow M, et al: Handbook of Pediatric Primary Care. New York, Wiley, 1979

Conger JJ: Adolescence and Youth: Psychological Development in a Changing World. New York, Harper & Row, 1973

Daniel WA Jr: Adolescents in Health and Disease. St Louis, CV Mosby, 1977

DeAngelis C: Pediatric Primary Care, 2nd ed. Boston, Little, Brown & Co., 1979

Gallagher JR, Heald F, Garrell D: Medical Care of the Adolescent, 3rd ed. New York, Appleton-Century-Crofts, 1976

Hymovich DP, Barnard MU: (Eds.) Family Health Care, vol. I. New York, McGraw-Hill, 1979

Hymovich DP, Chamberlin RW: Child and Family Development. New York, McGraw-Hill, 1980

Inman M: What teenagers want in sex education. Am J Nurs 74:1866–1967, 1974

Kaluger G, Kaluger MF: Human Development: The Span of Life, 2nd ed. St Louis, CV Mosby, 1979

Katchadourian H: The Biology of Adolescence. San Francisco, WH Freeman, 1977

Kohlberg L: Moral development and the education of adolescents. In Purnell RF (ed): Adolescents and the American High School. New York, Holt, Rinehart & Winston, 1970

Krozy R: Becoming comfortable with sexual assessment. Am J Nurs 78:1036–1038, 1978

Mancini M: Nursing, minors and the law. Am J Nurs 78:124–126, 1978

McCormick RM, Parkevich T: Patient and Family Education: Tools, Techniques and Theory. New York, John Wiley & Sons, 1979

Mercer RT: Perspectives on Adolescent Health Care. Philadelphia, JB Lippincott, 1979

Norris, CM: Self-care. Am J Nurs 79:486–489, 1979

Peach EH: Counseling sexually active very young adolescent girls. Am J Mat Child Nurs 5:191–195, 1980

Piaget J: To Understand Is to Invent: The Future of Education. New York, Grossman, 1973

Robbie M: Contraceptive counseling for the younger adolescent woman: A suggested solution to the problem. J Obstet Gynecol Neonatal Nurs 4:29–33, July–August 1978

Sahler OJ, McAnarney ER: The Child From Three to Eighteen. St Louis, CV Mosby, 1981

Tackett JJM, Hunsberger M: Family-centered Care of Children and Adolescents: Nursing Concepts in Child Health. Philadelphia, WB Saunders, 1981

Tanis JL: Recognizing the reasons for contraceptive non-use and abuse. Am J Mat Child Nurs 2:364, 1977

Taylor D: A new approach to contraceptive teaching for teens. Am J Mat Child Nurs 1:378, 1976

Tichy AM, Malasanos L: The physiological role of hormones in puberty. Am J Mat Nurs 1:384– 388, 1976

Torre C: Nutritional needs of adolescents. Am J Mat Child Nurs 2:118– 127, 1977

Vickery DM, Fries JF: Take Care of Yourself: A Consumer's Guide to Medical Care. Reading, Addison-Wesley, 1977

Wells, GM: Reducing the threat of a first pelvic exam. Am J Mat Child Nurs 2:3– 4, 307, 1977

Wold SJ: School Nursing: A Framework for Practice. St Louis, CV Mosby, 1981

Woods NF: Human Sexuality in Health and Illness, 2nd ed. St Louis, CV Mosby, 1979

Young CM: Adolescents and their nutrition. In Gallagher JR, Heald FP, Garell DC: Medical Care of the Adolescent. New York, Appleton-Century-Crofts, 1976

health problems of the adolescent   15

student objectives

The student successfully attaining the goals of this chapter will be able to

1 Define the following vocabulary terms:

amenorrhea   comedones   dependence   dysmenorrhea   gonorrhea
menorrhagia   mittelschmerz   obesity   overweight   polyphagia   sebum
syphilis

2 Describe factors that contribute to the development of obesity and discuss the importance of the early treatment of this problem during adolescence.

3 List the three principal psychological disturbances and the clinical manifestations of anorexia nervosa.

4 Describe the six categories of the most commonly abused drugs and discuss their effects.

5 Discuss the increasing problem of adolescent suicide and list six emotional factors that may alert the nurse that the adolescent may be in need of help.

6 List five signs of alcohol abuse.

Most adolescent health problems result from the rapid physiologic changes that are taking place, the individual's reaction to those changes, and the stress, conflict, and confusion that characterize adolescence. These young people are struggling with questions about identity, independence, career, sexuality, morality, and emotions, while alterations in their size and physical appearance make them uncomfortable and unfamiliar even with themselves. Coping with these changes and uncertainties is difficult for every adolescent, but for some, it is impossible. These troubled youngsters feel there is no solution but escape, and seek that escape through alcohol or other drugs, delinquent behavior, running away, or committing suicide. Between the ages of 15 and 24, suicide is the third leading cause of death.

The complex interrelationship of psychological well-being with physical health, though not completely understood, is evident throughout life, and particularly during adolescence. Emotions and attitudes affect nutrition and other health behaviors and can result in general or systemic disorders, which in turn can lead to further psychological stress. Therefore, this chapter is organized into the following three sections: nutritional disorders, psychological problems, and physiologic problems.

Nurses are assuming an increasingly important role in helping adolescents understand, manage, and, in some cases, prevent health problems. Fulfillment of this role demands an understanding of adolescent growth and development, the ability to listen and observe carefully, and to project an empathic, unjudging attitude.

nutritional disorders

OBESITY

Fat is a national problem in America, due largely to an overabundance of food and too little exercise. The thin figure, particularly for women, has become so idealized that being fat can handicap an individual socially and professionally, and severely damage self-esteem. *Obesity* occurs when an excessive accumulation of fat increases body weight; whereas, being *overweight* does not necessarily mean being obese, but that a person's weight is more than average for his height and body build.[1]

Obesity often begins in adolescence, and if not treated successfully, leads to chronic obesity in adult life. The obese adolescent often feels isolated from the peer group, normally a source of support during this period. Because of the obesity, the adolescent is embarrassed to participate in sports activities, thus eliminating one method of burning excess calories. Food is used as a means to satisfy emotional needs, establishing a vicious cycle (Fig. 15–1).

Some adolescents suffer from *polyphagia* (compulsive overeating). These persons lack control of their food intake, are unable to postpone their urge to eat, hide food for later secret consumption, eat when not hungry or to escape from worries, and expend a great deal of energy thinking about eating and securing food.[2] Not all compulsive eaters are overweight, and in some ways this disorder resembles *anorexia nervosa*.

Many factors contribute to the development of obesity: genetic, social, cultural, metabolic, and psychological. Children of obese parents are likely to share this problem, not only because of some inherited predisposition toward fat, but due to family eating patterns and the emotional climate surrounding food. Certain cultures equate being fat with being loved and being prosperous. If these values carry over into a modern family, the adolescent is torn between the standards of the peer group and those of the family.

Obesity is difficult to treat at any age but especially in adolescence. Much of teenage life centers around food, such as after-school snacks, the ice cream shop, the drive-in restaurant, the pizza parlor, fast-food restaurants serv-

---

DIET CLUBS

Diet clubs emphasize group support, sharing of both good and bad experiences, sound diet information, and recognition of dieting success. Members usually meet once a week and either pay a small fee or are asked to make a donation to help pay expenses.

Weight Watchers International, Inc.
800 Community Drive
Manhasset, NY 11030
(516) 627-9200

Trim Clubs, Inc.
1307 South Killian Drive
Lake Park, FL 33403
(305) 842-9411

The Diet Workshop, Inc.
111 Washington Street
Brookline, MA 02146
(617) 739-2222

Overeaters Anonymous World Service Office
2190 190th St.
Torrance, CA 90504
(213) 320-7941

TOPS (Take off pounds sensibly)
4575 S. 5th St.
P.O. Box 07489
Milwaukee, WI 53207
(414) 482-4620

Adapted from Overeaters anonymous: A self-help group. Am J Nurs 81:562, 1981

ing high-fat, high-calorie foods with low nutritional value. Diets that emphasize nutritionally sound meals and reduced calorie intake produce results too slow for impatient teenagers. Thus, the many quick weight loss programs, diet pills, and diet books find a ready market among adolescents.

Treatment must include a thorough exploration of the obese adolescent's food attitudes. Sometimes a team approach is necessary, using the skills of psychiatrist or psychologist, nutritionist, nurse, or other counselor. Many persons achieve better results from membership in self-help groups such as Weight Watchers, Overeaters Anonymous, and others. (See boxed material.)

Caregivers who work with obese adolescents should try to make these youngsters feel like worthwhile persons, and that obesity does not automatically make them unacceptable. Finding the support of a caring adult who will help the adolescent gain control of this aspect of his or her life can help give the necessary incentive to lose weight.

ANOREXIA NERVOSA

Preoccupation with reducing diets and the quest for the perfect (*i.e.*, thin) figure sometimes leads to *anorexia nervosa*, or self-inflicted starvation. This disorder generally occurs in adolescent girls, most often between the ages of 11 and 13, or between 19 and 20. These girls are usually intelligent, upper middle-class, with above-average performance in school. Although considered a psychiatric problem, it causes severe physiologic damage, and even death. Its incidence has increased since 1960, as has the professional literature discussing possible causes and approaches to treatment.

Etiology.   Opinions vary about the causes of this destructive disorder, and include psychodynamics, family interactions, distortions of perception, and behavioral, medical, and cultural factors.[3] Psychodynamic theories imply that the adolescent is regressing to an earlier developmental stage—the oral/anal stage—in an effort to avoid adolescent sexuality.

Problems with family interaction are thought to be a possible cause of anorexia nervosa. Focusing on the anorectic child reduces other internal conflict within the family. One high school senior whose development had been previously normal lost 20 pounds in 4 months after her father announced a decision to relocate to another part of the country.

Some authorities suggest that this disorder may be due to a malfunction of the hyopthalamus of the brain, but this theory is not as widely accepted as others.

Clinical Manifestations.   Anorexia is characterized by three principal psychological disturbances: (1) inability to correctly perceive body size; (2) absence of hunger or inability to perceive hunger; (3) feelings of ineffectiveness in everyday life. These girls are emaciated, almost skeletal, and yet they see themselves as overweight. They appear sexually immature, with dry skin, brittle nails, and often have lanugo (downy hair) over their backs and extremities. Other symptoms include amenorrhea (absence of men-

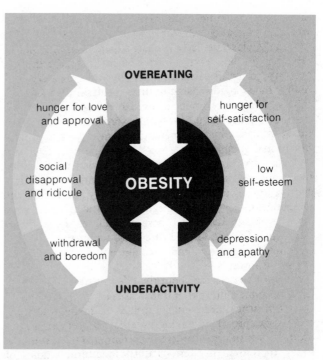

FIG. 15–1.   The vicious cycle in adolescent obesity. Many overweight teenagers withdraw from social interaction and develop feelings of inadequacy and inferiority. This reinforces the problems of obesity. (Reprinted by permission of the author and publisher, Szurek SA, Berlin IN: Psychosomatic Disorders and Mental Retardation in Children. Palo Alto, Science & Behavior Books, 1968)

struation), constipation, hypothermia, bradycardia, low blood pressure, and anemia.

Diagnosis.   Feighner and others have established the following diagnostic criteria for anorexia nervosa:[4]

- Age less than 25 years
- Anorexia with weight loss of 25% or more of total body weight
- Distorted perception of eating, food, and weight that includes denial of pleasure in eating, increased pleasure in losing weight, being thin, and hoarding food
- No known medical illness to explain anorexia or weight loss
- Often no other psychological disturbance
- Two or more of the following symptoms: *bulimia* (increased sensation of hunger); lanugo; amenorrhea; periods of overactivity; bradycardia; vomiting
- Bone age below normal

Treatment.   Adolescents diagnosed with anorexia nervosa are usually hospitalized to achieve the two goals of treatment: correction of the malnutrition, and identification and treatment of the psychological cause. Bruche, one of the pioneering authorities in this disorder, believes that when an individual's weight falls below a certain level, malnutrition causes an abnormal mental state.[5] Therefore, the nutritional state must be improved in order to deal with the psychological problems.

These adolescents have become experts in manipulating others and their environment. Once hospitalized, they may try to avoid gaining weight by ordering only low-calorie foods, by disposing of their meals in plants, trash, toilets, or in dirty linen, or by exercising in the hall or jogging in place in their room. In some cases nasogastric tube feedings or hyperalimentation is necessary to provide nutritional support.

Recent treatment has included behavior modification techniques. At the beginning of treatment, the patient is deprived of all privileges such as visitors, television, and telephone. Only when she begins to gain weight are privileges gradually restored. These techniques are effective only when the patient and caregivers understand the program and its purpose, and have agreed on individualized goals and rewards.

Authorities disagree about the effectiveness of behavior therapy; some believe that it increases the patient's feeling of powerlessness or loss of control. Some favor a multidisciplinary approach involving psychiatrist, pediatrician or internist, nutritionists, nurses, and family. This disorder is likely to remain mysterious until long-term studies of anorexia nervosa patients can offer additional insight.

CROHN'S DISEASE (GRANULOMATOUS ILEOCOLITIS)

Crohn's disease is a chronic recurrent inflammatory condition of the intestines that occurs most often in adolescents and young adults between the ages of 15 and 35. It is more common among persons of high income and educational levels living in urban areas.[6]

Clinical Manifestations. Signs and symptoms of this disorder vary widely, depending on the extent of the involvement. Regional ileitis is generally present in the terminal section of the large intestine but may affect several other areas of the intestinal mucosa. Acute episodes are characterized by sudden pain in the right lower abdominal quadrant. Fever is common, and joint pain and skin rashes occur often. Delayed growth and sexual maturation are common, indicating an endocrine-related etiology. Abscesses and strictures often form in the affected intestinal areas, sometimes requiring surgical resection.

Diagnosis. Chronic diarrhea, delayed growth, sexual immaturity, fever, weight loss, abdominal cramping and distention, are diagnostic criteria for Crohn's disease. Other symptoms may be present due to malnutrition or malabsorption, including iron-deficiency anemia, hypocalcemia, hypokalemia, macrocytic anemia, and hypoprothrombinemia. Diagnosis of more advanced cases also relies on radiographic findings that can reveal intestinal pockets, strictures, scars, and edema.

Treatment. The goal of treatment is to relieve the symptoms and discomfort of the client. Adequate rest, sleep, a well-balanced diet, and avoidance of stress and excitement are the cornerstone of treatment, seldom easy to implement in the life of today's adolescent. Special attention should be given to eliminating deficiencies of any nutrients, including iron. During acute episodes, a soft diet is recommended; high fiber foods are avoided at this time.

Treatment may include temporary use of steroids to reduce the inflammatory process. Dangerous side-effects can accompany long-term use of these drugs, including gastric ulceration and diabetes. For the adolescent, however, the most immediate and upsetting side-effect of steroids is acne; many adolescents stop taking their medication because of this effect.

Antidiarrheal agents, antispasmodics, and tranquilizers may also be used in treatment of symptoms. The use of immunosuppressive agents is being investigated.

psychological problems

SUBSTANCE ABUSE

Throughout history, people have used alcohol and other mood-altering drugs as a means of relieving the tensions and pressures of their lives. Many cultures, including our own, still sanction use of these substances, but object to their *abuse* (excessive use, or use in a way that is medically, socially, or culturally unacceptable). The unfortunate fact is that frequent use or abuse of these substances can lead to addiction or *dependence*, a compulsive need to use a substance for its satisfying or pleasurable effects. Dependence may be psychological, physical, or both. Psychological dependence means that the substance is desired for the effects or sensations it produces—alertness, euphoria, and so forth. Physical dependence results from drug-induced changes in body tissue function that require the drug for normal activity. Magnitude of physical dependence determines the severity of *withdrawal symptoms*, a pattern of cell malfunction caused by absence of the drug, including vomiting, chills, tremors, hallucinations, and other symptoms. The symptoms vary with the amount, frequency, and duration of drug use. Continued use of a substance results in *tolerance*, the ability of body tissues to endure and adapt to continued or increased use of a substance.

Use of alcohol and other drugs is considered adult behavior, and in this culture's ever-quickening thrust of children into adulthood, experiments with these substances begin at increasingly early ages. Drinking and the use of "recreational drugs" such as marijuana are considered by some young people to be sophisticated. Depending on peer-group attitudes, youngsters may be pressured to indulge in or abstain from the use of mood-altering substances.

Substances abused include alcohol and *controlled substances* (prescription drugs that can lead to dependence, and "street" drugs). Sale of alcohol is restricted to persons under age 18 in some states, and under age 21 in other states. Controlled substances are regulated by the Food and Drug Administration, and the Drug Enforcement Agency in the Department of Justice. Even though the legal availability of these substances is limited, particularly to adolescents, they are sufficiently accessible to create severe and chronic health problems and often lead to death at an early age.

Wieczorek and Natapoff classify adolescents who use alcohol and other drugs into three groups: experimenters, recreational users, and compulsive users.[7] Experimenters are casual users, and generally have no long-term dependence problems. Recreational users rely on drugs for rest and relaxation, but seldom use them in sufficient quantities to cause intoxication. Compulsive users are addicted to a substance, and their entire life centers on acquiring enough of the drug to function. They are unable to cope with personal relationships or intellectual activity, and often commit crimes to support their habit. These individuals have literally lost control of their lives, and require lengthy, intensive physical and psychological treatment to achieve rehabilitation.

The most effective and least expensive treatment for substance abuse is prevention, beginning with education in the early school years. Factual information about drugs and about coping with problems without drugs should be provided. Scare techniques are worse than useless because they arouse disbelief, aggression, and often add the tempting thrill of danger. The value of educational programs may be diluted if children come from a home where alcohol or other drugs are used by one or both parents.

Prevention includes understanding the reasons why adolescents abuse drugs. These include a poor self-concept, peer-group pressure, disturbed family interaction, boredom, curiosity, feelings of isolation (Table 15–1). In some instances, early identification of these factors by parents, teachers, counselors, or caregivers and prompt referral for treatment can help avoid the potential tragedy of substance abuse.

Nurses who care for adolescents in any setting need to be alert for signs of possible substance use and abuse: school absenteeism, poor academic performance, erratic behavior, dramatic swings in mood, needle marks on extremities, wearing dark glasses and long-sleeved shirts or blouses repeatedly, and an unkempt appearance. Again, it is important to maintain a nonjudgmental attitude of acceptance to enlist the trust and cooperation of the adolescent.

ALCOHOL ABUSE

In many areas of American cultures, drinking alcoholic beverages is considered acceptable and desirable social behavior. Although purchase of alcohol is legally restricted to adults, it is available in many homes and consequently the first drug most adolescents try has become the "drug of choice" among adolescents who use drugs. *Alcohol abuse* occurs when an individual ingests a quantity sufficient to cause intoxication (drunkenness). *Alcoholism* (chronic alcohol abuse or dependence) has reached epidemic proportions in America (an estimated 9 million persons), and increasing numbers of its victims are adolescents.

Drinking regularly now begins in the late school-age years and increases in frequency throughout adolescence. Some adolescents use alcohol in combination with

TABLE 15–1. SUMMARY OF PERSONALITY CHARACTERISTICS OF ADOLESCENT DRUG ABUSERS

Personality Characteristics	Manifestations Found in the Adolescent
Affect defense defect	Drugs are used as a defense against internal factors. Compulsive drug abuse is a means of self-treatment that has gotten out of hand. Drugs are abused by being used to lower feelings of intense rage, shame, guilt, disappointment, and loneliness.
Faulty ideal formation	Adolescents often have superego pathology or a lack of values or ideals. The high or pleasure obtained by the use of drug becomes the surrogate ideal. Parents are frequently not able to be effective role models. They may cope by cutting off their young teenager.
Hyposymbolization	This is an inability to symbolize which affects the teenager's inner self, emotions, and self-references. In general, abusers have difficulty articulating their feelings, wants, and desires. Some transfer this problem into somatic health problems.
Out-of-date object dependency	Adolescent drug abusers talk about their drugs with the "love" usually reserved for intimate partnerships. They frequently have excessively dependent personalities. The "single-minded" devotion to obtaining and using the drug can involve some fetishism. The focus on the drug object is totally out of proportion with reality.
Self-destructiveness	Adolescents who are drug abusers tend to be very self-destructive and self-punitive. Drugs may equate a suicide wish or an actual attempt.
Regressive gratification	Regressive gratifications attained with the abuse of drugs are an increase in self-esteem and narcissistic self-satisfaction.

(Wieczorek RR, Natapoff JN: A Conceptual Approach to the Nursing of Children: Health Care From Birth Through Adolescence. Philadelphia, JB Lippincott, 1981)

marijuana and other drugs, potentiating the effects of both substances, and increasing the probability for intoxication.

Alcoholism is costly in dollars and in damage to lives of victims and their families. During adolescence, alcohol abuse is closely linked with automobile accidents. A car is another symbol of adult status, and a means to escape adult supervision. Drinking with friends before or while driving often has tragic results. National Highway Traffic

Safety Administration statistics in 1976 showed that alcohol misuse caused 43% of nonpedestrian traffic fatalities, 38% of the young pedestrian fatalities, 14% of personal injury accidents, and 6.8% of property damage accidents.[8]

Signs of Alcohol Abuse. Wieczorek and Natapoff summarize the characteristics of "problem drinking" that precede alcoholism as follows:[9]

- Marked personality or behavior changes following alcohol consumption
- Frequent episodes of drunkenness
- Arrest or injury to self or others resulting from intoxication
- Family disturbances and impaired school or employment performance
- Alcohol ingestion before school or work

Adolescents who receive treatment and counseling for problem drinking are more likely to recover than adults who have been problem drinkers over a long period of time.

Alcoholism is characterized by

- The need for continually increasing amounts of alcohol to achieve the same effects as formerly caused by a few drinks
- Loss of control over drinking habits
- Psychological and physical reactions to withdrawal from alcohol
- "Blackouts" or drinking amnesia (inability to remember what happened while drinking).[10]

Treatment. Contrary to some opinions, alcoholism is not a weakness of character, but a major disease process that affects every organ of the body, the mental health status, and social competence of afflicted persons.[11] Treatment is lengthy, expensive, and has no chance for success until the alcoholic acknowledges the problem and his or her helplessness to deal with it.

Treatment begins with detoxification ("drying out") and management of withdrawal symptoms. After the initial period, nutritional support is essential; a well-balanced diet, high-potency vitamins, and plenty of rest help eliminate harmful side-effects of alcoholism.

Counseling to identify the problems that led to compulsive drinking and to help solve those problems is an essential part of treatment. Many counselors who work with alcoholic patients are persons who have conquered a drinking problem. This experience gives the counselor additional insight and empathy for the problem and the victim, and adds credibility to the counseling offered.

Alcoholics Anonymous (AA) is the best known of all self-help groups, and offers fellowship and understanding to the compulsive drinker. AA has chapters in every sizable community, and some areas have special programs for adolescents, as well as for families of alcoholics. Anyone who acknowledges having a drinking problem is welcome in AA and is helped to stay sober on the basis of taking "one day at a time."

Outcome. Recovery from alcoholism is a lifetime matter. The earlier the problem is diagnosed, the better the person's chances to respond to treatment. Ongoing support from health professionals, peers, family, and community is essential to successful treatment.

CONTROLLED SUBSTANCE ABUSE

Public recognition of rampant drug abuse during the 1960s led to the congressional enactment of the Comprehensive Drug Abuse Prevention and Control Act of 1970. Title II of this law is called the Controlled Substances Act (CSA) and replaces more than 50 former federal laws that sought to regulate narcotics and other harmful substances. Regulations issued in conjunction with CSA established five categories of controlled substances, according to the extent of their abuse potential and medical usefulness. These drugs are reclassified periodically, based on new research information. (See boxed material.)

Types of Drugs Abused. Other than alcohol, the mood-altering drugs commonly abused by adolescents can

---

SCHEDULES OF CONTROLLED SUBSTANCES

Schedule I   Drugs with a high potential for abuse and no currently accepted medical use in this country—such as heroin, LSD, PSP, and other hallucinogens, and marijuana.

Schedule II   Drugs that have recognized medical use but are considered dangerous because of their potential to create dependence—such as morphine, methadone, cocaine, amphetamines, and central nervous system depressants (amobarbital, pentobarbital, secobarbital, and methaqualone).

Schedule III   Drugs with less potential for abuse than those in Schedules I and II—such as products containing limited quantities of codeine and paregoric.

Schedule IV   Drugs with less abuse potential than those in I, II, and III—such as minor tranquilizers and hypnotics (meprobamate, chlordiazepoxide, and chloral hydrate).

Schedule V   Drugs with low abuse potential; mixtures of limited quantities of narcotic drugs with nonnarcotic medications—such as over-the-counter cough syrup with codeine.

Based on data from Rodman MJ, Smith DW: Pharmacology and Drug Therapy in Nursing, 2nd ed. Philadelphia, JB Lippincott, 1979

be grouped into six categories: narcotics, psychotomimetic (psychedelic) drugs, hypnotics, amphetamines, cocaine, and analgesics.[12]

The most commonly used *narcotics* are morphine and heroin. These drugs decrease anger, sex drive, and hunger by producing a dreamlike euphoric state. Highly addictive and extremely expensive, narcotics result in teenage prostitution, pushing (selling) drugs, and robbery as a means to support the drug habit.

Psychotomimetic (psychedelic) drugs, although not addictive in a physical sense, can create a psychological dependence from the hallucinations that result. This category of drugs includes LSD, PCP (angel dust), psilocybin, mescaline, marijuana, DMT, airplane glue, and STP. Effects can include intoxication, "bad trips," and overdosage.

Hypnotics are equal to narcotics in their addictive potential, and withdrawal from them must be carefully controlled to prevent delirium, seizures, or death. Barbiturates, glutethimide (Doriden), ethchlorvynol (Placidyl), and methaqualone (Quaalude) are the most commonly abused drugs in this group, and are sometimes used with alcohol, increasing the intoxicating effects, such as sleepiness, slurred speech, and impaired cognitive and motor function.

Amphetamines ("uppers") produce several effects on the central nervous system: increased alertness, wakefulness, and reduced awareness of fatigue, increased confidence and energy. Although not physically addicting they encourage psychological dependence and are abused by millions of Americans, many of whom become trapped in a destructive cycle of "uppers" and "downers" (barbiturates).

Cocaine is a stimulant that produces effects similar to amphetamines. Also called "coke" and "snow," the cocaine sold on the street is generally mixed with other substances of questionable origin. Sniffing cocaine has become a fashionable "recreation" in show-business circles, and other areas of society wealthy enough to afford it. Continued sniffing can lead to local ulceration of the nasal membranes and even to erosion of the nasal septum.

Analgesics, particularly those combining phenacetin, caffeine, and a hypnotic, are often abused by adolescents. Empirin and Fiorinal are two examples; their use often begins for relief of tension headaches, especially in women. Chronic abuse can result in blood and kidney disorders.

Treatment.   As mentioned earlier, the best treatment is prevention. When prevention is ineffective, emergency and long-term treatment become necessary. An overdose or a "bad trip" forces the adolescent to seek treatment. Emergency measures to restore normal respiration may include artifical ventilation and oxygenation.

Long-term treatment involves many health professionals such as psychiatric nurses, psychologists or psychiatrists, social workers, and community health nurses. The patient is also an important member of the treatment team, and must admit the problem, the need for help, and the willingness to take an active part in treatment.

DELINQUENCY

A *juvenile delinquent* is a person less than 16 years of age who repeatedly breaks laws. The juvenile court system was established during the early decades of the 20th century to provide more compassionate treatment and rehabilitation for these children. Prior to that time, children were tried as adults, imprisoned with hardened criminals, with no attempt made to understand their behavior. The system has been less than successful, however, and the rate of juvenile crime continues to rise, particularly violent crimes such as criminal homicide, forcible rape, robbery, and aggravated assault.

The causes of delinquency are not completely understood, but certain common characteristics have been identified. They are a sense of worthlessness, low self-esteem, poor family environment, peer pressure, unsuccessful school performance, delayed physical or intellectual development, lack of parental supervision. As stated earlier, some delinquent behavior is drug-related, but not all. Rebellion is a natural part of adolescence, but the majority of adolescents do not carry rebellion to such extremes.

Delinquent behavior develops easily among the large population of adolescent runaways. Estimates indicate that more than a million youngsters run away from home each year for various reasons. These children have no means of support, and are easy prey for adult criminals, particularly those connected with the sex industry.

Juvenile delinquents often have many physical health problems as well as the psychological disturbance that triggered their deviant behavior. Their nutritional state is usually poor, their development delayed, and substance abuse, venereal disease, or the results of physical abuse may further complicate their health. It is important for these youngsters to be able to reestablish trust with a caring adult who can make them feel worthwhile. It is equally important for caregivers to be able to set limits for these troubled young people and not to be manipulated by them. Surprisingly, they have a mature understanding of how to get their own way.

SUICIDE

Some adolescents are unable to cope with the crises of this developmental stage, and see death as the only solution to their many problems. Suicide is the third leading cause of death in persons between ages 15 and 24, and it is believed that many deaths reported as accidents are actually suicides. The adolescent suicide rate is higher among males than females, and is steadily increasing among members of both sexes.

Attempted suicide rarely occurs without warning, and is usually preceded by a long history of emotional problems, difficulty in forming relationships, feelings of rejection, and low self-esteem. Loss of one or both parents through death or divorce, a family history that includes suicide of one or more members, lack of success in academic or athletic performance are other frequent contributing factors. To this history is added one or more of the normal developmental crises of adolescence: difficulty in establishing independence, identity crisis, lack of intimate relationships, breakdown in family communication, a sense of alienation, and a conflict that interferes with problem solving. The adolescent's situation may be further complicated by an unwanted or unplanned pregnancy or drug addiction, leading to depression and a feeling of total hopelessness.

Health professionals involved with adolescents need to be aware of the factors that place an individual at risk for suicide, and also for the hints that signal an impending suicide attempt. Some of these desperate youngsters will verbalize their hopelessness with statements such as "I won't be around much longer" or "After Monday, it won't matter anyhow." They may begin giving away prized possessions, or appear suddenly elated after a long period of acting dejected. These behaviors should *never* be ignored, and an effort should be made to refer the adolescent for counseling and treatment. Nurses need to be aware of the resources within the adolescent's community: hot-lines and counselors who specialize in working with persons who have attempted suicide.

Suicide threats and attempts are usually a cry for help from a person who has lost all hope. If the cry is ignored, the attempt is likely to be repeated until success is achieved.

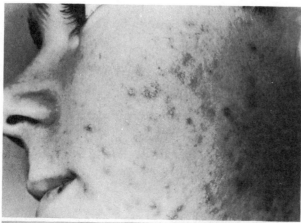
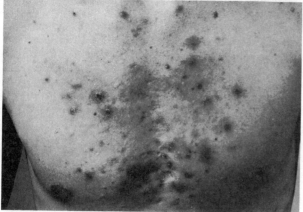

FIG. 15–2. Acne of face and chest. (Sauer GC: Manual of Skin Diseases, 4th ed. Philadelphia, JB Lippincott, 1980)

physiologic problems

ACNE VULGARIS

One of the most common health problems of adolescence, acne may be only a mild case of oily skin and a few blackheads, or a severe type with ropelike cystic lesions that leave deep scars, both physical and emotional. To adolescents who want to be attractive and popular, however, even a mild case of acne can cause great anxiety, shyness, and social withdrawal.

Characterized by the appearance of *comedones* (blackheads and whiteheads), papules or pustules on the face, and to some extent, on the back and chest, acne is caused by the endocrine imbalance that occurs during adolescence (Fig. 15–2). The sebaceous glands secrete *sebum* into skin follicles, which become impacted and irritated, causing the comedones of acne. Hereditary factors appear to be involved, as well as emotional conflicts, infection, poor hygiene, and diet. Untreated, the condition may become severe; therefore, early treatment is important.

Treatment. *Topical.* Scrupulous cleanliness is the most basic rule of treatment for acne. Vigorous scrubbing that causes irritation should be avoided. A soap substitute containing sulfur and salicylic acid may be more effective than soap.

Comedones should not be squeezed but removed by a comedone extractor, generally by a physician. Lotions containing sulfur and resorcin are useful for drying oily skin.

Severe acne that does not respond to normal skin care can be referred to a dermatologist. Systemic antibiotic therapy, ultraviolet light therapy, and topical application of vitamin A have been effective in many cases (Table 15–2).

General care. Sufficient sleep and exercise, recreation, and social activities are all beneficial. The role of diet varies with individuals, but such foods as chocolate, nuts, fried foods, and sea foods may exacerbate the condition. These can be eliminated from the diet, and then added one at a time to determine if there is a noticeable change in the skin condition.

Adolescents can be deeply troubled about acne and may be more willing to discuss its cause and treatment with a health professional than with parents. The importance of being a good listener cannot be overemphasized when working with adolescents.

MENSTRUAL DISORDERS

The beginning of menstruation, called *menarche*, normally occurs between ages 9 and 16, and for many girls this is a joyous affirmation of their femininity. Other adolescent girls may have negative feelings about this event, depending on how they have been prepared for menarche and for their roles as women. Irregular menstruation is common during the first year until a regular cycle is established.

PREMENSTRUAL TENSION

Women of all ages are subject to the discomfort of premenstrual tension, but the symptoms may be alarming to the adolescent. These symptoms include edema (resulting in weight gain), headache, increased anxiety, mild depression, or mood swings. The major cause of premenstrual tension is thought to be water retention following progesterone production after ovulation (Fig. 15–3).

Generally these discomforts are minor and can be relieved by reducing salt intake during the week prior to menstruation, and by the administration of mild analgesics and the local application of heat. When symptoms are more severe, physicians may prescribe a diuretic to relieve the edema and oral contraceptive pills to prevent ovulation.

DYSMENORRHEA

Many adolescent girls experience pain associated with menstruation (dysmenorrhea), including cramping abdominal pain, leg pain, and backache. This pain is caused by a disturbance in the secretion of prostaglandins, a substance that stimulates contraction of smooth muscle in the uterine wall.[13]

Severe dysmenorrhea necessitates examination to determine the possibility of pelvic abnormality. If none is present, the physician may prescribe estrogen and/or analgesics.

MITTELSCHMERZ

Some adolescent girls have dull aching abdominal pain at the time of ovulation (midcycle, hence the name mittelschmerz). The cause is not completely understood, but the discomfort usually lasts only a few hours and is relieved by analgesics, a heating pad, or a warm bath.

AMENORRHEA

The absence of menstruation is called *amenorrhea*. It can be *primary* (no previous menstruation) or *secondary* (missing three or more periods after menstrual flow has begun). Primary amenorrhea after age 16 warrants a diagnostic survey for genetic abnormalities, tumors, or other problems. Secondary amenorrhea can be a sign of pregnancy or the result of discontinuing oral contraceptives. Physical examination and complete gynecologic examination are necessary to help determine the cause.

MENORRHAGIA

Excessive, irregular, or protracted vaginal bleeding, called *menorrhagia*, is frequently due to an imbalance in the secretion of hormones. These cycles are usually anovulatory (not accompanied by the discharge of an ovum) and may be considered normal for the first 1 to 3 years after menarche, but complete physical examination should be made to rule out organic causes. If no lesions are found, a high protein diet should be given with iron and vitamin supplements.

INFECTIOUS MONONUCLEOSIS

Sometimes called "kissing disease," *infectious mononucleosis* ("mono") is thought to be viral in origin, probably

TABLE 15–2. FOUR METHODS OF TREATING ACNE VULGARIS

Type of Method	Description of Method
Topical agents	Cleansing agents that contain sulfur and salicylic acid are used because of their keratolytic properties. Agents that act as mild drying agents are used for peeling effects if the adolescent's skin is not hypersensitive. Topical lotions, creams, and gels are available. Some substances are tinted, so they may double as a cosmetic. Comedones and papulopustular acne are treated with benzoyl peroxide gels and vitamin A acid. Trade names are Desquam-X, Benzagel, Panxyl, and Retin A.
Systemic agents	Tetracycline and erythromycin are two antibiotics used in the therapy of papulopustular and cystic acne. Estrogen treatment is used cautiously for some female adolescents who experience premenstrual flare-ups of acne. The hazards of side-effects of hormone and antibiotic therapy should be considered beforehand. Risks should be explained to the client.
Physical agents	Ultraviolet light and cryotherapy may be employed. Radiation treatment is never used with acne in adolescents because the possible side-effects are too great.
Surgical treatments	The comedones of acne may be carefully incised and emptied. In cystic lesions corticosteroid may be injected into the cysts after drainage. Dermabrasion may minimize the scarring that has occurred. The client must wait until the acne condition is no longer active before a plastic surgeon can be consulted for this treatment.

(Wieczorek RR, Natapoff JN: A Conceptual Approach to the Nursing of Children: Health Care From Birth Through Adolescence. Philadelphia, JB Lippincott, 1981)

caused by the herpeslike Epstein-Barr virus. Additional research is needed to determine the mechanism of spread, but current information points to direct contact as the means of contagion. There is no immunization available, and treatment is symptomatic. Adolescents and young adults seem to be most susceptible to this disorder.

Clinical Manifestations. Infectious mononucleosis can present a variety of symptoms, some minor and some severe, that mimic hepatitis, neurologic disturbance, and cardiac disorders. These symptoms include sore throat, fever, palatine petechiae (red spots on the soft palate), swollen lymph nodes, and enlargement of the spleen, ac-

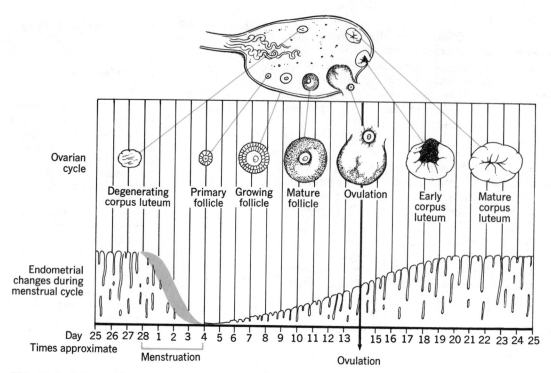

FIG. 15–3. Schematic representation of an ovarian cycle. Menstruation occurs with shedding of the endometrium. The follicular phase is associated with the rapidly growing ovarian follicle and the production of estrogen. Ovulation occurs midcycle, and mittelschmerz may occur. The secretory phase follows in preparation for the fertilized ovum. If fertilization does not occur, the corpus luteum begins to degenerate, estrogen and progesterone levels decline, and menstruation again occurs. (Chaffee EE, Lytle IM: Basic Physiology and Anatomy, 4th ed. Philadelphia, JB Lippincott, 1980)

companied by extreme fatigue and lack of energy. In some cases, headache, abdominal pain, and epistaxis are also present.

Diagnosis. Diagnosis of "mono" is based on clinical symptoms, laboratory evidence of lymphocytes in the peripheral blood with 10% or more abnormal lymphocytes present in a peripheral blood smear, and a positive heterophil agglutination test.[14] A recently developed slide test, Monospot, is proving valuable in diagnosis of this disorder. Rapid, sensitive, inexpensive, and simple to perform, it is capable of detecting significant agglutinins at lower levels, thus making possible earlier diagnosis.[15]

Treatment. No cure exists for infectious mononucleosis; treatment is based on symptoms. Aspirin is usually recommended for the fever and headaches. If staphylococci are present in the throat, penicillin is usually prescribed. Ampicillin is contraindicated because it often produces a maculopapular rash. Bedrest is suggested to relieve fatigue, but is not imposed for a specific amount of time. If the spleen is enlarged, the adolescent should be cautioned to avoid contact sports that might cause a ruptured spleen.

Outcome. The course of mononucleosis is usually uncomplicated. Fever and sore throat last from 1 week to 10 days. Fatigue generally disappears between 2 and 4 weeks

after appearance of acute symptoms, but may last as long as 1 year. The limitations that this disorder imposes on the teenagers' social life may cause depression, thereby prolonging the recovery time. In most cases, however, the adolescent is able to resume normal activities within 1 month after symptoms present.

SEXUALLY TRANSMITTED (VENEREAL) DISEASES

At one time, venereal diseases were thought to affect only depraved, delinquent persons. Today their incidence is second only to the common cold among American teenagers. Many sexually active youngsters are casual, permissive, and promiscuous about intercourse, but fearful and reluctant to seek treatment for the disease. Because the stigma remains, many cases go unreported and untreated, continuing the spread of infection.

Fear of parental discovery is a serious deterrent to seeking treatment. In some states doctors are legally barred from treating minors without their parents' consent; in others, however, this law has been changed to permit treatment for venereal disease without parental consent.

The number of diseases that can be sexually transmitted is growing. Gonorrhea and syphilis remain the most serious and the most prevalent, although genital herpes (type II) is increasing rapidly. This discussion will be limited to syphilis and gonorrhea (Table 15–3).

(Text continues on p. 286.)

TABLE 15–3. SEXUALLY TRANSMITTED INFECTIONS

Diagnosis and Causative Agent	Signs and Symptoms Perceived by Clients	Client's Presenting History	Signs and Symptoms on Physical Examination	Treatment	Nursing Intervention
Syphilis Treponema pallidum *Typology* A. Congenital B. Acquired 1. Primary 2. Secondary 3. Latent 4. Tertiary	*Primary* (8 d to 2 wk) Chancre at point of entry Regional lymphadenopathy *Secondary* Skin and mucosal lesions Generalized lymphadenopathy *Tertiary* Related to system affected (*e.g.,* central nervous system)	Sexual activity with partner(s) of opposite sex or same sex Previous history of syphilis or sexually related disease Persistent "pimple" at point of entry Untreated infected mother while child was *in utero*, 2nd or 3rd trimester	1. Observation of chancre 2. Lymphadenopathy *Lab tests* Darkfield exam positive Serologic tests positive (VDRL, RPR, FTA-abs)	*Syphilis of less than 1 yr's duration:* Benzathine penicillin G—2.4 million units total IM at one session or Aqueous procaine penicillin G—4.8 million units total IM (600,000 units IM daily for 8 d) *If the patient is allergic to penicillin:* Tetracycline—500 mg orally four times daily for 15 d (not recommended for pregnant or nursing women) or Erythromycin—500 mg orally four times daily for 15 d *Syphilis of more than 1 yr's duration or cardiovascular:* Benzathine penicillin G—7.2 million units total IM (2.4 million units IM weekly for 3 w) or Aqueous procaine penicillin G—9.0 million units total IM (600,000 units IM daily for 15 days *If the patient is allergic to penicillin:* Tetracycline—500 mg orally four times daily for 30 d (not recommended for pregnant or nursing women) or Erythromycin—500 mg orally four times daily for 30 d *Neurosyphilis:* Aqueous crystalline penicillin G—2 to 4 million units IV every 4 h for 8 to 10 d	1. A reportable disease 2. Case-finding and investigation 3. Atmosphere for individual client to ventilate feelings about the disease and willingness to confront that it is sexually transmitted May create anxieties with sexual partner(s) 4. Check for negative lab test after completion of the therapy 5. Periodic checks in pregnancy at 1st visit and in 3rd trimester

(continued)

TABLE 15–3. *(Continued)*

Diagnosis and Causative Agent	Signs and Symptoms Perceived by Clients	Client's Presenting History	Signs and Symptoms on Physical Examination	Treatment	Nursing Intervention
				Congenital syphilis with normal CSF: Benzathine penicillin G—500,000 units/kg IM in a single dose. *Congenital syphilis with abnormal CSF:* Aqueous crystalline penicillin G—50,000 units/kg IM or IV daily in two divided doses for at least 10 d or Aqueous procaine penicillin G—50,000 units/kg IM daily for at least 10 d	
Gonorrhea (GC) *Neisseria gonorrhoeae* Sites 1. Pharyngeal 2. Rectal site 3. Conjunctiva 4. Genital	White discharge Possible irritation and discomfort Possible burning on urination	Taking gyn history necessitates asking if client had previously been diagnosed with GC or other sexually transmitted conditions Sexual activity with partners of same or opposite sex	Observation of discharge, particularly at external cervical os Routine culturing of all female clients on pelvic exam—Cx anal and uretheral Gram stain positive for NG Culture of cervix in female and urethra in male	*Uncomplicated Genital, rectal and pharyngeal gonorrhea:* Procaine penicillin G—4.8 million units IM (2.4 million units into each of two sites) with 1 g probenecid orally, single dose or Ampicillin—3.5 g orally with 1 g probenecid orally, single dose (usually not effective in pharyngeal or rectal) or Tetracycline—1.5 g loading dose, followed by 0.5 g four times daily orally for 4 d or Spectinomycin—2 g IM, single dose (usually not effective in pharyngeal or rectal)	1. A reportable disease 2. Case-finding and investigation 3. Atmosphere for individual client to ventilate feelings about the disease and willingness to confront that it is sexually transmitted May create anxieties about relationship with the sexual partner 4. Check for negative culture 3–7 d after treatment is completed

TABLE 15–3. (*Continued*)

Diagnosis and Causative Agent	Signs and Symptoms Perceived by Clients	Client's Presenting History	Signs and Symptoms on Physical Examination	Treatment	Nursing Intervention

Pelvic Inflammatory Disease (PID)
 Most common offending organisms
 1. GC
 2. Non-GC
   a. *Streptococcus*
   b. *Staphylococcus*
   c. *E. coli*
   d. *Chlamydia trachomatis*
   e. *Mycoplasma hominis*
	Abdominal pain without the presence of GI signs and symptoms
	 Vaginal discharge
	 Temperature 37°C and up
		Previous history of venereal disease
		 Previous history of infection in vaginal or cervix areas
		 Question the use of IUD (indicates nongonococcal infection)
			Exquisite tenderness of pelvic exam; unilaterally or bilaterally
			 Cervix is painful on motion
			 Possible adnexal thickening
				PID
				 Treatment depends upon the organism cultured
				 Commonly seen schedules
				 If nonhospitalized: Procaine penicillin G—4.8 million units IM (2.4 million units into each of two sites) or ampicillin—3.5 g orally; with probenecid 1 g orally, single dose, followed by ampicillin 500 mg orally four times daily for 10 d
				   or
				 Tetracycline—1.5 g loading dose followed by 500 mg four times daily orally for 10 d
				 If hospitalized: Aqueous crystalline penicillin G—20 million units IV daily until improved, then ampicillin 500 mg orally four times daily to complete 10 d
				   or
				 Tetracycline—1 g or doxycycline 200 mg/d IV initially, followed by oral therapy to complete 10 d
					1. Acceptance of diagnosis
					 2. Confidentiality of client's diagnosis
					 3. Understanding of potential sequelae (*i.e.*, sterility risk for ectopic pregnancy)

SYPHILIS

Syphilis is a destructive disease caused by the spirochete *Treponema pallidum* that can involve every part of the body. Untreated, it can cause devastating long-term effects. Infected mothers are highly likely to transmit the infection to the unborn infants.

This infection is spread primarily by sexual contact and moist kissing. Symptoms usually appear about 3 weeks after exposure. If allowed to progress without treatment, syphilis has a secondary stage, a latent stage, and a tertiary stage.

Clinical Manifestations. The cardinal sign of primary syphilis is the *chancre*, a hard, red, painless lesion at the point of entry of the spirochete. This can appear on the penis in the male, or on the vulva or cervix of the female. The *secondary stage* is marked by rash, sore throat, and fever, appearing between 2 and 6 months after the original infection. Signs of both first and second stages will disappear without treatment, but the spirochete remains in the body.

The *latent stage* can persist for as long as 20 years without symptoms; however, blood tests are still positive.

In the *tertiary stage*, syphilis causes severe neurologic and cardiovascular damage, mental illness, and gastrointestinal disorders.

Treatment. Syphilis responds to penicillin therapy when it is carried through. A course of injections or oral dosages takes about 2 weeks.

Prevention. Even though syphilis represents only a small percentage of the venereal diseases found in adolescence, prevention is still the best treatment. Teenagers who are aware of the signs of syphilis may be able to avoid contact with an infected person. Use of a condom during intercourse is a partial protection as is washing the genital area with soap and/or using a vinegar douche immediately after intercourse. Factual information about the causes and consequences of venereal disease may be the best deterrent, but the facts need to be presented at an early age.

GONORRHEA

More than 1 million cases of gonorrhea are reported annually, making this disorder the most common venereal disease. Also called "the clap," "the drips," or "the dose," gonorrhea has mild primary symptoms, particularly in females, and often goes undetected and thus untreated until it progresses to serious pelvic disorders. This disease can cause sterility in the male.

Gonorrhea is transmitted by intimate physical contact with the genitals or rectum of an infected person. It is caused by *Neisseria gonorrhoeae*, a gram-positive diplococcus.

Appearance of symptoms (if any) varies between 1 day and 2 weeks after exposure, and may include dysuria with profuse yellow discharge, frequency and urgency of urination, and nocturia. Unfortunately a majority of cases are asymptomatic; therefore, gonorrhea should be considered a possible diagnosis in all sexually active adolescents.

Diagnosis is based on direct smear or culture techniques, and, in females, on newly available blood tests that can be performed in 2 minutes in the physician's office or clinic. This represents a real diagnostic breakthrough since the disease has always been more difficult to detect in the female.[16]

At one time penicillin was considered totally effective in the treatment of gonorrhea. Now, however, penicillin-resistant strains of gonorrhea have developed and in some areas physicians give penicillin only a 50–50 chance of curing the disease. If the adolescent is allergic to penicillin, erythromycin may be prescribed, but the outcome is not guaranteed.

TEENAGE PREGNANCY

A high rate of sexual activity among immature individuals has produced two tragic phenomena: epidemic venereal disease and a dramatic rise in teenage pregnancies, particularly in girls between 15 years and 17 years of age. More than 1 million teenage pregnancies were reported in 1977, a figure representing 10% of the teenage female population, and 59% of these resulted in live births.[16]

The pregnant adolescent is likely to be unmarried, with less than a high school education, and the recipient of inadequate prenatal care. Her future and that of her offspring are in jeopardy. Even if married, the girl is physically, emotionally, and socially at risk. She will probably be excluded from school, may be rejected by her family, and will have no adequate source of income during and after her pregnancy. A common reaction of adolescents to pregnancy is denial; thus, she is unlikely to seek prenatal care even if she is aware of the community resources.

Pregnancy holds its own developmental tasks, and these collide with the normal developmental tasks of adolescence, usually with disastrous results. As an adolescent, she is seeking independence; as an expectant mother without adequate resources she remains dependent. She is seeking identity; the only identity she gains is that of a young, confused, high-risk mother-to-be. Her acute awareness of body image must deal with the silhouette of pregnancy, certainly not in keeping with the slim figure desired by most adolescent girls.

Once pregnancy has been confirmed, the adolescent must decide whether to terminate the pregnancy by elective abortion, or to carry it to term. If she chooses to have the baby, she must then decide whether to keep it or relinquish it for adoption. These are difficult choices, particularly for a frightened, often unsupported, immature girl. Health professionals have an obligation to provide the facts and guidance that will enable the girl to make an informed choice. School nurses, social workers, teachers, and counselors may be her only resources.

In many areas of the country, school policy has been altered so that the pregnant adolescent is not forced to drop out of school. If this is not the case, the girl should be encouraged to continue her education elsewhere, even if it means relocation.

Adolescent clinics are beginning to play a particularly

important role in management of teenage pregnancy. Many of these clinics use a team approach to work with the girl, perhaps the young father, and the girl's parents; the physician, nurse clinician or nurse-midwife, nutritionist, and social worker offer understanding, supportive care, teaching, and counseling during the prenatal period and follow-up care after delivery. If the adolescent has chosen abortion, these clinics can also provide follow-up care and contraceptive counseling.

Nurses who work with pregnant adolescents need to resolve their own feelings to maintain a helpful, nonjudgmental attitude. These teenagers are very fragile emotionally and mentally during this crisis. With the right kind of care, however, the experience can become an opportunity for growth.

PULMONARY TUBERCULOSIS

Tuberculosis is present in all parts of the world, although many countries have shown a downward trend of mortality for several years. Prevalence of infection has declined rapidly in certain countries such as the United States and Japan.

The predominant cause of pulmonary tuberculosis is the human tubercle bacillus, *Mycobacterium tuberculosis*. The bovine type, caused by *M. bovis* in cattle and communicated to man through dairy produces, is now rare in the United States and a number of other countries. Mode of transmission is contact with bacilli in the sputum of infected persons. The bacillus is predominantly airborne.

Incubation period is about 4 to 6 weeks between exposure and development of a primary lesion. Relapse of a latent infection accounts for many of the active cases. Susceptibility is highest in children under 3 years of age and in adolescents and young adults. If sputum contains infectious tubercle bacilli, antimicrobial medications generally terminate the period of communicability in a few weeks.

Clinical Manifestations. In children with pulmonary tuberculosis there are usually general symptoms of chronic infection, such as fatigue and irritability. Some malnutrition may be present. Primary lesions in children generally go unrecognized.

Secondary lesions are more apt to occur in the adolescent period. Symptoms resemble those in an adult. Cough with expectoration, fever, loss of weight, malaise, and night sweats may be present.

Treatment. Medical treatment includes administration of isoniazid (INH). Bedrest for children is usually not indicated unless the child appears ill, and physical activity is not restricted. A well-balanced diet is important, but forced feedings are not indicated.

Identification and Preventive Treatment. Prevention requires correction of such undesirable social conditions as overcrowding and poverty. Health education; availability of medical, laboratory, and radiographic facilities for examination; and control of contacts and suspected individuals are all needed.

Children who demonstrate active tubercular lesions anywhere in the body, and children under the age of 4 years who have tuberculin-positive reactions are generally given a course of isoniazid for about 1 year. Older children who have recently become tuberculin-positive and who have been exposed to tuberculosis are treated in like manner whether or not they have a demonstrable infection.

Diagnostic tests include the intradermal Mantoux test using measured quantities of old tuberculin (OT). A commonly used test injects purified protein derivative (PPD) into the skin by use of the tine method. In the tine test PPD is inserted into four small puncture holes made in the upper arm with a four-pronged instrument.

Tuberculin testing is recommended when the child starts school and at adolescence. A positive reaction gives presumptive evidence but not proof of an active lesion. Radiographic screening of tuberculin-positive persons gives further evidence. Positive proof is obtained when tubercle bacilli are found in the sputum. For infants who swallow their sputum, gastric washings are indicated.

A vaccine called BCG is used in countries where the incidence of tuberculosis is high. It is given to tuberculin-negative persons, and is said to be effective for 12 years or longer. Mass vaccination is not deemed necessary in parts of the world where the incidence of tuberculosis is low.

summary

Adolescent life is beset by so many rapid, dramatic changes that it can be difficult for these individuals to gain a sense of perspective. Minor problems seem major, and major problems insurmountable. Adolescents with a positive sense of self-esteem and a supportive family environment are likely to weather this turbulence with fewer problems than youngsters with a poor self-image, fewer successes, and an unfavorable home environment.

Today's culture holds many options that have long-term implications for adolescents, their health and well-being. The choices they make related to nutrition, friends and associates, alcohol and other drugs, sexuality, and school and career plans can affect their entire adult life. Nurses and other health professionals have a critically important part in the care and education of these young people to help guide them toward intelligent, informed choices. Prevention of the health problems that characterize adolescence is the primary objective. Competent, compassionate care of those adolescents who do encounter physiologic and psychological problems is a second objective, and the third is to restore health as quickly and completely as possible.

review questions

1. Which factors contribute to the development of obesity?
2. What are the clinical manifestations of anorexia nervosa?
3. What is psychological dependence?
4. What is physical dependence?

5. What is the most effective and least expensive treatment for substance abuse?
6. What are the signs of alcohol abuse?
7. What is the best known self-help group for the treatment of alcoholism?
8. What is mittelschmerz?
9. Describe a chancre.

references

1. Whaley L, Wong D: Nursing Care of Infants and Children. St Louis, CV Mosby, 1979
2. Green RS, Rau JH: The use of diphenylhydantoin in compulsive eating disorders. In Vigersky RA (ed): Anorexia Nervosa, pp 377–382. New York, Raven Press, 1977
3. Richardson TF: Anorexia nervosa: An overview. Am J Nurs 80:1470–1471, 1980
4. Feighner JP, et al: Diagnostic criteria for use in psychiatric research. Arch Gen Psychiatry 26:57–63, 1972
5. Bruch H: The Golden Cage: The Enigma of Anorexia Nervosa. Cambridge, Harvard University Press, 1978
6. Daniel WA: Adolescents in Health and Disease. St Louis, CV Mosby, 1977
7. Wieczorek RR, Natapoff J: A Conceptual Approach to the Nursing of Children: Health Care From Birth Through Adolescence. Philadelphia, JB Lippincott, 1981
8. National Institute on Alcohol Abuse and Alcoholism: Alcohol and health. Second special report to U.S. Congress. Department of Health, Education and Welfare, Alcohol, Drug Abuse, and Mental Health Administration (ADM) 76-268, Washington, DC, U.S. Government Printing Office, 1976
9. Wieczorek RR, Natapoff J: A Conceptual Approach to the Nursing of Children: Health Care From Birth Through Adolescence. Philadelphia, JB Lippincott, 1981
10. Wieczorek RR, Natapoff J: A Conceptual Approach to the Nursing of Children: Health Care From Birth Through Adolescence. Philadelphia, JB Lippincott, 1981
11. Lenox Hill Hospital, Health Education Center. Alcoholism. New York, Lenox Hill Hospital, 1979
12. Wieczorek RR, Natapoff J: A Conceptual Approach to the Nursing of Children: Health Care From Birth Through Adolescence. Philadelphia, JB Lippincott, 1981
13. Henal MR, Buttram U, Segre EJ, Bessler S: The treatment of dysmenorrhea with naproxen sodium. Am J Obstet Gynecol 127:818–823, 1977
14. Wieczorek RR, Natapoff J: A Conceptual Approach to the Nursing of Children: Health Care From Birth Through Adolescence. Philadelphia, JB Lippincott, 1981
15. Whaley L, Wong D: Nursing Care of Infants and Children. St Louis, CV Mosby, 1979
16. Whaley L, Wong D: Nursing Care of Infants and Children. St Louis, CV Mosby, 1979
17. Jensen MD, Benson R, Bobak IM: Maternity Care: The Nurse and the Family, 2nd ed. St Louis, CV Mosby, 1981

bibliography

Bedger JE: Teenage Pregnancy: Research Related to Clients and Services. Springfield, Charles C Thomas, 1980

Block C: What you should know about mono. Better Homes and Gardens, 145–146, November, 1979

Bruch H: The treatment of eating disorders. Mayo Clinic Proceedings 51:262–272, May, 1976

Ciseaux A: Anorexia nervosa: The view from the mirror. Am J Nurs 80:1468–1470, 1980

Claggett MS: Anorexia nervosa: A behavioral approach. Am J Nurs 80:1471–1472, 1980

Coates TJ, Thoresen CE: Treating obesity in children and adolescents: A review. Am J Public Health 68, No. 2:143–149, 1978

Grollman EA: Suicide: Prevention, Intervention, Postvention. Boston, Beacon Press, 1975

Hart NA, Keidel GC: The suicidal adolescent. Am J Nurs 79:80–84, 1979

Harvey K: Caring perceptively for the relinquishing mother. Am J Mat Child Nurs 2:24–28, 1977

Howe J: Nursing Care of Adolescents. New York, McGraw-Hill, 1980

Kandell N: The unwed adolescent pregnancy: An accident? Am J Nurs 79:2112–2114, 1979

Kinney J, Leaton G: Loosening the Grip: A Handbook of Alcohol Information. St Louis, CV Mosby, 1978

Langford RW: Teenagers and obesity. Am J Nurs 81:556–559, 1981

Mercer RT: Perspectives on Adolescent Health Care. Philadelphia, JB Lippincott, 1979

Mercer R: Becoming a mother at sixteen. Am J Mat Child Nurs 1:44, 1976

Overeaters anonymous: a self-help group. Am J Nurs 81:560–563, 1981

Pannor R, Massarik F, Evans B: The Unmarried Father: New Approaches for Helping Unmarried Young Parents. New York, Springer-Verlag, 1971

Peach EH: Counseling sexually active very young adolescent girls. Am J Mat Child Nurs 5:191–195, 1980

Peoples MD, Barrett AE: A model for the delivery of health care to pregnant adolescents. JOGN 8:339, 1979

Smith PB, Mumford DM, Hamner E: Child-rearing attitudes of single teenage mothers. Am J Nurs 79:2115–2116, 1979

Teicher JP: Children and adolescents who attempt suicide. Pediatr Clin North Am 27:688–692, 1975

U.S. National Center for Health Statistics: Teenage child bearing. Monthly vital statistics report 26(5) HRA 77-1120. Washington, DC, U.S. Department of Health, Education and Welfare, September, 1977

Vourakis C, Bennett G: Angel dust: Not heaven sent. Am J Nurs 79:649–653, 1979

White JH, Schroeder MA: When your client has a weight problem: Nursing assessment. Am J Nurs 81:550–553, 1981

Wiley L: Nursing care of a suicidal adolescent. Nurs 80 10, No. 4: 56–59, 1980

Wold SJ: School Nursing: A Framework for Practice. St Louis, CV Mosby, 1981

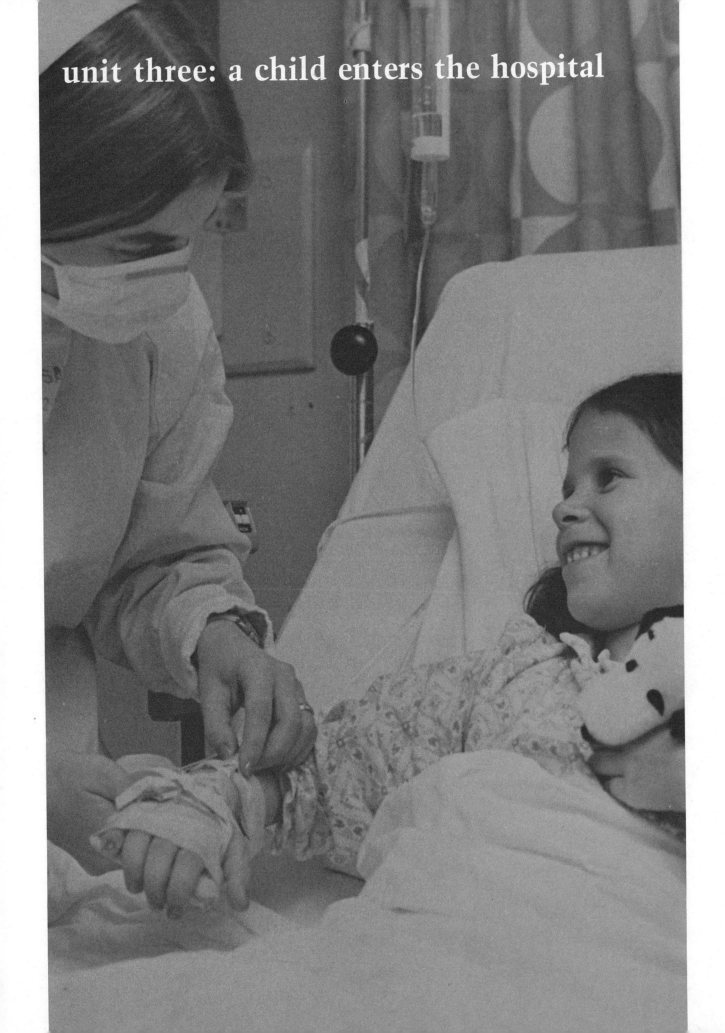

unit three: a child enters the hospital

admission and discharge

student objectives

The student successfully attaining the goals of this chapter will be able to

1 Define the following vocabulary terms:

child-life programs   denial   despair   directive play therapy
nondirective play therapy   protest

2 List four actions that many hospitals have taken to make the hospital a more attractive place for the child and to minimize parent–child separation.

3 List the five Cs, principles for communication with minority children and their families.

4 Describe the three stages of parent–child separation as formulated by Robertson.

5 Explain the differences between directive and nondirective play therapy.

6 List five items the nurse might include in the admission interview with the parents that would help to better familiarize her with the child.

learning about hospitals

The unknown frightens all of us, even intelligent, mature individuals. Until recently, hospitalization held countless unknowns for all patients, especially those too young or too afraid to ask questions. Small wonder that the littlest patients had bigger fears than anyone, except perhaps their parents.

Before children could learn about hospitals, however, hospitals had to learn more about children, especially their emotional needs. During the late 1950s and early 1960s, an increasing number of studies examined the effect of hospitalization on children's recovery and subsequent health. The concensus was that often the stress of hospitalization interfered with the healing process that was supposed to take place. The principal stress factor appeared to be separation of children and parents, compounded by the fear of entering an unknown, adultlike environment. Slowly but steadily these findings have begun to change hospital practices and procedures so that the ultimate goal of restoration of health can be reached as soon as possible with the least amount of trauma to children and families.

An important force in changing hospitals' approaches to care of children has been the organization formed in 1965, the Association for the Care of Children in Hospitals. Initiated by a group of recreational directors, play ladies, and child educators, it has grown rapidly to include representatives of pediatric medicine, surgery, nursing, social services, and other helping professions. Membership represents nearly all states in the United States and several Canadian provinces and foreign countries. Their annual conferences attract child-life specialists from around the world.

THE CHANGING SCENE IN CHILDREN'S HOSPITALS

Today, a growing number of hospitals have a *child-life program* to make hospitalization less threatening for children and their parents. These programs are usually under the direction of a child-life worker whose background is in psychology and early childhood development. This person works with nurses, physicians, and other health-team members to help them meet the developmental, emotional, and intellectual needs of hospitalized children, and also works with students interested in child health care to further their education.

The encouraging trend toward child-life programs has been fueled by the children's rights movement, which began to gain strength during the 1960s. This movement comprises persons who believe that the same standards of morality and behavior applied to adults must be adopted for children.[1] (See Children's Bill of Rights, Introduction.)

As hospital philosophy about the care of children has changed, so has the physical environment. Many children's departments and children's hospitals, once drab, bare, serious-looking places with starched, busy nurses doing "important" things, have relaxed and blossomed into bright, colorful settings populated by real and caring people (Fig. 16–1). Murals, paintings, and drawings (some

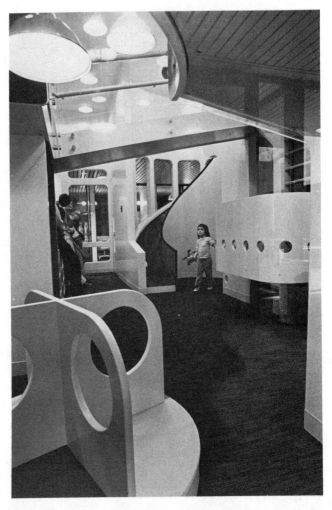

FIG. 16–1. Hospitals for children have taken on a new look; enclosed playgrounds such as this one acknowledge children's curiosity and need for activity. (Courtesy Boys' Town Institute for Communication Disorders in Children)

of them done by staff or patients), toys and books for waiting areas, and other homelike touches are apparent in patient rooms, treatment rooms, and playrooms.

Visiting hours and other hospital policies have been modified to minimize parent–child separation. In many hospitals, parents are free to visit their child at any time, and care by parents and rooming-in are encouraged, except in intensive care settings.

Hospitalized children are encouraged to dress in regular daytime clothes unless tests or treatments dictate otherwise; this helps maintain a link with their familiar world.

Another means of combating the loneliness that hospitalization can bring is to serve children's meals around a table, family-style. Eating is a social event, and food seems to taste better in company than alone. Children are more likely to eat what they have served to themselves than a premeasured, prearranged tray of food. Balanced diets are certainly desirable, but wholesome food placed on a child's tray and returned to the kitchen uneaten does little for the child's nutrition. Some hospitals offer children the opportunity to check their selection on menus; those too young to read can ask a parent to help them.

Although hospitals for children are more attractive in appearance and more relaxed in attitude, they remain a source of fear and anxiety. Learning about hospital policies and procedures can make children and parents more comfortable about hospitalization, and more cooperative in meeting the goals of treatment.

EARLY CHILDHOOD EDUCATION ABOUT HOSPITALS

Hospitals are part of the child's community just as police and fire departments are. When the child is capable of understanding the basic functions of these community resources and the people who staff them, it is time for an explanation. Many hospitals have Open House programs for well children on a monthly or biweekly basis. Children may attend with parents or in an organized community or school group. A room is set aside where children can handle equipment (Fig. 16–2), try out call bells, climb into cribs or hospital beds. Hospital staff members explain simple procedures and answer children's questions. A tour

of the pediatric department, including the playroom, may be offered. Some hospitals show slides or films about admission and care. Child-care workers, nurses, and volunteers help with these orientation programs.

School programs can help children feel more at ease and familiar with hospitals by providing books and films appropriate for various age groups. (See boxed material.) These materials show hospital routines as well as procedures such as roentgenography, injections, and physical examinations. Children are told that some things will hurt, but that doctors and nurses will do everything they can to make the hurt go away.

Parents can do their part in helping a child understand the purpose and use of hospitals, beginning at a very early age. Young children sometimes have the mistaken idea that the hospital is only a place where "mommies go to get babies;" older children may fear hospitals because they know of someone who has died in the hospital. Parents need to explain very carefully why the person died, making it clear that the hospital was not the reason.

PLANNED ADMISSIONS

Children who are candidates for admission to the hospital may attend the Open House programs or other special pro-

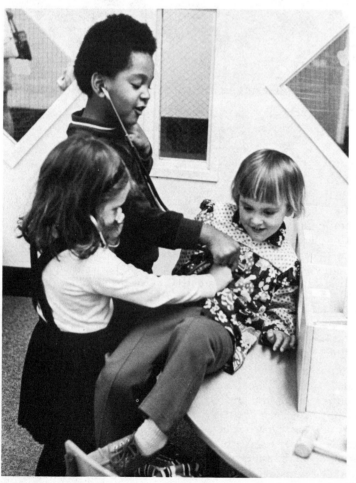

FIG. 16–2.   Listening to each other's heartbeat shows these children how the stethoscope works. (Photo by Marcia Lieberman)

BOOKS TO HELP CHILDREN UNDERSTAND HOSPITALS

Bemelmans L: Madeline. New York, Penguin Books, 1967

Chase FA: A Visit to the Hospital. New York, Grosset & Dunlap, 1977

Clarke B, Coleman LL: Going to the Hospital. New York, Random House, 1971

Rey M, Rey HA: Curious George Goes to the Hospital. Boston, Houghton-Mifflin, 1966

Shay A: What Happens When You Go to the Hospital? Chicago, Reilley and Lee, 1969

Sobol HL: Jeff's Hospital Book. New York, Henry Z Walck, 1975

Stein SB: A Hospital Story: An Open Family Book for Parents and Children Together. New York, Walker and Company, 1974

grams that are more detailed and specifically related to their expected experience. It is important for parents and siblings to attend the preadmission tour along with the future patient to reduce anxiety in all family members.

During the preadmission tour, children may be given surgical masks, caps, and shoe covers, and the opportunity to "operate" on a doll or other stuffed toy specifically designed for teaching purposes. Some hospitals have developed special coloring books to help prepare children for cardiac or other major surgery. These books are sent to children at home prior to admission. Once admitted, the children "operate" on a toy under the supervision of staff members (Fig. 16–3).

EMERGENCY ADMISSIONS

Emergencies such as poisoning or other accidental injury leave little time for explanation. The emergency itself is frightening to child and parents, and the need for treatment is urgent. Even though a parent tries to act calm and composed, the child can often sense the anxiety. If the hospital is still a great unknown, it will only add to the child's fear and panic. If the child has even a basic understanding about hospitals and what happens there, the emergency probably will seem a little less scary.

In an emergency, physical needs assume priority over emotional needs. The presence of a parent who can conceal his or her own fear usually comforts the child; however, the child may be angry that the parent does not "stop these people from hurting me more!"

admission procedures and discharge planning

The parent or other person bringing the child to the hospital should carefully explain to him where he is going and why. Any questions should be answered truthfully. Before or during the admission interview, the parent or other accompanying adult will be asked to provide information such as that requested in the questionnaire in Figure 16–4. On the form, the mother may be asked the child's nicknames, feeding habits, food likes and dislikes, sleeping schedule, toilet-training status, and any special words he understands to indicate needs or desires, such as words used for urinating and bowel movements. The nurse may choose to ask the questions and write down the answers herself, gaining the opportunity to observe the reactions of the child and parents as they answer. She must, however,

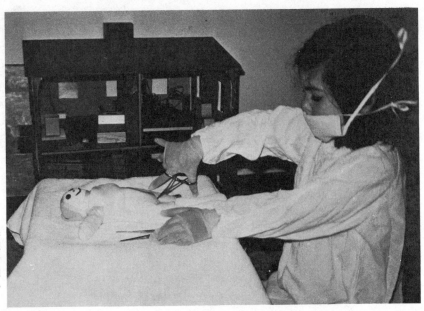

FIG. 16–3. Children who are going to have surgery can act out the procedures on toys, and thereby reduce some of their fear. (Photo by Sirgay Sanger; Petrillo M, Sanger S; Emotional Care of Hospitalized Children. 2nd ed., JB Lippincott, 1980)

Patient Name _____ Birth Date _____ Date _____

(THIS FORM TO BE COMPLETED BY PARENTS UPON ADMISSION)

A. Reason hospitalized _____

B. Recent exposures _____

A. PREGNANCY AND BIRTH

1. Did you have an illness during your pregnancy?   No   Yes
2. Did the baby come on time?   Yes   No
3. What was the birth weight?   _____
4. Did your baby have any trouble starting to breathe?   No   Yes
5. Did the baby have any trouble while in the hospital?   No   Yes

B. FEEDING AND DIGESTION

1. Was there severe colic or any unusual feeding problems the first 3 months?   No   Yes
2. Is your child's appetite usually good?   Yes   No
3. Is it good now?   Yes   No
4. Do any foods disagree with him/her?   No   Yes
5. Does he/she often have diarrhea?   No   Yes
6. Has constipation ever been much of a problem?   No   Yes
7. If on vitamins, what kind and how much?   _____
8. If still on formula, what one do you use?   _____

C. FAMILY HISTORY

Circle any of the following diseases that this child's parents, grandparents, aunts, uncles, brothers, sisters have had:

Seizures   cancer   inherited or family diseases   diabetes   asthma   tuberculosis   allergy   nervous breakdown   kidney   intestinal   arthritis

Are the child's parents both in good health?   Yes   No

List ages, sex, and general health of brothers and sisters:

_____

_____

_____

_____

Have any of your children died?   No   Yes

D. INFECTION, ILLNESSES, MISCELLANEOUS PROBLEMS AND DEVELOPMENT:

Has your child

1. Had as many as three attacks of ear trouble?   No   Yes
2. Had more than three colds or throat infections with fever a year?   No   Yes
3. Had any trouble with urination?   No   Yes
4. Ever had a convulsion?   No   Yes
5. Had any trouble with vision?   No   Yes
6. Had any trouble with hearing?   No   Yes

7. At what age did your child:
   Sit alone?   _____
   Walk alone?   _____
8. Did your child say any words by the age of 1½ years?   Yes   No
9. Does your child have any trouble sleeping?   No   Yes
10. Circle any of the following that your child has had:

"Red" measles   mumps   chickenpox   roseola   whooping cough   German or "3-day" measles   pneumonia   serious accidents   broken bones   removal of tonsils and adenoids

Other operations _____

Other diseases—what? _____

Hospitalizations—for what? _____

E. ALLERGIES

Has your child had:

1. Eczema or hives?   No   Yes
2. Wheezing or asthma?   No   Yes
3. Allergies or reactions to any medicine or injections?   No   Yes
4. Does he/she tend to have a stuffy nose or "constant cold"?   No   Yes

F. TESTS AND IMMUNIZATIONS:

Has your child had:

1. DPT?   _____ _____ _____ _____
2. Oral polio?   _____ _____ _____
3. Smallpox vaccination?   _____ _____
4. Mumps vaccine?   _____
5. Measles vaccine?   _____
6. German measles vaccine?   _____
7. Skin test for tuberculosis?   Yes   No
   Give date of last test   _____
8. Hearing tested?   Yes   No
9. Vision tested?   Yes   No

G. List any information which has not been asked but which you feel we should know.

FIG. 16–4.   Sample pediatric history questionnaire.

be nonjudgmental, refraining from comments such as "that was the wrong thing to do," or "there is a better way." The child's comments should be listened to attentively as well.

Through careful questioning, the interviewer tries to determine what the family's previous experience with hospitals and health-care providers has been. It is also important to ascertain how much parent and child understand about the child's condition and their expectations of this hospitalization, what support systems are available when the child returns home, and any disturbing or threatening concerns on the part of parent or child. These findings, in addition to a careful history and physical assessment, form the basis for the patient's total care plan while hospitalized.

During the interview, an identification bracelet is placed on the child's wrist. It is even important that the child be prepared for this simple procedure with an explanation of why it is necessary.

The nurse who receives the child on the pediatric unit should be friendly and casual, remembering that even a well-informed child may be shy and suspicious of excessive friendliness. The child who reacts with fear to well-meaning advances and clings to his mother is telling the nurse to go more slowly with the acquaintance process. Children who know that parents will stay with them are more quickly put at ease. After the child has been oriented to the new surroundings, perhaps clinging to mother's hand or carrying a favorite toy or blanket, the mother can undress him for the physical examination. Probably this procedure is familiar from visits to the pediatrician or clinic. If the mother feels confident about it, she can take the child's temperature and help obtain the urine specimen. If roentgenograms are required, the mother should be permitted to accompany the child to the radiology department.

The house physician in pediatrics will ask for a medical history and pertinent data, and may wish to do this without the child present. If the child is provided with some interesting activity while the nurse or play leader stays with him, this should not be greatly traumatic. He may accept the companionship of others in the playroom, or may be too shy and have to gradually work into a relationship.

Planning for discharge and care of the child at home begins early in the hospital experience. Nurses and other caregivers need to assess the child's and parents' level of understanding and ability to learn about the child's condition and about the care that will be necessary after the child goes home. Giving medications, using special equipment, enforcing necessary restrictions all must be discussed with the parent who will be the primary caregiver, probably the mother, and with one other person, usually the father. It is helpful to provide specific, written instructions for reference at home; the anxiety and strangeness of hospitalization can sometimes limit the amount of information retained from teaching sessions.

If the treatment necessary at home appears too complex for the parent to manage, it may be helpful to arrange for a visiting nurse to assist for a short period after the child is sent home.

Shortly before the child is discharged from the hospital, a conference can be arranged to review information and procedures with which the parents need to become familiar. This conference may or may not include the child, depending on his age and ability to understand. Questions and concerns need to be dealt with honestly, and a resource offered for questions that arise after discharge.

The return home can be a difficult period of adjustment for the entire family. Petrillo and Sanger offer some guidelines that can help parents.[2] (See boxed material.)

the child in the hospital environment

Earlier chapters have discussed the implications for hospital care for children in various developmental stages. Although the implications differ according to stage and to individual children, certain elements remain the same.

GUIDELINES FOR PARENTS DURING THE POSTHOSPITALIZATION PERIOD

1. Return the child to integrated family life as soon as possible. This means giving the child responsibilities equal to his abilities.
2. Acknowledge the child's bravery but refrain from making him the center of attention because of sickness. There is danger in his using symptoms for attention (secondary gains). Lots of hugs and kisses can be lavished when the hospital "veteran" does something that is cute or constructive, but is unrelated to his illness. Include pleasurable activities in his routines.
3. Be kind, firm and consistent, especially in the management of disciplinary problems.
4. Be truthful in order to preserve a child's trust.
5. Provide play materials such as clay, paints, doctor and nurse kits and equipment given to him in the hospital. Allow the child to play on his own.
6. Permit the verbal child to express his feelings regarding illness and hospitalization. Clarify distortions in his understanding. This expression of feelings helps the child integrate experiences into his life rather than to deny them.
7. Avoid leaving the child for long periods or overnight until he is well adjusted and trusting of his safety at home.
8. Allow the child to visit the staff in between admissions when in the hospital vicinity or after clinic appointments.

(Petrillo M, Sanger S: Emotional Care of Hospitalized Children: An Environmental Approach, 2nd ed. Philadelphia, JB Lippincott, 1980)

Any child who suddenly finds himself in a totally strange, perhaps dangerous situation will show distrust of everyone and everything he encounters. Not meaning to be willfully antagonistic, he is likely to be difficult because he is frightened. Impatience on the part of hospital staff, punishment in the form of restraints, scolding, or isolation, only reinforces the conviction that the hospital is indeed a bad place, and that he is being discriminated against. None of this is conducive to good health, either emotional or physical.

Hospitalized infants, toddlers, and preschoolers suffer great separation anxiety when it is not possible for parents to be with them. Older school-age children are easier to deal with because they can understand the reason for hospitalization and why cooperation is important. Adolescents worry about mutilation of their bodies and the possibility of death. Both school-age children and adolescents may find it difficult to express their attitudes and possible misconceptions about their illnesses.

THE NURSING CARE PLAN

Some nurses have found it helpful to make a nursing care plan, using pocket-size index cards that they can carry with them. One such plan is illustrated here.

First Cards

Name—Bobby S.	**Age—2**	**Diagnosis— Malnutrition**
Pertinent Background	*Development*	*Comparison to Average*
1. Place in family	Present weight	% weight for age
2. Type of home	Present height	% height for age
3. Birth weight	Motor development	
4. Birth height	Speech	
5. Pertinent background material	Adaptive behavior etc.	

Add symptoms of disease that the child exhibits, comparison with textbook pictures; medications ordered with effects desired and toxic reactions; treatments and procedures scheduled, as indicated.

Work Cards (Sample) First and Second Day

Objective	Anticipated problems	Anticipated solution	Evaluation
1. To foster security	1. Expect him to be shy, may not relate to me	1. Kindness, but let him make advances	1. Worked well, tomorrow will try. . . .
2.	2. May rebel against bed rest	2. Divert him by (suggest according to age)	2. Cried, would not be diverted will try. . . .
3.	3. May refuse food and drink	3. Plan a tea party	3. No problem NPO today

---

At the end of the first day, the nurse reviews and evaluates, notes new problems, discards those solved or that did not appear, and makes her work card for the next day.

Follow-Up Cards
Evaluation, Teaching, Long-Term Planning
1. Evaluation of results
2. Planning for future needs
3. Plans for parent, child, nurse teaching
4. Long-term home care
5. Community resource
6. Bibliography

This kind of care plan has proved valuable to the nurse. It is also taken to clinical conferences and serves as a basis for discussion. The nurse presents the knowledge and understanding she has acquired, shares her findings with the staff, and gains added insight through the discussion centered around her preliminary study.

This certainly is not an inflexible form, but a general guideline that can be helpful. The nurse no longer thinks of this child–patient as "the patient in room 415" or as "the child with malnutrition." Rather, she thinks of him as 2-year-old Bobby who has been taken from his home and put under her care.

The nurse can now care for him with some definite ideas about his needs and about how to meet them. In the course of the day, she may discover that he does not entirely conform to her expectations, and that perhaps her solutions were not entirely satisfactory, so she goes on from there. She has provided a measure of security for herself, however, before caring for Bobby, and her own confidence should provide strength for the child.

OBSERVING AND RECORDING

One of the most important parts of nursing care is continuous, careful observation of the patient's behavior, and recording those observations in clear, specific terms. Nurses' notes often provide vital clues to a child's condition, which physicians and other caregivers depend upon for further diagnosis and treatment.

Observation of behavior should include the factors that influenced the behavior and how often the behavior is repeated. Physical behavior as well as emotional and intellectual response should be noted, being aware of the child's age and developmental level, the abnormal environment of the hospital, whether the child has been hospitalized previously or otherwise separated from his parents. It is important to note whether his behavior is consistent or unpredictable, and any apparent reasons for changed behavior. These observations are considered in greater detail in the sections that follow.

THE INFANT

Activity. Healthy infants are constantly active, some more intense and curious than others. Illness modifies this activity, and the severity of the illness is directly related to the degree of impairment of activity. Does he lie quietly and manifest little or no interest in his surroundings? Is he in the same position each time you look at him?

State of Muscular Tension. The muscular state of an infant is tense, the grasp tight, the head raised when prone, and the kicks are vigorous. When the infant is supine, there is a space between the mattress and his back. How does this infant compare? Does he lie relaxed, with arms and legs straight and lax? Does he make any attempt to turn his head or raise it if placed in a prone position? Does he move about his crib?

Constancy of Reaction. A healthy infant shows a relative constancy of response and does not regress in his development. Was this child peppy and vigorous yesterday, but less so today? Did he respond to discomfort and painful procedures in an apathetic manner? Was he formerly interested in food, but now turns away? Does he respond to your presence or voice with his usual interest, or does he now turn his head and cry?

Behavior Indicating Pain. A healthy baby appreciates being loved and picked up. Does this child cry or protest when handled, and seem to prefer being left alone? Perhaps he cries when picked up, but stills after being held quietly for a time, thus indicating that something hurts when he is moved.

A healthy baby shows activity as distinguished from restlessness. Does this baby turn his head fretfully from side to side? Perhaps he pulls his ear or rubs his head. Perhaps he turns and rolls constantly, seeming to try to get away from pain. Is he indicating by these actions the discomfort that he cannot put into words?

A healthy baby shows activity in every part of his body. An infant may guard an arm or leg, or portion of the body, because it hurts to move it.

Physical Signs of Illness. Babies normally have a strong, vigorous cry. A weak, feeble cry, or a whimper indicates trouble. Nerve involvement may show in a high-pitched, shrill cry. If the infant appears to cry excessively, a cry chart is helpful to determine just how much he actually does cry. Observe the infant every ½ hour, and fill in the time period with various shadings of color for his activity at the time, such as sleeping, feeding, lying quietly awake, or crying. This makes your observations less subjective.

Skin Color. A healthy infant has a rosy tinge to his skin. Fingernails and toes are pink, mucous membranes pink-tinged. Does this baby show unusual pallor or blueness around the eyes and nose, or in the fingertips? Are the mucous membranes pale?

Appetite or Feeding Pattern. A healthy infant exhibits an eagerness and impatience to satisfy his hunger. The sick infant may show an indifference toward his formula, suck halfheartedly, vomit his feeding, or habitually regurgitate. He may take his feeding and subsequently exhibit discomfort.

Bizarre Behavior. Any kind of behavior that differs from that expected for the level of development should be noted. Is this child unusually good, or passive, in the face of strange surroundings, or does he respond with rejection to every overture, friendly or otherwise? Is he extremely clinging, never seeming satisfied with the amount of attention he receives?

It cannot be emphasized too strongly that any *one* manifestation in itself may not be significant. The important thing is whether or not this behavior is consistent with this particular child, or if it is a change from previous behavior. Perhaps he has always been pale or passive, or fussy in his feeding. Any such behavior needs to be noted, of course, but much significance depends greatly on the constancy of such behavior.

The nurse can tactfully, without alarming the parent, try to discover if he has always been a finicky eater, or been overactive, or an unusually quiet child.

THE OLDER CHILD

All of the previous observations are valid for the older child as well. In addition, there are a few somewhat different, or more mature reactions that may indicate an unhealthy state.

Covering up for Pain or Discomfort. A child seldom sees any enjoyment in illness or hospitalization. His burning desire is to get home again, and he will often go to great lengths to cover up any discomfort. Watch him sometimes when he does not know that you are. Is he limping, or holding one side of his abdomen, or showing any other sign of pain? If so, what does he do when he sees you watching him? Does he straighten up and say that he was just playing? Do you take his word for this, or do you report the behavior?

Extremes of Aggression or Passivity. How does this child behave? Does he resist any and all advances, and strike out against playmates or adults? Perhaps instead, he accepts everything. Even more important, is this a change in behavior? How can you know unless you have been consistently observant and have recorded behavior?

Reaction with Parents. Get a feeling of how a child reacts to his parents and they to him. How he reacts on the ward may be a reflection of his feelings toward his parents, or theirs to him. It may also reflect the parent's attitude to the situation of illness and hospitalization, or to the care that he now receives.

COMMUNICATION WITH CHILDREN

The nurse is constantly communicating with patients, even though they may not be able to understand her words or respond. Infants evaluate actions, not realizing that nurses who handle them abruptly and hurriedly may be rushed or insecure; these small patients feel only that these nurses are frightening and unloving.

The child who is old enough to distinguish between persons (generally some time after 6 months of age) tends to be frightened of strangers. Sudden, abrupt, or noisy approaches are almost certain to signal danger. It is important to let the child make an evaluation while still secure in mother's arms and wait for him to initiate the relationship.

Distrust of strangers may last through the first 3 or 4 years of life. A casual approach with reluctant children is usually more effective. Those children who show rejection or aggressive behavior are putting up a defense against their own fears, and the behavior should be ignored unless it threatens the child's own well-being or that of someone else. It is important to be firm without showing anger or disgust.

Some nurses have difficulty in accepting their own feelings while working with children. Each nurse brings personal feelings, fears, and conflicts to a new situation. Many feel a great inadequacy when beginning relationships with children. Perhaps they feel that they are not the all-knowing, all-powerful persons the child thinks they are, and are afraid that they are going to be found out; and so use aggression to cover their own insecurity. Nurses need to be willing to accept the fact that they are also human. A good nurse is self-accepting and self-confident, but she does not necessarily begin that way; she usually has to grow in maturity and insight.

After the nurse has honestly faced and accepted herself, she is no longer preoccupied with her own inner inadequacies and fears. Now she can consider the child's environment, background, and stage of development, and try to discover why the child behaves as he does. Is it a result of inconsistent handling at home, or is it the striving toward independence that his nature demands? It might even be a response to the nurse's authoritarian attitude; careful consideration should help modify the caregiver's expectations. Children who sense the nurse's genuine interest, eventually put forth some effort to respond.

DISCIPLINE, RULES, AND RESTRICTIONS

Hospitals, as facilities for the care and treatment of the sick, must have certain rules, probably different from those needed at home or school. Each child's physical condition may necessitate additional rules. Certainly no child in the hospital can be allowed conduct that would injure him or interfere with treatment. Being denied water or food just before surgery may seem like such a denial of human rights that the child will attempt to steal a drink from a faucet, or food from another child's tray. Often, also, his physical condition modifies activity. Unable to understand the "why" of prohibitions, he is apt to convince himself that "I could do that if the nurse would let me; she is just an old meany." The child may even convince parents that he has been treated unfairly, which of course points up the importance of total frankness between doctors, nurses, and parents.

Should children be allowed to be destructive as they work out their feelings? Aggression in speech, feelings, and symbolic actions should be permitted, as they help dissipate anger and feelings of helplessness. However, children should not be allowed to destroy or mutilate articles and toys belonging to others. Destroying their own toys in fits of anger may be a valuable lesson when they realize that a cherished possession has been ruined by their own actions. One important lesson children need to learn early in life is that they do not have the right to destroy or mutilate the possessions of others.

CULTURAL FACTORS IN COMMUNICATION

Each child is the product of a family, a culture, and a community. The culture determines not only the language but the health beliefs and practices of the family. Nurses who care for children need an understanding of the health practices and lifestyle of families from various cultures in order to plan culturally appropriate and acceptable care (Fig. 16–5).

In some cultures, family life is gentle, permissive, and loving; in others, unquestioning obedience is demanded; pain and hardship are to be stoically endured. The child may be from a cultural group that places high value on children, giving them lots of attention from many relatives and friends, or from a group that has taught the child that from early childhood he must fend for himself.

Cultural attitudes toward food, cleanliness, respect, and freedom are all important in planning care for the child while in the hospital and after returning home. The behavior and cooperation of child and family are essential to achieving restoration of good health.

Children from families who are new to this country or whose social contacts have been primarily with their own cultural group are likely to feel bewildered and antagonistic. Hospitals are strange to children raised in middle-class, white America. Is it any wonder that a Navajo Indian child reacts negatively to an atmosphere where food, language, people and surroundings are totally alien?

Respect for a child's cultural heritage and his individuality is an essential part of nursing care. The objective is to restore the health of the hospitalized child so that he can once again be a functioning part of his family and community, whatever the cultural background.

Dane Prugh suggests five principles, the five Cs, for dealing with minority children and their families:[3]

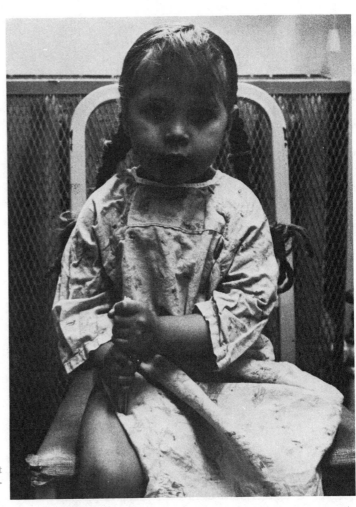

FIG. 16–5. Children whose cultural heritage is different from that of the hospital staff have special problems in adjustment. (Photo by Marcia Lieberman)

1. *Communication*—clear and direct between staff, patients, and families.
2. *Collaboration*—among various hospital disciplines, to give a consistency in communication with patients and parents.
3. *Continuity*—of relationships between staff, patients, and family.
4. *Consultation*—drawing on the expertise of medical, nursing, mental health, and other staff persons.
5. *Coordination*—in achieving an integrated plan of management, with a designated person responsible for its implementation.

COMMUNICATION WITH PARENTS

Routine conferences among the nursing staff, doctors, child-life workers, physical therapists, and other personnel concerned with children in the hospital are helpful in gaining an understanding of child patients. A clearer picture of the child is obtained, behavior better understood, and an opportunity presented to consider differing types of treatment and relationships. These can be rewarding to both patient and staff. When appropriate, parents can be invited to attend and gain valuable insights and understanding.

Some hospitals prefer to hold parent-group sessions. In either case, it is most important that parents are kept well-informed about what is going on and what is being planned for their sick child (Fig. 16–6).

Much can be done to make the parents feel welcome and important. When a procedure is planned, a parent can be told what is going to happen and be invited to help. However, no parent who is reluctant to help or observe a procedure should be urged to stay "because it is your duty as a parent." Some parents are so anxious and apprehensive that they communicate their concern to the child rather than provide support. The child thinks, "Even my mother is worried about what they are going to do to me." An overprotective mother may question or object to necessary procedures, thus giving the child an image of cruel, unfeeling hospital personnel.

An older child may feel self-sufficient, and be resentful of "being treated like a baby." However, it is normal to regress during illness, and most children of any age appreciate the presence of an assuring, self-controlled person during trying, uncomfortable times. The child needs to trust his environment. If, as frequently happens, the child regresses in order to handle the overwhelming distress, parents can offer support.

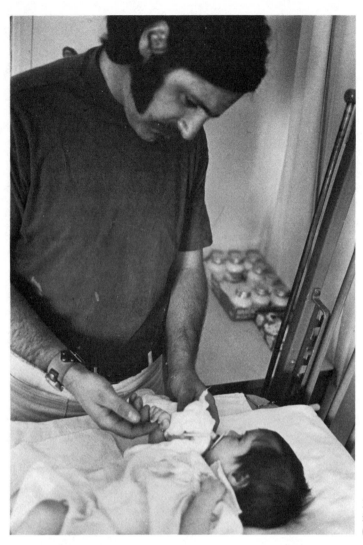

FIG. 16–6. Parents are under great stress when their child is hospitalized, particularly when the child is very young. (Photo by Marcia Lieberman)

CARE BY PARENTS AND ROOMING-IN

Research findings have proved beyond any reasonable doubt that separating young children from their parents, especially during times of stress, can have damaging effects.

Robertson, one of the early advocates of concern for hospitalized children, described the effects of separation from parents on young children.[4] He described three consecutive stages: protest, despair, and denial. In the first stage, protest, the young child cries, frequently refusing to be comforted by others, and constantly seeking his parent in every sight and sound. When his parent does not appear, he enters the second stage, despair, and becomes apathetic and listless. Caretakers often interpret this as a sign that the child is accepting the situation, but this is not the case; he has just given up.

In stage three, denial, the child begins taking interest in the surroundings and appears to accept the situation. However, the damage is revealed when his parents do visit him: he frequently turns away from them showing distrust and rejection. It may take a long time before he ac-

cepts them again, and even then, remnants of the damage linger. He may always have a memory of "when his parents walked away from him." Childhood impressions have a deep effect, regardless of how mistaken they may be.

The use of rooming-in now practiced in a large number of hospitals helps to remove the hurt and depression of the young hospitalized child. It is generally considered that separation from parents causes the greatest upset in children from 6 months of age to 3 or 4 years of age. However, all years of childhood should be considered when setting up a rooming-in system.

One advantage to the child whose parent is rooming-in is that the parent takes care of him, offering a measure of security. The parent may bathe, dress, and feed the child, prepare him for bed, and participate in his recreational activities. However, this should not be used to relieve staff shortages. If treatments are to be continued at home, rooming-in creates an excellent opportunity for the parent to observe and practice before leaving the hospital.

Rules should be clearly understood before admission, and facilities for parents should be clearly explained. The hospital may provide a folding cot in the child's room, or may only provide a reclining chair. Provision for meals should be explained.

Friction between parent and staff does occur at times. Parents who are overprotective or accustomed to being the authority figure may question or even interfere with treatments. Occasionally, parents will protest that they are paying for services and should not be expected to do more than entertain the patient.

Staff sometimes also create difficulties with rooming-in parents, particularly if they feel frustrated by the parent's presence or comments. Certainly some adults can be difficult to get along with, perhaps due to the parent's anxiety. Conferences between staff and parents are useful in straightening things out and creating a better atmosphere for everyone.

An occasional parent can hinder rather than help, especially with older children. One such mother who had a poor relationship with her 7-year-old son spent much of her time quarreling and arguing with him, but still insisted on rooming-in. Whether the child would have fared better had she been there only occasionally is difficult to determine.

THE INTENSIVE CARE UNIT

Seriously ill children who are admitted to the intensive care unit (ICU) or critical care unit (CCU) need constant monitoring with sophisticated electronic devices. Nurses in attendance must be constantly alert to each child's physical condition. Children's conditions change far more rapidly than adult conditions, so that effective nursing implies recognition of any impending threat to the child's physical progress. The nurse needs considerable training in using cardiac monitors, respirators, and the other technological equipment that has been so helpful in caring for the critically ill child.

Nurses understandably can become so involved in physical care that they cease to be concerned over the sick child's emotional needs. Yet, the emotional status of the child greatly influences physical progress toward health. Cheerful surroundings to brighten the department can lift a sick child's spirit. Toys such as dolls or stuffed animals, mobiles, and bright toys afford a comfortable feeling and may help remove the fear of strange surroundings and equipment. Soft music may be soothing. If the child's condition permits, being rocked or held lovingly in the arms of the nurse or attendant for periods each day will add greatly to his feeling of safety and comfort. All of this caring can boost morale and incentive toward health.

The parents' presence has a powerful effect on the child's will to survive. Intensive care units need to have visiting policies flexible enough to meet a child's need for parental presence. Comfortable lounging chairs contribute to the parent's comfort and enable a parent to stay longer and, if cots are not available, to sleep in the child's room at night if this seems to be helpful.

THE HOSPITAL PLAY PROGRAM

Play is the business of children and a principal way in which they learn, grow, develop, and act out feelings and problems. Playing is a *normal* activity, and the more it can be part of hospital care, the more normal and more comfortable this environment becomes.

In the playroom the children also can see their peer group and deal with illness. When they see that other children are playing who look worse than they do, then they can form relationships and talk about it or draw their feelings.[5]

Play helps children come to terms with the hurts, anxieties, and separation that hospitalization brings. No reprimand or punishment is called for when children bring out their hostilities, aggressions, and frustrations through play. Nurses should not say, "Now, Bobby, that's not nice." Bobby does not intend to be nice. He feels that people have not been nice to him and he is angry. The only way acceptable to others and to him is to express his hurts, fears, and even hatred through fantasy. Children who keep these negative feelings bottled up will suffer much greater damage than those who are allowed to let them out where they can be dealt with constructively. Children must feel secure enough in the situation to express "bad" feelings without fear of disapproval.

Children must not be allowed to harm themselves or others, however. While it is important to express feelings, acceptable or not, unlimited permissiveness is as harmful as excessive strictness. Children rely on adults to guide them and set limits for behavior because this means the adults care about them. When disapproval is necessary, it is important to make it clear that the disapproval is of the child's action, not the child himself.

TYPES OF PLAY THERAPY

Play therapy may be *directive* or *nondirective.* In directive play therapy, the person working with the child makes suggestions and interpretations of the child's words and actions. In nondirective play therapy, the adult allows the child to follow his own directions and reinforces his words and actions without showing rejection or acceptance. Generally nondirective therapy works best as the child then works through problems in his own way.

Play therapy means providing materials for the child to play with and opportunities for him to act out his feelings, observing him continually to gain a better understanding of his feelings about himself and his hospitalization.

Many people on the health team serve as *play therapists*: the child psychologist, the trained play leader, the child-life specialist, and the nurses. The psychologist, play leader, and child-life specialist are likely to concentrate their attention on seriously disturbed children, while nurses are responsible for children who are showing normal reactions to pain, fear, separation from home, and general bewilderment.

Rules for guidance of effective play are given by Petrillo and Sanger:[6]

Reflect only what the child expresses.
Supply materials that stimulate play.
Allow enough time without interruption.
Permit a child to play at his own pace.
Determine when it is appropriate to go beyond the child's expression.
Play for the child who cannot play for himself.
Allow direct play for the emotionally strong child. Be famil-

iar with some artistic material as a medium of expression. Have a knowledge of child growth and development because it guides the professional in clinical judgment.

THE HOSPITAL PLAY ENVIRONMENT

Although a well-equipped playroom is of major importance in any pediatric department, children can play out their fantasies and feelings in their own crib or bed if for some reason they cannot be brought to the playroom. Materials for their particular use can be brought to them, and someone, a nurse or student volunteer, should be available to give the necessary support and attention needed.

An organized and well-planned play area is of considerable importance in the overall care of the hospitalized child (Fig. 16–7). It should be large enough to accommodate cribs and wheelchairs, with a variety of play materials available to suit the ages and needs of all children. The child will choose the toy and the kind of play he needs or desires; thus, the selection and kind of play can usually be left unstructured. This does not, however, mean that the child should be ignored by the play leaders, or that nonparticipation is acceptable.

The needs of the timid child, or one who has been so strictly disciplined that he fears to step out on his own, must be taken into account. Even normally sociable children may carry their fears of the hospital environment into the playroom. It could be some time before timid, fearful or nonassertive children are able to feel free enough to take advantage of the play opportunities. Too much enthusiasm on the part of the play leader in trying to get the child to participate can defeat the play leader's purpose and make the child withdraw into himself. The leader must decide carefully whether to initiate an activity for a child or to let him advance at his own pace.

Often other children provide the best incentive by doing something interesting so the timid child forgets his apprehensions and tries for himself. Or a child will say, "Come and help me with this," and soon the other becomes involved. A fearful child will trust someone his own age before he will an adult who represents authority. Naturally, this does not mean ignoring the child's presence. The leader shows the child around the playroom, tells him that the children are free to play with whatever they wish, and that she is there to answer questions and to help when the child wishes or desires help.

When group play is initiated, the leader can invite the timid child to participate, but she does not insist. She can give him time to adjust and gain confidence.

Play Material.   One important function of a playroom is the provision of opportunities for the child patient to dramatize his hospital experiences. One section of the playroom containing hospital equipment, miniature or real, gives him opportunity to play out his feelings concerning his environment and treatments. Stethoscopes, simulated thermometers, stretchers, wheelchairs, examining tables, instruments, bandages, and other medical and hospital equipment are useful for this purpose.

Dolls dressed to represent the persons with whom he comes in contact daily—boy, girl, and infant patients, as well as parents, nurses, doctors, therapists, and other personnel, should be available. If nurses' caps and uniforms are worn in the hospital, replicas of the caps can be provided for children to use in acting out their hospital

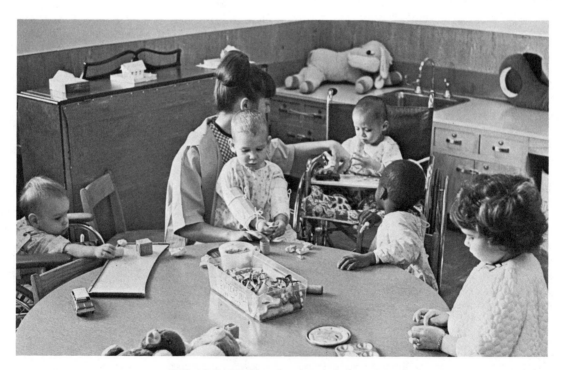

FIG. 16–7.   Children in a hospital playroom.

experiences. These simulated hospitals also serve an educational purpose; the child who is to have surgery, tests, or special treatments can be helped to better understand the projected procedures and why they are done.

Other useful materials for the child's play are listed here; these are only a few samples of the many possibilities:

Ingredients for homemade play dough. Allowing and helping a child to make his own play dough gives him greater satisfaction in using it than if the finished material is handed to him.

Finger paints, water colors, crayons, and colored pencils. Easels and drawing paper to use for his creations.

Cut-out books, scissors, paste. Pictures to paste on paper, perhaps to make the child's own scrapbook.

Games, blocks, jigsaw puzzles, building sets.

For children who can be more physically active: tricycles, small sliding boards, see-saws.

Miniature stores with scales, counters, play models of store products.

Books for all age groups are also important. Puppets play an important part in the children's department. The use of hand puppets does much to orient or assure a hospitalized child. The doctor or nurse puppet on the play leader's hand answers questions (and discusses feelings) that the puppet on the child's hand has asked. A child often finds it easier to express his feelings, fears, and questions through a puppet than to ask them directly. A child's ready sense of magic can let him half believe that the puppet is really expressing things that he hesitates to ask himself (Fig. 16–8).

OUTPATIENT PLAY FACILITIES

The pediatric clinic is a busy place. Growing knowledge of childhood diseases and their treatment has made possible the treatment of more children as outpatients, allowing them to live at home. Because they must also be treated as children, a properly equipped and adequately staffed playroom is needed in the pediatric outpatient area.

Many children with serious but chronic diseases become frequent visitors to the outpatient clinic. The provision of a playroom is not only enjoyable but helpful to children who are to undergo medical procedures, which can be frightening to the unprepared child. Play workers have an excellent opportunity to help an anxious child work through his fears.

Television programs and tape recorders are especially useful here, or a good storyteller. The one disadvantage, however, is that a child may be called for his treatment while a program is playing.

Some clinics allow the siblings of child patients in their playrooms as well. This is especially helpful when the mother has no one to care for them while she brings the child requiring observation and treatment to the clinic.

If for any reason a child must be left in the playroom

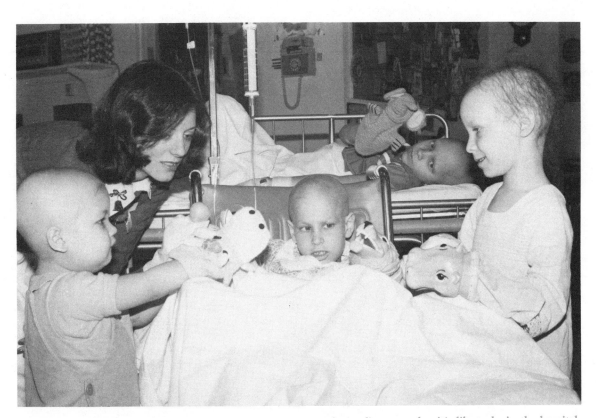

FIG. 16–8. A puppet play group led by a pediatric nurse oncologist discusses what it's like to be in the hospital. Group sessions inform children that others have similar feelings. (Photo by Terry Hanna)

without his parent, it is well to have name bands available, particularly for a new child or one unfamiliar to the staff.

Some children who have become engrossed in a play project may resent having to leave it when called for examination. It may be well to assure him that he can come back and finish his project, if his parent is willing or able to take the time.

THE SCHOOL PROGRAM IN THE HOSPITAL

The school program in children's hospitals has become quite well established in many areas. Convalescent hospitals and those for chronic diseases of children have had this service for children for some time. Occasionally, teachers or tutors have come into general hospitals to help an individual child. However, the idea of teachers regularly employed by the school system and working in the children's unit of a general hospital is relatively new.

Certainly being able to keep up with his classmates is a morale booster to a hospitalized child. However, such a program for the child with a short term illness has other values as well. In addition to his illness, the hospitalized child suffers from the strangeness of his surroundings. He is separated from all that is familiar in his life. The school atmosphere of teacher, books, and lessons gives him one familiar base on which to build security. The normal, everyday school experiences seem to be psychologically helpful to a child (Fig. 16–9).

A successful school program has been in operation for several years at Doernbacher Children's Hospital, division of the Medical School Hospital of the University of Oregon. Every school-age child is enrolled in this program

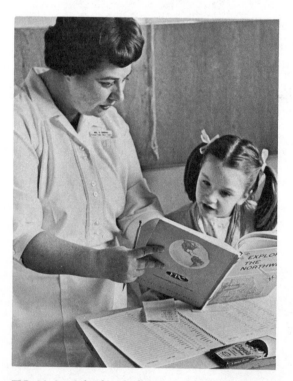

FIG. 16–9.   School in the hospital makes it seem like a more familiar place.

regardless of the length of his stay, unless his condition forbids such activity.

There are two regularly employed school teachers for a unit of about 30 children. As this hospital unfortunately does not have an adolescent unit, two additional teachers teach high school subjects to teenagers throughout the hospital. All children do regular schoolwork unless too ill. At 9 am, the teachers come around to each ward, bring the child's school bag to him, and get him started on his work for the day. Because of the diversity of ages and grades, individual study is the rule. Every effort is made to furnish the child with the same books and the same kind of instruction he has been receiving in school. Many children bring their school books with them. The school teachers go from child to child, moving on quietly when treatments are due. At noon, materials are collected, then after a rest period, the afternoon is given over to art work and crafts. Excellent rapport is established between nursing and educational personnel. The teachers are employed by the school system, thus school hours and holidays are observed. During the summer months, a play director and volunteers are with the children part of each day, although there is no regular school program.

summary

Tremendous progress has been made in recognizing and meeting the special needs of children and parents during hospitalization. In most hospitals, the environment is more cheerful, the rules more relaxed, and the approach more compassionate. Greater knowledge about disease and more advanced technological equipment have helped to vastly improve the physical care of young patients. Care of their emotional needs is not always so quickly achieved.

> The easiest thing for a hospital to provide is intensive care; the most demanding thing a hospital can give is the person. The need of all children is loving, supportive care. And *care* is more difficult to give than medicine.[7]

Although difficult, but nonetheless an integral part of nursing since its beginning, caring for and caring about children and their parents during the hospital experience can offer a wealth of personal and professional satisfaction.

review questions

1. What methods have hospitals used to reduce the loneliness of hospitalization?
2. Why is the nursing care plan an invaluable tool for providing the best possible individualized nursing care?
3. What are the five principles for dealing with minority children and their families?
4. How can the nursing staff gain an understanding of child patients?
5. Describe the effects on young children of parent–child separation.
6. How does play help the hospitalized child?
7. Describe "play therapy."
8. What types of play materials are useful for the hospitalized child?

references

1. Mendenwald NA: Children's liberation—in a hospital. Am J Mat Child Nurs 5:231–234, 1980
2. Petrillo M, Sanger S: Emotional Care of Hospitalized Children: An Environmental Approach, 2nd ed. Philadelphia, JB Lippincott, 1980
3. Prugh D: First Elizabeth M Straub memorial lecture. J Assoc Care Children Hosp 4, No. 2:8, 1975
4. Robertson J: Young Children in Hospitals, 2nd ed. New York, Basic Books, 1970
5. Francis S: In LaTour K: Little patients, big fears and hospitals that care. American Way, p 106. June 1980
6. Petrillo M, Sanger S: Emotional Care of Hospitalized Children: An Environmental Approach, 2nd ed. Philadelphia, JB Lippincott, 1980
7. Brookhouser P: In LaTour: Little patients, big fears and hospitals that care. American Way, p 106. June 1980

bibliography

Allmond B, Buckman W, Gofman H: The Family Is the Patient. St Louis, CV Mosby, 1979

Amdall M, et al: The evaluation of a child-life program and the impact on a pediatric inpatient service. J Assoc Child Care Hosp 5, No. 2:4, 1976

Baxter P: Frustration felt by a mother and her child during the child's hospitalization. Am J Mat Child Nurs 1:159–161, 1976

Farson F: Birthrights. New York, Macmillan, 1974

Frieberg KH: How parents react when their child is hospitalized. Am J Nurs 72:1270–1272, 1972

Green C: Understanding children's needs through play therapy. Nurs 74 4, No. 10:30–31, 1974

Hardgrove C: Living-in accommodations and practices for parents in hospital pediatric units: An update. J Assoc Child Care Hosp 4, No. 1:24–26, 1975

Hardgrove C, Dawson R: Ideas A to Z for personalizing pediatric units. Nurs 76 6, No. 4:57–65, 1976

Hilt NE: Pride, prejudice and parents. Pediatr Nurs 2, No. 3:32–35, 1976

Jackson PB, Bradham RF, Burnwell HK: Child care in the hospital: A parent–staff partnership. Am J Mat Child Nurs 3:104–106, 1978

Janovic F, Nierenberg J: The Hospital Experience. New York, Bobbs-Merrill, 1978

Johnson J, Kirchhoff KT, Endress MP: Easing children's fright during health care procedures. Am J Mat Child Nurs 1:206, 1976

Klinzing D, Klinzing G: The Hospitalized Child: Communication Techniques for Health Personnel. Englewood Cliffs, Prentice-Hall, 1977

Koss T, Teter M: Welcoming a family when a child is hospitalized. Am J Mat Child Nurs 5:51–55, 1980

McKeehan K: Continuing Care: A Multidisciplinary Approach to Discharge Planning. St Louis, CV Mosby, 1981

Norberta A: Caring for children with the help of puppets. Am J Mat Child Nurs 1:22–26, 1976

Plant EN: Working with Children in Hospitals. Chicago, The Press of Case Western Reserve University, 1971

Tealey A: Getting children to keep still during radiotherapy. Am J Mat Child Nurs 2:178, 1977

Zweig IK: A new way to get acquainted with the hospital: Pediatric open house for well children. Am J Mat Child Nurs 1:217–219, 1976

physical care of the sick child

student objectives

The student successfully attaining the goals of this chapter will be able to

1 Define the following vocabulary terms:

Body Surface Area (BSA)   Clark's rule   electrolytes   fractional dose
homeostasis   intermittent fever   interstitial   intravascular
Intravenous Pyelogram (IVP)   lysis   parenteral   remittent fever

2 List nine responsibilities of the nurse when administering medications.

3 Explain Clark's rule for computing pediatric dosages and discuss why the nurse would use it.

4 Describe the technique for administering oral medications to infants and young children.

5 Describe CPR techniques for an infant and for an older child.

6 Explain the differences between continuous, intermittent, and remittent fever patterns.

Caring for sick children challenges every nurse to function at the highest level of professional competence. Giving medications is one of the most important nursing responsibilities, calling for accuracy, precision, and considerable psychological skill. Monitoring vital signs, assisting with treatments, collecting specimens for diagnostic tests, and helping to maintain a safe environment are all part of nursing care. Meeting the challenge brings the satisfying reward of seeing children restored to health and returned to their family and friends.

medications for children

Giving medicines to small children is not easy. Even a nurse accustomed to preparing medications for adults experiences some anxiety when giving them to a child.

Certainly the importance of giving the right drug at the right dosage at the correct time to the right child cannot be overemphasized; however, administering medications involves much more than this. (See boxed material.) The nurse is responsible for (1) understanding the action of the drug and the responses of the patient; (2) being aware of potential adverse effects; (3) administering the correct dose (which is sometimes difficult if a child is uncooperative); and (4) understanding the metabolic systems of the different age groups of children—a factor that affects metabolism and the excretion of medications.[1]

The nurse prepares for administering medications, checking the reason for giving a particular medicine. Reference books and drug brochures are helpful, but information about recently approved drugs is not included in the standard references. In such cases, the nurse should check with the physician ordering the drug or the clinical pharmacist about new drugs.

The nurse observes the child for any unusual behavior following administration of medication. She records all unusual manifestations, noting that they had occurred during the period that a certain drug or drugs had been given. A reaction that is severe or unexpected should also be reported to the nurse in charge of the department.

Medicine vomited immediately after being swallowed can usually be repeated, if the nurse can be sure the full dose was vomited. It is well to check with the nurse in charge, however, as the child may have vomited because of a hypersensitivity to the drug. When medication is in the stomach for a short time, the nurse always seeks direction from the physician before repeating any or all of the dosage after vomiting.

Weeks suggests the following general guidelines for giving medication to children:[2]

- Approach the child with a positive attitude believing he will cooperate. Explain what you are doing.
- Allow the child to express his feelings; it is OK to be angry and afraid, but he must take his medication.
- When administering some oral medications the nurse may use liquids or soft foods to disguise a bad taste. But remember the child must eat or drink all of the food in order to get a full dose.
- Syringes are the most accurate way to deliver medication. Oral medications put into a cup may cling to the cup, and some of the dose will be lost.
- Do not use whole pills for children under 5 years. For preschoolers, crush pills between two spoons.
- Intramuscular injections are usually safer and easier if a second person restrains the child. A child may have difficulty cooperating with this painful procedure.

Always check the medicine card against the child's identification band. A hastily read card or quick recognition by sight can lead to error, particularly in a small child who doesn't understand enough to protest.

COMPUTING DOSAGES

Medications for children are seldom given in adult-size dosages. Instead the dosage is individually calculated according to the child's weight and/or body surface area (BSA). When ordering a drug, the physician considers the correct dose to be the amount required to safely bring about the desired action. Using the BSA method requires knowing the average dose per square meter (m^2) of a surface area:

$$BSA(m^2) \times Adult\ dose/m^2 = Child's\ dose$$

The nurse needs to know the approximate dosage for children of certain weight in order to validate her understanding of the physician's order, to detect any error in

---

RESPONSIBILITIES OF MEDICATION ADMINISTRATION

When administering any medication, the health professional must be responsible for the following:

1. Be licensed by the state to administer medication
2. Have knowledge of the medical condition, age, and development of the child who is to receive the medication
3. Have current knowledge of the expected drug action, recommended dose, route, possible side- and toxic effects
4. Prepare the proper dose and route in the proper manner
5. Verify the identity of the child

6. Approach the child in the proper manner by using speech, restraining techniques, and so on, as needed to administer the drug safely and with a minimum of trauma
7. Teach the child or parent how to store and administer the drug properly if it will be given at home; verify the parent's knowledge of the medication and side-effects
8. Record the medication administration process correctly on the child's medical record
9. Observe the child for drug effects

computation of fractional dosages, or to prevent misreading of an order. One estimated rule sometimes used to calculate approximate dosage is *Clark's rule*, applicable for children 2 years of age or older:

$$\frac{\text{Weight in lbs} \times \text{adult dose}}{150}$$

Calculating Fractional Dosage is necessary when full strength drugs must be diluted to achieve the concentration ordered by the physician. The simplest way to determine the amount needed of a full-strength drug is to divide the desired strength by the strength of the drug on hand. As most pediatric medications are administered in liquid form, the nurse simply gives the required fraction of the standard amount. The formula is

$$\frac{\text{desired dose}}{\text{dose on hand}} \times \text{diluent} = \text{amount to be given.}$$

For example, elixir of phenobarbital consists of 20 mg of phenobarbital in each 5 ml of the elixir. If the order reads "give 4 mg of phenobarbital," one would figure 4/20 × 5 ml (1/5 × 5) = 1 ml to be given (because this is an elixir it should be well diluted with water before giving it to a child).

After computing the dosage, the nurse should *always* have the computation checked by her instructor, the charge nurse, or someone in the department who is delegated for this purpose. Errors are easy to make, and easy to overlook. It is preferable for the second person to do the computation separately, then check both results.

Errors in medications can occur because nurses are not infallible. To admit an error is often difficult, especially if there has been carelessness concerning the rules. A person may be strongly tempted to adopt a "wait and see" attitude, the gravest error of all. It is much easier for a nurse to accept the censure of the doctor or the head nurse, whether deserved or undeserved, than to endure anxiety and guilt while waiting to see if there are to be any ill effects. Serious consequences for the child can possibly be avoided if the mistake is disclosed promptly.

ORAL MEDICATION

A small baby is not too particular about the taste of his food if he is hungry. Almost anything liquid can be sucked through a nipple, including liquid medicines, unless they are quite bitter. Medications that come in syrup or fruit-flavored suspensions are easily administered this way. Another method of administering oral medications is to

---

TECHNIQUE FOR ADMINISTRATING ORAL MEDICATION TO INFANTS AND YOUNG CHILDREN

Preparation

1. Compute a fractional dose if necessary; have the computation checked. (See Fractional Doses.)
2. Prepare according to the form of medication.
   a. *Tablet.* Crush it in a small amount of water. If the tablet is bitter crush it and mix it with honey or with corn syrup.
   b. *Suspension and syrup.* Shake well. Fruit flavored suspensions and syrups do not need dilution unless it is desired.
   c. *Elixir.* Alcohol base; these must always be diluted with an equal amount of water (or more to prevent aspiration).
3. Heart medication. Check the apical beat before administration, and compare it with the previous reading for the rate, quality, and rhythm. Report any significant deviation.

Administration

Infant

1. Identify the infant.
2. Pour the medication into a 1-ounce disposable bottle. Raise the infant's head or hold him and allow him to suck. Alternative—Raise the infant's head, administer the medication with a plastic medicine dropper or a 2½ – 3 ml syringe. Give it very slowly, and allow the infant to swallow before continuing.
3. See that the infant has swallowed all the medication before leaving. Look in his mouth.
4. Place the infant on his side to prevent aspiration.

Child

1. Identify the child.
2. Hold the child in an upright position. Allow the child to hold medicine cup if he wants. Give it slowly.
3. If the child resists, use firmness but do not force. Never hold the child's nose to force him to swallow. (He can aspirate liquid.)
4. Allow the child to swallow before continuing.
5. Check his mouth to be sure the medication has been swallowed before leaving.
6. If the child vomits, estimate the amount of emesis and report it. Do not repeat the medication unless so ordered.

Recording

Record the time, the dose, the route *e.g.,* (PO), and the child's reaction, if it is unusual.

drop them slowly into the baby's mouth with a plastic medicine dropper.

Elixirs contain alcohol and are apt to cause choking unless they are diluted. Syrups and suspensions do not need dilution, but are thick, and they may need dilution to ensure that the child gets the full dose.

If you have given a child a pill, make sure that he swallows it before you leave. Usually he opens up so wide that you can see back to his tonsils and look under his tongue.

It usually is best to give a small child his medicine in solution form. If you must use a tablet, dissolve it in water. Do not use orange juice for a solvent unless specifically ordered to do so. The child may associate the taste of orange juice with the unpleasant medicine for the rest of his life. If the medicine is bitter, honey or corn syrup can disguise the taste. He may come to dislike corn syrup, but that will not be as important to him as the inability to take orange juice.

There is little excuse for restraining a small child and forcing a medication down. The child can always have the last word if he chooses, and bring it up again. The danger of aspiration is very real. Of even greater importance is the antagonism and helplessness built up in the child by such a procedure. A child's dignity needs to be respected as much as that of an adult.

One does not offer a child a choice, of course, over whether to take his medicine when he really has no choice. Within limits, one can choose the most auspicious time. Small children waking from sleep are often bewildered and cross. Waiting a few minutes until the child becomes oriented to his surroundings may be all that is needed. Interrupting a child's meal is usually a poor practice. Enlisting a child's cooperation is important of course. However, the nurse must be the authority figure here, and show by her kind firmness and matter of fact approach that there is no reason for the child to refuse.

The older child deserves explanation about any treatment or medication. He may still lack the courage to cooperate, but he understands (even if unwillingly) the necessity for the procedure, and he does not lose his sense of self respect.

INTRAMUSCULAR MEDICATIONS

Children have the same fear of needles as adults. Students are reluctant to hurt the child, and frequently cause the very pain they are trying to prevent by inserting the needle slowly. A swift, sure jab is nearly painless, but the nurse must be prepared for the child's squirming and stay calm and sure. A second person is essential if the child is to be held firmly. (See boxed material.)

Always take time to explain to the child what you are going to do. He may be too small to understand all of the words, but tell him anyway. Children appreciate being treated honestly. A child who has been told that an injection or treatment will not hurt learns very quickly that he cannot trust adult promises. Neither does it boost the child's morale to be told "Oh, you're a big boy. Big boys don't cry." The child knows the needle does hurt. Moreover, he is *not* a big boy and there is nothing wrong in crying over a hurt anyway.

Too much time spent on preparation conveys the nurse's reluctance and children can be quick to take advantage with stalling tactics. They need firmness and prompt completion of the explained procedure.

PRINCIPLES

The point of the injection must be as far away as possible from the major nerves to avoid a serious injury to the child. Serious injury to the sciatic nerve, resulting in paralysis, has occurred following improperly placed injections in the buttocks.

The nurse giving intramuscular injections should have a basic knowledge of anatomy, particularly about nerve pathways and muscle placement. For example, the gluteal area actually extends to the anterior superior iliac spine—which should be taken into account when measuring the buttock for an injection site.

The muscular area chosen should be sufficiently developed to tolerate the injection. Infants under the age of 6 months have poorly developed gluteal muscles. The lateral aspect of the midanterior thigh is the preferred site for infants (Fig. 17–1). Some pediatricians prefer this site for young children as well.

The needle should be long enough to penetrate well within the muscle before depositing the medication. The plunger of the syringe should not be depressed until the needle is well within the muscle.

INTRAVENOUS FLUIDS

FUNDAMENTALS OF FLUID BALANCE

Maintenance of fluid balance in the body tissues is essential to health. Severe imbalance, when uncorrected will cause death, as exemplified in cases of serious dehydration resulting from severe diarrhea or vomiting, or from the loss of fluids in extensive burns. A brief review of fundamental concepts of fluid and electrolyte balance in body tissue will help the student understand the importance of adequate fluid therapy for the sick child.

Water. A continuous supply of water is necessary for life. At birth, approximately 70%–83% of body weight is water.[3] This proportion decreases to the adult level of approximately 60%, at about 1 year of age.

In health, the body's water requirement is met through the normal intake of fluids and foods. Intake is regulated by the person's thirst and hunger. Normal body losses of fluid occur through the lungs (breathing), the skin (sweating), in the urine and feces. In normal health, intake and output balance each other out, and the body is said to be in a state of *homeostasis*.

Homeostasis, meaning a uniform state, signifies biologically the dynamic equilibrium of the healthy organism. This balance is achieved by appropriate shifts in fluid and electrolytes across cellular membrane, and by elimination of end products of metabolism and excess electrolytes.

Body water, containing electrolytes, is situated within the cells, in the spaces between the cells, and in the plasma and blood. Failure to maintain homeostasis may be the result of some pathological process in the body. Imbal-

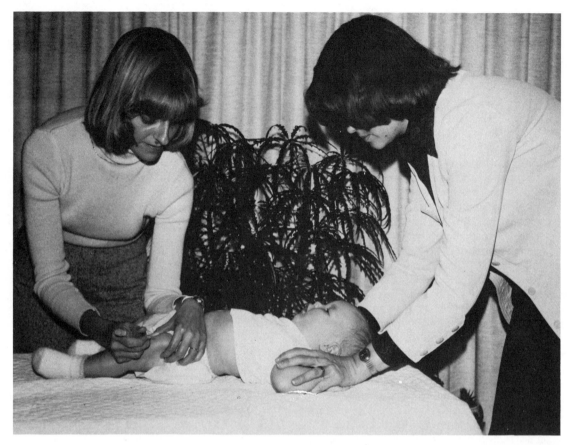

FIG. 17–1.   An intramuscular injection into the vastus lateralis muscle. One person restrains the upper torso while the other gives the injection. (Howry LB, Bindler RM, Tso Y: Pediatric Medications. Philadelphia, JB Lippincott, 1981)

ance is also the cause of disruption in water, electrolyte and acid–base balances found in many disorders. Some of the disorders associated with imbalance are pyloric stenosis, high fever, persistent or severe diarrhea and vomiting, and extensive burns.

Retention of fluid may occur through impaired kidney action or impaired metabolism.

Intracellular fluid is that fluid contained within the body cells. Nearly half the volume of body water in the infant is intracellular.

Each cell must be supplied with oxygen and nutrients to keep the body in health; also its water and salt levels must be kept constant within very narrow limits.

Cells are surrounded with semipermeable membrane which retains protein and other large constituents within the cell. Water, certain salts and minerals, nutrients and oxygen enter the cell through this membrane. Waste products and substances produced within the cell are diffused out into the surrounding spaces.

Extracellular fluid is situated outside the cells. It may be *interstitial*, situated within the spaces or gaps of body tissue, or *intravascular*, situated within the blood vessels

or blood plasma. *Blood plasma* contains protein within the walls of the blood vessels, and water and mineral salts that flow freely from the vascular system into the surrounding tissues.

Interstitial fluid has a composition similar to plasma except that it contains practically no protein. This reservoir of fluid outside the body cells decreases or increases easily in response to disease. An increase in interstitial fluid results in edema. Dehydration depletes this fluid before affecting the intracellular and plasma supply.

In the infant, about 25% body weight is due to interstitial fluid. In the adult, interstitial fluid accounts for only approximately 15% of body weight. Intracellular fluid accounts for about 45% of body weight in both infants and adults.

Infants and children become dehydrated much more quickly than adults. In part, this is because of a greater fluid exchange caused by the rapid metabolic activity associated with infants' growth, and in part because of the relatively larger ratio of skin surface area to body fluid volume; two or three times that of adults'.

Because of the above factors, the infant who is taking in no fluid will lose an amount of body fluid equal to his extracellular volume in about five days, or twice as rapidly

TECHNIQUE FOR INTRAMUSCULAR INJECTION

Equipment

A sterile syringe. A 2 ml Luer syringe; or a 2½ ml disposable syringe; or a 1 ml tuberculin syringe for a fractional dosage computed in one-hundredth of 1 ml.

A sterile injection needle 20 to 22 gauge, 1 inch in length.

A sterile container with skin preparation material. Bandaids.

Selection of the Site

A. Gluteal Area

Muscle: gluteus maximus. Area—upper outer quadrant of the gluteal area.

1. Place the patient on his abdomen with his toes turned in.
2. Using your thumb, define the anterior superior iliac spine (Fig. 17–2). (Site for IM injection into the gluteal muscle.)
3. Place your index finger on the head of the trochanter.
4. Define the quadrants of the gluteal mass.
5. Select the inner angle of the upper outer quadrant.
6. Inspect the area for induration and for trauma from previous injections. Rotate the sites as indicated.
   Note: if a suitable site cannot be found within acceptable boundaries, report this and seek instruction before giving, or use the anterior lateral aspect of thigh (or the deltoid, if approved).
7. A second person should help position, restrain, and divert the child. Explain that you are helping the child hold still, not punishing him.
8. Give the injection as explained in procedure.
9. Comfort the child. Apply a Bandaid as a comfort measure. The child may hold the Bandaid until ready. Allow the child to give an injection to a stuffed toy animal or a doll if he wishes, using a play syringe.

B. Vastus Lateralis Muscle

1. Place the infant on his back.
2. Measure the area from the greater trochanter to the patella. Select a site midway between the knee and the hip joint, using the lateral aspect of the thigh.
3. Give the injection as explained in procedure.
4. One nurse alone may give this injection to a small infant. Two nurses are preferable for an older infant.
5. Hold and comfort the infant following the injection.

C. Deltoid Muscle

The use of this area is limited because of the small space available, the undeveloped muscle in young children and painfulness of the procedure. It may be useful for older children, particularly for those who have limited availability for other sites.

Only a small area between the upper and lower portions of the deltoid muscle may be used to avoid the radial and axillary nerves (Fig. 17–3). Injections should not be made into the middle or the lower third of the upper arm. Permission should be obtained before using the deltoid area in children.

Procedure

1. Prepare the medication under sterile conditions and take it to the bedside.
2. Identify the patient from his identi-band.
3. Explain the procedure to the child.
4. Select the proper site and give the injection deep into the muscle. Withdraw the plunger slightly to check for blood in the syringe before injecting the medication.
5. Apply pressure over the site with sterile cotton, and withdraw the needle. Apply pressure and gentle massage. (Massage may be contraindicated if giving medication such as Imferon.)
6. Apply a Bandaid if there is any oozing.
7. Record the time, dose, route (IM), and the child's reaction if unusual.

as will the adult. The infant's relatively larger volume of extracellular fluid may be designed to partially compensate for this greater loss.

Electrolytes are chemical compounds (minerals) that break down into *ions* when placed in water. An ion is an atom having a positive or a negative electrical charge. Ions having a positive charge are called *cations*. Those having negative charge are called *anions*. Sodium (Na^+) is one example of a cation, chloride (Cl^-) is an example of an anion (Table 17–1).

Cations and anions must balance each other to function properly. This does not mean they are equal in amount, but rather in equilibrium. The chemical combining activity of cations and anions is expressed in milliequivalents. One milliequivalent of any cation reacts completely with any anion to produce activity.

Important cations in body fluids are sodium (Na^+), potassium (K^+), magnesium (Mg^{++}) and calcium (Ca^{++}). Important anions are chloride (Cl^-), phosphate (HPO_4^{---}), and bicarbonate (HCO_3^-). Electrolytes have the important function of maintaining acid-base balance. Each water compartment of the body has its own normal electrolyte composition.

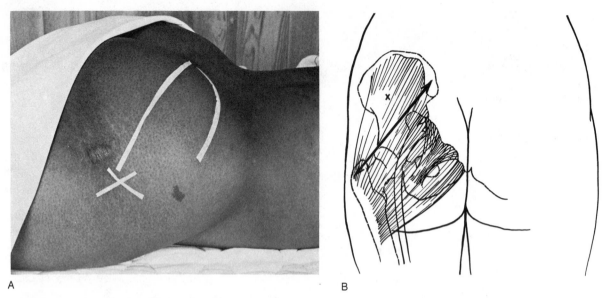

A   B

FIG. 17–2.   Site for an intramuscular injection into the upper quadrant of the gluteal muscle. (*A*) The crest of the ilium is outlined and the greater trochanter of the femur is marked with a large X. (*B*) The site of injection is lateral and slightly superior to the midpoint of a line drawn from the trochanter to the posterior superior iliac spine.

Acid–Base Balance.   The acidity of a solution is determined by the concentration of hydrogen (H^+) ions. Acidity is expressed by the symbol pH. Neutral fluids have a pH of 7.0, acid fluids below 7.0, and alkalines above 7.0. Normally, body fluids are slightly alkaline. Internal body fluids have a pH ranging from 7.35 to 7.45. Body excretions, however, are products of metabolism and become

acid in character. Normal pH of urine, for example, is 5.5 to 6.5.

Defects in the acid–base balance result either in acidosis or alkalosis. Acidosis may occur in such conditions as diabetes, kidney failure, or diarrhea. Hypochloremic alkalosis may occur in pyloric stenosis due to the decrease in chloride concentration and increase in carbon dioxide.

In normal health, the electrolyte and fluid balance is maintained through the intake of a well balanced diet. The kidneys play an important part in regulating concentrations of electrolytes in the various fluid compartments. In illness, the balance may be disturbed due to excessive losses of certain ions. Replacement of these minerals is necessary to restore health and to maintain life.

FLUID THERAPY

Fluid therapy consists of the administration of water, electrolytes, sometimes protein and calories to restore normal fluid balance. It may be needed to make up a body deficit, to replace abnormal losses, or to maintain normal fluid balance.

Fluids may be given orally, subcutaneously, or intravenously. When an illness is not serious and the child is able to take and retain fluids, oral feedings are usually sufficient. Accurate records of intake and output must be kept to ascertain whether the child's intake and output are well balanced. Normally, these should amount to approximately the same amounts.

Oral fluids may be mixtures of glucose, water and electrolytes, for the child who is able to retain fluids taken by mouth. The child can, of course, progress to formula or full liquids and on to solid foods as his condition permits. Certain conditions, such as acute diarrhea, may be aggra-

FIG. 17–3.   Site for a deltoid injection. It is important to inject into the belly of the deltoid muscle, about 2 to 3 finger breadths down from the acromion process on the outer aspect of the arm; the lower boundary is roughly opposite the axilla. The lower deltoid is dangerously close to the axillary nerve, which branches off from the radial nerve.

Deltoid muscle

Axillary nerve

Radial nerve

Redmann

TABLE 17–1. IMPORTANT ELECTROLYTES IN THE HUMAN BODY

Electrolyte	Symbol	Valence	Atomic Weight	Age	Normal Amounts in Human Plasma (mEq/liter)
Cations					
Calcium	Ca^{++}	2	40	Newborn	3.7– 7.0
				Infant	5.2– 6.0
				Child	5.0– 5.7
				Adult	4.5– 5.7
Magnesium	Mg^{++}	2	24	Newborn	1.4– 2.9
				Infant	1.2– 2.7
				Child	1.2– 2.6
				Adult	1.5– 3.0
Potassium	K$^+$	1	39	Newborn	5.0– 7.7
				Infant	4.1– 5.3
				Child	3.5– 4.7
				Adult	3.4– 5.6
Sodium	Na$^+$	1	23	Newborn	139– 162
				Infant	139– 146
				Child	138– 145
				Adult	135– 151
Anions					
Bicarbonate	HCO$_3^-$	1	61	All ages	24– 31
Chloride	Cl$^-$	1	35.5	Newborn	93– 112
				Infant	95– 110
				Child	101– 108
				Adult	98– 108
Phosphate	HPO$_4^{--}$	2	96	All ages	2.6– 3.2
	H$_2$PO$_4^-$	1	97		
Sulfate	SO$_4^{--}$	2	96.1	All ages	0.2– 1.3

(Howry LB, Bindler RM, Tso Y: Pediatric Medications, Philadelphia, JB Lippincott, 1981)

vated by oral intake. In such cases, *parenteral* fluids (fluids given other than by mouth) are indicated.

Parenteral fluids are commonly given intravenously. Occasionally subcutaneous infusions are given, but this is rarely practiced in children.

INTRAVENOUS INFUSIONS

Intravenous therapy may be used to correct electrolyte imbalance, as a medium for medication, or as a method of feeding when oral feeding is contraindicated.

Infants. Because an infant has small veins which are difficult to enter, a scalp vein may be used. Scalp veins are relatively easy to enter, and scalp-vein infusions are easier to manage. Special scalp-vein needles attached to small tubing are available. The area to be used needs to be shaved and cleansed with an antiseptic (Fig. 17–4). The baby should be mummied (Fig. 17–5) for the insertion, and the head held firmly against the treatment table. After insertion, the needle should be firmly taped in place, and

the plastic tubing taped to the side of the infant's head or cheek.

Sandbags are used to immobilize the head, and clove-hitch restraints (Fig. 17–6) are useful to prevent the infant from reaching the needle or catching his arm in the tubing. Observe for presence of pulse and check circulation frequently to be sure restraint is not too tight.

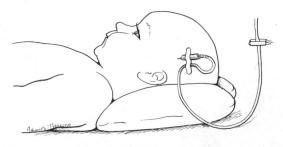

FIG. 17–4. A scalp vein infusion.

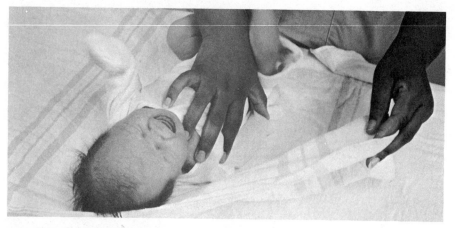
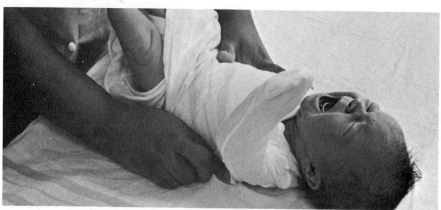
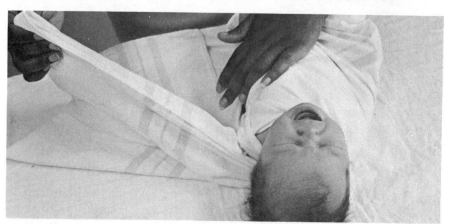
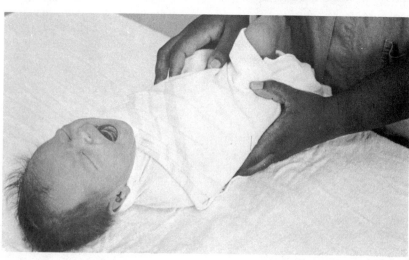

FIG. 17–5. Procedure for applying a mummy restraint. (King EM, Wieck L, Dyer M: Illustrated Manual of Nursing Techniques, 2nd ed. Philadelphia, JB Lippincott, 1981)

Other sites are on the back of the hand, the flexor surfaces of the wrist and the medial side of the ankle. The antecubital space is seldom used in small children because it is extremely difficult to restrain the child so that he cannot bend his arm.

Intravenous drip must be slow for the small child, in order to avoid overloading the circulation and inducing cardiac failure. It is extremely difficult to slow a regular intravenous drip to 4 or 6 drops per minute and still have it function properly. Various adapting devices are available that decrease the size of the drop to a "mini" or "micro" drop of 1/50 or 1/60 ml, thus delivering 50 to 60 mini- or micro-drops per cubic centimeter rather than the 15 drops of a regular set (Fig. 17–7). Many intravenous sets also contain a control chamber that is designed to deliver controlled volumes of fluid, avoiding the inadvertent entrance of too great a volume of fluid into the child's system.

None of these safeguards obviates the necessity of frequent inspection of the therapy. The drops are counted frequently and the site of injection examined. The child's movements frequently cause the infusion to slow up or to speed up, or may cause the needle to slip out of the vein. Routine recording of the rate and the amount of fluid is necessary.

The intravenous infusion therapy is uncomfortable, and the necessary restraints increase the child's frustration. If the nurse is reasonably careful, and if the needle is securely taped, the infant can frequently be held for comforting and relaxation.

When long-term intravenous therapy is contemplated, an intravenous cut-down is usually performed. This is accomplished by cutting down to the vein and threading in plastic tubing, with two or three silk sutures required to close the wound. This requires a sterile dressing and subsequent removal of the sutures.

A technique that modifies this surgical procedure is the use of an especially constructed needle through which tubing can be threaded into the vein and the needle then withdrawn, thus doing away with the dissection of a cut-down.

The infant needs careful restraint to avoid difficulties at the start of an intravenous infusion as well as to prevent him from dislodging the needle later. The mummy restraint is useful when attempting the scalp vein technique, or a modified mummy leaving an arm or a foot free if another site is used. A clove-hitch restraint for arms or legs gives the infant some freedom, and at the same time prevents interference with continuing therapy, or elbow restraints may be useful. Sandbags are necessary to immobilize the head if a scalp vein is used.

Older Children. *The older child* needs explanation and emotional support during intravenous therapy (Fig. 17–8). Threatening a child with a needle if he doesn't eat (or drink) is encouraging his fantasies of "badness" and punishment. Quite aside from the psychological harm, such treatment rules out any possibility of cooperation from a healthy-minded child. In an emotionally disturbed child, it deepens his despair over his self-convinced lack of worth.

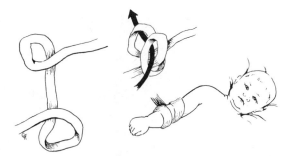

FIG. 17–6. The clove-hitch restraint keeps the infant or child from reaching an intravenous needle or interfering with dressings.

Explanations help clear the air of misunderstandings. For the child old enough to understand, an explanation in simple terms of the mechanism and purpose of the procedure will help greatly in obtaining the child's cooperation. Emotional support is of primary importance for any age.

An intravenous infusion does not necessarily interfere with play activities. When the needle is securely placed, children may usually be allowed up in a chair and into the playroom; activity is allowed or limited by children's understanding, cooperation, any necessary restrictions, and the presence of an informed and watchful attendant.

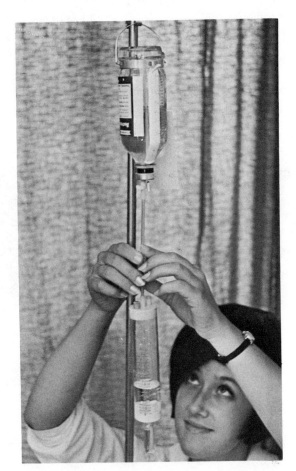

FIG. 17–7. Regulating intravenous flow.

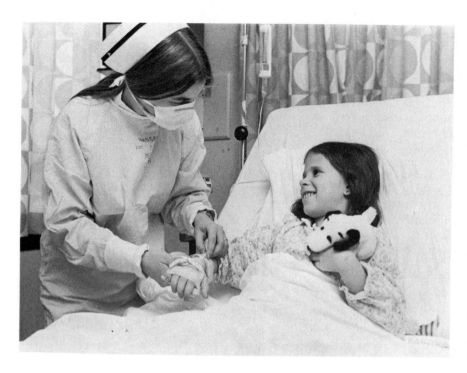

FIG. 17–8. Older children with intravenous infusions need honest explanations and emotional support. (J Practical Nurs, Sept, 1978)

regulating body temperature

The importance of maintaining normal body temperature has been discussed in the chapters on the newborn, and health problems of the infant. Significant alterations of body temperature can have severe consequences for all children. However, it should be noted that the so-called normal temperature is only an average and may vary in individuals. The child's temperature-regulating mechanism does not mature until about 8 years of age; thus, young children's temperatures may show wide swings unrelated to the seriousness of their disease condition.

Until age 5, temperatures should be taken rectally (Fig. 17–9); after that time they can be taken orally unless there is a risk that the child might harm himself, in which case the axillary method is used (Fig. 17–10). Depending

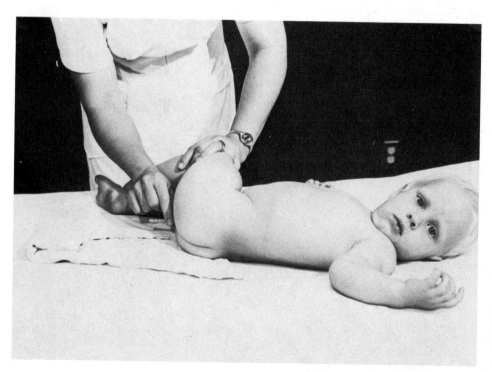

FIG. 17–9. When taking a rectal temperature, the nurse keeps one hand on the thermometer, and the other on the child's legs so he will not turn suddenly and break the thermometer. (King EM, Wieck L, Dyer M: Illustrated Manual of Nursing Techniques, 2nd ed. Philadelphia, JB Lippincott, 1981)

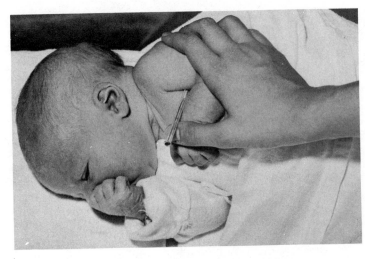

FIG. 17–10. Taking a child's temperature by axillary method requires holding the thermometer in place for 7 to 9 minutes in order to get an accurate reading. (King EM, Wieck L, Dyer M: Illustrated Manual of Nursing Techniques, 2nd ed. Philadelphia, JB Lippincott, 1981)

on the method used and the child's age, "normal" temperatures range from 99.7° F (37.7° C) at 1 year old to 98.6° F (37.0° C) at 5 years old; axillary temperatures are about two degrees lower. Inaccurate oral temperature readings can result if breathing is difficult and the child does not keep his mouth closed long enough. Use of electronic thermometers can alleviate this problem because they register temperatures much more rapidly and accurately. Rectal temperatures require that the thermometer be left in place for a full 3 minutes. Temperatures can vary from 0.5° to 2.0° during any 24-hour period, from a low point in the early morning to a peak in the late afternoon.

ELEVATED TEMPERATURE (FEVER, HYPERTHERMIA)

Fever is the body's signal of a problem; it is a symptom, not a disease. As mentioned earlier, the degree of fever does not correlate with the severity of the disease. A child is considered febrile when the rectal temperature measures 100° F, but treatment is often delayed until the temperature reaches 102° F.

Fever in children is most commonly caused by infection but can also indicate dehydration, inflammatory disease, tumors, and other pathologic conditions. Patterns of temperature are described as *continuous, intermittent,* and *remittent.*[4]

Continuous fever is characterized by consistent elevation of temperature with slight variation during the 24-hour cycle. In *intermittent fever,* the temperature is elevated during part of the day, but drops to normal or below normal levels within a 24-hour period. *Remittent fever* occurs when the temperature rises and falls dramatically, but never returns to normal during the 24-hour cycle.

Fevers that gradually recede to normal over a period of several days are said to resolve by *lysis.* Those that drop dramatically to normal within 36 hours do so by *crisis.*[5] In most infectious diseases, *diaphoresis* (sweating) accompanies fever.

The most important factor in care of the febrile child is to determine and treat the cause of the fever. Until the cause can be identified, measures must be taken to reduce the fever to make the child more comfortable, prevent dehydration, seizures, and the possible CNS damage that can result. Tepid sponge baths, maintaining hydration, and administering aspirin or acetaminophen are methods commonly employed. In some cases, the physician may order a hypothermia blanket or pad. Treatment with sponge baths or hypothermia should not be continued longer than 20–30 minutes, otherwise vasoconstriction will occur, resulting in further temperature elevation. The nurse should wait at least 30 minutes after the sponge bath to take the child's temperature because it will continue to decrease after the bath. Leaving the child uncovered, dressed only in lightweight pajamas, or diaper and shirt, also helps reduce body temperature.

LOWERED TEMPERATURE (HYPOTHERMIA)

Cold stress is most common in the newborn infant and is discussed in Chapter 2. In the very young infant, an abnormally low temperature can signal the presence of infection. A child suffering from prolonged exposure to cold temperature needs special attention to help regulate metabolism and increase comfort. A brief warm bath, warm pajamas, and a comfortably warm bed may be all that is necessary.

If local application of heat is prescribed, hot water bottles, heating pads, and hyperthermia pads (K-pads) may be ordered. Their use is described under Therapeutic Application of Heat.

THERAPEUTIC APPLICATION OF COLD

In addition to reducing body temperature, the local application of cold can also help prevent swelling, control hemorrhage, and provide an anesthetic effect. Intervals of approximately 20 minutes are recommended, both for dry cold (K-pads, ice bags, and commercial instant-cold preparations) and moist cold (compresses, soaks, and baths) treatments. Since cold decreases circulation, prolonged chilling can result in frostbite and gangrene. Detailed instructions for therapeutic application of cold and heat can be obtained in the procedure manuals of individual hospitals, and from manufacturers of commercial devices.

THEREPEUTIC APPLICATION OF HEAT

Local application of heat increases circulation by vasodilation, and promotes muscle relaxation, thereby relieving pain and congestion. It also speeds formation and drainage of superficial abscesses.

Artificial heat should never be applied to the skin of a patient without a physician's order. Tissue damage can occur, particularly in fair-skinned persons, or those who have suffered sensory loss or impaired circulation. These children should be closely monitored, and none should receive heat treatments longer than 30 minutes at a time, unless the physician's order so states.

Moist heat produces faster results than dry heat, and is usually in the form of hot compresses or soaks.

Dry heat can be applied by means of an electric heating pad, a K-pad (unit that circulates warm water through plastic enclosed tubing), or a hot water bottle. Many children have been burned because of improper use of hot water bottles; therefore, these are not recommended. Electric heating pads and K-pads should be covered with a pillowcase, towel, or stockinette.

assisting with diagnostic and treatment procedures

Many of the procedures in today's highly technologic hospitals can be frightening and painful to children. The nurse can be an important source of comfort to children who must undergo these procedures, even though it is difficult to assist with or perform procedures that cause pain

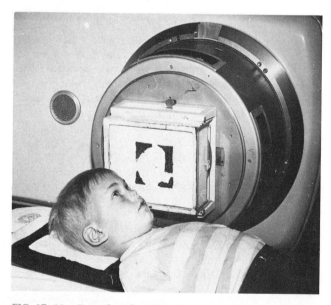

FIG. 17–11. Even though radiologic treatments are usually painless, the size and strangeness of the apparatus can be frightening to a child. This child is receiving cranial irradiation to destroy leukemic cells in the brain and spinal cord. Computerized tomography (CT) scanning can cause anxiety in children and parents unless they understand what will happen during this painless diagnostic test. (J Practical Nurs, Sept, 1978)

(Fig. 17–11A and B). It is a little less difficult if the child is old enough to understand the purpose of the procedure and the expected benefit. Infants can only be soothed and comforted before and after.

The nurse on the toddlers' ward has greater opportunity to explain than on the infants' division, but at best will only be imperfectly understood. Even if the toddler does grasp the words, they will have little meaning for him. The big reality is that he hurts.

Sometimes children's interest can be diverted so that they can forget their fright. They must be allowed to cry if necessary, and they should always be listened to, and their questions answered. It takes maturity and experience on the nurse's part to know exactly which questions are stalling techniques, which call for firmness and action. Children need someone to take charge in a kindly, firm manner that tells them the decision is not in their hands. They are really too young to take this responsibility for themselves.

Nurses have conflicting feelings about the merit of giving some reward after a treatment. Careful thought is necessary about this. Children given a lollipop or a small toy following an uncomfortable procedure tend to remember the experience as not totally bad. This has nothing to do with their behavior. It is not a reward for being brave, or good, or big; it is simply a part of the entire treatment. The unpleasant part is mitigated by the pleasant.

An older person can supply his own reward by contemplating the improvement in his health, but the child does not have sufficient reasoning ability to understand future benefits.

BLOOD TESTS

Blood tests are part of almost every hospitalization experience. Although the specimens are usually obtained by laboratory personnel or a physician, the nurse needs to be familiar with the general procedure in order to explain it to the child, and may be asked to help restrain him during the procedure. Blood specimens are obtained either by pricking the heel, great toe, earlobe, or finger, or by venipuncture. In infants, the jugular or scalp veins are most commonly used; at times, the femoral vein is used (Fig. 17–12A and B). In older children, the veins in the arm are used.

URINE TESTS

The procedures for collecting urine specimens are discussed in the chapter on Health Problems of the Infant.

STOOL TESTS

Stool specimens are tested for various reasons, including the presence of occult blood or excess fat. The nurse collects these specimens from a diaper or bedpan using a tongue blade, or directly from the patient using a rectal swab, and places them in clean cardboard receptacles. It is important that stool specimens not be contaminated with urine, and that they be labeled and delivered to the laboratory promptly.

CEREBROSPINAL FLUID TESTS

When analysis of cerebrospinal fluid is necessary, a lumbar puncture is performed. During this procedure the nurse must restrain the child in position as shown in Figure 17–13 until the procedure is completed. This position enlarges the intervertebral spaces for easier access with the aspiration needle. Children undergoing this procedure may be too young to understand the nurse's explanation, but are nonetheless entitled to honesty and understanding support.

ELECTRONIC TESTS

Electrocardiogram (ECG or EKG). This test measures the electrical impulses of the heart muscle and records the pattern of each phase of the cardiac cycle. The impulses are transmitted to the recording device by means of leads or electrodes placed on the skin. Although a technician generally performs the test, nurses need to be able to explain the procedure to the child. There is no pain involved; however, it is important that the child lie quietly during the test. The leads are attached by means of a rubber strap and an electrolyte lubricant is placed between the lead and the skin to increase conductivity.

Electroencephalogram (EEG). Similar in principle to the electrocardiogram, the electroencephalogram measures and records the electrical activity of the brain by means of leads or electrodes placed on the scalp. Although painless, the EEG can be frightening to the child and may necessitate sedation to maintain the quiet state necessary for the procedure. It is performed by a specially trained technician and takes about 1 hour.

RADIOLOGIC TESTS

Barium Enema. This procedure is used to help diagnose problems in the lower gastrointestinal tract, and requires specific preparation on the day preceding the test that may include laxatives, a cleansing enema, and a clear liquid diet. The nurse should consult the procedure manual of the employing hospital and physician's orders for precise details. While the patient is in the radiology department, radiologic personnel administer the barium enema, a portion of which is expelled immediately following the test. When the test is completed, another laxative or cleansing enema may be ordered. It is important to observe and record the child's bowel movements after this procedure.

Upper GI Series. Used to help identify problems in the stomach and small bowel, this test requires preparation and follow-up care similar to the barium enema.

Intravenous Pyelogram (IVP). This test is ordered to help diagnose problems in kidney function. A contrast medium is injected intravenously and roentgenograms are taken at 5, 10, and 15 minute intervals after injection to determine integrity of kidneys, ureters, and bladder. Preparation can include laxatives, withholding solid foods, and a cleansing enema; the individual hospital procedure manual should be consulted.

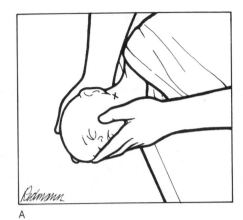

A

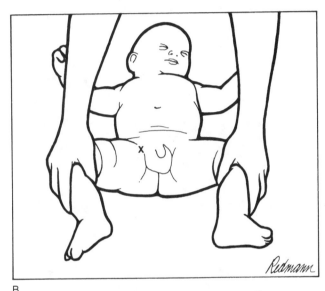

B

FIG. 17–12.   (*A*) Position of infant for jugular venipuncture. (*B*) Position of infant for femoral venipuncture.

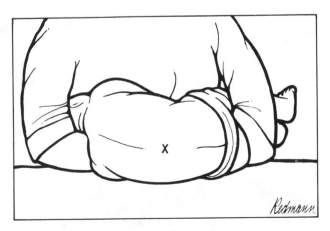

FIG. 17–13.   Position of infant for lumbar puncture.

Voiding Cystourethrogram. Used to determine the presence of reflux, this test involves the injection of contrast medium into the bladder through a urethral catheter, and taking roentgenograms before, during, and after voiding. Preparation includes withholding all food and fluids after midnight preceding the test.

safety in the children's department

Nurses who care for hospitalized children must guard against the kind of accidents that occur at home and also against those peculiar to the hospital situation. Parents whose children are accidentally injured at home generally

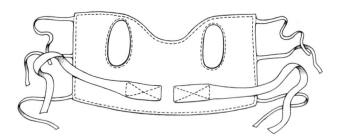

FIG. 17–14. (A) Jacket restraint to keep child in crib. Ties may be tied tightly to prevent child from standing in crib or climbing over sides. (B) Crib nets must be applied snugly over the top and sides of the crib and secured to the mattress strings. Children in a netted crib must not be left unobserved.

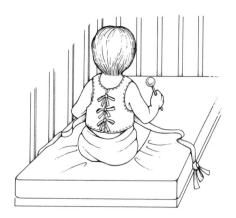

A

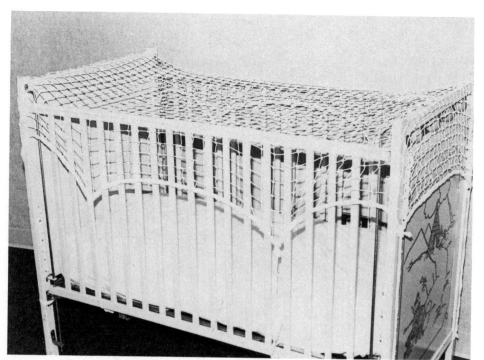

B

blame themselves, but when a child is injured in the hospital they are likely to wonder if nurses were watching the child carefully enough.

Highchairs in the children's department present a hazard for the child just learning to stand. Given the opportunity, the child will display the newly acquired ability to stand in his highchair; therefore, the simplest method of prevention is to abolish the use of highchairs in the hospital. Low chairs and tables are preferable for children who can sit without support; infant seats (Punkin' seats) are good for smaller children. Falls can still occur, but the consequences are not as serious.

Children love to climb, and an empty crib is fun to climb into but less fun to fall out of. A good rule is never to leave small children unattended while they are awake. Children can follow the nurse while she goes to the linen closet or the supply cupboard; when she goes to the tub room to bathe one child, the others can go along and play beside her during the bath. Keeping crib sides up, whether the crib is occupied or unoccupied, reduces the temptation to climb in. Clear, hard plastic domes are used on some cribs to keep children from falling out.

Restraints are sometimes necessary to keep an infant or young child from interfering with treatments. The child's instinct is to remove anything that makes him uncomfortable or interferes with his freedom. Thus, it is imperative that children in any kind of restraints be checked frequently. Children have strangled by getting their heads between the edge of a net crib-cover and the edge of the crib, or by becoming entangled in the ties of a jacket restraint (Fig. 17–14A and B).

Numerous examples verify this potential danger. One 2-year-old, after misbehaving in the playroom, was put in her crib and the restraint jacket fastened. In a fit of temper,

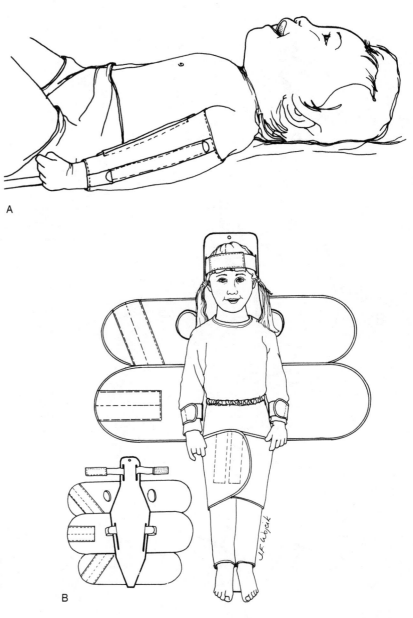

A

B

FIG. 17–15. (A) Elbow restraint. (B) Papoose board. (King EM, Wieck L, Dyer M: Illustrated Manual of Nursing Techniques, 2nd ed. Philadelphia, JB Lippincott, 1981)

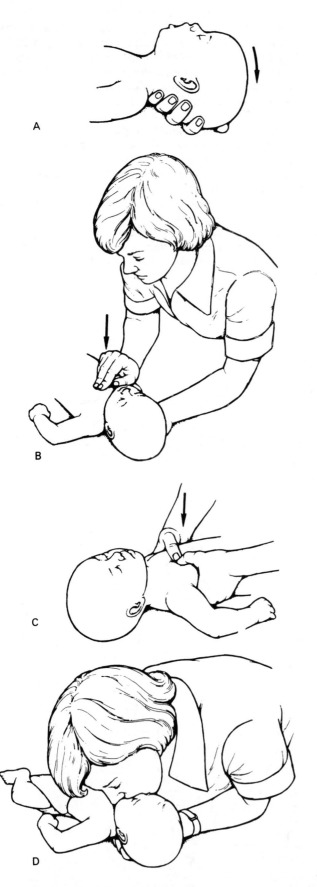

AIRWAY

- Clear the airway of mucus, if present. Use your finger in a sweeping motion.
- Tilt the infant's head backward *slightly*. Forceful extension of the neck may obstruct the infant's pliable breathing passages.

CIRCULATION

- Support the infant's back with your hand.
- Use the tips of your index and middle fingers to depress the mid-sternum about ½ to ¾ inches (B).
- Or, use alternate method (C). Circle chest with hands and compress sternum with both thumbs.
- Maintain a rate of 80 to 100 compressions per minute.
- Ventilate quickly, once after each five compressions.
- Do not interrupt compression during ventilation.

BREATHING

- Cover the infant's nose *and* mouth with your mouth.
- Use small breaths or puffs from cheeks to inflate the lungs once every three seconds.

FIG. 17–16. Techniques of cardiopulmonary resuscitation in an infant. (*A*) Position after clearing the airway. (*B*) Palpation of sternum. (*C*) Compression. (*D*) Ventilation. (Gildea JH: Techniques of cardiopulmonary resuscitation in an infant. Am J Nurs 78 No. 2:265, 1978; original art by Neil Hardy. Copyright © 1978, American Journal of Nursing Company. Reproduced with permission)

she climbed over the crib side and was found dangling over the side with the jacket pulled up around her neck. She could easily have strangled.

A toddler was told by his doctor that he could "go home today when his mommy comes." A little later he was found wandering the halls looking for his mother to take him home. Climbing over the side of his crib he had pulled the ties off his jacket restraint and reached the floor. Another child might have suffered a serious fall.

The nurse should remember that restraints are not to be used unless there is no other way of preventing damage to a child's health and safety. Figures 17–15A and B illustrate other kinds of restraint used in the hospital to prevent the young child from interfering with an important test or treatment.

Emergency procedures such as the Heimlich maneuver (see p 171) and cardiopulmonary resuscitation (CPR) (Fig. 17–16) should be part of every pediatric nurse's skills. Sudden death from cardiac disease occurs most often during the early months of life, but cardiac arrest can occur for any number of reasons in hospitalized children of all ages. Although the nurse in a hospital setting seldom needs to manage cardiac arrest alone, all nurses should know the location of emergency resuscitation equipment and how to initiate CPR.

Wieczorek and Natapoff offer the following guidelines for resuscitation of the infant, after the airway has been cleared:[6]

1. Place baby with head toward nurse, tilting it slightly downward.
2. Superimpose thumbs over the middle of the sternum (after quickly palpating sternal notch and xiphisternal junction). If pressure is applied on the xiphisternal junction rather than the sternum, liver damage can result.
3. Link fingers behind back of infant. Do not cover ribs.
4. Apply pressure on sternum ½ to ¾ inches downward and release rapidly at a rate of slightly more than 1 compression per second, producing 90 to 100 compressions per minute. Palpate the carotid pulse with each compression.
5. After 5 compressions, ventilate, giving one quick puff from air in resuscitator's cheeks. Be sure to cover both mouth and nose. (If ventilated once every 5 compressions, lungs will be inflated once every 3 to 4 seconds. If one person is doing CPR, ratio of ventilation to compression is 2 : 15; if two persons are performing the procedure, the ratio is 1 : 5).

When effective cerebral blood flow has been restored, pupils will constrict to normal size. Checking femoral pulses will indicate circulation to lower body.

CPR for older children is similar to that of the infant. The child is placed on a hard surface, and the airway is cleared. With children between 6 months of age and 3 years of age, the resuscitator places the heel of one hand on the lower third of the sternum and compresses the sternum downward approximately ¾ of an inch to 1 inch, 90–100 times per minute. The depth of compression for children over 6 years of age is 1½ to 2 inches; the rate is 80 compressions per minute. With children over 6 the resus-

citator places the heel of one hand over the lower third of the sternum and the other hand on top of the first. CPR should be continued until there are signs of recovery, then the child will probably be transferred to an intensive care unit for close observation.

summary

Whether a child is 6 months, 6 years, or 16 years old, illness and hospitalization make a significant impact on growth and development. Even with the most attractive, best equipped surroundings, and the most competent medical or surgical treatment, the child's recovery and rehabilitation will be incomplete without effective nursing care. Nurses are the child's continuing link with caring and understanding. Each nurse who gives competent, comforting care strengthens that link, and helps make hospitalization a positive growth experience for the child.

review questions

1. What are the general guidelines for giving medications to children?
2. Why must an intravenous drip for a small child be regulated slowly?
3. Why do older children need explanation and emotional support during intravenous therapy?
4. How soon after a tepid sponge bath should the nurse take the child's temperature?
5. How can the nurse maintain a safe and accident-free hospital environment?
6. Describe CPR for an infant and for an older child.

references

1. Weeks HF: Administering medication to children. Am J Mat Child Nurs 5:63, 1980
2. Weeks HF: Administering medication to children. Am J Mat Child Nurs 5:63, 1980
3. McGrath BJ: Fluids, electrolytes and replacement therapy in pediatric nursing. Am J Mat Child Nurs 5:58–62, 1980
4. Prior JA, Silberstein JS: Physical Diagnosis: The History and Examination of the Patient, 5th ed, p 60. St Louis, CV Mosby, 1977
5. Prior JA, Silberstein JS: Physical Diagnosis: The History and Examination of the Patient, 5th ed, p 60. St Louis, CV Mosby, 1977
6. Wieczorek RR, Natapoff, JN: A Conceptual Approach to the Nursing of Children: Health Care From Birth Through Adolescence. Philadelphia, JB Lippincott, 1981

bibliography

Birchfield ME: Nursing care for hospitalized children based on different stages of illness. Am J Mat Child Nurs 6:46–53, 1980
Carr JJ, et al: How to solve dosage problems in one easy lesson. Am J Nurs 76:, 1934, 1976
Chow M, Durand B, Feldman M, Mills M: Handbook of Pediatric Primary Care. New York, John Wiley & Sons, 1979
Evans M, Hansen B: Guide to Pediatric Nursing: A Clinical Reference. New York, Appleton-Century-Crofts, 1980

Fischbach F: A Manual of Laboratory Diagnostic Tests. Philadelphia, JB Lippincott, 1981

Gahart B: Intravenous Medications, 3rd ed. St Louis, CV Mosby, 1981

Howry LB, Bindler RN, Tso Y: Pediatric Medications. Philadelphia, JB Lippincott, 1981

Hughes WT, Buescher EC: Pediatric Procedures, 2nd ed. Philadelphia, WB Saunders, 1981

McCaffery M: Nursing Management of the Patient With Pain, 2nd ed. Philadelphia, JB Lippincott, 1979

McCormick RD, Gilson-Parkevich R: Patient and Family Education: Tools, Techniques, and Theory. New York, John Wiley & Sons, 1979

Metheny NM, Snively WD Jr: Nurses' Handbook of Fluid Balance, 3rd ed. Philadelphia, JB Lippincott, 1979

Rodman MJ, Smith DW: Pharmacology and Drug Therapy, 2nd ed. Philadelphia, JB Lippincott, 1979

Ryan SA, Clayton BD: Handbook of Practical Pharmacology, 2nd ed. St Louis, CV Mosby, 1980

Self TH, Srnka QM, Mauksch I: Systematic Patient Medication Record Review: A Manual for Nurses. St Louis, CV Mosby, 1980

Squire J, Clayton BD: Basic Pharmacology for Nurses, 7th ed. St Louis, CV Mosby, 1981

Strand MM, Elmer LA: Clinical Laboratory Tests: A Manual for Nurses, 2nd ed. St Louis, CV Mosby, 1980

Vestal KW: Critical Care Nursing. New York, John Wiley & Sons, 1981

Whitson BJ, McFarlane J: The Pediatric Nursing Skills Manual. New York, John Wiley & Sons, 1980

the child undergoing surgery

18

student objectives

The student successfully attaining the goals of this chapter will be able to

1 List five general aspects of preoperative care.

2 List three complications the nurse should observe the child for after surgery.

3 Explain the differences between gavage and gastrostomy feedings, and discuss the uses of each.

4 Describe the method for measuring the length of the tube used for gavage feeding.

5 Explain why a nasogastric tube is often used during and after abdominal surgery.

Surgery frightens most grownups, even though they can understand why it is necessary and how it will help correct their health problem. Very young children do not have this understanding and can become very frightened of even a minor surgical procedure. Older children and adolescents are capable of understanding the need for surgery and what it will accomplish, if they are properly prepared.

Many hospitals have outpatient surgery facilities ("surgicenters") that are used for minor procedures and can permit the patient to return home the day of the operation. These facilities help reduce or eliminate separation of parents and children, one of the most stressful factors in surgery for infants and young children. Whether hospitalized for less than a day or for several weeks, the child who has surgery needs understanding preoperative and postoperative care that is also thorough. When the child is too young to benefit from preoperative teaching, explanations should be directed to parents to help relieve their anxiety and prepare them to participate in the child's care after surgery.

preoperative care

Specific physical and psychological preparation of the child and the parents varies according to the type of surgery planned. General aspects of care include patient teaching, preparation of the skin, preparation of the gastrointestinal and urinary system, and preoperative medication.

PATIENT TEACHING

The child admitted for planned surgery will probably have had some pre-admission preparation by the physician and parents. Many parents, however, may have an unclear understanding of the surgery and what it involves, or may be too anxious to be helpful. It is up to the health professionals involved in the child's care to determine how much he knows and how much he is capable of learning, to help correct any misunderstandings, to explain the preparation for surgery and what the surgery will "fix," as well as how he will feel after surgery. This preparation must be based on the child's age, developmental level, previous experiences, and parental support. All explanations should be clear and honest, expressed in terms the child and his parents can understand. Questions should be encouraged to be sure all information is understood correctly. If at all possible, preoperative teaching should be done in short sessions, rather than trying to cover everything all at once.

As mentioned earlier, the use of puppets, dolls, or play with a miniature hospital is helpful in teaching children and allowing them to express their feelings, both before and after surgery. Making a sketch of a child's body, showing the part to be operated on gives the child some idea of what is to take place. The child may wonder how the doctor gets to the organ or part to "fix" it, and may decide that it must hurt very much to be cut open. Petrillo and Sanger suggest using less threatening words such as "opening" and "drainage," rather than "cutting" and "bleeding."[1]

Children should also be prepared for standard preoperative tests and procedures such as roentgenography and blood and urine tests. Nurses should explain the reason for withholding food and fluids prior to surgery so children do not feel that they are being neglected or punished when others receive trays.

Children sometimes interpret surgery as punishment and should be reassured that they did not cause the condition. They also fear mutilation or death, and need careful explanation that the doctor is only going to repair the affected body part.

It is important to emphasize that the child will not feel anything during surgery because of the special sleep that anesthesia causes. Describing the recovery room (wake-up room) and any tubes, bandages, or appliances that will be in place after surgery lets the child know what to expect. If possible the child should be able to see and handle the anesthesia mask (if this is the method to be used) and other equipment that will be part of the postoperative experience.

Role playing, adjusted to the child's age and understanding, is helpful. The child can be shown the stretcher he will ride on, and permitted to pretend to ride to the operating room, put on a mask, and go to sleep. If the nurse or play leader is asked to pretend to be the patient, she should do so.

The older child or adolescent may have a greater interest in the surgery itself, what is wrong and why, how it will be repaired, and how it will affect him after surgery. Model organs, such as a heart, are useful, or the patient may wish to make his own drawing.

A child needs to understand that several people will help to care for him before, during, and after surgery. If possible, staff from anesthesia, operating room, recovery room, or ICU should visit the child preoperatively. Explaining what the people will be wearing (caps, masks, and gloves), the equipment, and that the lights will be bright helps make the operating room experience less frightening. A preoperative tour of the recovery room or ICU is also helpful.

Most patients experience postoperative pain, and children should be prepared for this experience. They also need to know when they can expect to be allowed to have fluids and food after surgery.

Children should be taught to practice coughing and deep-breathing exercises. Teaching them to splint the operative site with a pillow helps reassure that the sutures won't break and let the wound open.

Children should be told where their parents will be during and after surgery, and every effort should be made to minimize parent–child separation. Parents should be encouraged to be with their child when he leaves for the operating room.

SKIN PREPARATION

Depending on the type of surgery, skin preparation may include a tub bath or shower, and will certainly include special cleaning and inspection of the operative site. Frequently the operative site is shaved the night before surgery, but this procedure may be delayed until immediately before the procedure. If fingers or toes are involved, the nails are carefully trimmed. The operative site may be painted with a special antiseptic solution as an extra precaution against infection; this depends on the physician's orders and the procedures of individual hospitals.

PREPARATION OF GASTROINTESTINAL AND URINARY SYSTEMS

The physician often orders a cleansing enema the night before surgery. This is an intrusive procedure and needs to be explained to the child before it is given. If the child is old enough, he should understand the reason for the enema.

Children usually receive nothing by mouth (NPO) 4 to 12 hours prior to surgery because food or fluids in the stomach might cause vomiting and aspiration, particularly during general anesthesia. The child should be told that food and drink are being withheld to prevent upset stomach. This period varies according to the age of the child; infants become dehydrated more rapidly than older children and thus require a shorter NPO period prior to surgery. Loose teeth are also a potential hazard and should be counted and recorded according to hospital policy.

In some cases, urinary catheterization may be performed preoperatively, but usually it is done while the child is in the operating room. The catheter is often removed immediately after surgery, but can be left in place for several hours or days. Children who are not catheterized prior to surgery should be encouraged to void prior to the administration of preoperative medication.

PREOPERATIVE MEDICATION

Depending on the physician's order, preoperative medications are ordinarily given in two stages: a sedative is administered about 1½ to 2 hours prior to surgery, and an analgesic–atropine mixture is administered immediately before the patient leaves for the operating room (Fig. 18–1). When the sedative has been given, the lights should be dimmed and noise minimized to help the child relax and rest. Parents and child should be aware that atropine can cause a blotchy rash and a flushed face.[2]

Preoperative medication should be brought to the child's room when it is time for administration. At that time, the child is told that it is time for medication and that another nurse has come along to help him hold still. Medication should be administered carefully and quickly because delays will only increase the child's anxiety.

If hospital regulations permit, parents should accompany the child to the operating room and wait with him until he is anesthetized. If this is not possible, the nurse who has been caring for the child can go with him to the operating room and introduce him to personnel there.

postoperative care

During the immediate postoperative period, the child will be cared for in the recovery room or the surgical ICU. Meanwhile the room on the pediatric unit should be prepared with appropriate equipment for the child's return. Depending on the type of surgery performed, it may be

	Atropine	Chlorpromazine	Diazepam	Meperidine	Morphine	Pentobarbital	Promethazine
Atropine	C	C	I	C	C	I	C
Chlorpromazine	C	C	I	C	C	I	C
Diazepam	I	I	C	I	I	I	I
Meperidine	C	C	I	C	C	I	C
Morphine	C	C	I	C	C	I	C
Pentobarbital	I	I	I	I	I	C	I
Promethazine	C	C	I	C	C	I	C

FIG. 18–1. Compatibilities of commonly used preoperative medications. C = compatible; I = incompatible. (Howry L, Bindler R, Tso Y: Pediatric Medications. Philadelphia, JB Lippincott, 1981)

necessary to have suctioning, resuscitation, or other equipment at the bedside.

When the child has been returned to his room, nursing care focuses on careful observation for any signs or symptoms of complications: shock, hemorrhage, or respiratory distress. Vital signs are monitored according to postoperative orders, and recorded. Dressings, IV apparatus, urinary catheters, and any other appliances are noted and observed (Fig. 18–2). An IV flow sheet is begun (Fig. 18–3). The first postoperative voiding is an important milestone in the child's postoperative progress because it indicates the adequacy of blood flow, and should be noted, recorded, and reported. Any irritation or burning should also be noted, and the physician notified if anuria (absence of urine) persists beyond 6 hours.

Postoperative orders may provide for ice chips or clear liquid to prevent dehydration; these can be administered with a spoon or in a small medicine cup. Frequent repositioning is necessary to prevent skin breakdown, orthostatic pneumonia, and decreased circulation. Coughing, deep breathing, paddling the feet, and position changes are done at least every 2 hours.

PATIENT TEACHING

Postoperative patient teaching is as necessary as teaching that helped prepare the patient. Some explanations and instructions given earlier may need to be repeated during postoperative care because the patient's earlier anxiety prevented thorough understanding. Now that tubes, restraints, and dressings are part of the child's reality, they need to be discussed again: why they are important and how they affect the child's activities.

Parents want to know how they can help care for the child and what limitations are placed on the child's activity. If parents know what to expect, and how to aid in their child's recovery, their cooperation can make life much more pleasant for patient and nurse.

As the child recuperates, he and his parents should be

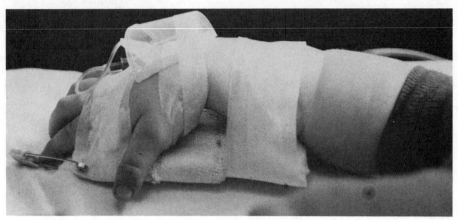

FIG. 18–2. Child's hand with IV infusion apparatus taped in place. (Howry L, Bindler R, Tso Y: Pediatric Medications. Philadelphia, JB Lippincott, 1981)

PEDIATRIC IV FLOW SHEET

Date and Time	Type and Amount of IV Fluid	Additives	Amount absorbed in ml (cumulative for each 8 hr shift)	Amount in volume control set in ml	Microdrops/ min	Remarks	Initials
2/4/80 0700	#1 IV: 250 ml D5⅓NS @ 25ml/hr	2.5 mEq KCl/250 ml	—	50	25	IV started in Ⓡ dorsal wrist	LH
" 0800			25	50	25		LH
" 0900			50	50	25		LH
" 1000			85	50	Rate ↓ to 15	IV has speeded up owing to arm position Rate ↓ to compensate	LH
" 1100			100	50	Rate ↑ to 25		LH
" 1200			125	50	25		LH
" 1300			150	50	25		LH
" 1400			175	50	25		LH
" 1500			(200)	50	25	8-hr cumulative total absorbed = 200 ml	LH
" 1600			25	50	25		RB
" 1700	#2 IV: 250 ml D5⅓NS @ 25ml/hr	2.5 mEq KCl/2½ ml	50	50	25		RB
" 1800			75	50	25		RB

Name: JOSEPHSON, CLARA
ID Number: 347291

FIG. 18–3. Sample of pediatric IV flowsheet recorded from 0700 to 1800 hours. The type and amount of IV fluid is recorded when it is hung. The amount absorbed is recorded every hour. The volume-control set (Volutrol) is filled from the IV bottle as needed and the amount in the Volutrol is recorded each hour. The rate of infusion in microdrops per minute is adjusted as necessary to meet ordered infusion rate and is recorded. The nurse also records any special remarks about the IV and signs her name or initials. (Howry L, Bindler R, Tso Y: Pediatric Medications. Philadelphia, JB Lippincott, 1981)

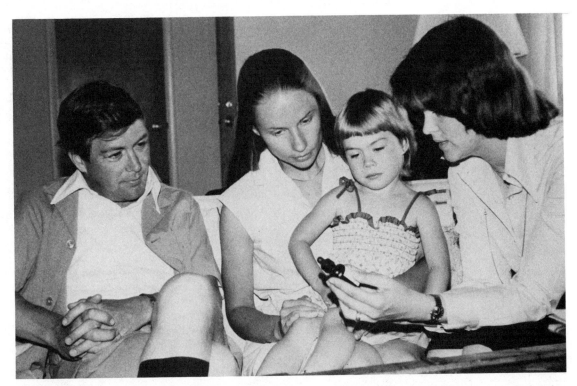

FIG. 18–4. Incorporating the entire family into the teaching process increases learning effectiveness. The family is being instructed about nasal medication administration. (Howry L, Bindler R, Tso Y: Pediatric Medications. Philadelphia, JB Lippincott, 1981)

encouraged to share their feelings about the surgery, any changes in body image, and their expectations for recovery and rehabilitation.

When it is time for the child's sutures to be removed, the nurse should reassure him that the opening has healed and his insides will not fall out when the sutures are removed. This is a common fear of children.

Before the child is discharged from the hospital, teaching focuses on home care, use of any special equipment or appliances, medications, diet, restrictions on activities, and therapeutic exercise (Fig. 18–4).

CHANGING SURGICAL DRESSINGS

Postoperative care includes close observation of any dressings for signs of drainage or hemorrhage, and reinforcement or changing dressings as ordered by the physician. Wet dressings can increase the possibility of contamination; clean, dry dressings increase the patient's comfort. If there is no doctor's order to change the dressing, the nurse is expected to reinforce the moist original dressing by covering it with a dry dressing and taping the second dressing in place.

Supplies needed for changing dressings vary according to the wound site and the physician's orders, which will specify sterile or antiseptic technique to be used. Detailed procedures for these techniques and the supplies to be used can be found in procedure manuals of individual hospitals.

As with all procedures, it is important to explain to the child what you are going to do and why, before beginning the dressing change. Some dressing changes may be painful; if so, the child should be told that it will hurt, and should be praised if his behavior shows courage and cooperation.

GAVAGE FEEDING

Sometimes children who have had surgery are too weak to tolerate adequate food and fluid by mouth and must receive nourishment by means of gavage feedings. This is particularly true of infants. If gavage feedings are not well tolerated, the nurse should report it and await alternate orders from the physician.

Whether the tube is inserted nasally or orally, the measurement is the same: from the tip of the child's nose to the earlobe and down to the tip of the sternum (Fig. 18–5). This length can be marked on the tube with tape or marking pen. The end of the tube to be inserted should be lubricated with sterile water or water soluble lubricating jelly, *never* an oily substance because of the danger of oil aspiration into the lungs.

To prepare the child for gavage feeding, elevate the head and place a rolled-up diaper behind the neck. Turn the head and align the body to the right.

After the tube is inserted, its position can be verified by aspiration of stomach contents or by inserting 1–2 cc of air (using a syringe with an adaptor) and listening with a stethoscope. If the tube is properly placed, gurgling or growling sounds can be heard as air enters the stomach. If

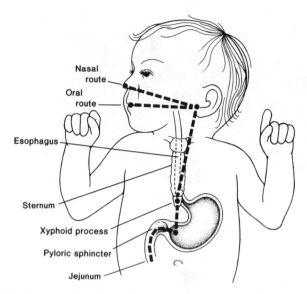

Nasal
route

Oral
route

Esophagus

Sternum

Xyphoid process

Pyloric sphincter

Jejunum

FIG. 18–5.   Dotted line indicates area to be measured for gastric intubation. (King EM, Wieck L, Dyer M: Illustrated Manual of Nursing Techniques, 2nd ed. Philadelphia, JB Lippincott, 1981)

stomach contents are aspirated, these should be measured and replaced, and, in very small infants, subtracted from the amount ordered for this feeding.

The nurse can hold the tube in place if it is going to be removed immediately after the feeding. If the tube will be left in position for further use, it should be secured with tape (Fig. 18–6). Correct position should be verified before each feeding.

The feeding syringe is inserted into the tube, and its plunger pushed gently to start the flow of formula, which has been warmed to room temperature. The plunger is

then removed and the feeding allowed to flow by gravity only. The entire feeding should take 15 to 20 minutes, after which the child will need to be burped, and positioned on the right side or abdomen for at least 1 hour to prevent regurgitation and aspiration.

The type and amount of contents aspirated by the nurse, the amount of formula fed, the infant's tolerance for the procedure, and the positioning of the infant after completion should be recorded on the chart. The feeding tube and any leftover formula should be discarded at the completion of the procedure.

GASTROSTOMY FEEDING

Children who must receive tube feedings over a long period of time may have a gastrostomy tube surgically inserted through the abdominal wall into the stomach. This procedure is performed under general anesthesia and is also used in children who have obstructions or surgical repairs in the mouth, pharynx, esophagus, or cardiac spincter of the stomach.

The surgeon inserts either a plain, a Foley, or a mushroom (Pezzer) catheter with the tip removed, and the catheter is left unclamped and connected to gravity drainage for 24 hours. Meticulous care of the wound site is necessary to prevent infection and irritation. Until the area has healed, it must be covered with a sterile dressing. Ointment, Stomadhesive, or other skin preparations may be ordered for application to the site. The child may need to be restrained to prevent pulling on the catheter that could cause leakage of caustic gastric juices.

Procedures for positioning and feeding the child with a gastrostomy tube are similar to gavage feedings. After each feeding, the child is placed on the right side or in Fowler's position. Depending on the child's condition, the tube may be left unclamped or clamped between feedings.

When regular oral feedings can be resumed, the tube is

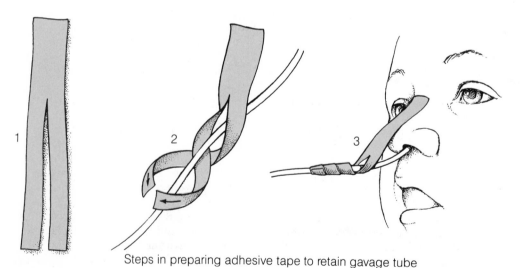

Steps in preparing adhesive tape to retain gavage tube

FIG. 18–6.   If the tube is left in place between feedings, it must be secured in place with adhesive tape. (King EM, Wieck L, Dyer M: Illustrated Manual of Nursing Techniques, 2nd ed. Philadelphia, JB Lippincott, 1981)

surgically removed, and the opening usually closes spontaneously.

IRRIGATION OF A NASOGASTRIC TUBE

In cases of abdominal surgery, nasogastric tubes are often inserted prior to the operative procedure in order to prevent vomiting (due to intestinal peristalsis caused by manipulation of the intestine during surgery) and decompress the intestine for easier handling during surgery. Decompression during the postoperative period helps relieve abdominal distention and the accompanying discomfort and tension on abdominal and intestinal wounds. If the tube becomes obstructed, the child can vomit and aspirate stomach contents into the lungs; thus nursing care is directed toward keeping the tube clear by irrigating every 2 hours with saline solution as ordered. If sterile technique has been ordered, the solution and other supplies must be sterile; otherwise clean technique is sufficient. Position of tube, flow, and contents returned must be documented in the patient's record, and any unusual fluctuations in the amounts for each period of time must be noted.

The indwelling tube is connected to the type of drainage ordered by the physician: intermittent machine suction, gravity drainage, or in-the-bed level drainage. Drainage or suction is discontinued for irrigation and the tubing disconnected. The end of the tube leading to the drainage or suction device is covered with a cap or hung from a support on the machine. The irrigating fluid is gently instilled into the tube inserted into the patient, and the tube reconnected to the drainage or suction apparatus; or the irrigating fluid may be withdrawn from the patient with a syringe.

The amount of fluid instilled is recorded, and any unsual circumstances noted and reported immediately (resistance to instillation or failure to drain normally). When the nurse is charting, the irrigating fluid is always subtracted from the gastric output at the end of each shift.

IRRIGATION OF AN URETHRAL CATHETER

Immobility or seriously restricted activity that follows surgery slows metabolism, resulting in nitrogen and calcium imbalance. This imbalance increases the potential for calcium deposits and other sediment in the urine that can clog catheter tubing. Irrigation of urethral catheters must be performed as ordered; this procedure requires sterile technique and supplies. The container of irrigating fluid should be at room temperature. The drainage tube is disconnected from the catheter, and the catheter allowed to drain into a drainage basin. The sterile end of the tube is covered with a sterile cap or placed in a sterile gauze square. The prescribed amount of irrigating solution is drawn into a sterile syringe and slowly injected into the catheter. The catheter is then pinched off, the syringe disconnected, and the solution allowed to drain into the basin by gravity. Catheter and drainage tubing are reconnected, and the procedure documented, including amount and characteristics of instilled solution, returned solution, the patient's reaction, and any difficulties encountered.

summary

Superb skills and technologic advances help today's surgeons achieve almost miraculous results in treating children's health problems. To the child facing surgery, however, and often to parents, the operating room is a never-never land filled with masked faces, sharp instruments, and countless nameless terrors. Teaching patients and parents what to expect, explaining what is going to happen before, during, and after procedures, helps reduce the fears and anxieties, and makes the patient part of the team working toward restoration of optimum health. Teaching is part of all nursing care and nowhere is it more important than for the child who must have surgery. Even the most remarkable surgical treatment is incomplete without nurses who offer skilled physical care and sensitive attention to the emotional needs of child and parents.

review questions

1. What is the role of the nurse concerning preoperative and postoperative patient and parent teaching?
2. What are the side effects of atropine?
3. Prior to gavage feeding how can the nurse be sure that the tube is in its proper position?

references

1. Petrillo M, Sanger S: Emotional Care of Hospitalized Children: An Environmental Approach, 2nd ed. Philadelphia, JB Lippincott, 1980
2. Evans M, Hansen B: Guide to Pediatric Nursing: A Clinical Reference. New York, Appleton-Century-Crofts, 1980

bibliography

Blos P Jr: Children think about illness: Their concepts and beliefs. In Gellert E (ed): Psychological Aspects of Pediatric Care. New York, Grune & Stratton, 1978

Brunner LS, Suddarth DS: The Lippincott Manual of Nursing Practice. Philadelphia, JB Lippincott, 1978

Brunner LS, Suddarth DS: Textbook of Medical-Surgical Nursing, 4th ed. Philadelphia, JB Lippincott, 1980

Hart LK, Reese JL, Fearing MO: Concepts Common to Acute Illness: Identification and Management. St Louis, CV Mosby, 1981

Hood GH, Dincher JR: Total Patient Care: Foundations and Practice, 5th ed. St Louis, CV Mosby, 1980

Hughes JG: Synopsis of Pediatrics, 5th ed. St Louis, CV Mosby, 1980

King EM, Wieck L, Dyer M: Illustrated Manual of Nursing Techniques. Philadelphia, JB Lippincott, 1981

Luciano K, Syumsky CJ: Pediatric procedures. Nurs 75, 5:49–52, Jan 1975

Marcinek MB: Stress in the surgical patient. Am J Nurs 77:1809–1911, 1977

McCormick R, Parkevich T: Patient and Family Education: Tools, Technique, Theory. New York, John Wiley & Sons, 1979

McEntyre RL: Practical Guide to the Care of the Surgical Patient. St Louis, CV Mosby, 1980

Scipien GM, et al: Comprehensive Pediatric Nursing, 2nd ed. New York, McGraw-Hill, 1979

Shirkey HC, et al (eds): Pediatric Therapy, 6th ed. St Louis, CV Mosby, 1980

Stephenson CA: Stress in critically ill patients. Am J Nurs 77:1806–1809, 1977

Treloar DM: Ready set—No! Something is missing from pediatric preoperative preparation. Am J Mat Child Nurs 3:50–51, 1978

Vaughan VC, III, McKay RJ, Behrman RE: Nelson's Textbook of Pediatrics, 11th ed. Philadelphia, WB Saunders, 1979

Whaley L, Wong D: Nursing Care of Infants and Children. St Louis, CV Mosby, 1979

Whitson J, McFarlane J: The Pediatric Nursing Skills Manual. New York, John Wiley & Sons, 1980

Wieczorek RR, Natapoff JN: A Conceptual Approach to the Nursing of Children: Health Care From Birth Through Adolescence. Philadelphia, JB Lippincott, 1981

Ziemer M, Carroll JS: Infant gavage feeding. Am J Nurs 78:1543–1544, 1978

the child with mobility problems 19

student objectives

The student successfully attaining the goals of this chapter will be able to

1 Define the following vocabulary terms:

Bryant's traction   compound fracture   decubitus ulcers   external fixation
halo traction   hypercalcemia   Milwaukee brace   paraplegia   quadriplegia
renal calculi   Russell's traction

2 List ten physical problems that can result from the prolonged restriction of mobility.

3 List six nursing measures that can help prevent physical problems in the child with a mobility problem.

4 Explain the differences between complete and incomplete, and simple and compound fractures.

5 List and describe the 5 Ps to be watched for after the application of a cast.

6 Describe three methods of treatment that may be used to correct scoliosis.

The human body is designed to move. When mobility is restricted because of illness or injury, the individual is affected physically and psychologically. Mobility is essential to a child's normal growth and development, and any limitations on that mobility make nursing care of that child more difficult.

Fractures, musculoskeletal disorders, and spinal cord injuries limit mobility of the young patient and require temporary or permanent use of special, often cumbersome equipment such as crutches, casts, braces, special beds, and wheelchairs. Care of these children includes teaching about the care and use of equipment and attention to the special physical and psychological needs created by limited mobility.

physical effects of limited mobility

The possibility of physical complications increases in direct proportion to the seriousness of the injury, the degree of immobilization necessary, and the length of time during which mobility will be restricted. Most children adapt quickly to the limitations imposed by a cast and crutches. Those who must undergo traction or other long-term treatment, however, require greater physical and emotional support to prevent complications.

Physical problems caused by prolonged restriction of mobility are primarily related to decreased muscle strength and mass, decreased metabolism, and bone demineralization.[1] These factors create the potential for loss of joint mobility, contractures, tissue breakdown and decubitus formation (pressure sores, pressure ulcers), orthostatic hypotension (lowered blood pressure when arising from a horizontal position, causing fainting), thrombus formation, pneumonia, constipation and fecal impaction, urinary infection and/or incontinence, formation of renal calculi, and neurosensory damage. Loss of appetite, feelings of fatigue and inertia can occur, further hindering healing and recovery.

psychological effects of limited mobility

Social, emotional, and developmental problems must be considered for the child immobilized by a cast or by traction. These devices interfere with normal developmental activities, and can permanently impair normal growth and development. The child of 2 or 3 who must use his large muscles is definitely frustrated. Early childhood is a time for learning balance, motor coordination, and similar physical developmental skills. Socially, a deformity or a defect may bring ridicule or teasing from other children, causing a loss of self-esteem.

The infant or toddler has not developed a body image and, uninhibited by emotional barriers, adapts more readily and makes maximum use of any opportunities for development. An older child is more likely to suffer emotionally from the inability to move freely and to control his own activities.

Children's normal response to stress is increased activity. Limited mobility hampers that reaction, intensifying the stress and anxiety. It also reduces the environmental stimulation available to the child, and can lead to feelings of isolation. Casts, traction, numbness or loss of feeling deprive the child of the psychological comfort of being touched.

Restricted mobility makes the child less independent, often resulting in regressive behavior. A toddler is likely to return to using diapers, especially if toilet training has just been completed. The child may have great difficulty using a bedpan after having just learned to sit on a potty chair, so diapers are likely to be indicated. Regression to a nursing bottle is also common, particularly when small children are hospitalized. For safety's sake, plastic bottles should be used for 2- and 3-year-olds who need the security of a nursing bottle.

Children sometimes feel that immobilization is a punishment and need to be repeatedly assured that it is not, but is necessary to help them get well. They may react to their condition and the limitations it imposes with anger and aggression or with submission and withdrawal. Often children who are immobilized become irritable and need a chance to act out their feelings.

nursing care

The goals of nursing care for the child with mobility problems are to prevent or minimize complications and help restore maximum function to the injured area.

Proper positioning including frequent changes of position whenever possible, range of motion exercises in unaffected extremities, care to keep sheets and clothing dry and free from wrinkles, monitoring bowel movements to prevent constipation and fecal impaction, and encouraging consumption of a protein-rich diet are important measures in preventing physical problems. Forcing fluids helps reduce the possibility of renal calculi and urinary tract infection, and aids bowel function. Meticulous skin care is essential, particularly over bony prominences (Fig. 19–1). When children are permitted to increase their mobility, activities must be increased gradually and carefully supervised because the child will be weakened, and may faint easily.

As often as possible, the child should be given a change of scene, using a wheelchair, stretcher, or stroller to move to the playroom or other new surroundings. Play activities, especially those with dolls, puppets, or art materials, offer the child an opportunity to act out anxieties, fears, and frustrations, and increase environmental stimulation.

Nurses and parents should encourage children to participate as fully as possible in their own care. Overprotection and oversolicitousness by the nurse can be a problem for the child, and may reinforce the child's tendency to regress to earlier developmental stages. Given the opportunity, children manage to feed and to help themselves in many difficult situations. They may need greater attention, understanding, and approval for a time to sustain their ego, but this should not be considered "spoiling." Careful observation will detect indications that a child is ready for greater independence.

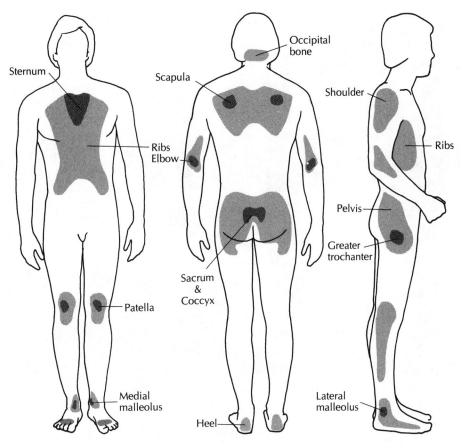

FIG. 19–1.   Skin care is particularly important over bony prominences. (King EM, Wieck L, Dyer M: Illustrated Manual of Nursing Techniques, 2nd ed. Philadelphia, JB Lippincott, 1981)

Nursing care also includes teaching patient and family to cope with the limited mobility. If the child is severely disabled, many health professionals may assist in care and teaching: social worker, orthotist, physical therapist, occupational therapist, and psychologist or psychiatrist. Severe disability affects every member of the child's family, and may require intensive, continuing support from several members of the health team in order to help the family cope.

fractures

A *fracture* is a break in a bone, usually accompanied by vascular and soft tissue damage, and characterized by pain, swelling, and tenderness. Children's fractures differ from those of adults in that they are generally less complicated, heal more quickly, and usually occur from different causes. The child has an urge to explore his environment, but lacks the experience and judgment to recognize possible hazards. In some instances, parents may be negligent in their supervision, but frequently the young explorer is simply too fast for them.

The bones most frequently fractured in childhood are the clavicle, femur, tibia, humerus, and wrist. Classification of fractures reflects the kind of bone injury sustained. If the fragments of fractured bone are separated, the frac-

ture is said to be *complete*. If fragments remain partially joined, the fracture is termed *incomplete*. *Greenstick* fractures are one kind of incomplete fracture common in children due to incomplete ossification. When a broken bone penetrates the skin, the fracture is called *compound*, or *open*. A *simple*, or *closed*, fracture is a single break in the bone without penetration of the skin. The types of fractures are shown in Figure 19–2. Fractures in the area of the growth plate (epiphyseal plate) can cause permanent damage and severely impair growth (Fig. 19–3).

Most childhood fractures are treated by realignment and immobilization, using either traction or closed manipulation and casting. A few patients with severe fractures or other injuries such as burns or other soft tissue damage may require surgical reduction and/or internal or external fixation. Internal fixation devices include rods, pins, screws, and plates made of insert materials that will not trigger an immune reaction. They make possible early mobilization of the child to wheelchair and crutches or a walker.

External fixation devices are used primarily in four conditions: massive open fractures with extensive soft tissue and/or neurovascular damage; infected fractures that fail to heal properly; acutely infected fractures; multiple trauma with a number of fractures, often accompanied by injuries to the head, chest, or abdomen, or burns.[2] These

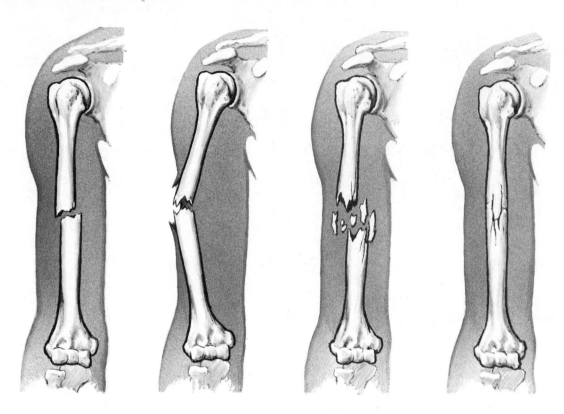

FIG. 19–2. Types of fractures.

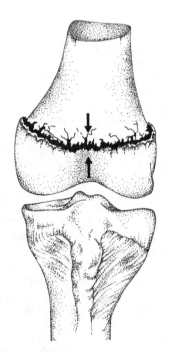

FIG. 19–3. One form of epiphyseal injury; a crushing injury (as might occur in a fall from a height) can destroy the layer of germinal cells of the epiphysis, resulting in disturbance of growth. (Redrawn from Specht E: Epiphyseal injuries in childhood. American Family Physician 10:102, 1974)

devices are applied under sterile conditions in the operating room and are augmented by soft dressings and elevation by means of an overhead traction rope (Fig. 19–4).

CASTS

The kind of cast used is determined by the age of the child, the severity of the fracture, the type of bone involved, and the amount of weight bearing. Common types of casts are shown in Figure 19–5. Most casts are formed from gauze strips impregnated with plaster of Paris or other material that is pliable when wet, but hardens with drying. Casts made of fiberglass, plastic, and other synthetic materials are being used with greater frequency for certain kinds of fractures, and offer the advantages of being lighter in weight and presenting a cleaner appearance because they can be sponged with water when soiled.

Child and parents should be taught what to expect after the cast is applied, and how to care for the casted area. Although the wet plaster of Paris feels cool on the skin when it is applied, evaporation soon causes a temporary sensation of warmth. The cast will feel heavy and cumbersome.

While the cast is wet, it should be handled only with open palms because fingertips can cause indentations and result in pressure points. If the cast has no protective edge, it should be petaled (see Fig. 4–20) with adhesive tape strips. If the cast is close to the genital area, plastic should be taped around the edge to prevent wetting and soiling the cast.

After the fracture has been immobilized, any complaints of pain signal complications and should be recorded and reported immediately. Webb recommends observation, documentation, and reporting the five Ps:[3]

> *pain*—Any sign of pain should be noted and the exact area determined.
> *pulse*—If an upper extremity is involved, brachial, radial, ulnar, and digital pulses should be checked; if a lower extremity, femoral, popliteal, posterior tibial, and dorsalis pedis pulses.
> *paresthesia*—Check for any diminished or absent sensation, or for numbness.
> *paralysis*—Check hand function by having the child try to hyperextend the thumb or wrist, oppose thumb and little finger, and adduct all fingers. Check function of the foot by having the child try to dorsiflex and plantarflex the ankles, and flex and extend the toes.
> *pallor*—Check the color of the extremity and the nail beds distal to the site of the fracture; pallor, discoloration, or coldness indicates circulatory impairment.

In addition to the five Ps, any foul odor or drainage, "hot spots" on cast (warm to touch), looseness or tightness, or any elevation of temperature should be noted, documented, and reported. Parents should be instructed to watch carefully for these same danger signals.

Children and parents should be cautioned *not* to put anything down inside the cast, no matter how much the casted area itches. Small toys should be kept out of reach until the cast has been removed.

When the fracture has healed, the cast is removed with a cast cutter. This can be a frightening experience for the child unless the person using the cast cutter explains and demonstrates that the device will not cut flesh but only the hard surface of the cast. The child should be told that there will be vibration from the cast cutter, but it will not burn.

After cast removal, the area that was casted should be soaked in warm water to help remove the crusty layer of skin that has accumulated. Application of oil or lotion may prove comforting. Parents and child must be cautioned against scrubbing or scraping this area as the tender layer of new skin underneath the crust may bleed.

TRACTION

Traction is a pulling force applied to an extremity or other part of the body. A system of weights, ropes, and pulleys is used to realign and immobilize fractures, reduce or eliminate muscle spasm, and prevent fracture deformity and joint contractures.

There are two basic types of traction: skin traction and skeletal traction. *Skin traction* pulls on tape, rubber, or plastic materials attached to the skin and indirectly exerts pull on the musculoskeletal system. *Skeletal traction* exerts pull directly on skeletal structures by means of a

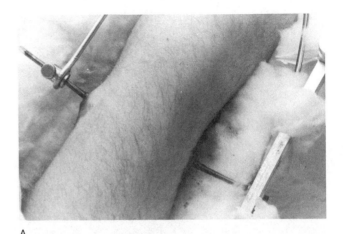

A

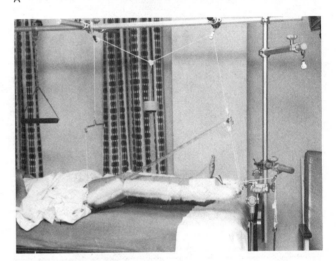

B

FIG. 19–4. (*A*) External fixation devices are applied surgically under sterile conditions. (*B*) The injured limb is supported with soft dressings and is elevated by means of overhead traction. (Farrell J: Illustrated Guide to Orthopedic Nursing. Philadelphia, JB Lippincott, 1977)

pin, wire, tongs, or other device surgically inserted through a bone.

Bryant's traction (Fig. 19–6) is often used for the treatment of a fractured femur in children under the age of 3. These fractures are frequently transverse or spiral fractures. The use of Bryant's traction entails some risk of compromised circulation and may result in contracture of the foot and lower leg, particularly in an older child.

To apply Bryant's traction, two overhead bars are passed horizontally over the crib, pulleys are attached to each bar, and the child's legs are suspended from the bar at right angles to the body. Weights are applied in sufficient amounts to keep the buttocks just clear of the bed. A solid Bradford frame aids in achieving additional countertraction and immobilization. The child's legs are wrapped with elastic bandages that should be removed at least daily for skin assessment and then rewrapped. Skin temperature and color of legs and feet must be checked frequently to

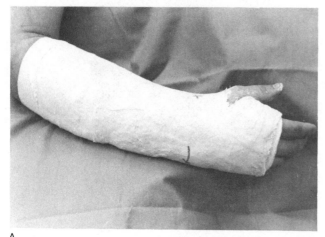

A

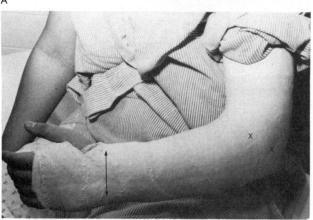

B

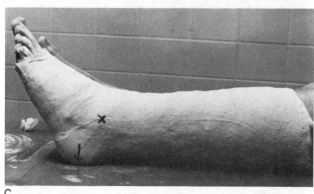

C

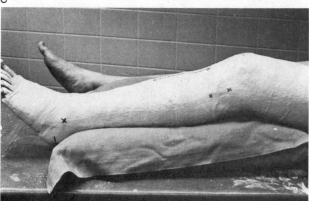

D

detect any circulatory impairment. Severe pain should be reported because it may indicate circulatory difficulty. When a child is in Bryant's traction, the nurse should be able to pass her hand between the child's buttocks and the sheet.

Russell's traction (Fig. 19–7) seems to be more effective for older children. A child in either type of traction, however, tends to slide down until the weights rest on the bed or the floor. He should be pulled up to keep the weights free, the ropes must be in alignment with the pulleys, and the alignment should be checked frequently. An older child may coax his roommate to remove the weights or the sandbags used as weights.

Side-arm traction (Fig. 19–8) is sometimes used for fractures of the humerus or the elbow.

Children in any kind of traction must be carefully monitored to detect any signs of neurovascular complications. Skin temperature and color, presence or absence of edema, sensation and motion should be assessed every hour for the first 24 hours after traction has been applied, and every 4 hours unless ordered otherwise.[4] Skin care must be meticulous. Alcohol should be used to toughen the skin rather than lotions or oils that soften the skin and contribute to tissue breakdown.

Patients in skeletal traction require special attention to pin tracts (Fig. 19–9). Any sign of infection (odor or local inflammation) should be recorded and reported at once.

EXTERNAL FIXATION DEVICES

Patients whose fractures are severe enough to require the use of external fixation also need special skin care at pin sites. The sites are left open to the air and should be inspected and cleansed regularly, at least twice a day in the immediate postoperative period and daily after that. Cleansing is done with a sterile cotton applicator dipped in hydrogen peroxide, and each pin site is rinsed separately with normal saline via syringe or applicator.[5] A nonocclusive antibacterial agent is applied with a sterile applicator and allowed to dry.

As early as possible, the patient (if old enough) or the parents should be taught to care for the pin sites. External fixation devices are sometimes left in place for as long as 1 year; therefore, it is important that the patient can accept this temporary change in body image and learn to care for the affected site. Patients with these devices will probably work with a physical therapist during the rehabilitation period and will have specific exercises to perform. Before discharge from the hospital, the patient should feel comfortable in moving about and should be able to recognize the signs of pin infection.

CRUTCHES

Children with fractures of the lower extremities and other lower leg injuries often must learn to use crutches to

---

FIG. 19–5. Types of casts. (*A*) Short arm cast. (*B*) Long arm cast. (*C*) Short leg cast. (*D*) Long leg cast. (Farrell J: Illustrated Guide to Orthopedic Nursing. Philadelphia, JB Lippincott, 1977)

avoid weight bearing on the injured area. Several types of crutches are available, the most common being *axillary* crutches, principally used for temporary situations. *Forearm*, or Canadian, crutches are usually recommended for children who will need crutches permanently, such as paraplegic children with braces. *Trough*, or platform, crutches are more suitable for children with limited strength or function in the arms and hands (Fig. 19–10).

Use of crutches is generally taught by a physical therapist, but it can be the responsibility of nurses. The type of crutch gait to be taught is determined by the amount of weight bearing permitted, the child's degree of stability, whether or not the knees can be flexed, and the specific goal of treatment for the individual child. The various gaits are shown in Figure 19–11, *A–D*.

scoliosis

Structural (idiopathic) scoliosis and nonstructural (functional) scoliosis are discussed in Chapter 13. The treatment for structural scoliosis includes correction of the curvature with braces or casts, followed, in severe curvatures, by internal fixation with rods, or spinal fusion to maintain the correction.

BRACES

The Milwaukee brace (Fig. 19–12) is considered the most effective spinal brace for treatment of scoliosis. It exerts lateral pressure and longitudinal traction, thus achieving vertical alignment.

The brace should be worn constantly except when bathing or swimming. It should be worn over a T-shirt or undershirt to protect the child's skin and the leather of the brace. The throat mold of the brace can be covered with soft cloth if sweating or irritation occurs.[6] Alcohol applied to pressure points will help toughen the skin.

Wearing the Milwaukee brace creates a distinct change in body image, usually in adolescence, a time when body consciousness is at an all-time high. Acceptance of the brace and its limitations may cause anger; the change in body image can cause a grief reaction. Working through these feelings successfully requires understanding support from nurse, family, and peers. Sometimes it is helpful for the patient in a Milwaukee brace to talk with other scoliosis patients and learn how they have coped. Understanding the disorder itself and the important benefits of treatment also can ease the adjustment.

CASTS

Curvatures that are too severe to respond to conservative treatment with the Milwaukee brace are treated by application of various kinds of casts. The most popular of these are the Risser localizer, or jacket cast (Fig. 19–13), the Risser turnbuckle cast, the Cotrel's E-D-F cast, and the surcingle cast. The localizer cast extends from the cervical area to the pelvis and allows the child to carry on with all normal activities except violent sports.

Before the cast is applied, the child should be given an explanation of the procedure and what the treatment is intended to accomplish. The adolescent female needs

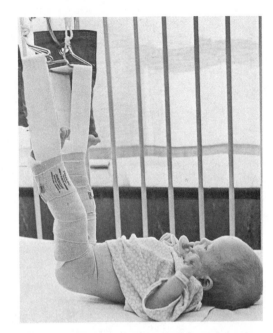

FIG. 19–6.   The small child who sustains a transverse or spiral fracture of the long bone may be placed in Bryant's traction.

reassurance that the cast will not interfere with breast development.

Care of the child in a localizer cast is similar to caring for a child in any kind of cast: regular observation and recording of color, temperature, presence or absence of edema, sensation and motion; proper positioning; meticulous skin care; and patient teaching. When the child goes home, he or she will need an understanding of cast care, a firm mattress (and probably a bed board), and family support. If return to school is not possible, ar-

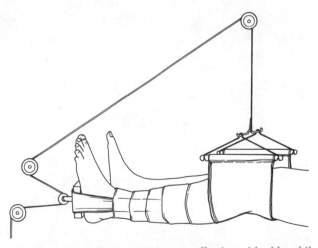

FIG. 19–7.   Russell's traction is more effective with older children who have femoral fractures. (King EM, Wieck L, Dyer M: Illustrated Manual of Nursing Techniques, Philadelphia, JB Lippincott, 1981)

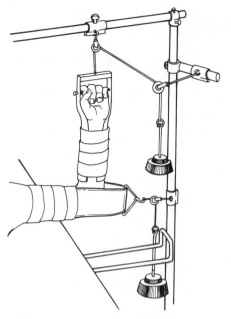

FIG. 19–8. Side-arm traction. (King EM, Wieck L, Dyer M: Illustrated Manual of Nursing Techniques, Philadelphia, JB Lippincott, 1981)

rangements need to be made for a tutor at home or a communication hook-up with the school. Casts need to be changed periodically to continue the correction as the child grows.

TRACTION

In some cases of severe scoliosis, halo traction is added to the body cast (Fig. 19–14). This form of skeletal traction uses stainless steel pins inserted into the skull and into the femurs. Weights are increased gradually to promote correction. When the curvature has been corrected, spinal fusion is performed.

The strange appearance of the halo traction apparatus magnifies the problems of body image, in addition to which, the head may need to be shaved. The child needs a thorough explanation of what will occur during the procedure, and if possible, should have the opportunity to talk with a child who has had this kind of traction.

Frequent shampooing, cleansing of the pin sites, and observation for signs of complications are critical in the care of children in halo traction. Any sign of infection, cyanosis, respiratory distress, diplopia, pupil irregularity, numbness, paralysis, or inability to void should be documented and reported at once. Particular care should

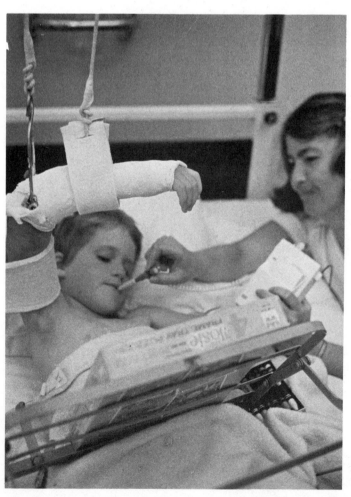

FIG. 19–9. Skeletal traction with olecranon pin and overhead suspension. (Photo by Marcia Lieberman)

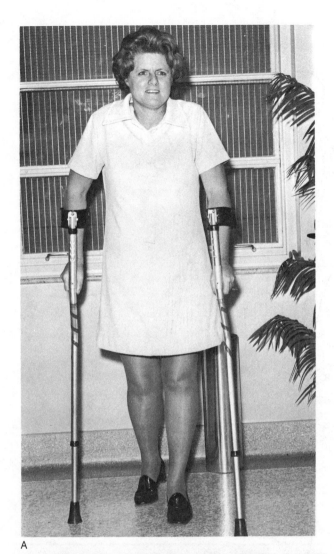

A

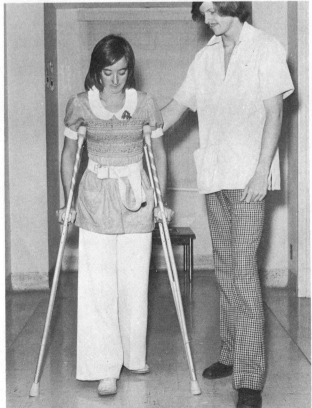

C

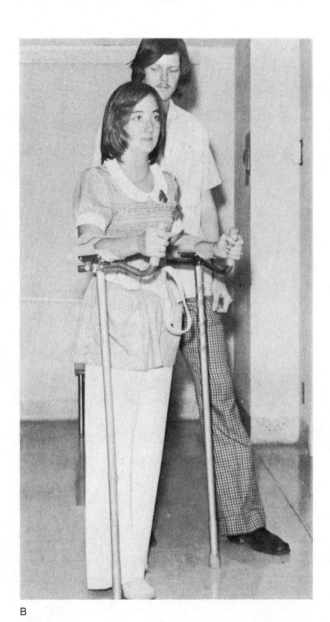

B

FIG. 19–10. Types of crutches. (*A*) Forearm or Canadian crutches. (*B*) Trough or platform crutches. (*C*) Axillary crutches. (Lewis LW: Fundamental Skills in Patient Care, 2nd ed. Philadelphia, JB Lippincott, 1980)

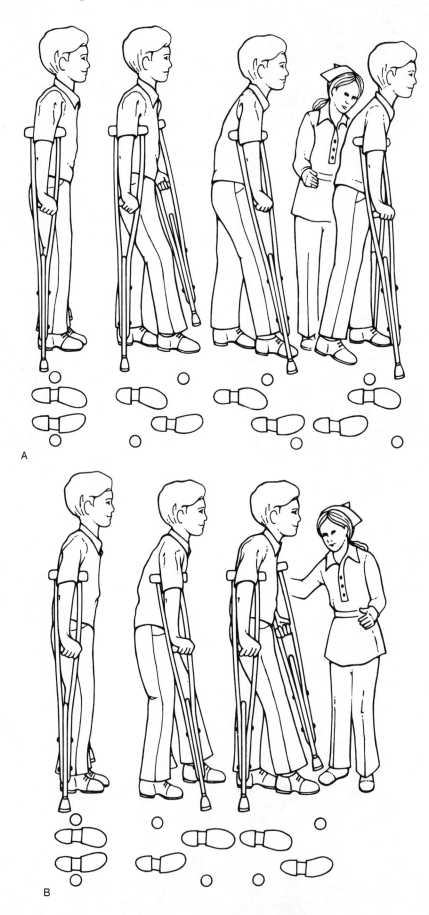

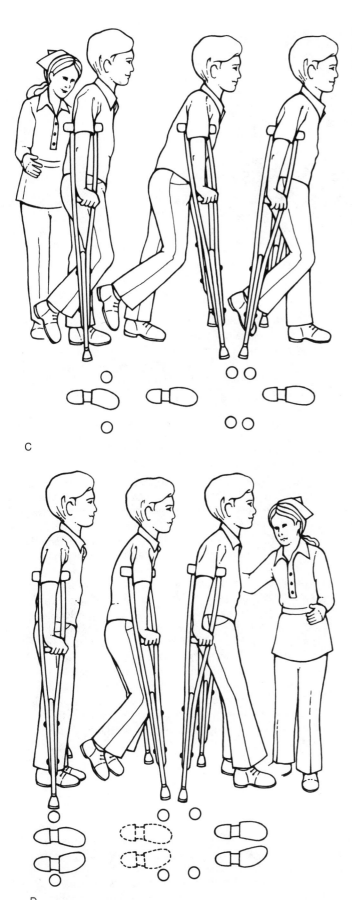

C

D

be taken to prevent bumping the halo since it magnifies sounds. Turning the child at least every 2 hours and skin care using alcohol every 4 hours help prevent tissue breakdown. Breathing exercises and range-of-motion activities reduce the possibility of complications.

juvenile rheumatoid arthritis

Each year about 5000 children in the United States develop juvenile rheumatoid arthritis (JRA), a crippling disorder of unknown causes.[8] Joint inflammation occurs first, and, if untreated, leads to irreversible changes in joint cartilage, ligaments, and menisci, and eventually to complete immobility.

The goal of treatment for JRA is to maintain mobility and preserve joint function. Treatment can include drugs, physical therapy, and surgery. Early diagnosis and drug therapy to control inflammation and the other systemic changes that occur in JRA can reduce the need for other types of treatment.

Enteric-coated aspirin is the drug of choice for JRA; an effective anti-inflammatory drug, it is inexpensive, easily administered, and has few side-effects when carefully regulated. When aspirin is no longer effective, nonsteroidal anti-inflammatory drugs (NSAID), indomethacin, gold preparations, antimalarials, steroids, penicillamine, and immunosuppressives may be used. All of these are toxic and must be closely monitored.

Physical therapy for JRA comprises exercise, application of splints, and heat. Implementing this program at home calls for the cooperation of nurse, physical therapist, and physician. Joints must be immobilized during active disease (accomplished by splinting), but gentle daily exercise is necessary to prevent alkalosis.[9]

Range-of-motion exercises, isometric exercises, swimming, and riding a tricycle or bicycle are an appropriate part of treatment for JRA, depending on the degree of disease activity. If exercise triggers increased pain, the amount of exercise should be decreased.

spinal cord injury

The patient with spinal cord damage is one of the greatest challenges confronting caregivers. In young children, the damage is most often the result of congenital conditions such as myelomeningocele; in adolescents and young adults, spinal cord injury results from automobile and other motor vehicle accidents. The neurologic sequelae of spinal cord injury are catastrophic, and the psychosocial

FIG. 19–11.   Types of crutch walking. (*A*) Four-point gait, taught when weight-bearing is permitted on both legs. (*B*) Two-point gait, taught when weight-bearing is permitted on both legs. (*C*) Three-point gait, taught when weight-bearing is permitted on only one leg and the other leg acts as a balance. (*D*) Swing-through gait, swing-to gait, or tripod gait, taught when weight-bearing is not possible on either leg. (King EM, Wieck L, Dyer M: Illustrated Manual of Nursing Techniques, Philadelphia, JB Lippincott, 1981)

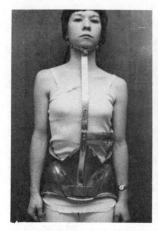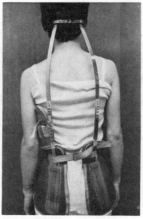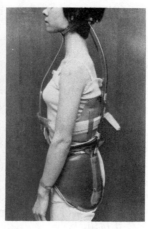

FIG. 19–12. The Milwaukee brace as seen from front, back, and side. (Farrell J: Illustrated Guide to Orthopedic Nursing. Philadelphia, JB Lippincott, 1977)

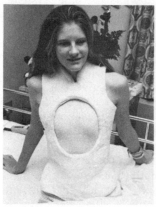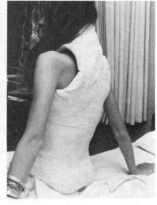

A   B

FIG. 19–13. Casting to correct scoliosis with the Risser localizer cast. (*A*) Front view. (*B*) Back view. (Farrell J: Illustrated Guide to Orthopedic Nursing. Philadelphia, JB Lippincott, 1977)

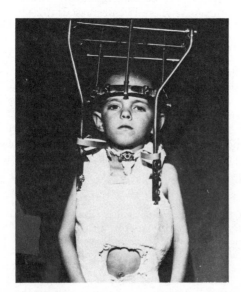

FIG. 19–14. Halo traction. (Perry J: The halo in spinal abnormalities. Orthop Clin North Am 3, No. 1:68, 1972)

adjustments of patient and family are painful and long-lasting.

Complete transection of the spinal cord (severing the cord from side to side) causes total loss of function. *Partial transection* (cross-section) results in severe disability. The ultimate outlook for the patient depends on the extent of the damage, the level of the injury, and the individual's access to and willingness to participate in a long-term rehabilitation program.

Spinal cord damage can cause *paraplegia* (paralysis of two extremities, usually the legs) or *quadriplegia* (absence of function in all four extremities). The higher the level of injury, the more serious the damage. Injuries to the cervical cord at about C4 results in loss of respiratory function and the patient dies unless immediate respiratory assistance is available. Injury to the thoracic area destroys bowel and bladder control.

Early care of the spinal cord injury patient is usually accomplished in an intensive care unit by highly trained staff. Treatment can include immobilization, cervical traction, or surgery. Long-term care is directed toward restoring maximum function, helping the patient and family cope with the profound sense of loss, and the necessary changes in lifestyle, and prevention of decubitus ulcers and other complications (Table 19– 1). Physical therapy, bladder and bowel training, temperature regulation, and skin care are all components of continuing care.

Tremendous advances have been made in the technology related to care of these patients. Special flotation beds, frames, and mobilization devices have dramatically improved the outlook for the severely disabled. Attitudes toward these patients are beginning to change, though slowly, and more of the world is accessible to disabled individuals each year.

summary

Health problems that affect children's mobility range from minor fractures to life-threatening trauma. The potential for physical and psychological complications resulting from long-term immobility is great. Meticulous physical care, including continuous observation for signs of problems,

TABLE 19–1. NURSING CARE FOR THE POSITION AND MOVEMENT OF THE CLIENT WITH SPINAL CORD INJURY

Task	Nursing Measures
Transfer of the child from the stretcher to a hospital bed	Check orders for type of bed needed, position, and movement activities allowed. Prepare the bed for the special needs of the client (*e.g.*, traction, bed board). Move client as a log from stretcher to bed with the assistance of 3 to 5 assistants.
Making occupied bed	Change sheets from head to toe and not from side to side. Avoid unnecessary movement of the client. When removing sheets avoid jerking the client.
Moving the client	Adjust bed foundation in regard to position desired. Place bolsters and pillows in position desired. Use a turning sheet. Support the body in correct alignment. Seek assistance from colleagues in the actual moving process. Check traction weights and pulleys.
Prevention of decubiti	Change position of client every 2 hours. Use air mattress. Use foam rubber under pressure areas (*e.g.*, elbows, head, heels). Use sheepskin when appropriate. Change linen frequently, check for wrinkles or food crumbs. Check for urine or stool incontinence. Skin care every 2 hours

(Wieczorek R, Natapoff J: A Conceptual Approach to the Nursing of Children: Health Care From Birth Through Adolescence. Philadelphia, JB Lippincott, 1981)

and sensitive attention and responses to the patient's emotional needs represent a unique contribution that nurses can make toward preventing complications and restoring optimum function.

review questions

1. What physical problems are created by prolonged restriction of mobility?
2. Why does restricted mobility result in regressive behavior?
3. What are the nursing goals for a child with mobility problems?
4. What nursing measures enable the nurse to fulfill the nurse's goals for mobility problems?
5. What are the different types of fractures?
6. Why is a compound fracture more serious that a simple fracture?
7. What are the five Ps the nurse observes for and documents after a cast application?
8. What are the two types of traction?
9. What is the drug of choice for the treatment of JRA?

references

1. Whaley L, Wong D: Nursing Care of Infants and Children. St Louis, CV Mosby, 1979
2. Kryschyshen P, Fischer D: External fixation for complicated fractures. Am J Nurs 80:256–259, 1980
3. Webb KJ: Early assessment of orthopedic injuries. Am J Nurs 74:1048–1062, 1974
4. Evans M, Hansen B: Guide to Pediatric Nursing: A Clinical Reference. New York, Appleton-Century-Crofts, 1980
5. Kryschyshen P, Fischer D: External fixation for complicated fractures. Am J Nurs 80:256–259, 1980
6. Hilt N, Schmitt W: Pediatric Orthopedic Nursing. St Louis, CV Mosby, 1975
7. Evans M, Hansen B: Guide to Pediatric Nursing: A Clinical Reference. New York, Appleton-Century-Crofts, 1980
8. Petty RE: Epidemiology of JRA. In Miller JJ, III (ed): Juvenile Rheumatoid Arthritis. Littleton, MA, PSG Publications, 1979
9. Wieczorek RR, Natapoff JN: A Conceptual Approach to the Nursing of Infants and Children: Health Care From Birth Through Adolescence. Philadelphia, JB Lippincott, 1981

bibliography

Anderson B: Carole: A girl treated with bracing. Am J Nurs 79:592–597, 1979

Anderson B, D'Ambra P: The adolescent patient with scoliosis. Nurs Clin North Am 11:697–708, 1976

Barrett MJ: Surviving adolescence in a back brace: Laura's experience. Am J Mat Child Nurs 2:160–163, 1977

Brunner N: Orthopedic Nursing: A Programmed Approach, 3rd ed. St Louis, CV Mosby, 1979

Deyerle WM, Crossland SA: Broken legs are to be walked on. Am J Nurs 77:1927–1930, 1977

Edmondson AS, Crenshaw AH (eds): Campbell's Operative Orthopedics, 6th ed. St Louis, CV Mosby, 1980

Farrell J: Illustrated Guide to Orthopedic Nursing, 2nd ed. Philadelphia, JB Lippincott, 1982

Hilt N, Cogburn S: Manual of Orthopedics. St Louis, CV Mosby, 1980

Hirschberg G, Lewis L, Vaughan P: Promoting mobility. Nurs 77 7, No. 5:42–27, 1977

Larrabee J: The person with a spinal cord injury: Physical care during early recovery. Am J Nurs 77:1320–1329, 1977

Larson CB, Gould M: Orthopedic Nursing, 9th ed. St Louis, CV Mosby, 1978

Lindsley CB: The child with arthritis. Issues Comp Pediatr Nurs 2, No. 4:23–32, 1977

Murray R, Kijek J: Current perspectives in rehabilitation. Nursing, Vol I. St Louis, CV Mosby, 1979

Nathan SW: Body image of scoliotic female adolescents before and after surgery. Mat Child Nurs 6:139–149, 1977

Ozonoff MB: Pediatric Orthopedic Radiology. Philadelphia, WB Saunders, 1979

Petrillo M, Sanger S: Emotional Care of Hospitalized Children: An Environmental Approach. Philadelphia, JB Lippincott, 1980

Rantz M, Courtial D: Lifting, Moving and Transferring Patients, 2nd ed. St Louis, CV Mosby, 1981

Sergil C: Current concepts in the management of scoliosis. Nurs Clin North Am 11:611–698, 1976

Wilson R: The MUD bed and its implication for nursing care. Nurs Clin North Am 11:725–730, 1976

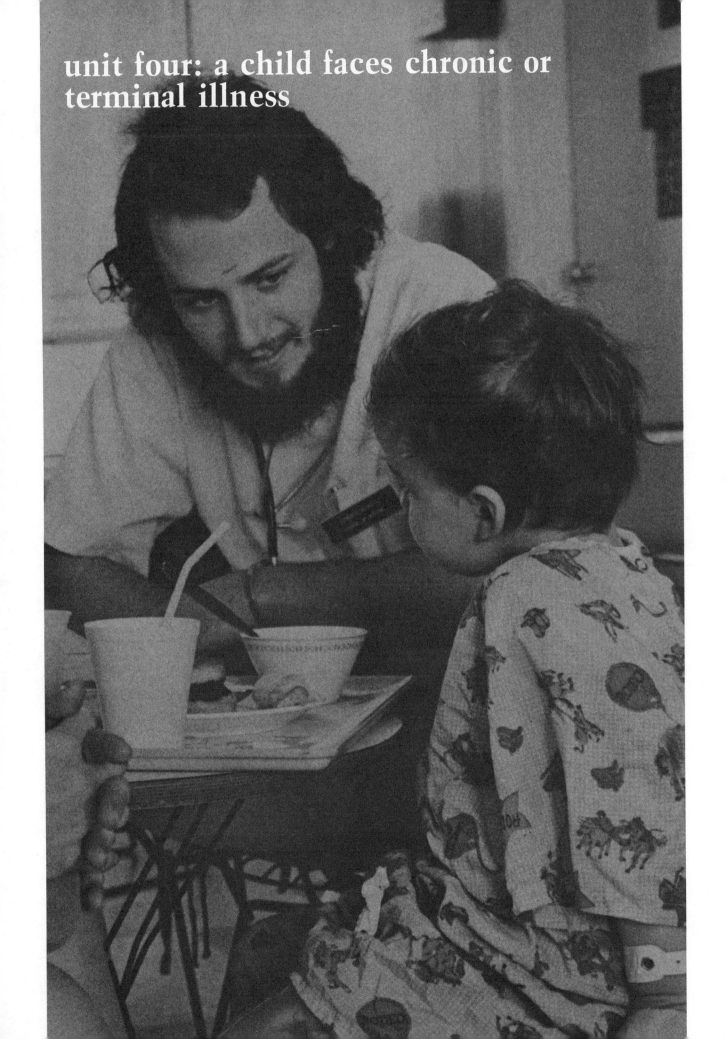

unit four: a child faces chronic or terminal illness

the child with a chronic health problem

20

definition of chronic illness
common problems in chronic illness
effects on the family
parents and chronic illness
the child with chronic illness
siblings and chronic illness
the nurse's role
prevention of chronic health problems
detection of chronic health problems
management of the child with chronic health problems
summary
review questions
references
bibliography

student objectives

The student successfully attaining the goals of this chapter will be able to

1 List seven childhood disorders that may be considered chronic health problems.

2 List the five characteristics common to all chronic health problems.

3 Describe the ten methods as identified by Juenker that children use to adapt to chronic health problems.

4 List seven key problems as defined by Strauss and Glaser that confront people with chronic health problems.

5 Describe two goals in the treatment of the chronically ill child and discuss the nurse's role in attaining those goals.

Chronic illness is the leading health problem in the United States. Not a specific disease, chronic illness is a collective term that includes such health problems as heart disease, cancer, stroke, arthritis, diabetes, mental retardation, and many others. Some of these problems are life-threatening, others are not. But all of them affect the lives of the patients, the families, and in some cases, the community. Chronic health problems must be *lived with*, because they cannot be cured, only controlled or managed.

Although the majority of children experience only brief, acute episodes of illness, a significant number are affected by chronic health problems. Estimates indicate that from 10% to 15% of children under age 18 have one or more chronic health problems.[1] Mental retardation and other handicapping birth defects, diabetes, leukemia, epilepsy, cystic fibrosis, hemophilia, asthma, allergies, vision or hearing impairment all have their beginnings in childhood, some on the first day of life. Other chronic diseases such as arteriosclerosis and cancer dramatically affect older people, but actually begin with health habits developed in early life.

definition of chronic illness

Chronic illness as defined by the National Commission on Chronic Illness is any impairment or deviation from normal that has one or more of the following characteristics:

- is permanent
- leaves residual disability
- is caused by nonreversible pathologic alteration
- requires special training of the patient for rehabilitation
- may be expected to require a long period of supervision, observation, or care.[2]

Although formulated in 1949 by a commission that is no longer in existence today, this definition is still considered appropriate.

common problems in chronic illness

Specific chronic health problems of children have been discussed in earlier chapters. Each requires individual management based on the disease process and the ability of patient and family to understand and comply with the treatment regimen. All chronic health problems, however, create some common difficulties for patients and families, and these are the focus of this chapter.

Strauss and Glaser define seven key problems that confront persons with chronic health problems and their families:[3]

1. Preventing medical crises and managing them when they do occur
2. Controlling symptoms
3. Carrying out prescribed regimens and managing problems related to carrying out the regimens
4. Preventing, or living with, social isolation caused by lessened contact with others

5. Adjusting to changes in the course of the disease, whether remissions or acute episodes
6. Attempting to normalize interaction with others and style of life
7. Searching for necessary money to pay for treatments or to survive despite partial or complete loss of employment

Dealing with these problems demands the joint effort of patient, family, friends, health professionals, and often, community resources. It requires that each person who works with the chronically ill child remembers that the ill child is a child first, with normal needs for love, attention, and discipline, and secondarily, a child with a health problem.

For many patients with chronic illnesses, the acute phases are the easiest to deal with because they often require hospitalization, and the burden of managing the illness shifts to health professionals. It is the ordinary business of day-to-day living that can drain patient and family of energy, hope, time, and money.

Nurses are in a uniquely favorable position to help patients and families deal with the problems of chronic illness because nursing has long emphasized the importance of caring rather than curing, and of considering the whole person within his total environment, not just the disease. Before nurses can begin to assist in managing these problems, however, it is necessary to have a solid understanding of how chronic health problems affect the patient, parents and siblings, peers, and the community at large.

effects on the family

The diagnosis of a chronic health problem causes a crisis in the family, whether it happens during the first few hours or days of the child's life or much later. Illness that is chronic strengthens some families, destroys others, and leaves many in a constant state of stress and anxiety just trying to survive.

> Being chronically ill is vastly different from being acutely ill. It stresses and drains the child and every family member over an infinite period of time. The wonderful resiliency of the human being is stretched almost beyond endurance, especially if there is no prospect of improvement, and even more if the child deteriorates with the passage of time.[4]

Many factors interact to affect the way a family copes with chronic illness, among them the age of the child at diagnosis, age, religious, cultural and educational background and income level of the parents, marital stability, number of children, support from extended family and the community. Generally speaking, families from lower socioeconomic and educational backgrounds are least likely to be able to cope satisfactorily with chronic illness; unfortunately, chronic illness occurs four times as often within this group.[5] Lawson has developed a tool for detecting families at risk for adapting poorly to chronic illness (Table 20–1).[6] Using this scale can help nurses identify families who will need extra support and guidance from health professionals.

TABLE 20–1.   SCALE FOR DETECTING FAMILIES AT RISK FOR ADAPTING POORLY TO CHRONIC ILLNESS

Factors	Rating				
	4	3	2	1	0
Age of parents (years)	<20	20–25	26–30	31–35	>35
Income ($)	<5000	5000–7500	7501–10,000	10,001–15,000	>15,000
Race	Black		Other		White
Years married	<2	2–4	5–7	8–10	>10
Strength of marriage	Weak		Average		Strong
Number of children	1	2	3	4	>4
Education level	<High school	High school	1–2 yr college	3–4 yr college	>4 yr college
Religious conviction	None		Average		Strong
Community involvement	None	One group	Two groups	>Three groups	Three groups
Support from maternal grandmother	None		Average		Strong
Husband/wife experiences with and feelings about chronic illness	Negative		Neutral		Positive

< = less than
> = greater than

Total*
Score

* The lower the score, the better the potential for the family adapting well to a chronic illness.

(Adapted from Lawson A: Chronic illness in the school-aged child: Effects on the total family. Am J Mat Child Nurs 2, No. 1:50, 1977. Copyright 1977, American Journal of Nursing Company)

PARENTS AND CHRONIC ILLNESS

Parents' reactions to the birth of a child with a defect are discussed in Chapters 3 and 4. The feelings of guilt, fear, and sorrow that intermingle during that experience also characterize later diagnosis of a chronic health problem (Fig. 20–1). Parents wonder what they might have done to cause the problem, may fear having other children, or if other children are present, may fear that they also have the disease.

> I had never felt so alone. No one had any advice to offer. My husband . . . had nothing to say. . . . Daily I turned over and over in my mind my choices, my guilty reasons, and my fears. . . . In my grief and frustration I came to hate my silent husband, never realizing that he was suffering too. His dreams were broken. It was his child too—and his unhappy marriage.[7]

Sorrow at the loss of the "perfect child" can last from a few weeks or months to an entire lifetime; Lawson suggests that this sorrow only dissolves with the death of the child.[8]

In the midst of the guilt, fear, and sorrow that surround chronic illness, parents must also deal with normal life problems such as marital stresses, finances, and social activities. Suicide and divorce rates appear to be higher in families with chronically ill children than in the population at large.

Treatments and changes in lifestyle necessitated by the child's chronic illness are often quite expensive. Many families are unaware of funding or other available assistance, information that can and should be supplied by health professionals. Some chronic health problems are so severe that they limit the parents' abilities to enjoy normal social activities. Exhausted financial and energy resources and embarrassment about the child's problem seriously hamper the family's social life. It can be difficult to find willing and qualified persons who can care for a child with a profound physical, mental, or emotional handicap.

THE CHILD WITH CHRONIC ILLNESS

FACTORS INFLUENCING ADAPTATION

The child's attitude toward his disease or handicap is a critical element in the long-term management and in the family's adjustment to the problem. The parent's attitude exerts a powerful influence on the child's attitude, as do the factors identified by Gingrich-Cross: developmental stage, experience, perception of the event, culture, support system, and the number and chronicity of stressors.[10]

Chronic illness that interrupts certain developmental stages can delay or prevent completion of important developmental tasks. A child who must be immobilized during the stage of industry versus inferiority is unable to complete the tasks of industry, such as helping with

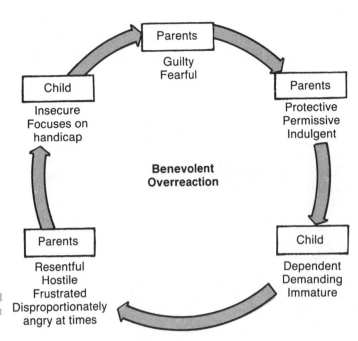

FIG. 20–1. Common cyclical response between parents and handicapped child. (Boone DR, Hartman BH: The benevolent over-reaction. Clin Pediatr 11, No. 5:268–271, May, 1972)

household chores, or working on special projects with siblings or peers.

Heredity and early environmental influences such as nutrition, parental attitudes, and previous illness also affect adaptation to chronic illness. Children who have been overnourished in infancy are likely to have chronic obesity, but may not perceive it as a problem if other members of the family are also obese.

Children often perceive any illness as punishment for a bad thought or action. Perception of chronic illness is subject to the same "magical thinking," depending on the child's developmental stage at the time of diagnosis. This perception is also influenced by attitudes of parents and peers, and by whether or not the dysfunctional body part is visible or invisible. Such problems as asthma, allergies, and epilepsy are difficult for children to understand because "what's wrong" is inside, not outside.

Cultural attitudes toward children and toward illness also influence the child's adaptation. If the child's disorder is nutritional, his therapeutic diet must be planned to be compatible with cultural food patterns.

The family, the peer group, and school personnel make up the support system that can affect adaptation. Meeting the child's physical needs sometimes leaves little time for meeting emotional needs. Children's adaptation to their illness or handicap is strongly influenced by the way able-bodied persons behave toward them. Too often parents and professionals treat children who have mild or moderate disabilities as though they were severely handicapped and much less capable of enjoying life. Persons who are blind, deaf, or crippled have reported that during the time they were growing up, they were made to feel that they had no right to experience sexual desire, and to do so was perverse.[11] Such attitudes add another loss to the multiple losses that confront the child with chronic illness.

Chronic illness introduces stressors into a young life that often continue to multiply as the disease process advances. The adolescent with Hodgkin's disease can be successfully treated for a time with chemotherapy and radiotherapy, but that means adding the side-effects of treatment (steroid-induced acne, edema, and alopecia) to the disease manifestations of night sweats, chronic fatigue, pruritus, and gastrointestinal bleeding. These stressors are often more than one young person can cope with for very long.

ADAPTIVE BEHAVIORS

The child's emotional adaptation to a chronic health problem is the most important determinant of physical adaptation. Children may use a variety of adaptive behaviors and nurses who work with these children need to be able to identify the behaviors in order to help the child and family. Juenker identified ten methods children use to adapt to chronic health problems:[12]

1. Choosing one aspect of a stressful event that they feel they can handle and focusing on it in order to prevent feeling overwhelmed
2. Denying the existence of the crisis to allow more time to assimilate the stressful event
3. Trying to escape by running away or avoiding confrontation
4. Consciously evaluating and accepting the stress
5. Seeking reassurance and security
6. Regressing to an earlier developmental level
7. Transforming the elements of a situation to make it more manageable, for instance, by reversing roles and playing "doctor."
8. Becoming depressed because they feel responsible for their illness
9. Manifesting hypochondriacal symptoms
10. Substituting a realistic goal for an unrealistic one

All of these behaviors are normal responses; some of them lead to healthy adaptation, others to chronic maladaptation. Nurses and parents need to be aware that these behaviors can appear and be ready to reinforce those that will prove beneficial to the child and the family on a long-term basis.

SIBLINGS AND CHRONIC ILLNESS

Some degree of sibling rivalry can be found in most families with healthy children, so it is not surprising that a child with a chronic health problem can seriously disrupt the lives of brothers and sisters. By necessity, much of the parents' time, attention, and money is directed toward management of the ill child's problem. This causes anger, resentment, and jealousy. Parents' failure to set limits for the ill child's behavior while maintaining discipline for the healthy siblings can cause further resentment. Some parents unknowingly create feelings of guilt in the healthy children by overemphasizing the ill child's needs. Families that seem to adapt most successfully to the presence of a child with chronic illness are those in which the parents find time for special activities with the healthy children, explain the ill child's condition as simply as possible, involve the healthy siblings in the care of the ill child according to their developmental ability, and set behavioral limits for all children in the family. This is a delicate balance that many families find impossible to sustain.

the nurse's role

PREVENTION OF CHRONIC HEALTH PROBLEMS

The causes of many chronic health problems such as diabetes, cystic fibrosis, arthritis, and epilepsy are not known; therefore, prevention is not possible. It is known, however, that many chronic diseases that manifest themselves in later life can be prevented by sound health habits in childhood and adulthood. In this regard, each nurse has an obligation to teach good health habits whenever the opportunity arises, particularly by being a positive role model in her own health habits. Children are most responsive to teaching by example, and nurses who smoke, or are seriously overweight, do not convey a healthy image to the children they care for.

Some chronic health problems can be prevented by adequate prenatal care. Good nutrition, regular prenatal checkups to detect any potential problems, and avoidance of smoking and alcohol and other drugs need to be part of every pregnant woman's preparation for birth. This does not mean that the child will be perfect, but only that the probability for a healthy child is greatly increased.

DETECTION OF CHRONIC HEALTH PROBLEMS

Some chronic health problems are not readily apparent and thus go untreated until they reach the acute stage.

NATIONAL ORGANIZATIONS RELATED TO CHRONIC HEALTH PROBLEMS

Parents and professionals can obtain information by writing to these organizations, many of which have local chapters. Organizations related to asthma and allergy are listed in Chapter 13.

American Cancer Society
777 Third Avenue
New York, NY 10017

American Heart Association
1 West 48th Street
New York, NY 10017

American Lung Association
1740 Broadway
New York, NY 10019

Arthritis Foundation
221 Park Avenue South
New York, NY 10003

Closer Look
National Information Center for the Handicapped
Box 1492
Washington, DC 20013

Easter Seal Society for Crippled Children and Adults
2023 West Ogden Avenue
Chicago, IL 60612

Leukemia Society of America, Inc
211 East 43rd Street
New York, NY 10017

National Aid to Retarded Citizens
2709 East Street
Arlington, TX 76011

National Association for Sickle Cell Disease, Inc
945 S Western Avenue, Suite 206
Los Angeles, CA 90006

National Cystic Fibrosis Research Foundation
3379 Peachtree Road NE
Atlanta, GA 30326

National Epilepsy League
6 N Michigan Avenue
Chicago, IL 60602

Parents of Down's Syndrome Children
11507 Yates Street
Silver Spring, MD 20902

United Cerebral Palsy Association
66 East 34th Street
New York, NY 10066

United Ostomy Association
1111 Wilshire Boulevard
Los Angeles, CA 90017

Youth-onset diabetes mellitus is one example. Nurses who are aware of the signs and symptoms of diseases and disorders (such as vision or hearing impairments) can recommend that the child be referred for treatment. Scoliosis is another chronic health problem often detected in screening tests performed by school nurses.

MANAGEMENT OF THE CHILD WITH CHRONIC HEALTH PROBLEMS

As mentioned earlier, when caring for the child with a chronic health problem, it is essential to consider the child first, and the problem second. Chronically ill children may have frequent periods of hospitalization, but familiarity with the experience can increase the child's anxiety rather than reduce it. It is important to consider the child's developmental stage and the tasks he is attempting, his fears, the adaptive behaviors he has learned, the family, and the symptoms that have necessitated hospitalization.

Yancy identifies the goals of treatment for the chronically ill child as follows: (1) to treat the disability/disease by correcting the defect, controlling the symptoms, or arresting progress of the disease, and (2) to prevent the disease, its treatment, and the people involved from interfering with the child's development or from disrupting the family.[13]

The nurse's role in accomplishing these goals can involve teaching patient and family, listening to their needs and feelings, helping them to accept their feelings as normal, acting as a resource person to put families in touch with self-help groups and other community resources, (see boxed material) and meeting the child's physical and emotional needs. This last aspect can prove quite challenging, and meeting the child's physical needs is often the easiest part. Meeting the child's emotional needs includes setting limits for behavior and seeing that those limits are observed, helping the child gain or maintain a sense of self-worth, and encouraging the child to participate as fully as possible in his own care. To allow the child complete freedom of behavior allows him to manipulate parents and staff; to do everything for the child reinforces the sick role instead of motivating recovery. When children must be disciplined, it is important to make it clear that the child's action was "bad," not the child himself. Sometimes both the behavior and appearance of a chronically ill child are most unattractive. The nurse who chooses to work with chronically ill children must be able to maintain a supportive and accepting attitude when caring for such children.

summary

Chronic health problems are increasing every day, with subtle to dramatic effects on the lives of millions of patients and families. Treatment of chronic illness is aimed at helping patients and families *live with* the illness and the problems it creates, so that all members of the family can realize their fullest potential. This treatment often requires a team of health professionals working closely with families to arrange treatments, transportation, and funding. Nurses are an essential part of that helping network, caring for children, counseling families, linking families with community resources, and teaching them what they need to know in order to continue to cope through the months and years ahead.

review questions

1. Define chronic illness.
2. What are the seven key problems that confront persons and families with chronic health problems?
3. Discuss how a chronic health problem affects the family.
4. Discuss why the child's attitude toward his disease or handicap is important.
5. What are the ten methods children use to adapt to chronic health problems?
6. What are the goals of treatment for the chronically ill child?

references

1. Pless IB, Douglas JWB: Chronic illness in childhood, Part I. Epidemiological and clinical characteristics. Pediatr 47, No. 2: 405–414, 1971
2. Anderson SV, Bauwens EE: Chronic Health Problems: Concepts and Application. St Louis, CV Mosby, 1981
3. Strauss A, Glaser B: Chronic Illness and the Quality of Life. St Louis, CV Mosby 1975
4. Battle CV: Symposium on behavioral pediatrics. Chronic physical disease: Behavioral aspects. Pediatr Clin North Am 22:525–531, Aug 1975
5. Roemer M, Kisch AI: Health, poverty, and the medical mainstream. In Bloomberg W, Schmant JJ (eds): Urban Poverty: Its Social and Political Dimensions. Beverly Hills, Sage Publications, 1970
6. Lawson BA: Chronic illness in the school-aged child: Effects on the total family. Am J Mat Child Nurs 2:49–56, 1977
7. Featherstone H: A Difference in the Family: Life With a Disabled Child. New York, Basic Books, 1980
8. Lawson BA: Chronic illness in the school-aged child: Effects on the total family. Am J Mat Child Nurs 2:49–56, 1977
9. Debuskey M (ed): The Chronically Ill Child and his Family. Springfield, Charles C Thomas, 1970
10. Gingrich-Crass J: Stress and crisis: Specific problems of adaptation. In Wold SJ: School Nursing: A Framework for Practice. St Louis, CV Mosby, 1981
11. Gliedman J, Roth W: The Unexpected Minority: Handicapped Children in America. New York, Harcourt Brace Jovanovich, 1980
12. Juenker D: Child's perception of his illness. In Steele S (ed): Nursing Care of the Child With Long-term Illness. New York, Appleton-Century-Crofts, 1977
13. Yancy WS: Approaches to emotional management of the child with a chronic illness. Clin Pediat, 11:64–67, 1972

bibliography

Allmond BW Jr, Buckman W, Gofman HF: The Family Is the Patient: An Approach to Behavioral Pediatrics for the Clinician. St Louis CV Mosby, 1979
Barnard KE, Erickson ML: Teaching Children With Developmental Problems: A Family Care Approach, 2nd ed. St Louis, CV Mosby, 1976
Chinn PC, Winn J, Walters RH: Two-way Talking With Parents of Special Children: A Process of Positive Communication. St. Louis, CV Mosby, 1978

Everson S: Sibling counseling. Am J Nurs 77:644–646, 1977

Holaday BJ: Achievement behavior in chronically ill children. Nurs Res 23:25, 1974

Holaday BJ: Parenting the chronically ill child. In Brandt TP, et al: Current Practice in Pediatric Nursing, Vol 2. St Louis, CV Mosby, 1978

Hymovich D: Assessment of the chronically ill child and family. In Hymovich D, Barnard M: Family Health Care. New York, McGraw-Hill, 1979

Jelneck LJ: The special needs of the adolescent with chronic illness. Mat Child Nurs J 6, No. 1:57–61, 1977

Lepler M: Having a handicapped child. Am J Mat Child Nurs 3:32–33, 1978

Mattson A: Long-term physical illness in childhood: A challenge to psychosocial adaptation. In Garfield CA (ed): Stress and Survival: The Emotional Realities of Life-threatening Illness. St Louis, CV Mosby, 1979

McKeever PT: Fathering the chronically ill child. Am J Mat Child Nurs 6:124–128, 1981

Safford PL: Teaching young children with special needs. St Louis, CV Mosby, 1978

Schulman JL: Coping With Tragedy: Successfully Facing the Problem of a Seriously Ill Child. Chicago, Follett, 1976

Sperling E: Psychological issues in chronic illness and handicapping. In Gellert E (ed): Psychosocial Aspects of Pediatric Care. New York, Grune & Stratton, 1978

Stewart JE: Home Health Care. St Louis, CV Mosby, 1979

Sultz HA, et al: Long-term Childhood Illness. Pittsburgh, University of Pittsburgh Press, 1972

Tudor M: Nursing intervention with developmentally disabled children. Am J Mat Child Nurs 3:25–31, 1978

Waechter EH: The adolescent with a handicapping or life-threatening illness. In Mercer R (ed): Perspectives on Adolescent Health Care. Philadelphia, JB Lippincott, 1979

the dying child

student objectives

The student successfully attaining the goals of this chapter will be able to

1. Define the following vocabulary terms:

   anticipatory grief   Candlelighters   Compassionate Friends
   empty-mother syndrome   hospice   thanatologist

2 List three factors that influence the child's understanding of death.

3 Describe anticipatory grief and discuss its possible effects on the grieving process.

4 List five guidelines for helping persons experiencing grief.

5 List twelve guidelines for helping children to cope with death.

6 Identify six factors that should be considered when families are deciding to care for the terminally ill child at home.

THE DYING PERSON'S BILL OF RIGHTS

I have the right to be treated as a living human being until I die.

I have the right to maintain a sense of hopefulness however changing its focus may be.

I have the right to be cared for by those who can maintain a sense of hopefulness, however changing this might be.

I have the right to express my feelings and emotions about my approaching death in my own way.

I have the right to participate in decisions concerning my care.

I have the right to expect continuing medical and nursing attention even though "cure" goals must be changed to "comfort" goals.

I have the right not to die alone.

I have the right to be free from pain.

I have the right to have my questions answered honestly.

I have the right not to be deceived.

I have the right to have help from and for my family in accepting my death.

I have the right to die in peace and dignity.

I have the right to retain my individuality and not be judged for my decisions which may be contrary to beliefs of others.

I have the right to discuss and enlarge my religious and/or spiritual experiences, whatever these may mean to others.

I have the right to expect that the sanctity of the human body will be respected after death.

I have the right to be cared for by caring, sensitive, knowledgeable people who will attempt to understand my needs and will be able to gain some satisfaction in helping me face my death.

(Created at a workshop on "The Terminally Ill Patient and the Helping Person," in Lansing, Mich., sponsored by the Southwestern Michigan Inservice Education Council and conducted by Amelia J. Barbus, Associate Professor Nursing, Wayne State University. American Journal of Nursing, 75:99, 1975; Copyright © 1975; American Journal of Nursing Co)

To care for a family facing the death of their child calls upon every personal and professional skill of the nurse. It means offering superb physical care and comfort measures for the child and continuing emotional support for child, parents, and siblings. This kind of caring demands an understanding of the nurse's own feelings about death and dying, knowledge of the grieving process that terminally ill patients and families experience, and a willingness to become involved.

Like chronic illness, terminal illness creates a family crisis with the potential for destroying or strengthening the family as a unit and as individuals. Nurses and other health professionals who can offer knowledgeable, sensitive care to these families help make the remainder of the child's life more meaningful and the family's mourning experience more healing. Helping a family struggle through this crisis and emerge stronger and closer can yield deep satisfaction.

The grieving process as described by Kubler-Ross and Lindemann is discussed earlier (see Fig. 3–12). Diagnosis of a fatal illness initiates that process in patient and family: denial and isolation, anger, bargaining, depression and acute grief, and, finally, acceptance. Not every patient or family will complete the process because each family as well as each death is personal and unique.

When death is expected, the family begins to mourn, a phenomenon called *anticipatory grief*. For some persons, this shortens the period of acute grief and loss after the child's death. Unexpected death offers no chance for preparation, and grief may last longer and be more difficult to resolve.

Death at an early age is a tragic reality for thousands of children each year. Accidents are the leading cause of death in children between the ages of 1 year and 14 years; cancer is the number one fatal disease in this age group. Nearly every one of these childhood deaths means at least one grieving parent, and perhaps brothers, sisters, and grandparents. Nurses who care for children and families need to be prepared for encounters with the dying and the bereaved.

the nurse's reaction to dying and death

I am a student nurse. I am dying. I write this to you who are, and will become, nurses in the hope that by my sharing my feelings with you, you may someday be better able to help those who share my experience. . . . You slip in and out of my room, give me medications and check my blood pressure. Is it because I am a student nurse, myself, or just a human being, that I sense your fright? And your fears enhance mine. Why are you afraid? I am the one who is dying!

I know you feel insecure, don't know what to say, don't know what to do. But please believe me, if you care, you can't go wrong. Just admit that you care. . . . Don't run away—wait—all I want to know is that there will be someone to hold my hand when I need it. . . . If only we could be honest, both admit of our fears, touch one another. If you really care, would you lose so much of your valuable professionalism if you even cried with me? Just person to person? Then it might not be so hard to die—in a hospital—with friends close by.*

Too often nurses and doctors make patients feel like this young student nurse was made to feel. They are so uncom-

* American Journal of Nursing, 70, No. 2, 1970; Copyright © 1970, American Journal of Nursing Co

fortable with dying patients that they avoid them, afraid the patients will confront them with questions they cannot or should not answer. These caregivers signal by their behavior that the patient should avoid the fact of his or her impending death and should keep up a show of bravery. In effect, they are asking the patient to meet their needs instead of trying to meet the patient's needs.

Death reminds us of our own mortality, not a pleasant thought for most of us. The thought that someone even younger than we are is about to die makes us feel more vulnerable. Every nurse needs to examine her own feelings about death, and why she has these feelings. How has she reacted to the death of a friend or a family member? When growing up, did she learn to avoid talking and thinking about death because of her parents' attitudes? Admitting that death is a part of life, and that patients should be helped to live each day to the fullest until death, is a step toward understanding and being able to communicate with those who are dying.

Learning to care for the dying means talking with other professionals, sharing concerns, and comforting each other in stressful times. It means reading the studies that have been done on death to discover how dying patients feel about their care, about their illness, about their families, about how they want to spend the rest of their lives. It also means being a sensitive, empathetic, unjudging listener to patients and families who need to express their feelings, even if they perhaps cannot express feelings to each other. Caring for the dying is usually a team effort involving nurse, physician, chaplain, social worker, psychiatrist, or *thanatologist* (a person trained especially to work with the dying and their families, sometimes a nurse), but often the nurse is the person who coordinates the care.

the child's understanding of death

How the child understands death depends on the developmental stage, cognitive ability, and experience with death such as the death of a family member or a pet. Even children who do not understand death are aware that they are dying.[1] Any attempts by parents or professionals to conceal the facts only destroy the child's sense of trust when it is needed most. However, nurses and other professionals are obligated to care for the child according to the parents' dictates about how much information is given or withheld.

DEVELOPMENTAL STAGE

Up until about age 8, children consider death to be reversible. Before the age of 3 they cannot comprehend the absence of life, and they have no concept of time, therefore, words such as "forever" have little meaning. Magical thinking lets them believe that they can cause death or illness by bad thoughts, and, therefore, they feel very guilty when a family member dies. During the preschool period, children begin to see the need for rituals when death occurs; if a pet dies, they prefer to mark the event with a "funeral" before burying the animal.

BOOKS TO HELP CHILDREN UNDERSTAND DEATH

Anders, Rebecca: A Look at Death. Minneapolis, Lerner Pub., 1977

Bancroft, Henrietta: Down Come the Leaves. New York, T Y Crowell, 1961

Bartoli, Jennifer: Nonna. New York, Harvey House, 1975

Brown, Margaret Wise: The Dead Bird. New York, Young Scott Books, 1958

Carrick, Carol: The Accident. Boston, Houghton Mifflin, 1976

Coutant, Helen: First Snow. New York, Alfred A Knopf, 1974

DePaola, Tomie: Nana Upstairs and Nana Downstairs. New York, Putnam, 1973

Fassler, Joan: My Grandpa Died Today. New York, Human Sciences Press, 1971

Gackenbach, Dick: Do You Love Me? Boston, Houghton Mifflin, 1975

Harris, Audrey: Why Did He Die? Minneapolis, Lerner Pub., 1965

Kohn, Bernice: One Sad Day. New York, Okpaku Communications, 1972

Mari, Iela and Mari, Enzo: The Apple and the Moth. New York, Pantheon Books, 1970

Martin, Patricia Miles: John Fitzgerald Kennedy. New York, Putnam, 1964

Miles, Miska: Annie and the Old One. Boston, Little, Brown, 1971

Ness, Evaline: Sam, Bangs and Moonshine. New York, Holt, Rinehart & Winston, 1966

Stein, Sarah B: About Dying. New York, Walker & Co., 1974

Tresselt, Alvin: The Dead Tree. New York, Parents Magazine Press, 1972

Tresselt, Alvin: Johnny-Maple-Leaf. New York, Lothrop, Lee & Shepard, 1948

Viorst, Judith: The Tenth Good Thing About Barney. New York, Atheneum Pub, 1971

Warburg, Sandol Stoddard: Growing Time. Boston, Houghton Mifflin, 1969

Wojciechowska, Maia: Hey, What's Wrong With This One. New York, Harper & Row, 1969

Wojciechowska, Maia: The Life and Death of a Brave Bull. New York, Harcourt, Brace & World, 1972

Young, Jim: When the Whale Came to My Town. New York, Alfred A Knopf, 1974

Zolotow, Charlotte: My Grandson Lew. New York, Harper & Row, 1974

As compiled in Davis AJ: *Please See My Need.* Charles City, Iowa, Satellite Continuing Education, 1981

School-age children are less egocentric than preschoolers and more responsive to logical explanation of their disease, its treatment, and expected outcome. By the age of 9 or 10, children begin to understand that death is final and inevitable. However, their feelings about death depend on the attitudes of the adults around them. These children are old enough to attend funerals if they have been prepared for what to expect and if they have the opportunity to leave should the experience become too upsetting.

Adolescents have the greatest difficulty coping with the idea of dying, even though they have intellectually reached an adult level of understanding about death. They feel that their "grown-up" lives are just beginning, they are just learning who they are; yet all their dreams and hopes will be unfulfilled when they die. Their concerns about body image and peer approval can mean that the effects of treatment (alopecia, steroid-induced acne and edema, and fatigue) may be more upsetting than the idea of dying.

EXPERIENCE WITH DEATH

Every death that touches the life of a child makes an impression that affects the way the child thinks about every other death, including his own. Attitudes of parents and other family members are powerful influences. It is important for parents to be able to discuss death with children when a grandparent, or other family member dies, even though the discussion may be painful. Otherwise, the child thinks that death is another one of those forbidden topics, which, undiscussed, leaves immeasurable room for fantasy and distortion in the child's imagination.

During the past two decades, much has been written to help all persons understand and cope with dying and death. In some schools, education about death is a part of general education about living, and a number of children's books help children of different ages relate the idea of death to familiar things, people, and experiences. (See boxed material.)

AWARENESS OF IMPENDING DEATH

Children know when they are dying.[2,3] Their play activities, their artwork, their dreams, and their symbolic language demonstrate this knowledge. Even though the youngster may not be able to place a name on it, he senses and fears what is going to happen. When parents insist that the child not learn the truth about the illness, they force professionals to work under a severe handicap, and deny their child the opportunity to talk about his fears and concerns.

Parents who permit openness and honesty in communication with dying children offer caregivers the opportunity to meet children's individual needs most effectively, to dispel misunderstandings that might prevent a peaceful death, and to see that the child and the family are left with little or no "unfinished business."

Openness does not mean that caregivers offer information not asked for by the child, but simply that the child be given the information he asks for using words that he can understand, in a gentle and straightforward manner. Truth can be kind as well as cruel. Honest, specific answers leave less room for the misinterpretation and distortion that are characteristic of children with cancer.[4]

the family's reaction to dying and death

Diagnosis of a potentially fatal disease such as leukemia, the most common childhood cancer, sends feelings of shock, disbelief, and guilt through every family member. Anticipatory grief begins then and continues until there are definite signs of remission.

PARENTS

Despite the fact that survival rates have improved dramatically for children with leukemia, the word still sounds the death knell in the hearts of most parents. They think it can't be happening to them; no parent ever expects to outlive his or her child. Most parents at first blame themselves, wondering if they overlooked some sign or symptom that should have been treated, questioning whether something in their genetic make-up is responsible. Some parents associate their child's illness with the belief that God is either punishing them or testing them in some way.

Nurses can offer effective support to parents by listening, helping to clarify misunderstanding, and encouraging parents to delay major changes in their family life until the child's condition has improved.

Anger, depression, ambivalence, and bargaining follow the initial shock of diagnosis. Parents can direct anger at hospital staff, themselves (because of guilt), at each other, or at the child. The nurse should reassure parents that this is a normal reaction, and avoid taking sides. If parents' anger at the caregiver appears to be justified, the nurse can suggest that they discuss the reasons for their anger with the specific person involved. Acceptance of anger is difficult, but to respond reciprocally with anger or fear only stifles communication.

Involving parents and child in the total plan for treatment and reinforcing that involvement with repeated teaching about procedures and why they are necessary can help parents overcome their feelings of ambivalence. Their depression usually is relieved when signs of a remission occur.

When the child has gone home from the hospital, parents are hopeful for a recovery, yet fear a relapse. It is very easy for parents to be overprotective toward a child in danger of dying, even though he is relatively well during periods of remission. As in chronic illness, this overprotective attitude reinforces the child's sick behavior and dependency, and is usually accompanied by a lack of discipline. Failure to set limits for the child accentuates his feeling of being different and creates problems for siblings. It allows the child to manipulate family members, a behavior that will probably not yield positive results when attempted with peers or caregivers.

When remission ends, the parents begin to grieve again, and may experience all phases of the grieving process. Hope for a recovery is gone and depression returns. Parents fear the imminent death, the thought that their child will suffer pain, and the possibility that the child may die when they are not there. Nurses can help relieve these fears by keeping parents informed about their child's condition, by making the child as comfortable as possible, and by being sure that parents are summoned when the child appears to be near death. When death comes, it is perfectly appropriate to share the parents' grief, to cry with the family, and then provide them with privacy to express their sorrow.

Death can begin another crisis for the family, even though they have had time to prepare for life without the child who has died. Parents need to feel that they did everything possible for the child. It may be helpful for them to know that caregivers are available for consultation later.

The death of a child who has been ill for months or even years can cause what Donna Wong has called *"the empty-mother syndrome."*[5] The child's illness probably consumed more of the mother's time and attention than that of any other family members, and once the funeral is over and family members begin to resume normal activities of school and work, the mother has a gaping void to fill. In addition to emptiness, she may experience a feeling of loneliness and even failure; the nurse can prepare her for these feelings and assure her that they are normal. Grieving for a child must include a kind of detachment from the lost child before the mother can reestablish emotional relations with her husband and her living children. She should be encouraged to seek involvement in new or former activities that draw on her individual interests and talents.

Fathers often have difficulty working through their grief because they feel they must be strong. Our culture emphasizes stoicism and control of emotion as definite masculine characteristics, and some fathers find it hard to break this taboo. This situation holds potential problems because the mother may interpret the father's behavior as lack of feeling. Nurses can encourage couples to share their feelings with each other honestly, and thus avoid the problems that lack of communication can foster.

Parents and families need to recognize that grief knows no time limit. A commonly held belief is that acute grief is usually completed within a year; in reality, grief may last 3 years or longer, particularly for the mother. Sometimes professional counseling is necessary to help parents work through grief. Many parents find comfort in sharing their feelings with others who have survived the same tragedy. Two national organizations were founded for that purpose and have local chapters in many cities. They are

Candlelighters
(Parents whose children have died or are dying of cancer)
123 C Street SE
Washington, DC 20003

Compassionate Friends
PO Box 1347
Oakbrook, IL 60521

Guidelines for helping children and others experiencing grief have been developed by

Grief Institute
PO Box 623
Englewood, CO 80151 (See boxed material)

CHILD

Living with cancer—or dying with it—is a painful experience. Treatments hurt the child, side-effects are unpleasant, and the child's natural reaction is anger, usually directed at parents. These children become uncooperative and hostile; some are aggressive, others withdrawn. Unless caregivers understand that this behavior is a signal that the child needs to talk about what's happening, the anger further isolates the child.

Chemotherapy and radiation therapy can cause *alopecia* (hair loss), an effect that is highly upsetting to some children depending on their developmental age. Children who are prepared for the possibility of hair loss and can help decide how to cope with it, perhaps by buying a wig before it is needed, seem to have less anxiety.

Every effort should be made to help the school-age child resume classwork in the usual setting. This requires care-

---

GUIDELINES FOR HELPING PERSONS EXPERIENCING GRIEF

Do

1. Remember that grief resulting from the loss of a beloved person often lasts several years.
2. Listen as they "retell it" over and over again. That is part of grief work.
3. Accept what may seem to be inappropriate anger, and guilt. They have to get it out through sharing.
4. Make every effort to put a family back in touch with the religious traditions of their childhood.
5. Discourage bereaved persons from making major decisions and changes in their lives during the first year.

Don't

1. Don't tell them not to cry. Cry with them. What most people are saying is that "you make me uncomfortable when you cry." That puts a burden on the people least able to carry a burden.
2. Don't be frightened when people act a "little bit crazy" soon after a death—comfort and protect them.
3. Don't shut children out of grief; share it with them.

(Courtesy Alice Demi, President, Grief Education Institute, PO Box 623, Englewood, CO 80151)

GUIDELINES FOR HELPING CHILDREN COPE WITH DEATH

Do

1. Know your own beliefs.
2. Begin where the child is.
3. Be there.
4. Confront reality.
5. Allow & encourage expression of feelings.
6. Be truthful.
7. Include the child in family rituals.
8. Encourage remembrance.
9. Admit when you don't know the answer.
10. Use touch to communicate.
11. Start death education early, simply, using naturally occurring events.
12. Recognize symptoms of grief and deal with the grief.
13. Accept differing reactions to death.

Don't

1. Praise stoicism.
2. Use euphemisms.
3. Be nonchalant.
4. Glamorize death.
5. Tell fairy tales and half truths.
6. Close the door to questions.
7. Be judgmental of feelings and behaviors.
8. Protect the child from exposure to experiences with death.
9. Encourage forgetting the deceased.
10. Encourage the child to be like the deceased.

(Courtesy Alice Demi, President, Grief Education Institute, PO Box 623, Englewood, CO 80151)

ful preparation and planning involving parents, child, teacher, and school nurse.

Chemotherapy can cause severe nausea and vomiting, making mealtime at home very difficult. It helps to offer small, frequent meals of the child's favorite foods. By contrast, steroid therapy causes a marked increase in appetite and parents need to be aware of this to avoid misinterpreting the change.

During the terminal phase of the child's illness, it is important to use all possible measures to make the child feel comfortable and loved. Frequent changes of position, gentle handling, and a soothing touch often reduce the need for pain medication.

Signs that death is near include loss of sensation and movement, loss of senses (vision first, then hearing), a feeling of heat, and minimal need for pain medication.[6] As these signs appear, the nurse should alert parents if they are not already present. The child's wishes should be respected: some children want to hold a parent's hand, others ask that no one touch them. As vision fails, the child may ask for bright light. Anyone with the child should be seated near the head of the bed.

Knowledge about the point at which hearing fails is uncertain; it is known that those who appear to be asleep or comatose can often hear everything that goes on around them. Caregivers and parents should talk to the dying child in a normal voice, and explain anything they are about to do to the child.

As death approaches, internal body temperature rises; thus, dying patients seem to be unaware of cold, even though their skin feels cool. Parents should understand this pheomenon so they do not think the child needs additional warmth.

In the period immediately before death, children who have remained conscious may experience restlessness followed by a time of peace and calm. Nurse and parents should be aware of these reactions and know that death is near.

SIBLINGS

Just as in chronic illness, siblings resent the attention given the ill child and are angry about the disruption in the family. Reaction varies according to developmental age and parental attitudes and actions. Younger children find it almost impossible to understand what is happening; it is even difficult for older children to grasp. Reaction to the illness and its accompanying stresses can cause problems for school-age siblings, which may be incorrectly labeled as learning disabilities or behavioral disorders unless school personnel are aware of the family situation.

When the child dies, siblings who are still prone to magical thinking may feel much guilt, particularly if a strong degree of rivalry existed before the illness. These children need continued reassurance that they did not cause or help to cause their sibling's death.

settings for care of dying children

Until the beginning of the 20th century, birth and death usually occurred at home with family members present. Development of new drugs to control infection, new surgical techniques, and life support systems gradually moved birth, death, and much of the health care in between those events into the hospital. By 1958, 50% of all deaths occurred in the hospital.

While dying in a hospital, a child may be afforded the latest technology and the most professional care, but this can also contribute to family separation, a feeling of loss of control, and a sense of isolation. After many interviews with dying patients, Samuel L. Feder stated, "In the patients I saw, the greatest threat was not so much death, whatever dying is, but rather the danger of progressive isolation and the development of a sense of 'aloneness.'"[8]

That pattern of care has begun to change; in many areas of the United States, patients can choose where they will die and who will be with them. Some still choose to die in the hospital; others, however, elect to be in a hospice or at home with their family.

HOSPICE CARE

In medieval times, the *hospice* was a refuge for travelers, not only those who traveled through the countryside, but those who were leaving this life for another, the terminally ill. Hospices were often operated by religious orders and became havens for the dying.

The modern hospice movement in health care began in England when Dr. Cicely Saunders founded St. Christopher's Hospice in London. This institution has become the model for others in the United States and Canada, with emphasis on sensitive, humane care for the dying. Hospice principles of care include relief of pain, attention to the needs of the total person, and absence of heroic life-saving measures.

The first hospice in the United States was the New Haven Hospice in New Haven, Connecticut. For the first 3 years of its existence, this hospice functioned on a home care basis. Other hospices operate as part of a hospital, but this has caused some controversy as to whether true hospice care can exist within a hospital environment.

HOME CARE

Many persons, young and old alike, find hospitals frightening, a fear that may or may not be justified. In addition, the costs of hospital care have risen dramatically during the last two decades. For these reasons, and because of the Patients' Rights movement, people are trying to exercise greater control over the major events in their lives. Earlier chapters discuss the home birth movement; some of the same principles underlie the movement toward home care of the dying.

The growing trend toward care of the dying at home, particularly children, has emerged spontaneously all across the country. Patients and families feel that it provides a more loving, caring environment, draws the family closer, and seems to help reduce the guilt that sometimes is part of bereavement.

A pioneering research project to study home care is being conducted at the University of Minnesota School of Nursing. Spearheaded by Dr. Ida Martinson, Home Care for the Child with Cancer (Grant CA 19460, awarded by the National Cancer Institute, DHEW) has found that families are capable of providing nursing care, and that pain *can* be controlled at home. In this program, parents have the option to take their child back to the hospital if care at home becomes too difficult. During a 2-year period, all but 12 of 58 children died at home. Eleven died in the hospital and one died in an ambulance.[9]

Home care dramatically reduces the high cost of dying. The Minnesota project showed that care at home had cost less than one third as much as hospital care.[10]

Care at home offers the patient a greater sense of security and control. Those who help care for a dying family member at home can perhaps reduce their own fear of death by learning that it does not have to be painful or traumatic.

Home care for the dying is not easy and is not for everyone. The Minnesota project identified six prerequisites for choosing home care:[11]

1. Treatment no longer seeks to cure; only to *care*
2. The child wants to be home
3. Parents, siblings, and/or significant others want to have the child at home
4. Parents, siblings, and/or significant others recognize their own ability to care for the ill child
5. A nurse is willing to be on call 24 hours a day for consultation and support
6. The physician agrees with the plan and is willing to be on call as consultant.

Families who choose home care and are able to manage it effectively benefit from the satisfaction of knowing that their child died as he had lived—as part of a family.

HOSPITAL CARE

Dying in the hospital has limitations and advantages. Both patient and family may find support from others in the same situation. Family members may not have the physical or emotional strength to cope with total care of the child at home, but they can participate in care that is supported by hospital staff. Hospital care is much more expensive, as mentioned earlier, but this fact is reassuring to some families. The hospital is still the culturally accepted place to die, and this is also important to some persons. Those who do choose hospital care need to know that they have rights and can exert some control over what happens to them and their families.

summary

Knowing that your child is dying, and being helpless to prevent it, is an agony unmatched by few other experiences. Caring for the dying child and the grieving family is a challenge that can be compared to few other nursing situations. The family's pain is emotional; the child's is emotional and physical. Trying to relieve the pain for both demands a sensitivity and a willingness to become involved. Involvement can be painful, too, but there is little true satisfaction without it.

review questions

1. What are the guidelines for helping persons experiencing grief?
2. What are the guidelines for helping children cope with death?
3. What is the leading cause of death in children between the ages of 1 through 14 years?
4. How can the nurse help the parents whose child is dying?

5. Why do many fathers have difficulty working through their grief?
6. What are the signs that death is near?
7. Discuss why there is a trend toward home care of the dying child.

references

1. Spinetta JJ, Rigler D, Karon M: Anxiety in the dying child. Pediatr 52:841–845, 1973
2. Solnit AJ, Green M: The child's reaction to the fear of dying. In Solnit AJ, Provence SA (eds): Modern Perspectives in Child Development. New York, Harper & Row, 1963
3. Koocher GP: Talking with children about death. Am J Orthopsychiatry 44, No. 3:404–411, 1944
4. Goggin EL, Lansky SB, Hassanein K: Personality characteristics of children with malignancies. 21st Annual Meeting of American Academy of Child Psychiatry, San Francisco, Oct 1974. In Sandoz Psychiatric Spectator 9:12, 1975
5. Wong DL: Bereavement: The empty-mother syndrome. Am J Mat Child Nurs 5:384–389, 1980
6. Gray VR: Some physiological needs. In Dealing With Death and Dying. Philadelphia, Intermed Communications, 1977
7. Martinson IM, Rude NV: Dying at home, hospice or hospital. In Anderson SV, Bauwens EE: Chronic Health Problems: Concepts and Application. St Louis, CV Mosby, 1981
8. Feder SL: Attitudes of patients with advanced "malignancy." In Shneidman ES (ed): Death: Current Perspectives. Palo Alto, Mayfield Publishing, 1976
9. Martinson IM, Rude NV: Dying at home, hospice or hospital. In Anderson SV, Bauwens EE: Chronic Health Problems: Concepts and Application. St Louis, CV Mosby, 1981
10. Martinson IM, Rude NV: Dying at home, hospice or hospital. In Anderson SV, Bauwens EE: Chronic Health Problems: Concepts and Application. St Louis, CV Mosby, 1981
11. Martinson IM, Rude NV: Dying at home, hospice or hospital. In Anderson SV, Bauwens EE: Chronic Health Problems: Concepts and Application. St. Louis, CV Mosby, 1981.

bibliography

Barton D (ed): Dying and Death: A Clinical Guide for Caregivers. Baltimore, Williams & Wilkins, 1977

Bouchard-Kurtz R, Speese-Owens N: Nursing Care of the Cancer Patient, 4th ed. St Louis, CV Mosby, 1981

Bradley B: Endings: A Book About Death. Menlo Park, Addison-Wesley, 1979

Bunch B, Bunch D: Dealing with death: The unlearned role: The grieving nurse. Am J Nurs 76:486–492, 1976

Cantor RC: And a Time to Live. New York, Harper & Row, 1978

Davis AJ (ed): Please See My Need. Charles City, Iowa, Satellite Continuing Education, 1981

Epstein C: Nursing the Dying Patient. Reston, Va, Reston Publishing, 1975

Garfield CA (ed): Stress and Survival: The Emotional Realities of Life-threatening Illness. St Louis, CV Mosby, 1979

Grollman E: Talking About Death: A Dialogue Between Parent and Child. Boston, Beacon Press, 1976

Grove S: Encounters with grief. Am J Nurs 78:414–424, 1978

Guylay JE: The Dying Child. New York, McGraw-Hill, 1978

Kastenbaum R: Death, Society and Human Experience, 2nd ed. St Louis, CV Mosby, 1981

Kruse LC, Reese JL, Hart LK: Cancer: Pathophysiology, Etiology, Management: Selected Readings. St Louis, CV Mosby, 1979

Kübler-Ross E: To Live Until We Say Goodbye. Englewood Cliffs, Prentice-Hall, 1978

Linger N: Understanding Bereavement and Grief. New York, Ktav Publishing House, 1977

Lund D: Eric. Philadelphia, JB Lippincott, 1974

Martinson IM: Home Care for the Dying Child: Professional and Family Perspectives. New York, Appleton-Century-Crofts, 1976

Martinson IM, Armstrong GD, Geis DP: Facilitating home care for children dying of cancer. Cancer Nurs 1:41–45, Feb 1978

Mills GC: Books to help children understand death. Am J Nurs 79:291–295, 1979

Moldow DG, Martinson IM: From research to reality: Home care for the dying child. Am J Mat Child Nurs 5:159–166, 1980

Rosenbaum EH, Rosenbaum IR: A Comprehensive Guide for Cancer Patients and Their Families. Palo Alto, Bull Publishing, 1980

Rudolph M: Should the Children Know? New York, Shocken Books, 1980

Sahler OJ (ed): The Child and Death. St Louis, CV Mosby, 1978

Schiff HS: The Bereaved Parent. New York, Penguin, 1978

Schulman JL: Coping With Tragedy: Successfully Facing the Problem of a Seriously Ill Child. Chicago, Follett, 1976

Sharkey F: A Parting Gift. New York, St Martins Press, 1982

Spinetta JJ, Spinetta P: Living With Childhood Cancer. St Louis, CV Mosby, 1981

Stein SB: About Dying: An Open Family Book for Parents and Children Together. New York, Walker & Co., 1974

Stoddard S: The Hospice Movement: A Better Way of Caring for the Dying. New York, Stein and Day, 1977

Ufema J: The dying patient. In Reinhardt AM, Quinn MD (eds): Family Centered Community Nursing: A Sociocultural Framework, Vol 2. St Louis, CV Mosby, 1980

Waechter EH: Children's awareness of fatal illness. Am J Nurs 71:1168, 1971

appendix a: united nations declaration of the rights of the child

preamble

Whereas the peoples of the United Nations have, in the Charter, reaffirmed their faith in fundamental human rights, and in the dignity and worth of the human person, and have determined to promote social progress and better standards of life in larger freedom.,

Whereas the United Nations has, in the Universal Declaration of Human Rights, proclaimed that everyone is entitled to all the rights and freedoms set forth therein, without distinction of any kind, such as race, color, sex, language, religion, political or other opinion, national or social origin, property, birth or other status,

Whereas the child, by reason of his physical and mental immaturity, needs special safeguards and care, including appropriate legal protection, before as well as after birth,

Whereas the need for such special safeguards has been stated in the Geneva Declaration of the Rights of the Child of 1924, and recognized in the Universal Declaration of Human Rights and in the statutes of specialized agencies and international organizations concerned with the welfare of children,

Whereas mankind owes to the child the best it has to give,

now therefore the general assembly proclaims

This Declaration of the Rights of the Child to the end that he may have a happy childhood and enjoy for his own good and for the good of society the rights and freedoms herein set forth, and calls upon parents, upon men and women as individuals and upon voluntary organizations, local authorities and national governments to recognize these rights and strive for their observance by legislative and other measures progressively taken in accordance with the following principles:

PRINCIPLE 1

The child shall enjoy all the rights set forth in this Declaration. All children, without any exception whatsoever, shall be entitled to these rights, without distinction or discrimination on account of race, color, sex, language, religion, political or other opinion, national or social origin, property, birth or other status, whether of himself or of his family.

PRINCIPLE 2

The child shall enjoy special protection, and shall be given opportunities and facilities, by law and by other means, to enable him to develop physically, mentally, morally, spiritually and socially in a healthy and normal manner and in conditions of freedom and dignity. In the enactment of laws for this purpose the best interests of the child shall be the paramount consideration.

PRINCIPLE 3

The child shall be entitled from his birth to a name and a nationality.

PRINCIPLE 4

The child shall enjoy the benefits of social security. He shall be entitled to grow and develop in health; to this end special care and protection shall be provided both to him and to his mother, including adequate prenatal and postnatal care. The child shall have the right to adequate nutrition, housing, recreation and medical services.

PRINCIPLE 5

The child who is physically, mentally or socially handicapped shall be given the special treatment, education and care required by his particular condition.

PRINCIPLE 6

The child, for the full and harmonious development of his personality, needs love and understanding. He shall, wherever possible, grow up in the care and under the responsibility of his parents, and in any case in an atmosphere of affection and of moral and material security; a child of tender years shall not, save in exceptional circumstances, be separated from his mother. Society and the public authorities shall have the duty to extend particular care to children without a family and to those without adequate means of support. Payment of state and other assistance toward the maintenance of children of large families is desirable.

PRINCIPLE 7

The child is entitled to receive education, which shall be free and compulsory, at least in the elementary stages. He shall be given an education which will promote his general culture, and enable him on a basis of equal opportunity to develop his abilities, his individual judgment, and his sense of moral and social responsibility, and to become a useful member of society.

The best interests of the child shall be the guiding principle of those responsible for his education and guidance; that responsibility lies in the first place with his parents.

The child shall have full opportunity for play and recreation, which shall be directed to the same purposes as education; society and the public authorities shall endeavor to promote the enjoyment of this right.

PRINCIPLE 8

The child shall in all circumstances be among the first to receive protection and relief.

PRINCIPLE 9

The child shall be protected against all forms of neglect, cruelty and exploitation. He shall not be the subject of traffic, in any form.

The child shall not be admitted to employment before an appropriate minimum age; he shall in no case be caused or permitted to engage in any occupation or employment which would prejudice his health or education, or interfere with his physical, mental or moral development.

PRINCIPLE 10

The child shall be protected from practices which may foster racial, religious and any other form of discrimination. He shall be brought up in a spirit of understanding, tolerance, friendship among peoples, peace and universal brotherhood and in full consciousness that his energy and talents should be devoted to the service of his fellow men.

appendix b: joint statement on maternity care (1971), supplementary statement (1975), and statement on parent and newborn interaction (1977)

joint statement on maternity care (1971)

The American College of Obstetricians and Gynecologists, The Nurses Association of The American College of Obstetricians and Gynecologists and the American College of Nurse-Midwives recognize the increasing needs for general health care and, more specifically, the deficits in availability and quality of maternity care. The latter, which are not confined to any social class, can best be corrected by the cooperative efforts of teams of physicians, nurse-midwives, obstetric registered nurses and other health personnel. The composition of such teams will vary and be determined by local needs and circumstances. The functions and responsibilities of team members should be clearly defined according to the education and training of the individuals concerned.

To achieve the aims of providing optimal maternity care for all women the following recommendations are made:

1. The health team organized to provide maternity care will be directed by a qualified obstetrician-gynecologist.
2. In such medically directed teams, qualified nurse-midwives may assume responsibility for the complete care and management of uncomplicated maternity patients.
3. In such medically directed teams, obstetric registered nurses may assume responsibility for patient care and management according to their education, training and experience.
4. In such medically directed teams, other health personnel who have been trained in specific areas of maternity care may participate in the team functions according to their abilities and within the definitions of responsibility established by the team.
5. Written policies describing the specific functions of each of the team members should be prepared. They should be reviewed and revised periodically according to changing needs.

In endorsing the above statement, The American College of Obstetricians and Gynecologists, The Nurses Association of The American College of Obstetricians and Gynecologists and the American College of Nurse-Midwives recognize as their common goal the need for improvement and expansion of health services now being provided for women.

In order to maintain a continuing evaluation of the health services being provided for women and to plan for needed improvements and expansion, a mechanism for continued communication between all the organizations responsible for their provision is being developed.

The American College of Nurse-Midwives
1000 Vermont Avenue NW
Suite 500
Washington, DC 20005

The American College of Obstetricians and Gynecologists
One East Wacker Drive
Chicago, IL 60601

The Nurses Association of The American College of Obstetricians and Gynecologists
One East Wacker Drive
Chicago, IL 60601

supplementary statement (1975)

Many questions have arisen concerning the meaning of the recommendation in the Joint Statement on Maternity Care (1971) that the health care team be "directed by a qualified obstetrician-gynecologist." These questions are justified and are accentuated by other developments in the speciality of obstetrics-gynecology which include the changing birth rate, formalization of new roles for personnel, emphasis on preventive care, HMOs, plans for national health insurance, PSROs, and regionalization of health services.

It is recognized that the obstetrician-gynecologist cannot under all circumstances be physically present to direct the health team; therefore it is essential that mechanisms of communication be clearly established for him or her to provide direction. Thus, the nature of the direction of the health team indeed becomes crucial.

The obstetrician-gynecologist working within a team giving health care to women has many responsibilities. These range from the direct provision of services to community health efforts and include:

a. The supervision of the medical care provided by all team members.
b. The direct provision of care for complications of pregnancy and for complex medical and surgical gynecological conditions.
c. The setting of medical care standards.
d. The provision of consultation to other team members.
e. The surveillance of task distribution within the team.
f. Participation in the ongoing educational activities of the team.
g. The introduction of new medical techniques as they become available.
h. The development of medical research.*

In view of the diversity of health care systems in which the obstetric-gynecologic health team currently functions, no universal systems model can be applied. Generally, however, the team is found in the following broad contexts:

1. Urban (intramural, on site, immediate referrals)
2. Rural (with institutional affiliation)
3. Rural (without institutional affiliation but with obstetric consultation available)
4. Private office (urban or rural)

The logistics of consultation and referral may vary with geographic and climatic conditions, but the following basic principles of team interaction are valid regardless of these conditions:

1. There must be a written agreement among members of the team clearly specifying consultation and referral

* From "Medical Practice in the Obstetric-Gynecologic Health Care Team," Interorganizational Committee on Ob/Gyn Health Personnel, Sept 1973.

policies and standing orders. The representatives of each practice discipline should participate in the development of and be signatory to the agreement.
2. The obstetrician-gynecologist, upon signing protocols, must accept full responsibility for direction of medical care rendered by the team in accordance with his or her orders.
3. In circumstances wherein the functions of the team leader are necessarily performed by physicians without specialty training in obstetrics-gynecology, medical direction should be provided through a formal consultative arrangement with a qualified obstetrician-gynecologist who is available to team members for continuing consultation and assurance of quality care.

statement on parent and newborn interaction (1977)†

> Mothers separated from their young soon lost all interest in those whom they were unable to nurse or cherish.
>
> *Pierre Budin* (1907)

Since the above 1907 statement of concern about the psychosocial cost of interference with parent and newborn interaction, increasing evidence has accumulated to support the concept of an "attachment and bonding" process in the human race. The major components of very early contact are touching, eye contact between mother and infant and parallel facial positioning (*en face*). Coincident with the development of that concept, the family-oriented birth process has received increasing acceptance by the providers of perinatal care. A more sophisticated public awareness, with emphasis on smaller families, has intensified the desire of mothers and fathers for greater involvement in all aspects of the birth and nurturing process in their families. Disruptions of the service and/or increased cross infection have not been reported when hospitals and professional staff have encouraged early parent-newborn interaction.

It is timely to review all hospital procedures and professional practices for their appropriateness and thereby encourage the hospitals to reassess their policy in support of the bonding principle. Such a review should include: public health regulations, hospital admission policies, labor and delivery practices, and nursery and postpartum care. Reevaluation of existing practices must preserve the significant technological advances which have resulted in improved obstetrical and newborn care. Innovative alternative setting for birth in the hospital with adequate professional support should be explored and evaluated.

The Committee on Maternal and Child Care encourages medical staffs to continue to review hospital practices and, when necessary, to develop and formulate appropriate policies respecting all aspects of professional support for the birth and nurturing processes.

† American Medical Association House of Delegates, Chicago, December 4–7, 1977.

appendix c: statements of policy for the care of children and families in health-care settings

preamble

Advancement of technology and medical science has permitted more children to live, to live longer and in most cases, to live more fully. In the process, other dangers to children's healthy development have arisen or come to light. These problems have in turn stimulated the current progress in the behavioral sciences.

Threats posed to the emotional security and development of many children and their families by serious illness, disability, disfigurement, treatment, interrupted human relationships and nonsupportive environments have been clearly demonstrated by worldwide research studies. The outcomes can range from temporary but frequently overwhelming anxiety and emotional suffering to long-standing or permanent developmental handicaps. Such interference with the fullest possible development and expression of individual potential is an unacceptable price to pay.

Closer contact with the emotional life of children, increased parent involvement and communication amongst professionals have also contributed to greater understanding as well as to improvements of care. Whereas there is still much to learn regarding the inter-relatedness of such factors as age, type of illness, length of hospitalization, critical developmental periods and vulnerability, sufficient knowledge now exists to direct action toward both minimizing and preventing such harm.

The Association for the Care of Children in Hospitals endorses the following policies:

ALL PEDIATRIC HEALTH CARE SETTINGS SHOULD:

1. Have a stated philosophy of care which is specific, easily understood by, and made available to patients and families, and which applies in a coordinated manner to all disciplines and departments.
2. Assist or provide programs of prevention and restorative care which respond to emotional, social and environmental causal factors of accidents and illness.
3. Create and maintain a social and physical environment which is as welcoming, unthreatening and supportive as possible, and which fosters open communication, encourages human relationships, and invites involvement of children, their families and community in decisions affecting their care.
4. Avoid hospitalizing children whenever possible through the development of alternatives.
5. Develop and utilize ambulatory, day and home care programs which are financially and geographically accessible.
6. Minimize the duration of unavoidable hospital stays, while recognizing discharge planning needs.
7. Provide for and encourage the presence and participation in the hospital of persons most significant to the child, to approximate supportive home patterns of interactions and routines.
8. Provide consistent, emotionally supportive nurturing care for young children during the absence of their parents.
9. Respect the unique care-taking role of parents as well as their individual responses, and provide ongoing understandable information and support which will enable them to utilize their strengths in supporting their child.
10. Provide a milieu which is responsive to the uniqueness of each child and adolescent, their ethnic and cultural backgrounds and developmental needs.
11. Provide readily accessible, well designed space, equipment and programs for the wide range of play,

educational and social activities which are essential to all children and adolescents, particularly those who have been deprived of normal opportunities for development.

12. Provide child care professionals who are skilled at assessing emotional, developmental and academic needs, communicating with and fostering the involvement of patients and their families in activities appropriate to their needs.

13. Ensure that children and their parents are informed, understand and are supported prior to, during, and following experiences which are potentially distressing.

14. Carefully select all staff and volunteers according to their commitment to the foregoing policies. Those in direct contact, however limited, with children, youth, and families should be sensitive, perceptive and compassionate. Professionals involved in more extended, intimate and responsible positions of child care should have special training in child development, family dynamics and the unique psychological needs of children when ill and under stress.

15. Facilitate orientation, continued learning, and consultation in relation to all of the above, and provide support which recognizes the emotional demands of staff.

16. Encourage and foster the inclusion of the above educational focus in the basic curriculum and field experiences of the various professional and technical personnel preparing for careers in pediatric settings.

17. Support the evolvement of resources for early detection, and of attitudes and facilities for ongoing care of children with health and/or developmental problems.

18. Provide for ongoing evaluation of policies and programs by the recipients of care and staff at all levels.

19. Support and disseminate research which clarifies and pertains to the above.

20. Promote education within the community about the health and developmental needs of children.

Endorsed by the Association for the Care of Children in Hospitals, 1977

appendix d: abbreviations commonly used

Abbreviations	Meaning	Derivation
aa	of each	ana (Greek)
ac	before meals	ante cibum (Latin)
ad lib	as desired	ad libitum (Latin)
AP	apical pulse	
bid (or 2 id)	two times daily	bis in die (Latin)
BP	blood pressure	
C	Celsius	
c̄	with	
cc	cubic centimeter	
cm	centimeter	
DC	discontinue	
F	Fahrenheit	
fl	fluid	
g	gram	
gtt	drop, drops	guttae (Latin)
(H)	hypodermically	
hs	at hour of sleep	hora somni (Latin)
IM	intramuscularly	
IV	intravenously	
kg	kilogram	
L	liter (1000 ml, or 1 qt approx)	
mg	milligram	
ml	milliliter	
mm	millimeter	
OD	right eye	oculus dexter (Latin)
OS	left eye	oculus sinister (Latin)
OU	both eyes	oculus unitas (Latin)
oz, or ℥	ounce	
p̄	after	
pc	after eating	post cibum (Latin)
PO	by mouth	per os (Latin)
prn	as necessary	pro re nata (Latin)
q	every	

Abbreviations	Meaning	Derivation
qid (or 4 id)	four times daily	quater in die (Latin)
qs	as much as necessary	quantum satis (Latin)
RBC	red blood cell count	
s̄	without	
s̄s̄	one-half	
tid (or 3 id)	three times daily	tres in die (Latin)
WBC	white blood cell count	
×	times	
ʒ	dram	

appendix e: metric doses with approximate apothecary equivalents*

LIQUID MEASURE

Metric		Apothecary
4000	ml	1 gallon
1000	ml	1 quart
500	ml	1 pint
30	ml	1 fluid ounce
4	ml	1 fluid dram
0.06	ml	1 minim

Note: a milliliter (ml) is the approximate equivalent of a cubic centimeter (cc).

EQUIVALENT WEIGHTS IN METRIC AND IN APOTHECARY SCALES

Metric		Apothecary
30	g	1 ounce
15	g	4 drams
1	g	15 grains
60	mg	1 grain
30	mg	1/2 grain
15	mg	1/4 grain
1	mg	1/60 grain
0.4	mg	1/150 grain
0.25	mg	1/250 grain
0.2	mg	1/300 grain
0.12	mg	1/500 grain

*When prepared dosage forms such as tablets, capsules, and pills are prescribed in the metric system, the pharmacist may dispense the corresponding approximate equivalent in the apothecary system, and vice versa.

CONVERSION OF AVOIRDUPOIS BODY WEIGHT TO METRIC EQUIVALENTS

lb	kg	kg	lb
10	4.5	10	22
20	9.1	20	44
30	13.6	30	66
40	18.2	40	88
50	22.7	50	110
60	27.3		
70	31.8		
80	36.4		
90	40.9		
100	45.4		

One pound = 0.454 kilograms
One kilogram = 2.2 pounds

CONVERSION OF HEIGHT TO METRIC EQUIVALENTS

Inches	Centimeters
18	46
24	61
30	76
36	91
42	107
48	122
54	137
60	152
66	168

One inch = 2.54 cm
One cm = 0.3937 inch

EQUIVALENT CENTIGRADE AND FAHRENHEIT TEMPERATURE READINGS

Celsius	Fahrenheit
35	95.0
36	96.8
37	98.6
38	100.4
39	102.2
40	104.0
41	105.8

To convert Celsius readings to Fahrenheit, multiply by 1.8 and add 32.

To convert Fahrenheit readings to Celsius, subtract 32 and divided by 1.8.

glossary

Achylia—absence of pancreatic enzymes, causing intestinal malabsorption and severe malnutrition; typical of cystic fibrosis.

Acidosis—disturbance of acid–base balance in body fluid, characterized by drowsiness, dry skin, flushed cheeks and lips, acetone breath with fruity smell, and hyperpnea. If untreated, leads to coma.

Allergen—substance causing an allergic or sensitive reaction in body organs and tissues. Pollen, mold, certain foods, and drugs are the most common.

Amenorrhea—absence or abnormal cessation of menstruation.

Amniocentesis—procedure in which a sample of amniotic fluid is withdrawn for prenatal diagnosis of possible problems such as mental retardation, blood disorders, or respiratory problems.

Anorexia nervosa—self-inflicted starvation, generally occurring in adolescent girls, most often between the ages of 11 and 13, or 19 and 20.

Anticipatory grief—mourning that occurs when death is expected, as in the diagnosis of terminal illness.

Apgar score—evaluation for newborns, developed by Dr. Virginia Apgar; administered 60 seconds after birth and 5 minutes later.

Apnea—temporary interruption of breathing.

Archetypes—predetermined patterns of human development, which, according to Carl Jung, replace instinctive behavior of other animals.

Associative play—engaging in a common activity but without a sense of belonging.

Asthma—reversible, obstructive airway disease caused by a hyperreactive response.

Astigmatism—vision disorder caused by unequal curvatures in the cornea of the eye, producing a blurred image.

Ataxia—failure of muscular coordination; used to describe least common type of cerebral palsy, characterized by lack of coordination due to disturbances of kinesthetic and balance senses.

Athetosis—type of cerebral palsy marked by involuntary, incoordinate motion with varying degrees of muscle tension.

Atresia—absence of a normal body opening, or abnormal closure of a body passage.

Attachment—originally called "bonding;" process in which infant and parents get to know each other beginning in the first moments after birth.

Aura—a sensation signaling an impending epileptic seizure.

Autism—psychological disorder of children, characterized by: inability to relate to and interact with others; inability to communicate; obsession with preservation of sameness; preoccupation with objects instead of people.

Autograft—skin taken from one area of a patient's body for grafting on another area of same patient.

Birthing room—homelike birth setting within a hospital or birth center, which permits father, mother, and new baby to be together during labor and after birth.

Bryant's traction—type of skin traction commonly used to treat fractured femur in children under 3 years of age.

BSA—body surface area

Candlelighters—national organization of parents whose children have died or are dying of cancer.

Caries—cavities in the teeth.

Castration—removal of the testes; boys in the preschool-age group often fear this kind of mutilation.

Celiac crisis—acute phase of celiac syndrome, marked by copious vomiting; large, watery stools; drowsiness; and severe dehydration.

Cephalhematoma—collection of blood between the periosteum and the skull of the newborn.

Child-life programs—programs designed to make hospitalization less threatening for children and parents, usually directed by a child-life worker with a background in psychology and early childhood development.

Chordee—cordlike anomaly extending from the scrotum to the penis, pulling the penis downward in an arc.

Chromosomes—small, threadlike structures within each cell that contain genes, the units that carry genetic instructions.

Circadian rhythms—innate mechanisms that regulate human biologic functions, the most obvious of which is sleep.

Clark's rule—formula or rule for calculating the approximate dosage for children 2 years of age or older:

$$\frac{\text{weight in lbs} \times \text{adult dose}}{150}$$

Classification—the ability to group objects into a hierarchical arrangement.

Comedones—blackheads and whiteheads on the skin caused by excessive secretion of sebum into skin follicles; common among adolescents.

Compassionate Friends—national organization of parents who have experienced the death of their child.

Compound fracture—a fracture in which the broken bone penetrates the skin.

Conductive hearing loss—hearing impairment caused by failure of middle ear structures to carry sound waves to inner ear.

Conservation—the principle of continuous quantity (*i.e.*, the volume of liquid does not change when poured from one container to another of different shape or size).

Controlled substances—prescription drugs that can cause dependence, and "street drugs;" regulated by the Food and Drug Administration and the Drug Enforcement Agency of the Department of Justice.

Cooperative play—play in which children cooperate with one another, as in team sports.

Cryptorchidism—failure of one or both testes to descend into the scrotum.

Curling's ulcer—also called a "stress ulcer;" gastric or duodenal ulcer that frequently occurs following severe burns.

Dawdling—delaying tactic used by children, sometimes because they are unable to choose between their own desires and those of parents.

Decentration—being able to see several aspects of a problem at once and understanding the relationship of parts to a whole; a change from the egocentric thinking of early childhood.

Deciduous teeth—"baby" teeth, gradually replaced by permanent teeth beginning about age 6.

Decubitus ulcer—pressure sore; tissue breakdown due to prolonged immobility, infrequent position changes, and inadequate skin care.

Denial—the third stage of behavior in a child separated from parents; preceded by protest and despair; when parents visit, the child in the denial stage turns away, showing distrust and rejection.

Dependence—compulsive need to use a substance for its satisfying or pleasurable effects; may be psychological, physiologic, or both.

Despair—second stage of behavior in child separated from parents; preceded by protest and followed by denial; child becomes apathetic and listless.

Diaphoresis—sweating

Diplopia—double vision

Directive play therapy—person working with hospitalized children makes suggestions and interprets play activities, unlike nondirective play therapy, in which the child follows his own impulses and the adult shows neither rejection nor acceptance.

Discipline—to train or instruct so as to produce a particular behavior pattern, especially moral or mental improvement and self-control.

Down's syndrome—mongolism; the most common chromosomal abnormality causing mental retardation; characterized by almond-shaped eyes; shortness of head; retarded body growth; short, flattened bridge of nose.

Dysmenorrhea—pain associated with menstruation, including cramping, abdominal pain, leg pain, and backache.

Ecchymosis—accumulation of blood under the skin and outside of vessels; "black eye;" bruising of the tissue surrounding the eye.

Echolalia—"parrot" speech; echoing words of others without indication of understanding.

Egocentric—unable to put oneself in another's place or to see another's point of view.

Ejaculation—sudden expulsion of semen

Electrocardiogram (ECG, EKG)—a test measuring and recording the electrical impulses of the heart.

Electroencephalogram (EEG)—electronic measurement of brain's electrical activity.

Electrolytes—chemical compounds (minerals) that break down into ions when placed in water. An *ion* is an atom bearing either a positive or negative electrical charge. Electrolytes maintain acid–base balance of body fluids.

Embryo—a growing organism that has become implanted in the uterine lining.

Empty-mother syndrome—Wong's description of the feelings of a mother whose child dies after a long illness.

Encopresis—involuntary fecal soiling beyond the age when control is expected (about age 3).

Engrossment—father's absorption and interest in his newborn infant.

Enterobiasis—oxyuriasis; pinworm infestation of the cecum that may enter the appendix.

Enuresis—involuntary urination beyond the age when bladder control should have been achieved. Nocturnal enuresis (bedwetting) may persist in many children until age 7.

Epiphyses—growth centers at the ends of long bones and at the wrist.

Erythroblastosis fetalis—hemolytic disease of the newborn in which the infant's red blood cells are broken down and destroyed, producing severe anemia and hyperbilirubinemia.

Extended family—one or more nuclear families plus other kinsmen.

External fixation—method used to stabilize severe fractures that cannot be casted.

Failure to thrive—failure to gain weight and develop normally with no apparent physical cause; thought to result from emotional deprivation.

Fractional dose—dilution of full-strength drugs to concentration ordered by physician:

$$\frac{\text{desired dose}}{\text{dose on hand}} \times \text{diluent} = \text{amount to be given}$$

Fetus—growing organism that has assumed a human likeness, generally about the 8th week of life.

Fontanel—triangular space at the juncture of the bones of the newborn's skull.

Galactosemia—recessive hereditary metabolic disorder due to absence of enzyme that converts galactase into glucose. Unless milk is eliminated from the infant's diet, cataracts, liver and spleen damage, and mental retardation result.

Gastrostomy feeding—administering nutrients through a tube that has been surgically inserted through the abdominal wall into the stomach.

Gavage feeding—administering nutrients through a tube inserted nasally or orally and passed into the stomach.

Genotype—each person's individual set of genes.

Gonorrhea—the most common sexually transmitted (venereal) disease; also called "the clap," "the drips," or "the dose." Caused by *Neisseria gonorrhoeae*, a gram-positive diplococcus.

Glycosuria—abnormally high level of sugar in the urine; symptom of diabetes mellitus.

Halo traction—form of traction used with body cast to correct severe scoliosis; uses stainless steel pins inserted in skull and femurs.

Head Start—federally funded program to enrich the environment of preschool children in families with limited social, cultural, and economic resources.

Hemophilia—hereditary disorder resulting from inborn errors of metabolism that delay coagulation of blood.

Hirschsprung's disease—congenital aganglionic megacolon, characterized by obstinate constipation.

Homeostasis—a balanced state of the body; dynamic equilibrium of an organism.

Hordeolum, external—a sty, a purulent infection of an eyelash follicle, generally caused by *Staphylococcus aureus*.

Hospice—an institution and concept devoted to sensitive, humane care of the dying.

Hyaline membrane disease—respiratory distress syndrome (RDS), affecting about one-half of all preterm infants.

Hydrocephalus—an excess of cerebrospinal fluid within the ventricular and subarachnoid spaces of the cranial cavity.

Hyperbilirubinemia—abnormally high levels of bilirubin in the blood that can cause jaundice and brain damage.

Hypercalcemia—elevated levels of calcium in the blood.

Hyperopia—farsightedness; common condition of young children, sometimes persisting into first grade and beyond.

Hypocalcemia—deficiency of calcium in the blood.

Hyposensitization—immunization against allergies by injection.

Hypospadias—congenital condition of the male child in which the urethra terminates on the ventral (under) side of the penis instead of at the tip.

Hypothermia—lowering the body temperature, a technique used in cardiac surgery to increase the time circulation can be stopped without causing brain damage.

Imperforate anus—congenital disorder in which the rectal pouch ends blindly above the anus and there is no anal orifice.

Insulin—substance secreted by the pancreas responsible for burning and storage of sugar. Inadequate supply of insulin causes diabetes mellitus. Children with this disorder must receive insulin by injection.

Intermittent fever—temperature that is elevated during part of a 24-hour period, but drops to normal or below normal within a 24-hour period.

Interstitial—situated within body tissue spaces, rather than within a vessel (intravascular).

Intimacy—mutual sharing of deep feelings with another person.

Intravascular—situated within the blood vessels or blood plasma.

Intravenous pyleogram (IVP)—a test used in diagnosing problems in kidney function.

Intussusception—telescoping of one portion of the bowel into a distal portion, occurring most frequently at the juncture of the ileum and the colon.

Ipecac—an over-the-counter preparation used to induce vomiting.

Karyotype—a photograph of matched and grouped pairs of chromosomes, used to locate chromosomal malformations and translocations.

Ketone bodies—compound containing β-hydroxybutyric acid, acetoacetic acid, and acetone; formed when glucose is unavailable for cellular metabolism.

Kussmaul breathing—paroxysms of dyspnea or labored breathing, occurring in diabetic coma.

Kwashiorkor—protein–calorie malnutrition; characterized by swollen abdomen, retarded growth, muscle wasting, edema, apathy, and irritability.

Lacto-ovo-vegetarian diet—diet that includes dairy products, eggs, fruits, vegetables, and grain products.

Lanugo—fine, downy hair covering the skin of the fetus, normally absent in a full-term infant.

Legg-Calvé-Perthes disease—osteochondrosis of the hip; an aseptic necrosis of the head of the femur; cause usually unknown.

Logan bar—a wire bow used in the treatment of cleft palate to prevent tension on the corrective sutures.

Lordosis—"swayback;" abnormally concave curvature of the spine when viewed from the side; usually corrected with skeletal maturation.

Lysis—fevers that gradually recede to normal over a period of several days.

Magical thinking—belief that words and thoughts can make things real; difficulty in separating fantasy and reality.

Masturbation—stimulation of the genitalia by means other than intercourse.

Meconium—sticky, greenish black substance found in the intestine of the newborn; composed of bile, mucus, cellular waste, intestinal secretions, fat, hair, and other materials swallowed during fetal life.

Menarche—beginning of menstruation

Meningitis—inflammation of the meninges, most commonly caused by *Hemophilus influenzae* bacillus.

Meningocele—congenital defect in which a portion of the spinal meninges protrudes through a bony defect in the spinal column and forms a sac.

Menorrhagia—excessive, irregular or prolonged vaginal bleeding.

Milia—pearly white cysts appearing on faces of many newborn infants.

Miliaria rubra—prickly heat; rash or pinhead-size reddened papules.

Milwaukee brace—spinal brace used to correct structural scoliosis.

Minimal brain dysfunction (MBD)—characterized by hyperactivity, perceptual motor impairment, coordination difficulties and language and symbolic impairments.

Mittelschmerz—dull, aching abdominal pain at the time of ovulation (mid-cycle).

Molars—teeth used for grinding on both sides and at the back of the jaw.

Molding—compression of the bones of the infant skull as the head moves through the birth canal, causing them to overlap at the suture lines, giving the head an asymmetrical or elongated appearance.

Mutation—fundamental change in the structure of a gene, resulting in transmission of a trait different from that normally carried by that particular gene.

Myelomeningocele—protrusion of the spinal cord and the meninges through a bony defect in the spine.

Myopia—nearsightedness

Negativism—when the response to everything is "no." Typical behavior for toddlers, usually an assertion of individuality rather than an intent to disagree.

Nocturnal emissions—"wet dreams;" involuntary ejaculation of semen during adolescence.

Noncommunicative language—egocentric language, used by children under age 4 simply for the pleasure of saying and hearing words.

Nuclear family—also called *conjugal family*; comprises a man, his wife, and their children (biologic or adopted), who share a common household.

Obesity—increased body weight due to an excessive accumulation of fat.

Oedipal stage—a stage in child development when the child is attracted to the parent of the opposite sex (usually age 5 years to 6 years).

Oliguria—producing an abnormally small amount of urine.

Omphalocele—rare congenital anomaly in which some of the contents of the abdomen protrude through the root of the umbilical cord and form a sac on the abdomen.

Orchiopexy—surgery to correct undescended testes (cryptorchidism), securing the gonads in the scrotum.

Orthoptics—therapeutic exercises to correct vision problems.

Orthotist—a specialist skilled in orthotics, the field of knowledge related to the use of orthopedic appliances.

Overweight—weight that is greater than average for a particular height and body build.

Parallel play—play alongside another but done independently, such as a craft group in which each member is working on an individual project.

Paraplegia—paralysis of two extremities, usually the legs.

Parenteral—route for administering nutrients, fluids, and/or medications that does not involve the alimentary canal; usually intravenous injection.

Paresthesia—abnormal sensation such as burning, tingling, numbness.

Patent ductus arteriosus—congenital heart disorder in which the ductus arteriosus fails to close and allows blood to be shunted from the aorta into the pulmonary artery, flooding the lungs and overloading the left heart chambers.

Pediculosis—lice infestation of the scalp or other hairy parts of the body.

Pellagra—nutritional disorder resulting from lack of niacin in the diet; causes gastrointestinal and neurologic symptoms.

Phenylketonuria—congenital absence of the enzyme necessary for metabolism of phenylalanine, an essential amino acid. Untreated, it causes mental retardation.

Phimosis—adherence of the foreskin to the glans penis, preventing retraction.

Phototherapy—exposure of newborns to fluorescent lights to prevent bilirubin concentration from reaching dangerous levels.

Pica—the ingestion of non-food substances such as laundry starch, clay, tissue paper, and paint.

Placenta—afterbirth; organ that links mother and unborn infant and provides oxygen, nutrients, and protection for the infant, while eliminating waste products.

Plaque—a film formed on the teeth as a result of bacterial interaction with sugar.

Plumbism—lead poisoning

Polydipsia—abnormal thirst, one symptom of diabetes mellitus.

Polygamy—having more than one spouse at a time.

Polyphagia—abnormal increase in food consumption, one symptom of diabetes mellitus; compulsive overeating.

Polyuria—dramatic increase in urinary output, usually with enuresis; symptom of diabetes mellitus.

Postmature—any infant born after completion of the 42nd week of gestation, regardless of birth weight.

Premature—any infant of less than 37 weeks' gestation.

Priapism—perpetual abnormal erection of the penis.

Protest—first stage of behavior in child separated from parents; precedes despair and denial. Child cries and refuses to be comforted, constantly seeking his parent.

Puberty—age of reproductive maturity

Pyelonephritis—pyuria; pyelitis; the most common urinary tract infection in childhood.

Pyloric stenosis—congenital disorder involving severe narrowing of pyloric lumen, causing stomach dilation.

Quadriplegia—absence of function in all four extremities.

Remittent fever—dramatic rise and fall of temperature without return to normal during a 24-hour period.

Renal calculi—kidney stones; hardened deposits of calcium and other mineral salts.

Regression—progress in reverse; reversion to an earlier stage of development or behavior.

Retrolental fibroplasia—blindness caused by damage to the immature retina due to high blood concentrations of oxygen.

Reversibility—the ability to think in either direction, allowing one to count forward or backward, or to add and subtract.

Rickets—nutritional disorder caused by lack of vitamin D; affects the growth and calcification of bones.

Ritualism—following or repeating certain routines, making rituals of simple tasks.

Rumination—voluntary regurgitation

Russell's traction—type of traction used for treatment of femoral fractures in children age 3 and older.

Schizophrenia (childhood)—late-onset psychosis; developing in children between the ages of 6 and 10, manifesting characteristics similar to autism: poorly developed speech, self-stimulating behaviors, absence of a sense of self.

School phobia—reluctance to go to school due to fear of the school situation or to fear of leaving home and parents, or both.

Scoliosis—lateral curvature of the spine; *non-structured* (functional) *scoliosis* is caused by poor posture, muscle spasm due to trauma or unequal leg length; *structural* (idiopathic) *scoliosis* is caused by rotated and malformed vertebrae.

Scurvy—nutritional disorder resulting from deficiency of vitamin C; characterized by irritability, loss of appetite, and digestive disturbances.

Seborrheic dermatitis—"cradle cap;" characterized by yellowish, scaly, or crusted patches on the scalp.

Sebum—thick, semi-fluid substance secreted by the sebaceous glands, causing blackheads and whiteheads, particularly during adolescence.

Sensorineural hearing loss—hearing impairment caused by damage to nerve endings in the cochlea or to nerve pathways to the brain. Generally severe and unresponsive to treatment.

Small for gestational age (SGA)—term infants or low birth weight.

Snellen chart—vision testing chart in which letters in each line are smaller than the line above.

Socialization—the process by which a child learns the rules of the society and the culture in which he lives.

Strabismus—crossed eyes; the failure of the two eyes to focus on the same object simultaneously, resulting in double vision (diplopia).

Sublimation—redirecting unacceptable urges into more acceptable outlets and behaviors.

Sudden infant death syndrome (SIDS)—also known as "crib death;" a sudden and unexpected death of an infant that cannot be explained even after autopsy.

Superego—an individual's sense of moral responsibility.

Surfactant—biochemical compound that reduces surface tension inside the air sacs of the lungs, keeping them partially expanded after each breath. Premature infants' lungs are deficient in surfactant, leading to hyaline membrane disease.

Synovitis—inflammation of a synovial membrane; in children commonly affects the hip or knee.

Syphilis—second only to gonorrhea in occurrence, this veneral disease is caused by the spirochete *Treponema pallidum.*

Talipes equinovarus—clubfoot; a congenital disorder in which the entire foot is inverted, the heel drawn up, and the forefoot adducted.

Teratogenesis—disruption in prenatal growth processes that results in a child with a physical defect.

Tetralogy of Fallot—common congenital heart defect involving four disorders: pulmonary stenosis, ventricular septal defect, overriding aorta, and right ventricular hypertrophy.

Thanatologist—person trained to work with the dying and their families.

Tinea (ringworm)—fungal infection of the skin. Occurs as *tinea capitis* or *tinea tonsurans* (ringworm of the scalp), *tinea corporis* (ringworm of the body), *tinea pedis* (ringworm of the feet), all commonly caused by *Microsporum.*

Urticaria—hives; bright red, itchy swellings on various parts of the body; usually an allergic reaction to food or drugs.

Vernix caseosa—greasy, cheeselike substance that protects the skin during fetal life.

Viability—the earliest gestational age at which a fetus can survive outside the uterine environment.

Wilms' tumor—an adenosarcoma in the kidney region; one of the most common abdominal neoplasms of early childhood.

Witches' milk—pale milky fluid sometimes secreted from the breasts of newborns as a result of maternal estrogens in the bloodstream.

Withdrawal—an ineffective method of contraception in which the male withdraws his penis from the female's vagina immediately prior to ejaculation, not realizing that pre-ejaculation secretions often contain sperm.

Zygote—a fertilized ovum, produced by the union of sperm and egg.

index

Numbers followed by an *f* indicate a figure; *t* following a page number indicates tabular material.